McGraw-Hill SPECIALTY BOARD REVIEW

Seventh Edition

Anesthesiology
Examination & Board Review

Edited by

Mark Dershwitz, M.D., Ph.D.
Professor and Vice Chair of Anesthesiology
Professor of Biochemistry & Molecular Pharmacology
University of Massachusetts Medical School

and

J. Matthias Walz, M.D.
Associate Professor of Anesthesiology and Surgery
University of Massachusetts Medical School

McGraw-Hill
New York

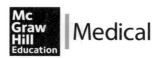 Medical

New York   Chicago   San Francisco   Athens   London   Madrid   Mexico City
Milan   New Delhi   Singapore   Sydney   Toronto

McGraw-Hill Specialty Board Review:

Anesthesiology Examination & Board Review, Seventh Edition

1 2 3 4 5 6 7 8 9 0   DOW/DOW   18 17 16 15 14 13

ISBN 0-07-177076-3

Notice

Medicine is an ever-changing science. As new research and clinical experience broaden our knowledge, changes in treatment and drug therapy are required. The authors and the publisher of this work have checked with sources believed to be reliable in their efforts to provide information that is complete and generally in accord with the standards accepted at the time of publication. However, in view of the possibility of human error or changes in medical sciences, neither the authors nor the publisher nor any other party who has been involved in the preparation or publication of this work warrants that the information contained herein is in every respect accurate or complete, and they disclaim all responsibility for any errors or omissions or for the results obtained from use of the information contained in this work. Readers are encouraged to confirm the information contained herein with other sources. For example and in particular, readers are advised to check the product information sheet included in the package of each drug they plan to administer to be certain that the information contained in this work is accurate and that changes have not been made in the recommended dose or in the contraindications for administration. This recommendation is of particular importance in connection with new or infrequently used drugs.

This book was set in Palatino by Cenveo® Publisher Services.
The production supervisor was Richard Ruzycka.
The editors were Brian Belval and Brian Kearns.
Project management was provided by Vastavikta Sharma, Cenveo Publisher Services.
RR Donnelley was printer and binder.

This book is printed on acid-free paper.

Cataloging-in-Publication Data for this book is on file with the Library of Congress.

Contents

Contributors

Salahadin Abdi, M.D., Ph.D.
Professor and Chair
Department of Pain Medicine
Division of Anesthesiology and Critical Care
University of Texas MD Anderson Cancer Center
Houston, TX

Rae M. Allain, M.D.
Associate Director of Surgical Critical Care
Department of Anesthesiology & Pain Medicine
St. Elizabeth's Medical Center
Associate Professor of Anesthesiology
Tufts University School of Medicine
Boston, MA

Theodore Alston, M.D., Ph.D.
Department of Anesthesia, Critical Care and Pain
  Medicine
Massachusetts General Hospital
Assistant Professor of Anesthesia
Harvard Medical School
Boston, MA

John G. Antonakakis, M.D.
Staff Anesthesiologist
Portsmouth Regional Hospital
Portsmouth, NH

Mark Dershwitz, M.D., Ph.D.
Professor and Vice Chair of Anesthesiology
Professor of Biochemistry & Molecular
  Pharmacology
University of Massachusetts Medical School
Worcester, MA

Eleanor M. Duduch, M.D.
Residency Program Director
Clinical Associate Professor of Anesthesiology
University of Massachusetts Medical School
Worcester, MA

Renée M. Goetzler, M.D., M.P.H.
Associate Program Director
Carney Hospital
Associate Clinical Professor of Medicine
Tufts University School of Medicine
Boston, MA

Robin K. Guillory, M.D.
Co-Medical Director of the Neuroscience ICU
University of Louisville Hospital
Assistant Professor of Anesthesiology
Department of Anesthesiology and Perioperative
  Medicine
University of Louisville School of Medicine
Louisville, KY

John J. A. Marota, M.D., Ph.D.
Department of Anesthesia, Critical Care and Pain
  Medicine
Massachusetts General Hospital
Assistant Professor of Anesthesia
Harvard Medical School
Boston, MA

Stavros G. Memtsoudis, M.D., Ph.D., F.C.C.P.
Clinical Professor of Anesthesiology and Public
  Health
Weill Cornell Medical College
Director of Critical Care Services
Hospital for Special Surgery
New York, NY

Christian Müller, M.D.
Director of Cardiac Anesthesia
Assistant Professor of Anesthesiology
University of Massachusetts Medical School
Worcester, MA

Ronald B. Rubin, M.D., F.A.C.O.G.
Assistant Professor of Anesthesiology
University of Massachusetts Medical School
Worcester, MA

Brian D. Sites, M.D.
Associate Professor of Anesthesiology and
 Orthopedic Surgery
Director of Regional Anesthesiology
Geisel School of Medicine at Dartmouth College
Hanover, NH

J. Matthias Walz, M.D.
Associate Professor of Anesthesiology and Surgery
University of Massachusetts Medical School
Worcester, MA

Rebecca M. Zanconato, M.D.
Assistant Professor of Anesthesiology and
 Pediatrics
University of Massachusetts Medical School
Worcester, MA

Preface to the 7th Edition

The 7th edition of *The McGraw-Hill Board Review of Anesthesiology* is timed to coincide with the most substantial changes ever made by the American Board of Anesthesiology in the certification examination process. Beginning with the group of residents that begin anesthesiology training in 2013, the written examination is being divided into two parts. Residents will take the examination on Basic Topics following the first year of residency training, and will take the examination on Advanced Topics two years later following completion of the residency. Thus, this book has been completely redesigned and rewritten to conform to these changes implemented by the Board.

Once again, the subspecialty areas within anesthesiology were written by colleagues with special expertise in these fields. We are pleased by the addition of several new contributors. Drs. Brian Sites and John Antonakakis wrote the chapters on regional anesthesia, Dr. Stavros Memtsoudis on respiration, Dr. Christian Müller on cardiothoracic anesthesia, Dr. Rebecca Zanconato on pediatric anesthesia, Dr. Salahadin Abdi on acute and chronic pain, and Dr. Eleanor M. Duduch on a new chapter on anesthesia for miscellaneous procedures. As in the last edition, Dr. Ronald Rubin, one of the few physicians in the United States fully trained and certified in both anesthesiology and obstetrics & gynecology wrote the chapter on anesthesia for obstetrics, Dr. Ted Alston on circulation, Dr. John Marota on the nervous system, Dr. Renée Goetzler, an internist, on the hepatic, renal, metabolic, and hematologic systems, and Dr. Rae Allain on critical care, this time accompanied by Dr. Robin Guillory.

The reference list was expanded and most of the references are also available online via the website AccessAnesthesiology (www.accessanesthesiology.com). Because of the supreme importance of pharmacology to the practice of anesthesiology, we believe every anesthesiologist should own a comprehensive reference. In the United States, the clear choice is Goodman and Gilman, now in its 12th edition and edited by Brunton, et al. Thus the majority of the pharmacological questions in this book are referenced to it. Pediatric and obstetric anesthesia remain important parts of every resident's training and a large portion of many persons' practices. Because the pediatric and obstetric sections in the major references are abbreviated, many of the pediatric and obstetric questions are referenced to the textbooks edited by Coté, et al. and Chestnut, et al., respectively.

For this edition, the Introduction was also extensively rewritten to include new information from the American Board of Anesthesiology on the aforementioned changes in the certification process as well as on the Maintenance of Certification in Anesthesiology (MOCA) process. MOCA is mandatory for diplomates with time-limited certificates issued after 2000 who wish to maintain their certification.

This book contains 1500 questions and answers and many more references. There will be errors despite the best efforts of the authors and the editors to prevent them. We are very grateful to those persons who previously contacted us to report errors they had found in previous editions. Once again, we would very much appreciate having any and all mistakes brought to our attention, and we have listed our email addresses below to facilitate communication.

We would like to acknowledge the contributors to previous editions of this book: Drs. Paul Alfille, Thomas Beach, William Denman, Peter Foley, Philippa Groves, Grace Harrell, and Bobbie Jean Sweitzer. We would also like to thank our families for tolerating our absences necessitated by the preparation of this latest edition.

Mark Dershwitz
mark.dershwitz@umassmed.edu
J. Matthias Walz
matthias.walz@ummassmemorial.org
Worcester, Massachusetts
April, 2013

Introduction

If you are planning to prepare for the American Board of Anesthesiology (ABA) written examinations, including MOCA (see below), then *The McGraw-Hill Board Review of Anesthesiology*, 7th edition, is designed for you. Here, in one package, is a comprehensive review resource with 1,500 Board-type multiple-choice questions with referenced, paragraph-length discussions of each answer.

Organization of this Book

The *McGraw-Hill Board Review of Anesthesiology*, 7th edition, is divided into two parts, covering the material that will appear on the Basic and Advanced written examinations, respectively. The Basic examination is taken after completion of the first (CA-1) year of anesthesiology residency training, while the Advanced examination is taken after completion of the third and final (CA-3) year of residency training. Successful passage of the Basic examination is required before a candidate can register for the Advanced examination. Successful passage of the Advanced examination is required before a candidate can register for the Applied (formerly called the oral) examination. Both the Basic and Advanced examinations are computer-based examinations taken at a standardized testing center. Complete information on the ABA examination process is found in the *Booklet of Information* published yearly by the ABA. While the Booklet was formerly available in hard copy, it is currently only available via download in PDF format from the ABA website, www.theaba.org.

Question Types

There are three different types of questions found on the Basic and Advanced examinations. Each of these question types is also found in this book. In testing parlance, they are referred to as A-type, G-set, and R-type questions.

A-type (single-best answer) questions. This type of question presents a problem or asks a question and is followed by four or five choices, only one of which is entirely correct. The directions preceding this type of question will generally appear as:

DIRECTIONS (Question 1): Each of the numbered items or incomplete statements in this section is followed by answers or by completions of the statement. Select the ONE lettered answer or completion that is BEST in each case.

An example for this item type is

1. A previously healthy 22-year-old male is undergoing surgical removal of a loose body in his knee under general anesthesia. Approximately one hour after beginning anesthesia, the patient becomes severely hypertensive. The most likely cause of the hypertension is

    (A) pheochromocytoma
    (B) malignant hyperthermia
    (C) light anesthesia
    (D) thyroid storm
    (E) drug overdose

In this type of question, choices other than the correct answer may be partially correct, but there can only be one best answer. In the question above, the key word is "most." Although all of the options listed may cause intraoperative hypertension, and all must be considered in the differential diagnosis, the most likely etiology of intraoperative hypertension is light anesthesia, or answer (C).

G-set questions. A G-set begins with a case presentation, a figure, a diagram, or a related item. This is then followed by a series of A-type questions that all pertain to the case, figure, diagram, etc. An example of this item type is

TABLE 1. STRATEGIES FOR ANSWERING SINGLE-BEST ANSWER QUESTIONS*

1. Remember that only one choice can be the correct answer.
2. Read the question carefully to be sure that you understand what is being asked.
3. Quickly read each choice for familiarity. (This important step is often not done by test takers.)
4. Go back and consider each choice individually.
5. If a choice is partially correct, tentatively consider it to be incorrect. (This step will help you lessen your choices and increase your odds of choosing the correct choice/answer.)
6. Consider the remaining choices and select the one you think is the answer. At this point, you may want to quickly scan the stem to be sure you understand the question and your answer.
7. Click on the correct answer on the computer screen. (Even if you do not know the answer, you should at least guess; you are scored on the number of correct answers, so do not leave any blanks.)

*Note that steps 2 through 7 should take an average of about a minute. The actual examination is timed for an average of about one minute per question.

Directions: use the following scenario to answer Questions 1-2:

A 55-year-old woman presents to the pain clinic with the complaint of intermittent episodes of electric shock-like pain over the right side of her nose and cheek. These episodes are most likely to occur when she is applying makeup, although they might also be precipitated by a strong breeze blowing on her face.

1. The most likely diagnosis is

(A) occipital neuralgia
(B) trigeminal neuralgia
(C) meralgia paresthetica
(D) facial neuralgia
(E) glossopharyngeal neuralgia

2. The drug of choice for managing her symptoms is

(A) diazepam
(B) morphine
(C) carbamazepine
(D) fluoxetine
(E) chlorpromazine

R-type (extended matching) questions. These are multiple-choice questions organized into sets that use one list of options for all items in the set. An example of an R-set is

DIRECTIONS (Questions 1-3): Each group of items below consists of lettered headings followed by a list of numbered phrases or statements. For each numbered phrase or statement, select the ONE lettered heading or component that is most closely associated with it. Each lettered heading or component may be selected once, more than once, or not at all.

(A) α_1-adrenoceptor agonist
(B) α_1-adrenoceptor antagonist
(C) α_2-adrenoceptor agonist
(D) α_2-adrenoceptor antagonist
(E) β_1-adrenoceptor agonist
(F) β_1-adrenoceptor antagonist
(G) β_2-adrenoceptor agonist
(H) β_2-adrenoceptor antagonist

For each medication, select the most accurate description of its receptor activity.

1. atenolol
2. albuterol
3. clonidine

Answers, Explanations, and References

At the end of each chapter, there is a section containing the answers, explanations, and references to the questions. This section (1) tells you the answer to each question; (2) gives you an explanation/review of why the answer is correct, background information on the subject matter, and why the other answers are incorrect; and (3) tells you where you can find more in-depth information on the subject matter in other reference books. We encourage you to use this section as a basis for further study and understanding.

If you choose the correct answer to a question, you can then read the explanation (1) for reinforcement and (2) to add to your knowledge about the subject matter (remember that the explanations usually tell not only why the answer is correct, but also why the other choices are incorrect). If you choose the wrong answer to a question, you can read the explanation for a learning/reviewing discussion of the material in the question. Furthermore, you can note the reference cited (e.g., 5:345), look up the full source in the References on page 431 (e.g., Longnecker DE, et al., eds. *Anesthesiology*, 2nd ed. New York: McGraw-Hill, 2012), and refer to the page cited (p. 345) for a more in-depth discussion.

Practice Tests

In the two 150-question Practice Tests at the end of Parts I and II, the questions cover all of the topics in the preceding chapters in that Part. This format mimics the actual exam and enables you to test your skill at answering questions in all of the areas under simulated examination conditions.

How to Use this Book

There are two logical ways to get the most value from this book. We shall call them Plan A and Plan B.

In Plan A, you go straight to the Practice Test and complete it according to the instructions. Analyze your areas of strength and weakness. This will be a good indicator of your initial knowledge of the subjects and will help to identify specific areas for preparation and review. You can now use the preceding chapters to help you improve your relative weak points.

In Plan B, you go through the first nine chapters in Parts I or II checking off your answers, and then comparing your choices with the answers and discussions in the book. Once you have completed this process, you can take the Practice Test to see how well prepared you are. If you still have a major weakness, it should be apparent in time for you to take remedial action.

In Plan A, by taking the Practice Test first, you get quick feedback regarding your initial areas of strength and weakness. You may find that you have a good command of the material indicating that perhaps only a cursory review of the preceding chapters is necessary. This, of course, would be good to know early in your exam preparation. On the other hand, you may find that you have many areas of weakness. In this case, you could then focus on these areas in your review, not just with this book, but also with the cited references and with your current textbooks and journals.

It is, however, unlikely that you will not do some studying prior to taking the ABA exam (especially since you have this book). Therefore, it may be more realistic to take the Practice Test after you have reviewed the first nine chapters in Parts I or II (as in Plan B). This will probably give you a more realistic type of testing situation since very few of us just sit down to a test without studying. In this case, you will have done some reviewing (from superficial

to in-depth), and your Practice Test will reflect this studying time. If, after reviewing the preceding chapters and taking the Practice Test, you still have some weaknesses, you can then go back to the preceding chapters and supplement your review with your texts.

The American Board of Anesthesiology

History

Anesthesiology is a relatively new specialty, and therefore the ABA is also relatively young.

The American Society of Anesthesiologists had its beginnings in 1911 in the New York area when two groups merged to form the New York Society of Anesthetists. The group grew and by 1935 was national in scope. In 1936 the name was changed to the American Society of Anesthetists, and the society was incorporated.

The American Society of Anesthesiology, Inc. grew out of a committee representing the American Society of Anesthetists, Inc., the American Society of Regional Anesthesia, Inc., and the Section on Surgery of the American Medical Association. In 1937, the American Board of Anesthesiology, Inc., was formed as an affiliate of the American Board of Surgery, Inc. In 1941, the board was approved as a separate entity.

"The ABA mission is to advance the highest standards of the practice of anesthesiology. The ABA exists in order to:*

A. Advance the highest standards of practice by fostering lifelong education in anesthesiology, which the ABA defines as the practice of medicine dealing with but not limited to:
    (1) Assessment of, consultation for, and preparation of, patients for anesthesia.
    (2) Relief and prevention of pain during and following surgical, obstetric, therapeutic and diagnostic procedures.
    (3) Monitoring and maintenance of normal physiology during the perioperative or periprocedural period.
    (4) Management of critically ill patients.
    (5) Diagnosis and treatment of acute, chronic and cancer related pain.

(6) Management of hospice and palliative care.

(7) Clinical management and teaching of cardiac, pulmonary, and neurologic resuscitation.

(8) Evaluation of respiratory function and application of respiratory therapy.

(9) Conduct of clinical, translational and basic science research.

(10) Supervision, teaching and evaluation of performance of both medical and allied health personnel involved in perioperative or periprocedural care, critical care, pain management, and hospice and palliative care.

(11) Administrative involvement in health care facilities and organizations, and medical schools as appropriate to the ABA's mission.

B. Establish and maintain criteria for the designation of a Board certified and subspecialty certified anesthesiologist as described in the ABA's Booklet of Information.

C. Inform the Accreditation Council for Graduate Medical Education (ACGME) concerning the training required of individuals seeking certification as such requirements relate to residency and fellowship training programs in anesthesiology.

D. Establish and conduct those processes by which the Board may judge whether a physician who voluntarily applies should be issued a certificate indicating that the required standards for certification or maintenance of certification as a diplomate of the ABA in anesthesiology or its subspecialties have been met.

A Board certified anesthesiologist is a physician who provides medical management and consultation during the perioperative period, in pain medicine and in critical care medicine. At the time of application and at the time of initial certification, a diplomate of the Board must possess knowledge, judgment, adaptability, clinical skills, technical facility and personal characteristics sufficient to carry out the entire scope of anesthesiology practice independently, without accommodation or with reasonable accommodation. An ABA diplomate must logically organize and effectively present rational diagnoses and appropriate treatment protocols to peers, patients, their families and others involved in the medical community. A diplomate of the Board can serve as an expert in matters related to anesthesiology, deliberate with others, and provide advice and defend opinions in all aspects of the specialty of anesthesiology. A Board certified anesthesiologist is able to function as the leader of the anesthesiology care team.

Because of the nature of anesthesiology, the ABA diplomate must be able to manage emergent life-threatening situations in an independent and timely fashion. The ability to independently acquire and process information in a timely manner is central to assure individual responsibility for all aspects of anesthesiology care. Adequate physical and sensory faculties, such as eyesight, hearing, speech and coordinated function of the extremities, are essential to the independent performance of the Board certified anesthesiologist. Freedom from the influence of or dependency on chemical substances that impair cognitive, physical, sensory or motor function also is an essential characteristic of the Board certified anesthesiologist.

E. Serve the public, medical profession, health care facilities and organizations, medical schools, and licensing boards by providing the names of physicians certified by the Board.

Certification Requirements*

At the time of certification by the ABA, the candidate must:

A. Hold an unexpired license to practice medicine or osteopathy in at least one state or jurisdiction of the United States or province of Canada that is permanent, unconditional and unrestricted. Further, every United States and Canadian medical license the applicant holds must be free of restrictions. Candidates for initial certification and ABA diplomates have the affirmative obligation to advise the ABA of any and all restrictions placed on any of their medical licenses and to provide the ABA with complete information concerning such restrictions within 60 days after their imposition or notice, **whichever first occurs**. Such information shall include, but not be limited to, the identity of the State Medical Board imposing the restriction as well as the restriction's duration, basis, and specific terms and conditions. Candidates and diplomates discovered not to have made disclosure may be subject to sanctions on their candidate or diplomate status.

B. Have fulfilled all the requirements of the continuum of education in anesthesiology.

C. Have on file with the ABA a Certificate of Clinical Competence with an overall satisfactory rating covering the final six-month period of clinical anesthesia training in each anesthesiology residency program.

D. Have satisfied all examination requirements of the Board.

E. Have a professional standing satisfactory to the ABA.

F. Be capable of performing independently the entire scope of anesthesiology practice without accommodation or with reasonable accommodation.

Although admission into the ABA examination system and success with the examinations are important steps in the ABA certification process, they do not by themselves guarantee certification. The Board reserves the right to make the final determination of whether each candidate meets all of the requirements for certification, including A, E and F above, after successful completion of examinations for certification. ABA certificates in anesthesiology issued on or after January 1, 2000 are valid for 10 years after the year the candidate passes the examination for certification. ABA certificates are subject to ABA rules and regulations, including its Booklet of Information, all of which may be amended from time to time without further notice. A person certified by the ABA is designated a diplomate in publications of the American Board of Medical Specialties and the American Society of Anesthesiologists.

Maintenance of Certification in Anesthesiology Program*

The ABA issues a certificate that is valid for 10 years to diplomates certified on or after January 1, 2000. They must satisfactorily complete the requirements of MOCA before their time-limited certificate expires to maintain diplomate status in the specialty. MOCA is a 10-year program of ongoing self-assessment and lifelong learning, continual professional standing assessment, periodic self-directed assessments of practice performance and quality improvement, and an examination of cognitive expertise. A diplomate's MOCA cycle begins the day after the ABA awards initial certification or maintenance of certification in the specialty. The ABA awards a certificate for Maintenance of Certification in the specialty of Anesthesiology when a diplomate has completed all MOCA program requirements within the preceding 10 years. At the time of completion of maintenance of certification, the diplomate must be capable of performing independently in the specialty or subspecialty, without accommodation or with reasonable accommodation.

Although admission into the MOCA program and success with components of the program are important steps in the ABA maintenance of certification process, they do not by themselves guarantee maintenance of certification. The Board reserves the right to make the final determination of whether each diplomate meets all of the requirements for maintenance of certification, including Professional Standing and the ability to perform independently in the specialty or subspecialty, without accommodation or with reasonable accommodation, before awarding maintenance of certification. ABA maintenance of certification certificates are subject to ABA rules and regulations, including its Booklet of Information, all of which may be amended from time to time without further notice.

Physicians should maintain competency in the following general areas: patient care, medical knowledge, practice-based learning and improvement, interpersonal and communication skills, professionalism, and systems-based practice. The MOCA requirements for Professional Standing, Lifelong

---

*The American Board of Anesthesiology, Inc., Booklet of Information, February, 2013.

Learning and Self-Assessment (LLSA), Cognitive Expertise, and Practice Performance Assessment and Improvement (PPAI) are designed to provide assessments of these six general competencies.

A. PART I: PROFESSIONAL STANDING ASSESSMENT

ABA diplomates must hold an active, unrestricted license to practice medicine in at least one jurisdiction of the United States or Canada.

The ABA assesses a diplomate's Professional Standing continually. ABA diplomates have the affirmative obligation to advise the ABA of any and all restrictions placed on any of their medical licenses and to provide the ABA with complete information concerning such restrictions within 60 days after their imposition. Such information shall include, but not be limited to, the identity of the medical board imposing the restriction as well as the restriction's duration, basis, and specific terms and conditions. Diplomates discovered not to have made disclosure may be subject to sanctions on their diplomate status. Professional Standing acceptable to the ABA is a prerequisite qualification for cognitive examination and for maintenance of certification.

B. PART II: LIFELONG LEARNING AND SELF-ASSESSMENT

ABA diplomates should continually seek to improve the quality of their clinical practice and patient care through self-directed professional development. This should be done through self-assessment and learning opportunities designed to meet the diplomate's needs and the MOCA requirement for Lifelong Learning and Self-Assessment (LLSA).

LLSA requirements by certification year are available on the ABA website at www.theABA.org.

The LLSA requirement for maintenance of certification is 250 credits for continuing medical education (CME) activities.

(1) All 250 credits must be Category 1 credits for ACCME-approved programs or activities.

(2) From 2006 to 2012, no more than 70 credits for CME programs and activities may be completed in the same calendar year. Effective as of 2013, no more than 60 credits for CME programs and activities may be completed in the same calendar year. MOCA participants will have to complete some CME activity in at least five years of each 10-year MOCA cycle and are encouraged to complete some CME activity in each of the six general competencies for physicians.

Self-Assessment CME Credit Requirements

(1) All newly certified diplomates and non-time limited diplomates who enrolled in the MOCA program from January 1, 2008, to December 31, 2009, are required to complete 60 Category 1 credits of ABA-approved self-assessment activities once during their 10-year MOCA cycle. A list of the approved activities is available on the ABA website at www.theABA.org.

(2) All diplomates certified on January 1, 2010, or after and non-time limited diplomates who enroll in the MOCA program after January 1, 2010, are required to complete 90 Category 1 credits of ABA-approved self-assessment activities once during their 10-year MOCA cycle. A list of the approved activities is available on the ABA website at www.theABA.org.

Patient Safety CME Credit Requirements

(1) All newly certified diplomates and non-time limited diplomates who enroll in the MOCA program after January 1, 2008, are required to complete 20 Category 1 credits of Patient Safety CME. A list of the approved activities is available on the ABA website at www.theABA.org.

CME sponsors may submit CME activities and credits to the ABA electronically for ABA diplomates. ABA diplomates may self-report their CME activities and credits to the

ABA electronically. Whereas provider-reported CME activities do not require verification by the ABA, self-reported CME activities are subject to audit and verification by the ABA within three years of their submission. **Therefore, diplomates must keep documentation of every self-reported CME activity for at least three years after they submit it to the ABA for LLSA credit.**

C. PART III: COGNITIVE EXPERTISE ASSESSMENT

Diplomates who participate in MOCA must demonstrate their cognitive expertise by passing an ABA examination administered via computer under secure, proctored, standardized testing conditions. About 75% of the test items are based on general anesthesia topics, and the remainder of the examination is approximately evenly distributed among the following areas: pediatric anesthesia, cardiothoracic anesthesia, neuroanesthesia, obstetric anesthesia, critical care medicine and pain medicine.

Diplomates may satisfy the examination requirement no earlier than the seventh year of their 10-year MOCA cycle. Examination prerequisites for the purpose of satisfying the MOCA program requirement are:

(1) Professional standing acceptable to the ABA.

(2) Practice Performance Assessment and Improvement (PPAI) participation acceptable to the ABA.

(3) Diplomates must complete half (125 credits) of the total CME requirement. Requirements by certification year are available on the ABA website at www.theABA.org.

There is no limit to the number of times diplomates may take the MOCA examination to satisfy the maintenance of certification requirement. The ABA will inform registered examinees of the procedure for making an examination appointment approximately four months prior to the examination date.

The MOCA Cognitive Examination is administered twice each year. Test dates are available on the last page of the Booklet of Information. However, for the most current test dates please visit the ABA website at www.theABA.org, which is the official source of ABA test dates and deadlines.

The ABA must receive all documentation it requires to make a decision about a diplomate's eligibility for examination by October 31 of the preceding year for the winter examinations and by April 30 of the examination year for the summer examinations.

These deadlines are absolute, and the ABA must have documentation that the diplomate has met all of the prerequisites by the appropriate deadline. When the ABA does not have the required documentation by the appropriate deadline, it will evaluate the diplomate's eligibility for the next MOCA examination. **It ultimately is the responsibility of the diplomates to assure that the ABA receives documentation in a timely manner that they have met all of the MOCA examination prerequisites.**

D. PART IV: PRACTICE PERFORMANCE ASSESSMENT AND IMPROVEMENT

ABA diplomates should be continually engaged in a self-directed program of Practice Performance Assessment and Improvement (PPAI).

The PPAI requirement consists of the following activities:

(1) Case Evaluation: A four-step process where diplomate's assess their practice and implement changes that improve patient outcomes. A case evaluation may be completed in a specialty or subspecialty of anesthesiology. Instructions and examples are available on the ABA website at www.theABA.org.

(2) Simulation Education Course: A contextual learning opportunity to assess and improve one's practice in areas such as crisis management in a simulation setting at an ASA-endorsed center. A simulation education course may be completed in a specialty or subspecialty of anesthesiology. Information on ASA-endorsed simulation centers

Practice performance assessment and improvement requirements by year in MOCA cycle										
Year certified	1	2	3	4	5	6	7	8	9	10
2000-2003					Attestation				Attestation	
2004-2007					Attestation	Case evaluation or simulation				
2008 or later	*Case evaluation or simulation					*Case evaluation or simulation				
						Attestation				

*Complete <u>both</u> a case evaluation and simulation course during your 10-year MOCA cycle.
One activity must be completed between years 1 to 5, and the second between years 6 to 10.

is available on the Maintenance of Certification page of the ABA website at www.theABA.org.

(3) Attestation: The ABA solicits references to verify diplomate's clinical activity and participation in practice improvement activities.

During their 10-year MOCA cycle, diplomates must complete the PPAI activities as defined in the above chart, based on the year they were certified.

Diplomates certified between January 1, 2001 and December 31, 2007, have the option of completing a Simulation Course in lieu of completing an Attestation.

Diplomates certified between January 1, 2004 and December 31, 2007 who elect to complete a Simulation Course in lieu of an Attestation must complete a Case Evaluation in years 6-10.

Evidence of one PPAI activity acceptable to the ABA is a prerequisite for the MOCA Cognitive Examination.

Additional information about the ABA's PPAI process and requirements by year certified can be found on the ABA website at www.theABA.org.

Reciprocity For Diplomates:

Diplomates may complete one Part IV activity through any other ABMS Board and submit it to the ABA to fulfill the MOCA Part IV Case Evaluation requirement. Documentation of completion of the activity must be submitted with diplomates' requests for Part IV credit. All diplomates enrolled in MOCA must complete a Simulation Education Course and an Attestation as defined by their specific program requirements.

E. MOCA CYCLE DURING AND AFTER TRANSITION PERIOD

The transition from a voluntary recertification examination program to MOCA began in January 2004. The voluntary recertification examination ended with the administration of the December 2009 Recertification Examination.

(1) Diplomates certified before 2000 have a certificate that is not time-limited. They do not have to complete the MOCA program to maintain certification. They may, however, voluntarily participate in the MOCA program. The first time they apply for MOCA they may complete the program in as soon as two years. They may complete the expedited MOCA program only once; thereafter, the 10-year MOCA program is their only option.

Diplomates certified before 2000 who choose to complete their first MOCA program within five years of their enrollment must complete two PPAI activities, an attestation and either a case evaluation or simulation education course; those who choose to complete the program within 6-10 years of their enrollment must complete all three PPAI activities. The Professional Standing assessment is continual. They can satisfy LLSA requirements on the basis of CME activities completed after certification and within the past 10 years. They can take a secure examination when they have satisfied all of the prerequisite requirements by the appropriate deadline.

(2) The MOCA program is the only option to maintain certification for ABA diplomates certified in or after 2000. The ABA automatically enrolls diplomates in MOCA when they are awarded time-limited certification or when they successfully complete each MOCA cycle. They have to maintain Professional Standing acceptable to the ABA and satisfy the Cognitive Examination requirement. Additionally,

a. Diplomates certified in 2000, 2001, 2002, or 2003 were issued a time-limited certificate before the MOCA program was available. For these diplomates, the LLSA requirements for the secure examination prerequisite and for the awarding of maintenance of certification are prorated, and, the PPAI requirement consists of the ABA obtaining attestations and evidence of the candidate's clinical activity and ongoing practice performance assessment and improvement in Years 5 and 9 of their MOCA cycle.

b. The MOCA program was available when diplomates were issued a time-limited certificate in 2004, 2005, 2006, and 2007. For these diplomates, the LLSA requirements for the secure examination prerequisite and for the awarding of maintenance of certification are not prorated. For PPAI, the ABA will obtain attestations and evidence of the candidate's clinical activity and ongoing program of practice performance assessment and improvement in Year 5 of the candidate's MOCA cycle, and they have to complete one of two PPA I activities (case evaluation or simulation education) in Years 6 through 10.

c. Diplomates enrolled in MOCA from 2000 through 2007 may complete a simulation course in place of providing references to support their attestations. In order for the diplomate to receive PPAI credit for the course, the simulation course must be completed at an American Society of Anesthesiologists (ASA) endorsed simulation center and all follow-up must be completed within the required timeframe. Once all portions of the simulation course are complete, the ASA will report the completion to the ABA on behalf of the diplomate.

d. The LLSA requirements for the secure examination prerequisite and for the awarding of maintenance of certification are not prorated for diplomates issued a time-limited certificate in or after 2008. For PPAI, these diplomates have to complete three PPAI activities (case evaluation, simulation education, and an attestation).

Diplomates may visit the ABA website at www.theABA.org or contact the ABA office for additional information regarding their MOCA program requirements.

F. ENROLLMENT APPLICATION PROCEDURE

Diplomates are automatically enrolled in MOCA when they are awarded time-limited primary certification in anesthesiology and again when they successfully complete each MOCA cycle, including an expedited MOCA cycle. The ABA automatically enrolls diplomates with a non-time limited primary certificate in MOCA upon their completion of the MOCA program in 2005 or thereafter. **All other ABA diplomates have to apply to the ABA to enroll in MOCA.**

Diplomates not automatically enrolled in MOCA may electronically enroll at any time via the ABA website at www.theABA. org. Exceptions to this requirement will be considered upon written request. Written requests are to be addressed to the ABA Secretary and must include the basis for the requested exception.

Applicants must provide information about all their medical licenses and current contact information (e.g., postal address) to complete the application process. **It ultimately is the responsibility of every applicant to assure that the ABA receives all required information**."

Information concerning the Board and its requirements may be obtained from

The American Board of Anesthesiology, Inc.
4208 Six Forks Road, Suite 900
Raleigh, NC 27609-5735
Telephone: (866) 999-7501
FAX: (866) 999-7503
Web: www.theABA.org

Examination Preparation

Ideally, preparation for the examination should begin during training. During this period, time spent in a systematic approach to the body of knowledge will be well rewarded.

A Content Outline of the In-Training Examination, by the American Board of Anesthesiology and the American Society of Anesthesiologists, covers the knowledge that should be gained during residency training. It serves as a grid for the questions to be covered in the examination and was used by all of this book's authors to choose topics to be covered by each chapter's questions. A copy of the most current Content Outline may be obtained from the ABA's website at www.theABA.org.

Textbooks provide a good background of information. Popular comprehensive texts include those edited by Longnecker, et al., and Miller, et al. Many subspecialty texts are available in the areas of pain management, critical care, cardiothoracic, obstetric, and pediatric anesthesia.

The best sources of current information are journals and meetings. The newest data and latest techniques are reported in these two sources, and one should be familiar with them. An invaluable source of information is the Annual Refresher Course given each year in conjunction with the ASA meeting in October. Lectures are given throughout the meeting. A syllabus is available covering all the lectures and is supplied electronically to attendees.

Format of Examinations

The Basic and Advanced examinations of the American Board of Anesthesiology are of the objective, multiple-choice form employing the same question types used in this book. They are computer-based examinations taken at a standardized testing center.

PART I
Basic Topics in Anesthesiology

CHAPTER 1

Physics, Chemistry, and Mathematics
Questions

DIRECTIONS (Questions 1-34): Each of the numbered items or incomplete statements in this section is followed by answers or by completions of the statement. Select the ONE lettered answer or completion that is BEST in each case.

1. A patient with severe pulmonary fibrosis wishes to travel on an airplane. What amount of supplemental oxygen will be needed to maintain the arterial oxygen concentration at about 70 mm Hg? Assume the airplane cabin is pressurized at 580 mm Hg and that the patient's alveolar-arterial oxygen gradient is 150 mm Hg.

   (A) 40%
   (B) 50%
   (C) 60%
   (D) 70%
   (E) 80%

2. A clinician wishes to perform a single-breath induction with sevoflurane and exceed the maximum sevoflurane concentration supplied by the vaporizer. She fills a 3-L reservoir bag with oxygen and adds 2 mL of sevoflurane liquid to the bag. What will the concentration of sevoflurane vapor be in the reservoir bag? Assume the operating room is at sea level and the room temperature is 20°C. The ideal gas constant is 0.082 L-atm-$°K^{-1}$-$mole^{-1}$, the specific gravity of sevoflurane is 1.52, and its molecular weight is 200 g/mol.

   (A) 12.2%
   (B) 13.5%
   (C) 14.8%
   (D) 16.1%
   (E) 18.5%

3. In the typical operating room, patients lose heat via all of the following mechanisms EXCEPT

   (A) sublimation
   (B) conduction
   (C) convection
   (D) radiation
   (E) evaporation

4. An anesthesiologist plans a clinical study comparing a new antiemetic with ondansetron. 100 women undergoing elective laparoscopic tubal ligation will be randomized to receive either the new antiemetic or a standard 4-mg dose of ondansetron. The primary outcome variable is the number of women that vomit postoperatively in each group. In all likelihood, the best statistical test to compare the two treatments will be

   (A) Student's t-test for unpaired data
   (B) Student's t-test for paired data
   (C) analysis of variance
   (D) chi squared
   (E) Wilcoxon rank-sum test

DIRECTIONS: Use the following scenario to answer Questions 5-7:

The standard extension cord used in a particular hospital is 15 feet long and has a capacitance of 0.05 µF. The capacitive reactance of each extension cord when used with 60 Hz power is 53 kilohms. Three of these extension cords are plugged into a circuit protected by the same circuit breaker and line isolation monitor. Assume that the three extension cords are the only sources of capacitance and capacitive reactance on the circuit.

5. What is the value of the capacitance in the circuit?

   (A) 0.0167 μF
   (B) 0.025 μF
   (C) 0.05 μF
   (D) 0.10 μF
   (E) 0.15 μF

6. What is the value of the capacitive reactance in the circuit?

   (A) 17.7 kilohms
   (B) 26.5 kilohms
   (C) 53 kilohms
   (D) 106 kilohms
   (E) 159 kilohms

7. Will the line isolation monitor alarm?

   (A) No, because the leakage current is less than 1 mA.
   (B) No, because the leakage current is less than 5 mA.
   (C) No, because the leakage current is less than 10 mA.
   (D) Yes, because the leakage current is greater than 5 mA.
   (E) Yes, because the leakage current is greater than 10 mA.

8. In order to perform a meta-analysis, a researcher

   (A) must show significance at a very high probability level (e.g., p < 0.001)
   (B) combines the results from several similar studies
   (C) needs to enroll at least 1,000 patients in a study
   (D) designs a study that takes place at numerous (e.g., > 100) independent clinical sites
   (E) studies numerous independent parameters that evaluate an intervention (e.g., drug treatment)

9. The electrical current, often called the "let-go current," above which contraction of the finger flexors is unable to be overcome by voluntarily contracting the finger extensors is approximately

   (A) 0.15 mA
   (B) 1.5 mA
   (C) 15 mA
   (D) 150 mA
   (E) 1.5 A

DIRECTIONS: Use the following table to answer Questions 10-12:

Gas or vapor	Viscosity (centipoises)	Molecular weight (g/mol)	Density (kg/m³)	Boiling point (C)
Argon	0.022	39.9	1.66	−186
Carbon dioxide	0.0145	44	1.82	−57
Diethyl ether	0.00075	74	3.08	35
Helium	0.0188	4	0.166	−269
Nitrogen	0.0175	28	1.16	−196
Nitrous oxide	0.0133	44	1.83	−88
Oxygen	0.020	32	1.33	−183
Xenon	0.022	131	5.46	−108

10. Due to an allergic reaction, a patient has severe tracheal edema that uniformly narrows the trachea from the vocal cords to the carina. Compared with breathing 100% oxygen, for a given inspiratory force, airflow will be increased to the greatest degree by diluting the oxygen with

    (A) helium
    (B) nitrogen
    (C) argon
    (D) nitrous oxide
    (E) xenon

11. A patient with an intraluminal tracheal tumor has severe narrowing of the airway resulting in an air passage resembling a pinhole. Compared with breathing 100% oxygen, for a given inspiratory force, airflow will be increased to the greatest degree by diluting the oxygen with

(A) diethyl ether

(B) carbon dioxide

(C) helium

(D) xenon

(E) nitrous oxide

12. Ordinarily it is not permissible to use a rotameter designed for one gas to control the flow of another gas. In a military field hospital without spare parts, a biomedical engineer wishes to cannibalize other equipment to replace a broken oxygen flowmeter. Although not a perfect match, the best replacement for the broken oxygen rotameter would be one designed to control the flow of

(A) argon

(B) helium

(C) nitrogen

(D) nitrous oxide

(E) carbon dioxide

13. Regarding the critical temperature of nitrous oxide in an E cylinder attached to an anesthesia machine in an operating room, the critical temperature

(A) is not relevant in an operating room environment

(B) is the temperature in the tank that permits nitrous oxide to exist as a liquid

(C) cannot be exceeded without risking tank rupture

(D) is the temperature above which nitrous oxide cannot exist as a liquid

(E) is the temperature at which nitrous oxide liquid becomes a gas

14. An anesthesia tech accidentally left the oxygen flowmeter set at 15 L/min on a Friday afternoon and the oxygen flowed at this rate through the absorber all weekend. On Monday morning, when 10% desflurane in 100% oxygen is administered, the patient may be exposed to a toxic concentration of

(A) ozone

(B) phosgene

(C) carbon dioxide

(D) carbon monoxide

(E) fluoride

15. A cylinder of oxygen has an internal volume of 6 L and a pressure of 1700 psi. How many liters of oxygen will this tank supply at sea level?

(A) 660 L

(B) 680 L

(C) 694 L

(D) 706 L

(E) 716 L

16. A patient is undergoing operative repair of an arm fracture. The anesthesiologist is standing four feet from the patient's arm. The surgeon is using fluoroscopy to visualize the fracture. Assume the amount of radiation to which the anesthesiologist is exposed is x. If the anesthesiologist moves to a new position eight feet from the arm, then the amount of radiation exposure will decrease to approximately

(A) 0.75x

(B) 0.5x

(C) 0.33x

(D) 0.25x

(E) 0.125x

17. The absorption of one molecule of carbon dioxide by soda lime causes the net production of how many molecules of water?

(A) 0

(B) 1

(C) 2

(D) 3

(E) 4

18. The current delivered to the patient by an electrocautery device differs from the current supplied by an electrical utility in its

(A) capacitance

(B) frequency

(C) amperage

(D) voltage

(E) power

19. A solution of intravenous fluid has the following composition:

    100 mM glucose
    120 mM sodium chloride
    10 mM potassium chloride
    5 mM calcium chloride
    4 mM magnesium chloride

The osmolality of this solution is approximately

    (A) 239 mOsm/kg H_2O
    (B) 278 mOsm/kg H_2O
    (C) 287 mOsm/kg H_2O
    (D) 378 mOsm/kg H_2O
    (E) 387 mOsm/kg H_2O

DIRECTIONS: Use the following figure to answer Question 20:

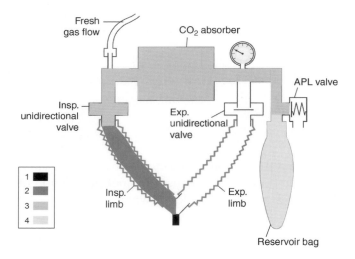

20. In an intubated patient connected to an anesthesia machine, mechanical dead space consists of the volume of the endotracheal tube proximal to the teeth plus which one (or more) of the volumes indicated in the figure? The different volumes are indicated by the different shadings as shown in the legend in the lower left of the figure.

    (A) 1
    (B) 1 + 2
    (C) 1 + 2 + 3
    (D) 1 + 2 + 3 + 4

21. The protection device known as a ground fault interrupter is rarely used in operating rooms because it

    (A) protects against microshock but not macroshock injury
    (B) does not function well in a wet environment
    (C) disconnects power to life support equipment
    (D) cannot be tested by the user for proper functioning
    (E) does not have an audible alarm

22. The Doppler effect is the principle behind numerous monitoring devices. When the source of an audio wave moves toward the observer, the sound

    (A) amplitude decreases
    (B) frequency decreases
    (C) frequency increases
    (D) phase decreases
    (E) phase increases

23. If two different tissues have the same partial pressure of an anesthetic gas, the concentration of the gas in the tissues will

    (A) differ according to each tissue's blood flow
    (B) differ according to each tissue's partition coefficient
    (C) vary according to the atmospheric pressure
    (D) not depend on body temperature
    (E) be the same

24. When the relative humidity is 100% then

    (A) relative humidity and absolute humidity are equal
    (B) relative humidity and specific humidity are equal
    (C) the relative humidity will decrease if the temperature decreases
    (D) a patient's perspiration will not evaporate

25. The National Fire Protection Association mandates which one of these standards for operating rooms?

(A) Isolated power is required in all operating rooms

(B) Isolated power is required in areas designated as wet locations

(C) In the event of a power failure, emergency power must become operative within 1 second

(D) When isolated power is present, a line isolation monitor must also be present

DIRECTIONS: Use the following scenario to answer Questions 26-27.

A university endocrinology clinic diagnosed pheochromocytoma in seven patients in the preceding year. The mean arterial pressures (MAP), in mm Hg, of the seven patients at initial presentation were 120, 130, 135, 145, 150, 150, and 164.

26. The median of the MAP values is

(A) 130

(B) 142

(C) 145

(D) 150

(E) 155

27. The sample standard deviation of the MAP values is

(A) 3.8

(B) 7.2

(C) 11.1

(D) 14.7

(E) 22.4

28. Which one of the following intravenous solutions is a colloid?

(A) lactated Ringer solution

(B) 0.9% saline

(C) 7.5% saline

(D) 5% albumin

(E) 5% glucose

29. Of the following intravenous solutions, the one whose osmolality is most different from that of plasma is

(A) lactated Ringer solution

(B) 5% glucose

(C) 2.5% glucose + 0.45% saline

(D) 0.9% saline

(E) 5% glucose + 0.45% saline

30. If the skin resistance between a person's arms is 6000 ohms, and the person's right arm is connected to an earth ground, and 120 V are applied to his/her left arm, the current flowing from arm to arm will be

(A) nearly 0 if the 120 V are supplied by a grounded electrical system

(B) 20 mA if the 120 V are supplied by a grounded electrical system

(C) 20 mA if the 120 V are supplied by an isolated electrical system

(D) 50 mA if the 120 V are supplied by an isolated electrical system

(E) 50 A if the 120 V are supplied by an isolated electrical system

DIRECTIONS (Questions 31-34): Each group of items below consists of lettered headings followed by a list of numbered phrases or statements. For each numbered phrase or statement, select the ONE lettered heading or component that is most closely associated with it. Each lettered heading or component may be selected once, more than once, or not at all.

(A) Volt

(B) Ampere

(C) Joule

(D) Henry

(E) Farad

(F) Ohm

(G) Coulomb

(H) Watt

(I) Sievert

(J) Gray

(K) Hertz

(L) Newton

(M) No unit

For each measurement, select the appropriate unit.

31. The amount of radiation to which a patient is exposed while undergoing a CT scan.

32. The baricity of a local anesthetic solution for spinal anesthesia.

33. The electrical power used by a warming blanket.

34. The electrical impedance of an anesthesiologist measured from the person's left hand to right hand.

Answers and Explanations

1. **(B)** The patient's alveolar oxygen concentration is estimated from the alveolar gas equation:

$$P_{AO_2} = F_{IO_2} \times (P_{atm} - P_{H_2O}) - P_{aCO_2}$$
$$\times \left(F_{IO_2} + \left(\frac{1 - F_{IO_2}}{RQ} \right) \right)$$

Assuming a value of 0.8 for the respiratory quotient, the patient's alveolar oxygen concentration would be approximately 222 mm Hg when breathing 50% oxygen. The patient's arterial oxygen concentration would therefore be approximately 72 mm Hg. *(5:459)*

2. **(A)** A volume of 2 mL of sevoflurane liquid has a mass of 3.04 g corresponding to 0.0152 moles. The volume of an ideal gas, V, is $nRT/P = (0.0152) \times (0.082) \times (273 + 20) = 0.365$ L. A volume of 0.365 L of sevoflurane vapor in the 3-L reservoir bag represents a concentration of 12.2%. *(5:627)*

3. **(A)** The four mechanisms of heat loss are conduction, convection, radiation, and evaporation. Sublimation is the phase transition between a solid and a gas. *(5:259)*

4. **(D)** Of the tests listed, only the chi squared text compares proportions (in this case, the proportion of patients vomiting) in two populations. Student's t-test and analysis of variance compare means in two populations, while the Mann-Whitney test is a nonparametric test that assesses whether one population has larger values than another. *(4:1202-11)*

5. **(E)** The three extension cords represent capacitors connected in parallel. When capacitors are connected in parallel, their capacitances are added. *(5:372)*

6. **(A)** The three extension cords represent reactances connected in parallel. When three identical reactance values are connected in parallel, the resulting reactance value is one-third that of each individual unit. *(5:372)*

7. **(D)** The leakage current due to the extension cords will be given by Ohm's law, $I = E/Z$, where I is current in amperes, E is voltage in volts, and Z is impedance in ohms. In this circuit, since the only contribution to impedance is capacitive reactance, the potential leakage current is 6.8 mA at 120 V. Since the typical line isolation monitor will alarm when the potential leakage current is above 5 mA, the line isolation monitor will indeed alarm. *(5:376-8)*

8. **(B)** In a meta-analysis, several studies that measured similar outcome variable(s) are combined, typically to increase the statistical power that is derived from a larger number of study subjects. *(www.cochrane.org/handbook/915-what-does-meta-analysis-entail)*

9. **(C)** When electrical currents of 10-20 mA are applied to the upper extremity, sustained muscle contraction occurs of a magnitude that cannot be overcome. If the individual is holding onto a wire, he or she probably will not be able to let go. *(5:374-5)*

10. **(D)** Laminar flow in a tube is governed by Poiseuille's law that relates laminar flow to the 4th power of the radius:

$$\text{Flow} = \frac{\pi p r^4}{8vl}$$

where p is the pressure, r is the radius of the tube, v is the viscosity of the gas, and l is the length of the tube. Since flow is inversely proportional to viscosity, the flow will be increased to the greatest degree by diluting oxygen with nitrous oxide, the gas that has the lowest viscosity among the choices. (5:622)

11. **(C)** Gas flow through a pinhole results in turbulent flow that is inversely proportional to density. Thus, helium, the least dense gas of those listed, would provide the greatest increase in flow when used to dilute oxygen. (5:622)

12. **(B)** The proper functioning of a rotameter tube depends on laminar flow in the tube that is governed by Poiseuille's law. Therefore the closest replacement rotameter would be for helium, the gas with the viscosity closest to that of oxygen. (5:623)

13. **(D)** The critical temperature of nitrous oxide is the temperature at which it boils into a gas, regardless of the pressure in the tank. For nitrous oxide, that temperature is 36.5°C, a temperature that could easily be reached in an operating room without air conditioning. (5:618, 622)

14. **(D)** Desflurane, but not sevoflurane, may react with dry soda lime to yield a potentially toxic concentration of carbon monoxide. The reaction of trichloroethylene, an obsolete anesthetic agent, yielded phosgene. (5:614)

15. **(C)** At constant temperature, the product of the pressure and volume of a gas is constant (Boyle's law). Thus, the volume of gas at sea level where the atmospheric pressure is 14.7 psi will be (1700 psi) × (6 L)/(14.7 psi) = 694 L. (5:618)

16. **(D)** Radiation intensity decreases as a function of the square of the distance. Thus, by doubling the distance between the patient and the anesthesiologist, the amount of the radiation exposure will decrease to one-fourth its previous value. (5:385)

17. **(B)** A molecule of carbon dioxide reacts with one molecule of water to form carbonic acid. The reaction of one molecule of carbonic acid with two molecules of sodium hydroxide produces two molecules of water. Therefore, there is the net production of one molecule of water. (5:641)

18. **(B)** The standard frequency used by electrical utilities in the United States is 60 Hz, while the current delivered by an electrocautery device is in the range of $10^5 – 10^6$ Hz.

19. **(E)** Osmolality is the concentration of osmotically active particles per kilogram of solvent. At both room and body temperatures, the difference between 1 L of water and 1 kg of water can be ignored. Glucose does not dissociate in solution so its osmotic concentration is its molar concentration. Sodium chloride and potassium chloride each dissociate into two osmotically active particles, while calcium chloride and magnesium chloride each dissociate into three osmotically active particles. The total osmolality is therefore approximately $100 + 240 + 20 + 15 + 12 = 387$ mOsm/kg H_2O. (5:511)

20. **(A)** Mechanical dead space in this patient is the sum of the volume of the endotracheal tube proximal to the teeth plus the volume of the arm of the Y-connector. None of the other volumes in the circle system contribute to mechanical dead space.

21. **(C)** A ground fault interrupter provides excellent protection against injury from macroshock (but not microshock). It has a "test" button to confirm proper functioning. Although it does not have an audible alarm, that is not the reason why it is rarely used in operating rooms. A ground fault interrupter protects the user by disconnecting power to the devices

connected to it. These devices may include life support equipment in an operating room. *(5:379)*.

22. **(C)** The definition of the Doppler effect is that when the source of an audio wave moves toward the observer, the frequency of the sound increases. *(5: 430)*

23. **(B)** The definition of partition coefficient is the ratio of the concentrations of a substance in two contiguous compartments at steady state (i.e., when the partial pressure of the substance is equal in both compartments). Partition coefficients vary according to temperature but not according to atmospheric pressure. *(5:600)*

24. **(D)** Absolute humidity is the amount of water vapor in air, in units of mass/volume. Specific humidity is the ratio of the mass of water vapor in a volume of air to the mass of that volume of air. Relative humidity is the ratio of the partial pressure of water vapor in air to the saturated (maximum) partial pressure of water vapor at the same temperature and pressure. Since the maximum water vapor content of air increases with temperature, if the temperature of a saturated volume of air is decreased, water vapor will condense into droplets forming fog, but the relative humidity will remain 100%. When a patient is placed in an atmosphere of 100% relative humidity, perspiration will not evaporate and there will be no evaporative heat loss (as long as the volume of the saturated air is large enough such that the patient's body temperature does not raise the air temperature by conduction or convection).

25. **(B)** Isolated power is required only in wet areas. Line isolation monitors are not required, nor is the instantaneous (i.e., < 1 sec) availability of emergency backup power. *(5:378, 380)*

26. **(C)** The median value is the value that falls in the middle of the subjects' values. In this group of seven patients, the median value is

145 because there are three values lower (120, 130, and 135) and three values higher (150, 150, and 164).

27. **(D)** The sample standard deviation, s, is given by the following equation:

$$s = \sqrt{\frac{\sum_{i=1}^{N}(x_i - \bar{x})^2}{N-1}}$$

where N is the number of observations, $\bar{x}$ is the mean, and x_i represents each individual observation. The sum of the squares of the differences is 1298, thus the sample standard deviation is 14.7.

28. **(D)** Colloid solutions contain solutes of high molecular weight (e.g., > 30 kDa). *(5:200)*

29. **(E)** The osmolality of 5% glucose + 0.45% saline is approximately 50% greater than that of plasma. The other four solutions have approximately the same osmolality as plasma. *(5:535)*

30. **(B)** Current will flow only if both the patient and the electrical system are grounded. The magnitude of the current is given by Ohm's law that states that current (in amps) equals the voltage (in volts) divided by the resistance (in ohms). Thus, the current will equal 120 V/6000 ohms or 0.02 A, that is 20 mA. *(5:362-3, 376-8)*

31. **(I)** The unit of radiation exposure is the Sievert. *(5:385)*

32. **(M)** Baricity is the ratio of the specific gravity of the local anesthetic solution to the specific gravity of spinal fluid at the same temperature. Since it is a ratio, it has no units. *(5:794)*.

33. **(H)** The unit of electrical power is the Watt. *(5:372)*

34. **(F)** The unit of electrical resistance is the Ohm. *(5:372)*

Anesthesia Equipment
Questions

DIRECTIONS (Questions 35-75): Each of the numbered items or incomplete statements in this section is followed by answers or by completions of the statement. Select the ONE lettered answer or completion that is BEST in each case.

35. An anesthesiologist is administering isoflurane via a variable bypass vaporizer in Denver (altitude 1,609 m). The fresh gas flow rates are 1 L/min oxygen and 2 L/min nitrous oxide. When the vaporizer is set to deliver 2% isoflurane, the concentration of isoflurane present at the common gas outlet is approximately

    (A) 1.1%
    (B) 1.6%
    (C) 2%
    (D) 2.7%
    (E) 3.4%

36. A patient is being monitored with a bispectral index (BIS) monitor. When the value for BIS is 60, it means that the patient

    (A) has about a 60% probability of being awake
    (B) has a very small (less than 1%) probability of having recall of intraoperative events
    (C) does not require additional opioid
    (D) if not pharmacologically paralyzed, will not move in response to surgical incision
    (E) is less likely to be awake than if the BIS value were 50

37. An open waste-gas scavenging system

    (A) must have a negative pressure relief valve
    (B) must have a positive pressure relief valve
    (C) must be connected to a source of vacuum
    (D) does not need a reservoir
    (E) cannot be simultaneously connected to the APL and ventilator relief valves

38. Which one of the following statements is TRUE regarding blood pressure cuffs?

    (A) The bladder length should be 50% of the limb circumference.
    (B) The bladder width should be 40% of the limb circumference.
    (C) A cuff designed for a thigh cannot be used on a large arm.
    (D) A cuff designed for an arm cannot be used on a small thigh.
    (E) A cuff whose bladder is too narrow for the limb will give an erroneously low blood pressure.

DIRECTIONS: Use the following figure to answer Questions 39-40:

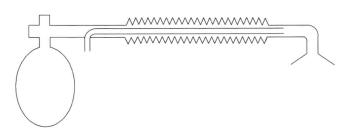

39. The system depicted in the figure is the

    (A) Georgia valve
    (B) Jackson–Rees system
    (C) T-piece
    (D) Bain circuit
    (E) Mapleson A system

40. A disadvantage of the circuit in the figure is the

    (A) inability to use spontaneous ventilation with the system
    (B) requirement for low flow
    (C) inability to scavenge waste gases
    (D) presence of overflow valve farther from the patient
    (E) kinking of inner delivery tube

41. A resident notices an increasing discrepancy between the $Paco_2$ and the end-tidal carbon dioxide. Factors that increase this difference include ALL of the following EXCEPT

    (A) mismatch of ventilation and perfusion
    (B) wheezing
    (C) high fresh gas flow rates
    (D) high cardiac output

42. An anesthesia technician is transporting several Aladin isoflurane vaporizer cassettes on a cart. After one of the cassettes accidentally tips over onto its side

    (A) the wick will become saturated
    (B) the cassette must be returned to the factory
    (C) the concentration of the vapor will be higher than calculated
    (D) the cassette should be flushed with oxygen at 10 L/min for 10 min
    (E) the cassette may be put into use immediately

43. Which one of the following situations regarding intraoperative monitoring is mandated by the American Society of Anesthesiologists' Standards for Basic Intraoperative Monitoring?

    (A) A patient having an inguinal herniorrhaphy under local anesthesia with monitored anesthesia care must have a resident or attending anesthesiologist or nurse anesthetist present in the operating room at all times during the surgical procedure.
    (B) A patient who underwent a thoracotomy and wedge resection yesterday and who is receiving a continuous epidural infusion of 0.1% bupivacaine must have his heart rate taken and recorded every five minutes.
    (C) A patient having a total knee replacement under spinal anesthesia must have the expired carbon dioxide measured.
    (D) A patient having intraoperative radiation therapy under general anesthesia must have a resident or attending anesthesiologist or nurse anesthetist present in the operating room at all times during the procedure.
    (E) A woman in labor with an indwelling epidural catheter and receiving a continuous epidural infusion of local anesthetic must have her blood pressure taken and recorded every five minutes.

44. An anesthesia circuit is connected to a circle system and the combined volume of both is 6 L. The fresh gas flow is 3 L/min. After isoflurane 2% is turned on, how long will it take the concentration in the circuit to reach 1.96% isoflurane (i.e., 98.1% of the concentration set on the vaporizer?)

    (A) 0.5 min
    (B) 1 min
    (C) 2 min
    (D) 4 min
    (E) 8 min

45. A negative-pressure leak test

    (A) is accomplished by having the clinician apply mouth suction to the tubing connected to the common gas outlet
    (B) reliably finds leaks in the carbon dioxide absorber

(C) is only appropriate for anesthesia machines containing a check valve downstream from the vaporizers

(D) must be performed with the anesthesia machine's master switch turned on

(E) may detect internal vaporizer leaks

46. All anesthesia machines approved for current use have check valves located at the

(A) common gas outlet

(B) expiratory connection on the circle system

(C) vaporizer outlet

(D) waste gas scavenging outlet

47. A 56-year-old woman with breast cancer metastatic to the spine needs an MRI to evaluate the metastases. Because she cannot lie flat comfortably, general anesthesia is planned. Anesthesia equipment that is UNSAFE to use in a room containing a functioning magnetic resonance imaging machine includes

(A) laryngeal mask airway

(B) fiberoptic oximeter probe

(C) blood pressure cuff

(D) Macintosh laryngoscope with plastic handle

(E) end-tidal carbon dioxide sampling tubing

48. The major component, by weight, in currently used carbon dioxide absorbents is

(A) barium hydroxide

(B) calcium hydroxide

(C) pH indicator

(D) potassium hydroxide

(E) sodium hydroxide

49. The formation of carbon monoxide in a carbon dioxide absorber is facilitated by the presence of ALL of the following compounds EXCEPT

(A) desflurane

(B) potassium hydroxide

(C) sodium hydroxide

(D) water

50. A patient is being ventilated with a traditional anesthesia machine ventilator using the following set parameters:

Tidal volume = 500 mL
Ventilatory rate = 10/min
I:E ratio = 1:3
Oxygen flow = 1 L/min
Nitrous oxide flow = 2 L/min

The resulting minute ventilation is approximately

(A) 5 L/min

(B) 5.25 L/min

(C) 5.5 L/min

(D) 5.75 L/min

(E) 6 L/min

51. The tubing that connects the APL (adjustable pressure limiting, or pop-off) valve to the waste gas scavenging system is the same diameter as the tubing or the connector that is connected to the

(A) circle system

(B) common gas outlet

(C) endotracheal tube

(D) reservoir bag

(E) ventilator pressure relief valve

52. The anesthesia machine checkout instructions published by the American Society of Anesthesiologists in 2008 include ALL of the following steps EXCEPT

(A) assessment of the competency of the unidirectional valves in the breathing circuit

(B) calibration of the oxygen analyzer

(C) confirmation that the carbon dioxide absorbent is not exhausted

(D) determination that the vaporizers can deliver agent

(E) determination of the internal pressure of the attached oxygen cylinder

53. The typical automatic noninvasive blood pressure measuring device most accurately determines

   (A) cessation of Korotkoff sounds
   (B) diastolic blood pressure
   (C) mean arterial pressure
   (D) systolic blood pressure

54. The device used to reduce the pressure of a gas from a compressed gas cylinder to a usable, nearly constant pressure is

   (A) a gauge
   (B) a flowmeter
   (C) an indicator
   (D) a regulator
   (E) a check valve

55. The position best tolerated by the surgical patient is the

   (A) lithotomy position
   (B) prone position
   (C) horizontal supine position
   (D) Trendelenburg position
   (E) Fowler position

56. If a nitrous oxide tank is contaminated with water vapor, ice will form on the cylinder valve as a result of the

   (A) latent heat of vaporization
   (B) specific heat
   (C) vapor pressure
   (D) low pressure of the nitrous oxide
   (E) ambient temperature

57. The indicator in carbon dioxide absorbent is

   (A) methylene blue
   (B) ethyl violet
   (C) bromthymol blue
   (D) phenolphthalein
   (E) cresol purple

DIRECTIONS: Use the following figure to answer Question 58:

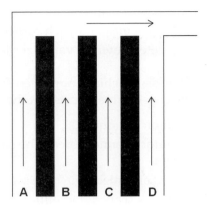

58. The oxygen flowmeter should be at position

   (A) A
   (B) B
   (C) C
   (D) D
   (E) position is not critical

59. An anesthesiologist is using an anesthesia machine equipped with an oxygen proportioning system, as well as an extra flowmeter that is supplied by a helium tank. A hypoxic gas mixture may be administered to the patient in any of the following situations EXCEPT

   (A) the gas supplied by the wall oxygen outlet is not oxygen
   (B) there is a leak in the oxygen flowmeter
   (C) the helium flowmeter is adjusted to an excessively high flow rate
   (D) the nitrous oxide flowmeter is adjusted to an excessively high flow rate

60. A resident is teaching a medical student to intubate for the first time. She hands her a laryngoscope handle with a Macintosh blade and tells her that in order to use the Macintosh blade properly, the

   (A) tip is advanced into the vallecula
   (B) epiglottis is lifted directly
   (C) laryngoscope is held in the right hand
   (D) patient should be told to say, "Ah."
   (E) blade enters the mouth on the left side

61. A nitrous oxide tank contains gas at a pressure of 750 psi. When the last drop of liquid nitrous oxide evaporates

    (A) the pressure will fall rapidly
    (B) the rate of pressure fall is dependent on the rate of flow
    (C) the pressure will begin to rise as the gas expands
    (D) the pressure will be zero
    (E) the pressure will remain at 750 psi until the tank is empty

62. A patient with a prior history of awareness under anesthesia is to be monitored with a BIS monitor. This monitor most reliably indicates the depth of anesthesia when the patient is anesthetized with

    (A) oxygen plus high-dose fentanyl
    (B) ketamine
    (C) nitrous oxide
    (D) xenon
    (E) propofol

63. When the oxygen flush valve is pressed

    (A) oxygen at the pressure of the compressed oxygen cylinders is applied to the breathing system
    (B) the oxygen flow rate is accurately displayed by the oxygen rotameter
    (C) excessive agent concentration may be applied to the breathing system if the vaporizer is on
    (D) barotrauma may result if the APL valve is open and connected to an open scavenging system
    (E) the ventilator should not be in the inspiratory phase of positive pressure ventilation

64. The diameter index safety system (DISS)

    (A) prevents attachment of gas-administering equipment to the wrong type of gas
    (B) prevents incorrect yoke-tank connections
    (C) consists of quick-connectors typically mounted on the wall or hanging from the ceiling

    (D) is found on the wall end, but not the machine end, of gas hoses connected to anesthesia machines
    (E) is prohibited on the outlet connections of portable gas tanks

65. In the supine position, all of the following areas should be padded EXCEPT

    (A) occiput
    (B) elbows
    (C) antecubital fossae
    (D) heels
    (E) popliteal fossae

66. The TRUE statement regarding ECG lead placement is

    (A) lead I displays the ECG signal recorded from the left arm and right arm.
    (B) lead II displays the ECG signal recorded from the left arm and right leg.
    (C) lead III displays the ECG signal recorded from the left leg and right leg.
    (D) lead V1 displays the ECG signal recorded from a unipolar electrode placed in the 2nd intercostal space at the right midaxillary line.
    (E) lead V6 displays the ECG signal recorded from a unipolar electrode placed in the 4th intercostal space at the anterior axillary line.

67. The laryngeal mask airway

    (A) protects against aspiration as well as an endotracheal tube
    (B) can be used to prevent airway obstruction during monitored anesthesia care
    (C) permits positive pressure ventilation
    (D) requires a flexible fiberoptic laryngoscope for proper placement
    (E) is more easily placed when an assistant applies cricoid pressure

68. Viewing the waveform of the capnograph may detect all of the following scenarios EXCEPT

    (A) disconnection of wall oxygen supply
    (B) exhaustion of carbon dioxide absorbent
    (C) pulmonary embolus
    (D) wheezing
    (E) esophageal intubation

69. All of the following are true of the lithotomy position EXCEPT

    (A) the back is supine
    (B) the knees are flexed
    (C) the hips are flexed
    (D) the legs are internally rotated
    (E) there are few hemodynamic disadvantages to the position

70. The isolated power supply system used in operating rooms requires that

    (A) the metal portions of the operating table be connected to earth ground
    (B) the patient be insulated from the metal portions of the operating table
    (C) the anesthesia machine and anesthesia monitors be connected to different electrical circuits than electrocautery devices
    (D) conductive flooring be used in the operating room
    (E) a transformer be connected between electrical equipment in the operating room and the electric power supplied by the utility company

71. A fiberoptic bronchoscope is useful for airway management of the patient with a difficult airway, and the suction channel of the scope may facilitate intubation by facilitating all of the following actions EXCEPT

    (A) administer oxygen
    (B) ventilate the patient during bronchoscopy

    (C) advance the scope over a wire inserted percutaneously through the larynx
    (D) spray local anesthetic
    (E) aspirate tracheal secretions

72. Pulse oximeters

    (A) are based on the Bernoulli principle
    (B) can differentiate carboxyhemoglobin from oxyhemoglobin
    (C) cannot differentiate methemoglobin from oxyhemoglobin
    (D) use a single wavelength of red light

73. Gases and vapors that may be measured by infrared spectrometry include ALL of the following EXCEPT

    (A) halothane
    (B) isoflurane
    (C) carbon dioxide
    (D) nitrogen
    (E) nitrous oxide

74. The fail-safe valve on an anesthesia machine

    (A) prevents delivery of a hypoxic mixture
    (B) prevents nitrous oxide flow unless the oxygen flowmeter is on
    (C) prevents high pressure in the breathing circuit from reaching the vaporizers
    (D) requires that oxygen tanks be full
    (E) is open if oxygen pressure is present

75. Venous air embolism may be rapidly detected by ALL of the following methods EXCEPT

    (A) alteration in heart sounds detected by a precordial Doppler
    (B) decrease in expired carbon dioxide on the capnometer
    (C) increase in expired nitrogen measured by mass spectroscopy
    (D) decrease in oxygen saturation indicated by the pulse oximeter

Answers and Explanations

35. **(D)** At the reduced barometric pressure in Denver (about 630 mm Hg), the concentration of isoflurane delivered by a variable bypass vaporizer will be slightly higher than the vaporizer setting. *(5:599)*

36. **(B)** The BIS monitor measures the depth of hypnosis and the BIS value can be used to predict the probability that a patient will be awake and responsive or will have recall at a given point in time. The BIS value is not a measure of the likelihood of movement or of the magnitude of noxious stimuli requiring opioid therapy. During surgery, the typical BIS target value is between 40 and 60. At a BIS value of 60, the probability of responsiveness to verbal command is about 20%, while the probability of recall is less than 1%. *(5:482, 692)*

37. **(C)** An open waste-gas scavenging system requires a reservoir but no valves. It must be connected to a source of vacuum to actively withdraw waste gases. It is usually connected to both the APL and ventilator relief valves via a "Y" connector. *(5:655-6)*

38. **(B)** The bladder length should be at least 80%, and the width 40%, of the limb circumference. If the bladder is too small, a larger pressure will be needed to occlude flow and an erroneously high blood pressure reading will result. The labeling of a cuff as "adult" or "thigh" is a general guideline; the cuff size should be chosen to match a particular limb size, regardless of whether the limb is the arm or leg. *(Circulation 1980; 62:1146A-1155A)*

39. **(D)** The circuit shown is a Bain circuit that is a modification of the Mapleson D system. *(5:639)*

40. **(E)** The inner tube may become disconnected or it may kink, leading to excessive rebreathing of exhaled gases or disruption of fresh gas flow. The Bain circuit permits spontaneous ventilation, requires relatively high fresh gas flows, permits easy waste gas scavenging, and positions the pop-off valve away from the patient for easier adjustment. *(5:639)*

41. **(D)** The difference between arterial and measured end-tidal carbon dioxide will be increased by ventilation-perfusion mismatch (e.g., emboli, decreased cardiac output), prolonged expiratory phase (e.g., wheezing), and high fresh gas flow rates that dilute expired carbon dioxide. *(5:465-7)*

42. **(E)** The Aladin vaporizer is not of the variable bypass type. When the cassette is disconnected from the vaporizer, it may be transported in any position without hazard. *(5:635)*

43. **(A)** Standard I of the ASA Standards for Basic Intraoperative Monitoring mandates that "qualified anesthesia personnel shall be present in the room throughout the conduct of all general anesthetics, regional anesthetics, and monitored anesthesia care. In the event there is a direct known hazard (e.g., radiation) to the anesthesia personnel that might require intermittent remote observation of the patient, some provision for monitoring the patient must be made." The standards "are not intended for application to the care of the obstetric patient in labor or in the conduct of

pain management." The patient having spinal anesthesia may have his or her ventilation "evaluated by continual observation of qualitative clinical signs," according to Standard II. *(5:88-90)*

44. **(E)** The time constant of the system is the volume divided by the fresh gas flow, i.e., 6 L ÷ 3 L/min, or 2 min. Since $1 - e^{-\frac{t}{\tau}} = 1 - e^{-1} = 0.63$, after one time constant the isoflurane concentration will be 63% of the value set on the vaporizer. After two time constants, the percentage is 85%; after three time constants, 95%; after four time constants, 98%; and after five time constants, 99.3%. *(5:601)*

45. **(E)** The negative-pressure leak test is a universal test for leaks in the low-pressure circuit of anesthesia machines, regardless of whether the low-pressure circuit contains a check valve. Performing the test requires applying negative pressure with a suction bulb to the common gas outlet (from which the carbon dioxide absorber has been disconnected) with the machine's master switch turned off. With the suction bulb collapsed, each vaporizer is individually turned on and reinflation of the suction bulb indicates an internal leak in that vaporizer. *(5:659-60)*

46. **(B)** Unidirectional check valves are required on the inspiratory and expiratory connections on the circle system to prevent rebreathing of exhaled gas. Some anesthesia machines have check valves at the common gas outlet or at vaporizer outlets, but they are not necessary. *(5:636-7, 640)*

47. **(D)** Administering anesthesia and/or monitoring a patient during an MRI scan is a challenge. Laryngeal mask airways are safe. An oximeter probe with a fiberoptic cable to the monitor is safe, while an oximeter probe connected with an electrical cable may cause a burn at the probe site. Blood pressure cuffs are safe as long as the tubing connectors are not ferromagnetic and plastic gas sampling tubing is safe. While plastic laryngoscope blades are readily available, the light sources require batteries that are ferromagnetic and should not be brought into the room containing the MRI machine. *(5:1273; Anesthesiology 2009; 110:459-79.)*

48. **(B)** While some absorbents have low percentages of sodium or potassium hydroxide, most of the absorbent consists of calcium hydroxide. Barium hydroxide is no longer used. *(5:641)*

49. **(D)** The formation of carbon monoxide results when desflurane reacts with a strong base (i.e., sodium or potassium hydroxide, but not calcium hydroxide) in the absence of water, i.e., in absorbent that has been dried by being flushed with dry gas. *(5:641)*

50. **(D)** In a typical anesthesia ventilator, during inspiration, the pressure relief valve is closed so that the tidal volume delivered to the patient is the sum of the set tidal volume plus the fresh gas flow that occurs during inspiration. In this case, the total fresh gas flow is 3,000 mL/min or 50 mL/sec. With a ventilator rate of 10/min, each breath lasts for 6 sec. With an I:E ratio of 1:3, the inspiratory phase lasts for 1.5 sec. Therefore, the set tidal volume is augmented by fresh gas flowing for 1.5 sec, or 75 mL/breath. *(5:650)*

51. **(E)** The waste gas scavenging system is connected to the APL valve and the ventilator pressure relief valve with 19- or 30-mm tubing. The circle system connectors and the connection for the reservoir bag are 22 mm, while the common gas outlet and endotracheal tube connections are 15 mm. All of these measurements are internal diameter (ID). *(5:655)*

52. **(D)** Confirmation of the ability of the vaporizers to deliver volatile agent is not one of the listed steps. *(5:662)*

53. **(C)** Automatic noninvasive blood pressure devices use oscillometry and directly measure mean arterial pressure that is the pressure at which the cuff pressure fluctuations are maximal. Each manufacturer employs its own, and unique, algorithm to estimate systolic and diastolic pressures. These devices do not listen for Korotkoff sounds. *(5:406)*

54. **(D)** The mechanism to reduce pressure of a gas to a useful pressure is a regulator. A gauge is a device to measure the pressure. The flowmeter is a device to measure the flow being delivered. A check valve is a device to allow flow in one direction only. *(5:619)*

55. **(C)** The horizontal supine position is the one best tolerated, but even that one has its problems. Merely because the patient does not have to be moved should not cause one to be complacent with positioning. Pressure points should be padded, the superficial nerves protected, and the eyes protected. *(5:362-3)*

56. **(A)** The nitrous oxide tank contains a liquid, and in order for it to become vaporized, heat must be supplied. As the cylinder is opened, heat is removed from the cylinder and from the air in the immediate vicinity. The temperature falls, causing condensation. *(5:626)*

57. **(B)** The indicator in carbon dioxide absorbent is ethyl violet. *(5:641)*

58. **(D)** Placement of the oxygen flowmeter in the position nearest to the common gas outlet will avoid delivery of a hypoxic mixture should a crack occur in the flowmeter tubing. If a leak occurs in this position, all components of the gas will leak out the crack in the tubing. *(5:622)*

59. **(D)** An oxygen proportioning system mechanically connects the oxygen and nitrous oxide flow controls so that as the nitrous oxide flow is increased, or the oxygen flow is decreased, the flow of the other gas is changed to maintain a minimum oxygen concentration of 25%. The system depends upon oxygen being correctly supplied to the oxygen flow control. Therefore, increasing the nitrous oxide flow will not, by itself, result in a hypoxic mixture. Any additional flow controls (e.g., helium, air, carbon dioxide) are not linked to the oxygen flow control, and increasing their flow could lead to a hypoxic mixture. Oxygen leaking from the oxygen flowmeter is not detected by the proportioning system and could also result in a hypoxic mixture. *(5:624)*

60. **(A)** The Macintosh blade is used by placing it in the vallecula (the space between the base of the tongue and the epiglottis). The laryngoscope is held in the left hand, and the blade enters the mouth on the right. Because of the widespread availability of fiberoptic laryngoscopes, it is now uncommon to use a Macintosh blade for an awake intubation. *(5:563)*

61. **(B)** When the last drop of nitrous oxide liquid evaporates, the tank is approximately 16% full. The pressure fall will depend on the size of the tank and the rate of flow. *(5:622)*

62. **(E)** The BIS monitor has been validated primarily with anesthetic techniques based exclusively or primarily on propofol or volatile anesthetics. It does not reliably indicated depth of anesthesia when the anesthetic technique is based exclusively or primarily on ketamine, nitrous oxide, xenon, or opioids. *(5:610)*

63. **(E)** The oxygen flush valve can apply oxygen to the breathing system at the pressure of the pipeline supply (e.g., approximately 50 psi) possibly causing barotrauma. If the APL valve is open and the scavenging system is of the open type, barotrauma is minimized. If oxygen is being supplied by the gas cylinders mounted on the anesthesia machine, the cylinder pressure is decreased to approximately 45 psi in the anesthesia machine, and this pressure is applied to the breathing circuit when the oxygen flush valve is pressed. During the inspiratory phase of positive pressure ventilation, both the ventilator relief and pop-off valves are closed, and pressing the oxygen flush valve will apply high pressure to the breathing circuit. The oxygen flush valve is positioned distally to the rotameters and vaporizers in an anesthesia machine. *(5:621, 631)*

64. **(A)** The system is based on matching specific bores and diameters that are assigned to the specific gases. The DISS should prevent attachment of gas administration equipment to the wrong gas. This is not the protective system for cylinder-yoke attachments that use the pin index safety system (PISS). DISS connectors

must be screwed on and are therefore not considered "quick-connectors." They are required on the machine end, and are optional on the wall end, of hoses connecting anesthesia machines to the wall. A gas-specific "quick-connector" is an alternative for the wall connection. DISS connectors are also sometimes found on the gas outlets of portable gas tanks. *(5:619)*

65. **(C)** Pressure damage may occur on the occiput, elbows, and heels after prolonged procedures. Padding the popliteal fossae may decrease postoperative stiffness and back pain. There is little indication to pad the antecubital fossae. *(5:362-3)*

66. **(A)** Lead I is described correctly. Lead II is left arm and left leg, lead III is right arm and left leg, V1 is placed in the 4th intercostal space to the right of the sternum, and V6 is placed in the 5th intercostal space at the mid-axillary line. *(6:1832)*

67. **(C)** The laryngeal mask airway permits positive pressure ventilation if the fit and seal of the airway are adequate for a particular patient. It is positioned blindly in a patient under general anesthesia. If anesthesia depth is inadequate, laryngospasm may result. There is no protection against aspiration. *(5:555-6)*

68. **(A)** Exhaustion of the carbon dioxide absorbent will increase the amount of rebreathing of exhaled gas and increase the inspired carbon dioxide concentration. This result would be displayed as an increasing baseline on the capnometer waveform. A pulmonary embolus typically produces a sudden decrease in end-tidal CO_2. Wheezing appears as a prolonged approach to plateau during expiration. An esophageal intubation results in no (or minimal) measured carbon dioxide. If the wall oxygen supply is disconnected, oxygen will be supplied by the gas cylinders on the anesthesia machine, if their valves are open. If the cylinders are closed or empty, all fresh gas flow from the common gas outlet will cease. *(5:465-6)*

69. **(D)** In the lithotomy position, internal rotation of the legs stretches the common peroneal nerve around the head of the fibula causing a nerve palsy to be more likely. Hemodynamic stability is preserved because the legs are elevated above the heart. *(5:363-5)*

70. **(E)** In an isolated power supply system, an isolation transformer is connected between the electric power supplied by the utility company and the electrical outlets in the operating room. The safety provided by this system depends on the patient and any wires or metallic objects in contact with the patient not being connected to earth ground. Conductive flooring was used in the past to avoid static electricity sparks that could cause fires or explosions in the presence of flammable anesthetics. *(5:375-8)*

71. **(B)** The suction port of a fiberoptic bronchoscope is designed primarily to aspirate secretions. However it may also be used to administer oxygen to a spontaneously breathing patient or to spray local anesthetic in the airway or on the vocal cords. It may also be used to pass the scope over a retrograde wire. The patient cannot be ventilated via this port. *(5:567-9)*

72. **(C)** Pulse oximeters use two wavelengths of light—one red and the other infrared—to estimate the percentage of hemoglobin in the oxygenated form by applying Beer's law that relates absorbance of light by a chemical to its concentration. Both carboxyhemoglobin and methemoglobin are misinterpreted as oxyhemoglobin by pulse oximeters. *(1:670-1; 4:877-9; 5:1213-4, 1448-9)*

73. **(D)** Nitrous oxide and all of the volatile anesthetics absorb infrared light. Nitrogen and oxygen may be determined by mass spectroscopy or Raman spectroscopy. Oxygen may also be measured by electrochemical or galvanic detectors. *(1:669-70; 4:869-70; 5:1213, 1454)*

74. **(E)** The fail-safe valves on anesthesia machines are on if oxygen pressure is present. It is important to understand that this valve is strictly pressure-related. As long as there is oxygen pressure in the machine, the valves will be on,

permitting flow of other gases such as nitrous oxide, carbon dioxide, air, helium, nitrogen, etc. It is therefore possible to still deliver a hypoxic mixture to the patient even with a functioning fail-safe valve. In contrast, newer machines have proportioning systems that ensure a minimum concentration of oxygen delivered at the common gas outlet. *(1:569-70; 4:1014; 5:277)*

75. **(D)** A decrease in oxygen saturation may be a late manifestation of venous air embolism, and should not be the method upon which detection is relied. The precordial Doppler, capnometer, and mass spectrometer will all indicate the presence of a venous air embolism quickly and with high sensitivity. *(1:766; 4:1635-7; 5:2290)*

CHAPTER 3

Circulation
Questions

DIRECTIONS (Questions 76-149): Each of the numbered items or incomplete statements in this section is followed by answers or by completions of the statement. Select the ONE lettered answer or completion that is BEST in each case.

76. A hypertensive woman is well controlled by amlodipine and quinapril, and she is planned for cholecystectomy. According to the American College of Cardiology/American Heart Association (ACC/AHA) Guidelines for Perioperative Cardiovascular Evaluation and Care for Noncardiac Surgery, her antihypertensive medications should be

    (A) continued during the perioperative period
    (B) held on the morning of surgery
    (C) held for 24 h before surgery
    (D) replaced by intravenous medications on day of surgery
    (E) reduced by 50% for 24 h before surgery

77. A 62-year-old woman is seen in the preoperative clinic prior to undergoing a total knee replacement. Routine laboratory results include a serum potassium concentration of 5.7 mEq/L. This could be an effect of which one of these medications?

    (A) hydrochlorothiazide
    (B) bumetanide
    (C) ethacrynic acid
    (D) triamterene
    (E) chlorthalidone

78. A 58-year-old woman has a preoperative B-type natriuretic peptide (BNP) level of 200 pg/mL four years after aortic valve replacement. This substance

    (A) decreases urine production
    (B) is produced by the kidneys
    (C) is often at a normal level despite heart failure
    (D) is a product of immunological B-cells
    (E) is a marker of inflammation and myocardial damage in heart failure

79. A 43-year-old woman is in the PACU following facial cosmetic surgery when suddenly her cardiac rhythm changes to supraventricular tachycardia. The PACU resident decides to administer adenosine. The effects of this medication usually last for just a few seconds, but may be prolonged by the prior administration of

    (A) caffeine
    (B) theobromine
    (C) epinephrine
    (D) dipyridamole
    (E) ketamine

80. A 70-year-old man underwent coronary surgery with the aids of cardiopulmonary bypass and heparin. His chance of postoperative heparin-induced thrombocytopenia (HIT) is approximately

    (A) 2%
    (B) 20%
    (C) 50%
    (D) 80%
    (E) 99%

81. A 72-year-old woman takes aspirin and clopidogrel because of the recent insertion of a drug-eluting coronary stent. She has a reducible ventral hernia that will require repair at some point, but the surgeon wants her to stop the clopidogrel a week prior to the surgery. Based on the 2007 advisory from the American College of Cardiology and the American Heart Association, it is recommended that she delay elective repair of her hernia until how long after her stent procedure?

   (A) 1 month
   (B) 3 months
   (C) 6 months
   (D) 12 months
   (E) 24 months

82. High saturation of hemoglobin with oxygen is planned in a patient with sickle cell disease. A factor that tends to increase the affinity of hemoglobin for oxygen is

   (A) acidosis
   (B) hyperthermia
   (C) carbon monoxide
   (D) hypercarbia
   (E) diphosphoglycerol

83. A 70-year-old man with a palpable pulsatile abdominal mass underwent CT evaluation and was found to have an aortic aneurysm 4.5 cm in diameter. His approximate annual risk of rupture is

   (A) 0.5-5%
   (B) 10-20%
   (C) 20-40%
   (D) 30-50%
   (E) 50-70%

84. A 25-year-old man has suffered hemorrhagic trauma in a motor vehicle accident. He bears blood group A and can receive

   (A) whole blood of type AB
   (B) red cells of type A or O
   (C) FFP of any type
   (D) red cells of any type
   (E) whole blood of type O

85. A 30-year-old man has fainted several times and has familial hypertrophic obstructive cardiomyopathy. Hemodynamic goals during anesthesia for inguinal hernia repair include

   (A) decreased preload
   (B) decreased afterload
   (C) decreased contractility
   (D) increased heart rate
   (E) low hematocrit

86. A 60-year-old patient with aortic valve area of 0.8 cm^2 is planned for laparoscopic cholecystectomy. In an effort to optimize hemodynamics in aortic stenosis, the goals generally include

   (A) low preload
   (B) low afterload
   (C) low heart rate
   (D) low hematocrit
   (E) high pulmonary vascular resistance

87. A 60-year-old man with mean arterial pressure of 50 mm Hg is considered for intraaortic balloon counterpulsation. The device can be beneficial in the following conditions EXCEPT

   (A) aortic regurgitation
   (B) mitral regurgitation
   (C) ventricular septal defect
   (D) myocardial ischemia
   (E) myocardial stunning

88. A preoperative patient is noted to have elevated mean red cell volume. This could indicate the following EXCEPT

   (A) aplastic anemia
   (B) anemia of chronic liver disease
   (C) iron deficiency anemia
   (D) anemia of folate or vitamin B12 deficiency
   (E) chemotherapy

89. A 50-year-old with von Willebrand disease requires thyroidectomy. Hemostatic aids might include the following EXCEPT

   (A) desmopressin (DDAVP)
   (B) cryoprecipitate
   (C) aminocaproic acid

(D)   tranexamic acid

(E)   vitamin K

90.   A critically ill patient is monitored with the aid of a dorsalis pedis arterial catheter after failure of a femoral catheter. As the pressure monitoring site moves distally from the aorta the

(A)   pulse pressure increases

(B)   upstroke is sooner

(C)   mean pressure decreases

(D)   diastolic pressure increases

(E)   dicrotic notch is earlier

91.   A 65-year-old man has a type II aortic aneurysm. In the Crawford classification of thoracoabdominal aortic aneurysm extent, the following are true EXCEPT

(A)   type I does not involve the renal arteries

(B)   the renal arteries are involved in types II, III, and IV

(C)   type IV involves the entire descending thoracic aorta

(D)   type II arises near the left subclavian and reaches the abdominal bifurcation

(E)   type III arises in the midportion of the descending thoracic

92.   Hypoxia general elicits vasodilation in patients. However, hypoxic vasoconstriction is prominent and clinically important in the

(A)   lungs

(B)   brain

(C)   heart

(D)   liver

(E)   skin

93.   A 64-year-old male with a past medical history significant for coronary artery disease and peripheral vascular disease is found unresponsive in his bed. It is two days since he underwent right femoro-popliteal bypass grafting, and his postoperative course had been complicated by ventricular arrhythmias. Upon arrival of the rapid response team, the airway is secured, and an ECG is obtained that shows a polymorphic tachycardia that is oscillating

around the baseline, and intermittent sinus rhythm with T-wave alternans. This arrhythmia

(A)   may be elicited by procainamide

(B)   is a type of supraventricular tachycardia

(C)   can be caused by hypermagnesemia

(D)   is characterized by a short QT interval

(E)   is more frequent in men than women

94.   Pain control fails to improve the tachycardia of a patient in the PACU. At equianalgesic doses, the opioid most likely to increase heart rate is

(A)   morphine

(B)   meperidine

(C)   fentanyl

(D)   sufentanil

(E)   hydromorphone

95.   A 60-year-old man is suspected of acute coronary syndrome. Myocardial oxygen demand may be decreased by

(A)   tachycardia

(B)   decreased preload

(C)   increased afterload

(D)   increased contractility

(E)   increased wall tension

96.   A 70-year-old woman is under anesthesia in preparation for coronary surgery. Coronary perfusion pressure is increased as a result of

(A)   increased diastolic blood pressure

(B)   increased left ventricular end-diastolic pressure

(C)   systolic hypertension

(D)   tachycardia

(E)   hypocapnia

97.   A patient with mild aortic stenosis is undergoing splenectomy. At a constant stroke volume, cardiac output is

(A)   proportional to resistance

(B)   a linear function of heart rate

(C)   dependent on blood volume

(D)   related to potassium concentration

(E)   inversely proportional to arterial blood pressure

98. Your patient is in normal sinus rhythm. The intrinsic rate of the sinoatrial node is generally

(A) 20 to 40 beats per minute
(B) 40 to 60 beats per minute
(C) 70 to 80 beats per minute
(D) 80 to 100 beats per minute
(E) 100 to 120 beats per minute

99. Electrocardiographic monitoring is indicated during anesthesia to detect all of the following EXCEPT

(A) efficacy of pump function
(B) arrhythmias
(C) ischemia
(D) electrolyte disturbance
(E) pacemaker function

100. Your patient has a history of deep venous thrombosis and pulmonary embolism. An endogenous inhibitor of intravascular coagulation is

(A) factor V Leiden
(B) activated protein C
(C) bradykinin
(D) Hageman factor
(E) argatroban

101. A 40-year-old skier is hypotensive after a femur fracture and is suspected of fat embolus. Other clinical manifestations of fat emboli include the following EXCEPT

(A) petechiae
(B) hypoxemia
(C) confusion
(D) bradycardia
(E) cyanosis

102. A preoperative patient is noted to have a low platelet count. The minimum number of platelets needed for surgical hemostasis is approximately

(A) 10,000/mm^3
(B) 50,000/mm^3
(C) 80,000/mm^3
(D) 120,000/mm^3
(E) 1,000,000/mm^3

DIRECTIONS: Use the following figure to answer Questions 103–106:

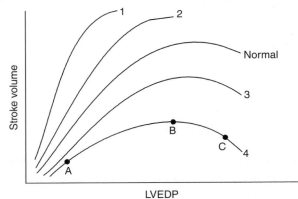

103. Left ventricular end-diastolic pressure is most closely approximated by

(A) arterial blood pressure
(B) central venous pressure
(C) pulmonary artery systolic pressure
(D) pulmonary capillary wedge pressure
(E) right atrial pressure

104. The curves marked 3 and 4 in the graph shown could be seen in patients

(A) with increased contractility
(B) on digoxin or epinephrine
(C) who are in heart failure
(D) who have been treated with glucagon
(E) who respond to increased left ventricular end-diastolic pressure (LVEDP) with increased stroke volume

105. If a patient's status is represented by point A on curve 4 in the graph shown, then administration of intravenous fluid may

(A) shift the patient to the normal curve
(B) shift the patient to point B or C
(C) take the patient to point B only
(D) have no effect
(E) shift the patient to curve 2

106. Administration of an inotrope to a patient at point B on curve 4 is intended to

(A) shift the patient to curve 3
(B) shift the patient to point A
(C) shift the patient to point C
(D) maintain the patient at point B
(E) shift the patient to curve 1

107. A 5-foot, 7-inch, 40-year-old man weighing 320 pounds is planned for laparoscopic gastric bypass. Morbid obesity is associated with

(A) decreased cardiac output
(B) hypertension
(C) decreased pulmonary artery pressure
(D) decreased blood volume
(E) decreased cardiac workload

108. A newborn has persistent patency of the ductus arteriosus. This may close in response to

(A) hypoxemia
(B) alprostadil (prostaglandin E_1)
(C) heparin
(D) indomethacin
(E) nitrous oxide

109. You are hyperventilating a neurosurgery patient to an arterial Pco_2 value of 28 mm Hg. The coronary circulation responds to hyperventilation with

(A) no change
(B) an increase in flow
(C) a decrease in flow
(D) a transient increase followed by an intense vasodilatation
(E) intense vasoconstriction

110. Your patient's blood pressure is 160/100. The mean pressure is approximately

(A) 110 mm Hg
(B) 120 mm Hg
(C) 130 mm Hg
(D) 140 mm Hg
(E) 150 mm Hg

111. A small bubble is noted in the saline-filled plastic tubing connected to an arterial catheter of your patient. The bubble

(A) is not significant
(B) leads to an artificially high reading
(C) affects only the diastolic pressure
(D) leads to a damping of the tracing
(E) has a greater effect on the mean blood pressure

112. Under normal circumstances, the plasma protein (colloid) osmotic pressure is

(A) 0 mm Hg
(B) 5 mm Hg
(C) 20 mm Hg
(D) 50 mm Hg
(E) 100 mm Hg

113. Pulmonary edema may result from all of the following EXCEPT

(A) altered permeability
(B) decreased pulmonary capillary pressure
(C) decreased oncotic pressure
(D) increased negative airway pressure
(E) head injury

114. You encounter a cyanotic patient. Net right-to-left shunt is a feature of

(A) atrial septal defect
(B) ventricular septal defect
(C) patent ductus arteriosus
(D) tetralogy of Fallot
(E) increased ventricular filling pressure

115. You notice an increase in heart size before revascularization of a patient undergoing coronary surgery. If the size of the ventricle increases

(A) wall tension needed to pump the same amount of blood is less
(B) less oxygen is needed to pump blood
(C) the heart becomes more efficient
(D) wall tension will increase proportionally with the radius
(E) wall tension will be proportional to wall thickness

116. Your goal is to maintain coronary blood flow while a patient with coronary disease undergoes cholecystectomy. The flow

    (A) is independent of the systolic pressure
    (B) is not affected by humoral agents
    (C) is increased by a slow heart rate
    (D) is increased by a fast heart rate
    (E) occurs almost entirely in systole

117. You are monitoring a patient with the aid of a pulmonary artery catheter. Pulmonary artery pressure

    (A) increases passively with increases of cardiac output
    (B) remains constant with change of cardiac output
    (C) is not important to pulmonary vascular resistance
    (D) is not dependent on the radius of the vessels
    (E) depends entirely on cardiac output

118. You are evaluating the degree of congestive heart failure in a preoperative patient with dyspnea on exertion. Increased sympathetic tone in congestive heart failure may be indicated by

    (A) memory loss
    (B) weakness
    (C) fatigue
    (D) confusion
    (E) anxiety

119. A 56-year-old female is undergoing left pneumonectomy for lung cancer. A few hours after the surgery, the patient is noted to have progressive hypoxemia, and hypotension requiring vasopressor support. A stat transthoracic echocardiogram obtained at the bedside is suggestive of right-heart failure. The next best step in management would be

    (A) administration of selective pulmonary vasodilators
    (B) afterload reduction with infusion of intravenous nicardipine

    (C) endotracheal intubation and high levels of positive end-expiratory pressure (PEEP)
    (D) a reduction in F_{IO_2}
    (E) endotracheal intubation and permissive hypercarbia

120. Cardiopulmonary bypass is initiated in a 70-year-old man planned for coronary surgery. Unexpected hypotension (mean aortic pressure of 30 mm Hg) is rapidly encountered and may be due to all of the following EXCEPT

    (A) hemodilution
    (B) decreased catecholamines
    (C) aortic stenosis
    (D) persistent systemic to pulmonary shunt
    (E) aortic dissection

121. Your patient requires cardiopulmonary bypass. Myocardial preservation during that procedure may include all of the following EXCEPT

    (A) maintaining the ventricle in a distended state
    (B) cardioplegia
    (C) nearly continuous perfusion
    (D) avoidance of ventricular fibrillation
    (E) maintaining the heart at a low temperature

122. Following breast surgery under general anesthesia, your patient in the recovery room exhibits elevated blood pressure readings of about 190/110 mm Hg. Your approach should be

    (A) treat the blood pressure with small doses of an antihypertensive medication
    (B) do nothing, but wait to see if the hypertension is a transient problem associated with emergence from anesthesia
    (C) examine the patient for evidence of hypoxia or hypercarbia
    (D) recheck the blood pressure yourself to make sure the cuff is the correct size
    (E) arrange a cardiology consultation

123. A 97-year-old woman undergoes bowel resection under general anesthesia. Cardiovascular changes that occur with advancing age are

(A) decreasing blood pressure
(B) increase in cardiovascular reserve
(C) loss of elasticity of the vascular tree
(D) increased number of myofibrils
(E) increase in cardiac output

124. Poor right ventricular contractility is noted in the operating room soon after mitral valve replacement. The right ventricle

(A) has little function in the adult patient
(B) is very easily cooled in the patient undergoing cardiopulmonary bypass
(C) can overcome pulmonary vascular resistance very effectively, and, therefore, is not of concern in terminating cardiopulmonary bypass
(D) is more likely to be injured by intracoronary air than is the left ventricle during cardiopulmonary bypass
(E) is unaffected by PEEP

125. A preoperative patient is planned for surgery prompted by workup of hypertension. A cause of systemic hypertension that is amenable to surgical correction is

(A) essential hypertension
(B) secondary aldosteronism
(C) renal parenchymal disease
(D) pheochromocytoma
(E) long-standing renal artery stenosis

DIRECTIONS: Use the following scenario to answer Questions 126–127. A 24-year-old female is admitted for evaluation of chest pain. The pain is sharp and aggravated by breathing. A chest x-ray shows an enlarged heart, ECG shows decreased voltage, and there is a pericardial friction rub. Pericardiocentesis demonstrates purulent fluid. Serial x-rays show widening of the cardiac shadow, and the patient is scheduled for pericardial drainage.

126. On physical examination, you would expect to find

(A) a water-hammer pulse
(B) an increased cardiac output
(C) distended neck veins that flatten in the sitting position
(D) decreased arterial pressure
(E) low central venous pressure

127. A pulsus paradoxus is a pulse that has the following properties EXCEPT that it

(A) reduces in amplitude >10 mm Hg on inspiration
(B) can occur in hemorrhage and in severe obstructive lung disease
(C) is an exaggeration of the normal respiratory effect on the arterial pulse
(D) is stronger on inspiration
(E) is associated with tamponade, pulmonary embolism, and tension pneumothorax

128. A 68-year-old is noted to have an abnormal Allen test before cardiac surgery. The test is

(A) used to assess adequacy of radial artery perfusion
(B) of little predictive value
(C) positive if good flow occurs
(D) negative if good flow occurs
(E) independent of hand position

129. Central venous cannulation is indicated in all the following procedures EXCEPT

(A) a surgical procedure in which there is an unusual position, e.g., head-down position
(B) patients in shock
(C) total parenteral hyperalimentation
(D) intravenous administration of vasopressors
(E) inadequate venous access in a patient with extensive burns

130. A 42-year-old patient with a past medical history of insulin dependent diabetes mellitus and end-stage renal disease requiring hemodialysis is admitted to the intensive care unit with signs and symptoms of septic shock secondary to community acquired pneumonia. The patient has very poor peripheral access, and a decision for placement of a central venous catheter, as well as an arterial catheter for blood pressure monitoring, is made. With respect to potential sites of vessel cannulation it is true that

(A) chylothorax is common with right internal jugular cannulation

(B) brachial plexus trauma is common with the antecubital approach for central venous cannulation

(C) the risk of pneumothorax is low with the subclavian approach

(D) the Allen test rules out ischemic complications related to a radial arterial catheter

(E) the dorsalis pedis is not the artery of choice for blood pressure monitoring in a patient with diabetes

131. You are asked by a member of the orthopedic team to do a preoperative evaluation on an 87-year-old female admitted from the emergency department for left femur fracture. The patient has a heart murmur, and an echocardiogram obtained by the medical consultant shows aortic stenosis with a valve area of 0.6 cm². The patient with severe aortic stenosis usually has

(A) a rapidly deteriorating course once symptoms are present

(B) a large left ventricular cavity

(C) low voltage criteria on the electrocardiogram

(D) protection against ischemia due to the large ventricle

(E) a very compliant ventricle

132. A bridge-to-transplant patient with biventricular heart failure is stabilized by placement of a left ventricular assist device and by administration of inhaled nitric oxide. The inhaled drug has the following properties EXCEPT that it

(A) may cause methemoglobinemia

(B) often lowers mean pulmonary artery pressure

(C) exhibits virtually no systemic vasodilation

(D) often decreases systemic oxygenation

(E) increases vascular smooth muscle cyclic GMP

133. Following cardiac surgery, a patient is noted to exhibit equalization of diastolic filling pressures (central venous, right ventricular diastolic, pulmonary artery diastolic, pulmonary capillary wedge) that tends to occur in

(A) mitral stenosis

(B) pulmonary embolus

(C) tricuspid regurgitation

(D) cardiac tamponade

(E) atrial fibrillation

134. Vitamin K

(A) is required for synthesis of functional clotting factors VII, IX, X, and II (prothrombin)

(B) antagonizes heparin

(C) potentiates warfarin

(D) antagonizes protamine sulfate

(E) is a prominent citrus product

135. A patient in renal failure is receiving erythropoietin in preparation for cardiac surgery. This substance

(A) is normally produced by the liver

(B) increases platelet production

(C) increases red blood cell production

(D) increases white blood cell production

(E) is a breakdown product of heme

136. A 20-year-old tachycardic patient improves following an intravenous dose of adenosine. The drug

(A) inhibits phosphodiesterase

(B) is inactivated by catechol O-methyltransferase

(C) decreases atrioventricular conduction

(D) is a β-adrenergic agonist

(E) is primarily cleared by the kidneys

137. A preoperative 3-year-old exhibits "tet spells." An agent that may reduce right-to-left shunt in tetralogy of Fallot is

(A) sodium nitroprusside

(B) labetolol

(C) propranolol

(D) phenylephrine

(E) diltiazem

138. Seven years after heart transplantation, a 60-year-old woman is planned for appendectomy. The transplanted, denervated heart responds to

(A) circulating catecholamines

(B) circulating acetylcholine

(C) neuromuscular blocking agents

(D) vagal stimulation

(E) muscarinic blocking agents

139. A 58-year-old man with chest pain exhibits elevation of the ST segments of precordial ECG leads. This finding can occur in all of the following conditions EXCEPT

(A) Prinzmetal's angina (coronary spasm)

(B) acute pericarditis

(C) myocardial infarction

(D) myocardial contusion

(E) during normal exercise in an individual without coronary disease

140. You consider verapamil for a tachycardic patient. The drug may exacerbate all of the following diseases or symptoms EXCEPT

(A) sick sinus syndrome

(B) atrial fibrillation

(C) atrioventricular block

(D) Wolff–Parkinson–White syndrome

(E) congestive heart failure

141. You measure cardiac output in order to calculate systemic vascular resistance in a septic patient. Cardiac output is

(A) identical in the left and right heart

(B) usually 2 to 3 L/min in a 70-kg man

(C) unaffected by blood volume

(D) the product of heart rate and stroke volume

(E) the product of heart rate and mean arterial pressure

142. You consider reduction of myocardial contractility in a cardiac patient. Contractility is decreased by

(A) sympathetic stimulation

(B) parasympathetic tone

(C) milrinone administration

(D) norepinephrine

(E) epinephrine

DIRECTIONS: Each group of items below consists of lettered headings followed by a list of numbered phrases or statements. For each numbered phrase or statement, select the ONE lettered heading or component that is most closely associated with it. Each lettered heading or component may be selected once, more than once, or not at all.

(A) atrial fibrillation

(B) hypertrophic obstructive cardiomyopathy

(C) pericarditis

(D) aortic regurgitation

(E) pulmonary embolism

(F) Eisenmenger syndrome

(G) tricuspid regurgitation

(H) myocardial infarction

For each patient with a cardiac symptom or sign, select the most likely mechanism causing the symptoms or sign.

143. A 50-year-old man has dyspnea on mild exertion, bounding pulses, and a diastolic murmur.

144. A 40-year-old woman with a long-standing heart murmur has shortness of breath, cyanosis, and a systolic heart murmur

145. A 20-year-old man becomes profoundly hypotensive after modest intraoperative bleeding.

146. A 70-year-old woman with an irregular pulse suffers sudden loss of the right lower quadrant of the visual field.

147. A 25-year-old heroin user has peripheral edema.

148. A 70-year-old woman develops acute dyspnea one week after hip replacement. She is tachypneic and cyanotic. A chest x-ray is unremarkable.

149. A 20-year-old man has chest pain, a friction rub on chest auscultation, and J-point elevation on most ECG leads.

Answers and Explanations

76. **(A)** Antihypertensives are recommended to be continued. In particular, beta-blockers and clonidine are continued because of the potential for significant withdrawal syndromes. *(5:743)*

77. **(D)** Hyperkalemia is associated with amiloride, spironolactone, and triamterene. The other choices tend to decrease potassium. *(5:743)*

78. **(E)** A low BNP level might be useful to select out high-risk patients who do not need echocardiograms to rule out ventricular dysfunction. Preoperative levels may predict myocardial injury and hospital length of stay. It may be a useful marker of perioperative deterioration. *(5:109)*

79. **(D)** Dipyridamole blocks reuptake of adenosine, delaying its clearance and potentiating its effects. Caffeine and theobromine are competitive inhibitors of adenosine action. *(5:765)*

80. **(A)** The frequency of HIT after cardiac surgery is about 2%. However, 25-50% of patients develop heparin-dependent antibodies postoperatively over the first 5-10 days after exposure. If this immunological response strongly activates platelets and coagulation, it causes the prothrombotic disorder known as HIT. Antibody assays do not necessarily indicate HIT, but negative assays are helpful to rule out the problem. *(5:900)*

81. **(D)** Antiplatelet therapy is more important than time between stent placement and surgery in reducing stent thrombosis. Although dual antiplatelet continuation for 12 months is mandatory, clopidogrel treatment beyond 12 months may not be necessary. *(5:106)*

82. **(C)** The other factors facilitate release of oxygen from hemoglobin. *(5:460)*

83. **(A)** The first four percentages are respectively for 4.0-4.9, 6.0-6.9, 7.0-7.9, and >8 cm. *(5:1024)*

84. **(B)** A patient bearing blood group A can receive whole blood type A, red cells of type A or O, plasma of type A or AB, any cryoprecipitate or platelets of any type. *(6:951)*

85. **(C)** Intraoperative hemodynamic goals include increased pre-, and, afterload, and decreased contractility, and heart rate. *(5:910)*

86. **(C)** High pre- and afterload and low heart rate can be salutary, as long as the low rate does not compromise cardiac output. *(5:910)*

87. **(A)** The balloon worsens aortic regurgitation. *(6:2235-6)*

88. **(C)** The anemia of iron deficiency is microcytic. *(5:199)*

89. **(E)** The von Willebrand factor is not sensitive to vitamin K. The sensitive factors are II, VII, IX, X, C, and S. *(5:205, 6:980-1)*

90. **(A)** The mean pressure is fairly uniform throughout the arterial tree, but the pulse pressure is higher in the foot than in the wrist or aorta. *(5:406-7)*

91. **(C)** Type IV arises at the level of the diaphragm. *(5:917-8)*

92. **(A)** The vasoconstrictor response of the pulmonary circulation differs from that of other tissues in order to match lung perfusion to ventilation. *(5:967-9)*

93. **(A)** The description of the arrhythmia is consistent with torsades des pointes. The phrase was taken from a ballet-dancing maneuver. It is a type of polymorphic ventricular tachycardia characterized by a long QT interval. Procainamide can prolong the QT interval and elicit torsade. Magnesium can be therapeutic. The arrhythmia occurs more frequently in women than in men. *(6:54, 175-6, 1884, 1891)*

94. **(B)** Meperidine tends to decrease cardiac output and increase heart rate. Other μ-receptor agonists tend to decrease heart rate. *(1:715-6)*

95. **(B)** Myocardial oxygen consumption is increased by tachycardia. It causes increased demand for oxygen at the same time that it leads to decreased oxygen supply by decreasing coronary blood flow. Increased afterload leads to increased wall tension, both of which require more oxygen. Increases in contractility require more oxygen. *(5:903)*

96. **(A)** Coronary perfusion (CPP) occurs mostly during diastole. CPP = DBP − LVEDP, where DBP is diastolic blood pressure and LVEDP is left ventricular end-diastolic pressure. As DBP rises or LVEDP falls, the flow will increase. Tachycardia decreases time of perfusion, since diastole is shortened. Systolic hypertension decreases perfusion, since the ventricle contracts harder, allowing less perfusion during systole. *(5:902)*

97. **(B)** At a constant stroke volume, cardiac output is a linear function of heart rate. The other factors are important in the generation of cardiac output, but they are direct or indirect determinants of stroke volume: resistance (afterload), arterial pressure, and blood volume (preload). Cardiac output is not directly related to potassium concentration. *(6:1856)*

98. **(C)** The intrinsic rate of the sinoatrial node is generally 70 to 80 beats per minute. Since it has a faster rate, it is the dominant pacemaker. The more caudal a pacemaker cell is located in the conduction system, the slower its intrinsic rate. The atrioventricular node hasan intrinsic rate of 40 to 60 beats per minute. *(6:1867-71)*

99. **(A)** The ECG cannot detect efficacy of pump function. The ECG may show a normal sinus rhythm during pulseless electrical activity (electromechanical dissociation) when the pump is not working effectively at all. The ECG can also be observed for changes indicative of electrolyte disturbance, especially of calcium and potassium. Ischemia may be detected by changes in the tracing. Pacemaker function may be checked by observing the tracing while turning the pacemaker on and off (e.g. with a magnet). Arrhythmias are detected by the ECG. *(5:89)*

100. **(B)** Endothelial thrombomodulin converts intravascular thrombin from a clotting enzyme into an activator of protein C. The activated protein C has anticoagulant activity through its destruction of factors V and VIII. Factor V Leiden is a single point mutation that makes the molecule resistant to destruction by activated protein C and therefore increases the risk of intravascular thrombosis. Argatroban is a synthetic inhibitor of thrombin. Activated Hageman factor initiates the intrinsic blood clotting cascade and activates prekallikrein to produce bradykinin. *(1:860, 883)*

101. **(D)** Fat emboli may be seen with fractures. Fat embolism syndrome is associated with petechiae, hypoxemia, confusion and cyanosis. Tachycardia is often present. *(5:1203)*

102. **(B)** The minimum number of platelets needed for normal coagulation is controversial, but is frequently cited as $30,000–50,000/mm^3$. *(5:1446)*

103. **(D)** Pulmonary capillary wedge pressure is the best estimate of left ventricular end-diastolic pressure. By measuring changes in cardiac output and pressures, a ventricular function

curve can be drawn and therapeutic interventions evaluated. Right heart pressures do not necessarily provide accurate estimates of left heart pressures and function. Therefore, central venous pressure gives the worst approximation of left side function. *(5:414-5)*

104. **(C)** The curves are representative of patients who are not responding to increases in LVEDP with increases in stroke volume. These do not show any effect of increased contractility or any effect of inotropic intervention. In such a patient, inotrope administration may be the next logical step. *(1:792)*

105. **(B)** A patient on such a low curve may respond to fluid by advancing to point B, but the patient may also react adversely and fall even farther down on the curve. This would be represented by point C. *(1:792)*

106. **(A)** The inotrope ought to improve contractility. *(1:792)*

107. **(B)** Severe hypertension is seen in 5% to 10% of patients with morbid obesity. Moderate hypertension is seen in 50% of patients. The cardiac output is increased, as is the pulmonary artery pressure. Blood volume is increased, and the cardiac workload is increased. *(5:305)*

108. **(D)** The ductus normally closes in response to elevated arterial oxygen tension and patency may be maintained deliberately with alprostadil (PGE$_1$). *(5:1181)*

109. **(C)** Coronary circulation reacts to carbon dioxide in a manner similar to cerebral circulation. Although this may be salutary in the instance of head trauma, in the patient with chest pain and ischemia, hyperventilation may lead to further decrease of coronary flow. The magnitude of the decrease is not large. *(5:902)*

110. **(B)** An estimate for mean arterial pressure is: MAP = diastolic + (systolic − diastolic)/3. *(5:1369)*

111. **(D)** The pressure waveform may be affected by the presence of even small bubbles. The bubble,

being very compliant, leads to a damping of the trace and a reading that hovers around the mean. Both systolic and diastolic pressure will be affected. *(5:407)*

112. **(C)** The plasma oncotic pressure is important in maintaining the fluid balance in the capillaries. The balance between the driving pressure and the oncotic pressure prevents tissue edema. The delicate balance can be disturbed by either increases or decreases in pressure or increases or decreases in oncotic pressure. *(5:338-9)*

113. **(B)** Pulmonary edema results from an increase in pulmonary capillary pressure. Pulmonary edema may also result from neurological injury. Negative airway pressure pulmonary edema has been reported in the patient with airway obstruction who is breathing against a closed glottis or an occluded endotracheal tube. *(5:422-3)*

114. **(D)** There is increased pulmonary blood flow in the other lesions. *(5:928-32)*

115. **(D)** As the size of the ventricle increases, the radius increases, and the wall tension increases. The law of LaPlace states that more tension is needed to generate the same pressure as the radius increases. This makes the heart more inefficient and requires more oxygen to pump blood. *(1:749)*

116. **(C)** Coronary perfusion is improved by slow heart rates, since most perfusion occurs during diastole. The coronary flow is not independent of systolic pressure, since areas of the subendocardium are poorly perfused during systole. *(6:1998)*

117. **(A)** As the cardiac output increases, pulmonary artery pressure increases. Other factors also are involved in pulmonary artery pressure, e.g., the radius of the vessels. Vasoconstriction and vasodilatation of the pulmonary vessels occur with changes of cardiac output to regulate pulmonary vascular resistance. *(5:412-15, 932, 969)*

118. **(E)** The anxiety seen in patients with congestive heart failure is due to increased sympathetic activity. The increased sympathetic activity is a compensatory mechanism, and it is not directly related to the low flow state, as are the other options. Memory loss, weakness, fatigue, and confusion are directly caused by low output. *(6:1904-5)*

119. **(A)** Hypoxia, hypercarbia, and PEEP increase the afterload of the failing right heart. After pneumonectomy, a healthy right ventricle may fail when suddenly challenged with increased afterload due to the decrease in cross-sectional area of the pulmonary vasculature, and resulting pulmonary hypertension. Selective pulmonary vasodilators such as inhaled nitric oxide or inhaled epoprostenol can be useful to reduce PVR. *(5:1005)*

120. **(C)** Hypotension persisting after initiation of bypass may be a sign of aortic insufficiency. The initial hemodilution may cause decreased catecholamines and decreased viscosity. These should be transient. If persistent, one must look for other problems, e.g., a persistent shunt or aortic dissection. *(5:923)*

121. **(A)** Allowing the ventricle to become overdistended can be detrimental, and most centers use a ventricular vent to decompress it. The ventricle should be kept in a nonbeating state and kept cold to lower oxygen consumption. Fibrillation should be avoided, since the oxygen cost is great. *(5:908)*

122. **(C)** The recovery room patient with hypertension should be examined to rule out hypoxia or hypercarbia. If present, these must be treated, and this takes precedence over other considerations. After you have ruled out those problems, you can proceed with a methodical assessment of the problem: retake the pressure, and if it is not life threatening, you may want to watch it or treat it with a drug. In some cases, a consultation may be in order. *(5:1281, 1291-2)*

123. **(C)** The vascular tree becomes less elastic with age. Blood pressure rises with age that may be a reflection of the loss of elasticity. The number of myofibrils decreases, and the cardiac output decreases. The cardiovascular reserve decreases as a reflection of the other changes. *(5:279-80)*

124. **(D)** Right ventricular function is receiving much more attention, and the interdependence of the two ventricles is being appreciated to a greater degree. Blood flow occurs during systole and diastole. Since there is good collateral flow, it is harder to cool the right ventricle. Pulmonary vascular resistance is hard to overcome, since the ventricle muscle is not as well developed. PEEP will be transmitted to the right ventricle, decreasing venous return. *(5:924; 6:2076)*

125. **(D)** Pheochromocytoma is often amenable to surgical correction. Other causes of secondary hypertension, secondary aldosteronism and renal parenchymal disease, may not be so amenable. The patient with renal artery stenosis may be treated surgically if the condition is diagnosed early. If later, surgery may be of no help. *(5:1125)*

126. **(D)** A water-hammer pulse is seen in the patient with aortic insufficiency. The patient with pericardial effusion will exhibit pulsus paradoxus. The cardiac output is decreased. The neck veins are distended and stay distended in the supine position, since little drainage can occur. Blood pressure will decrease. *(6:2221)*

127. **(A)** Pulsus paradoxus is an exaggeration of the normal variation in the pulse with inspiration. The pulse reduces in amplitude on inspiration. *(6:1824-5)*

128. **(B)** The Allen test is used to assess the adequacy of ulnar artery flow when cannulating the radial artery. Studies have shown poor correlation with subsequent problems. The reason for this is that many of the problems are embolic in nature that cannot be predicted with an Allen test. In addition to the lack of data showing correlation, there is confusion as to what is positive or negative. It is better to

describe the result of the test. Since the position of the wrist is important, one must ascertain that the wrist is not hyper extended when performing the test. *(5:409)*

129. **(A)** A central venous line is not indicated because the patient is in an abnormal position. It is indicated in patients with shock. Hyperalimentation, inotropic drugs, and irritating solutions should be infused through a central venous catheter. Patients with lack of peripheral large bore IV access, who are expected to require substantial fluid resuscitation, such as burn patients, should undergo placement of a central venous catheter. *(5:412)*

130. **(E)** Pneumothorax is a common problem with subclavian cannulation. Chylothorax is a complication of left internal jugular cannulation. There should be no brachial plexus trauma with the antecubital approach. Allen's test is not a foolproof method to determine the patency of the ulnar arch. The dorsalis pedis artery should be avoided in the patient with diabetes or peripheral vascular disease. *(5:408-9)*

131. **(A)** The patient with aortic stenosis has a rapidly deteriorating course once angina, syncope, and congestive heart failure occur. The size of the ventricular muscle mass increases, but the cavity size does not change. The increased size also renders the muscle more prone to ischemia. Fast heart rates will cause a low cardiac output, since ventricular filling will be compromised. In addition, coronary perfusion will suffer. Low heart rates can also be devastating, since the stroke volume is fixed. The most common problem is that of tachycardia. *(5:63)*

132. **(D)** Inhaled nitric oxide (NO) dilates blood vessels in ventilated regions of the lungs and can thereby improve the matching of perfusion to ventilation. While intravenous vasodilators can worsen ventilation:perfusion matching and so worsen systemic arterial oxygenation, inhaled nitric oxide often improves systemic oxygenation. Inhaled nitric oxide exhibits little or no systemic vasodilation because the molecule is rapidly destroyed in the systemic circulation. Reaction

with heme is one mechanism of NO destruction, and hemoglobin oxidation occurs concomitantly. In most clinical situations, NO benefits occur at doses that do not cause significant methemoglobin levels. *(1:558-9; 5:969)*

133. **(D)** The filling pressures are elevated and tend to equalize in pericardial constriction and pericardial tamponade. *(5:458)*

134. **(A)** The synthesis of vitamin K-dependent clotting factors is inhibited by warfarin. Protamine antagonizes heparin. *(1:860-1)*

135. **(C)** The anemia of chronic renal failure stems from diminished production of erythropoietin, a protein available for therapeutic purposes. *(1:1068-70)*

136. **(C)** Adenosine may normally regulate coronary blood flow. It may interrupt reentrant supraventricular tachycardia. It is not an adrenergic catechol. It is inactivated by adenosine deaminase. *(1:834)*

137. **(D)** Increased peripheral resistance may reduce cyanosis in tetralogy of Fallot. *(5:928)*

138. **(A)** Because of esterase activities of the blood, there is no circulating acetylcholine. β-adrenoceptor antagonists slow the transplanted heart, but antimuscarinic agents do not speed the transplanted heart. *(5:1093)*

139. **(E)** With the exception of normal exercise, all of the conditions listed can cause ST elevation. In the case of transmural ischemia and infarction, this may be followed by the occurrence of Q-waves. Electrocardiographic changes associated with normal exercise may include downward displacement of the J point. *(6:1831, 1836, 1971)*

140. **(B)** Verapamil may increase the heart rate in case of supraventricular tachycardia due to WPW syndrome. *(1:833)*

141. **(D)** Cardiac output is a function of many components of the circulatory system. The typical output is 5 L/min in a healthy resting adult.

Output is affected by blood volume. Cardiac output is the product of heart rate and stroke volume. Communications of the bronchial artery capillaries with those of the pulmonary veins is a reason for left ventricular output exceeding the right. Left-to-right shunting through an atrial septal defect could increase right output over left. *(5:418-22, 604)*

142.   **(B)** Myocardial contractility is affected by both neural and humoral factors. Parasympathetic tone and myocardial ischemia both decrease contractility, whereas sympathetic stimulation and inotrope administration increase contractility. *(1:178; 6:1804)*

143.   **(D)** The patient might have regurgitation caused by an ascending aortic aneurysm. *(6:2061-3)*

144.   **(F)** The cyanosis indicates a right-to-left shunt. This could be the result of increased pulmonary vascular resistance in response to a lesion initially causing right-to-left shunting. Examples include septal defects and patent ductus. *(6:1923-4)*

145.   **(B)** In this cardiomyopathy, ventricular obstruction is worsened by hypovolemia and by sympathetic tone and can be relieved by beta-adrenergic blockers, phenylephrine, and/or volume administration. *(6:1968-9)*

146.   **(A)** Thrombi often form in the left atrium during fibrillation, and these can embolize. *(6:3274-5)*

147.   **(G)** The tricuspid valve may have been damaged by endocarditis. *(6:1930, 1948)*

148.   **(E)** The embolic source is likely venous thrombi of the legs. *(6:2090, 2173)*

149.   **(C)** The problem can follow respiratory infections and may respond to COX inhibitors. *(6:1830, 1971-3)*

CHAPTER 4

Respiration
Questions

DIRECTIONS (Questions 150-235): Each of the numbered items or incomplete statements in this section is followed by answers or by completions of the statement. Select the ONE lettered answer or completion that is BEST in each case.

150. At functional residual capacity (FRC)

(A) no further inspiration is possible
(B) chest wall elastic forces are greater than the lungs elastic recoil
(C) the pressure difference between the alveoli and the intrapleural space is zero
(D) the total pulmonary vascular resistance is very high
(E) the pressure difference between the alveoli and atmosphere is zero

151. All statements in regard to the sensation of dyspnea are correct EXCEPT dyspnea may be:

(A) influenced by chemoreceptors that are located in the medulla
(B) mediated by J-receptors during pulmonary edema
(C) due to hyperinflation of the lung
(D) mediated by metaboreceptors located in muscle
(E) due to low cardiac output in individuals with obesity

152. During mechanical ventilation proximal airway pressure will increase with

(A) decreases in tidal volume
(B) increases in lower respiratory system compliance
(C) increases in respiratory flow
(D) decreases in PEEP
(E) decreases in airway resistance

153. A 60-year-old man with COPD and an 80-pack-year smoking history is scheduled to undergo pulmonary function testing. Measurements that can be obtained by spirometry include all of the following EXCEPT

(A) tidal volume
(B) residual volume
(C) expiratory reserve volume
(D) inspiratory reserve volume
(E) vital capacity

154. A double-lumen tube is used for anesthesia in patients with severe

(A) asthma
(B) hemoptysis
(C) emphysema
(D) heart failure
(E) tracheal stenosis

155. Carbon dioxide transport involves all of the following EXCEPT

(A) water
(B) bicarbonate ion
(C) carbonic anhydrase
(D) hemoglobin
(E) carboxyhemoglobin

156. In the normal upright lung

(A) the blood flow is greatest at the apex
(B) the ventilation is greatest at the apex
(C) the ventilation/perfusion (V/Q) ratio is higher at the apex
(D) ventilation is uniform
(E) the P_{O_2} is lower at the apex compared to the base

157. A 57-year-old woman is undergoing thoracotomy for resection of her left lower lobe because of a small-cell tumor. She has a right-sided double-lumen endotracheal tube in place. All of the following are effective ways to improve oxygenation during one-lung ventilation EXCEPT

   (A) lung recruitment maneuver in the dependent lung
   (B) decrease blood flow in the dependent lung, i.e., placement of a ligature on the pulmonary artery
   (C) increase blood flow and perfusion to the dependent lung
   (D) increase Pao_2 in the nondependent lung
   (E) PEEP to the dependent lung

158. If one measured pleural pressure in a standing human, one would find that the pressure was

   (A) highest at the apex of the lung
   (B) highest at the base of the lung
   (C) equal at all levels
   (D) unrelated to body position
   (E) completely unpredictable from one level to another

159. The LaPlace law is important in pulmonary physiology because it describes

   (A) the properties of gas mixtures
   (B) the angles of the bronchi
   (C) the bucket handle movement of the ribs during ventilation
   (D) the pressure relationships within the alveoli
   (E) resistance in large airways

160. Surfactant is a substance that

   (A) is produced in the liver of the newborn
   (B) is important in newborns but has little importance in the adult
   (C) is produced by the basement membrane of the lung
   (D) lowers surface tension in the alveoli
   (E) is a long-chained carbohydrate molecule

161. The functional residual capacity (FRC) is defined as the combination of

   (A) tidal volume and residual volume
   (B) tidal volume and expiratory reserve volume
   (C) tidal volume and inspiratory reserve volume
   (D) residual volume and expiratory reserve volume
   (E) vital capacity less the closing volume

162. A 16-year-old girl with asthma is to undergo routine pulmonary function testing. In order to measure the FEV_1 during spirometry, she

   (A) is asked to inhale forcefully
   (B) exhales forcefully from total lung capacity to residual volume
   (C) is asked to breathe slowly at normal tidal volumes
   (D) forcefully exhales from total lung capacity to respiratory reserve volume
   (E) is asked to forcefully exhale for 1 second

163. A previously healthy 46-year-old man developed gallstone pancreatitis and then required mechanical ventilation to maintain adequate oxygenation. The ICU team decided that his case of adult respiratory distress syndrome was best managed with high-frequency jet ventilation. This ventilatory mode

   (A) can provide ventilatory support only when a tightly sealed airway is established
   (B) cannot be applied for surgical procedures
   (C) can be used to provide emergency ventilation after cricothyroid cannulation
   (D) creates a jet drag effect, preventing secondary gases from entering the airway
   (E) is only necessary during rigid bronchoscopy

164. Factors contributing to increased airway pressure under anesthesia include all of the following EXCEPT

(A)   muscle paralysis of the chest wall

(B)   a decrease in functional residual capacity

(C)   the supine position

(D)   the presence of an endotracheal tube

(E)   controlled ventilation

165.   Distribution of ventilation in the lung is such that

(A)   the apical portions are better ventilated

(B)   the dependent areas are better ventilated

(C)   the central or hilar areas are better ventilated

(D)   all areas are ventilated equally

(E)   ventilation is not affected by position

166.   The level of arterial Pco_2 ($Paco_2$)

(A)   depends on minute ventilation only

(B)   is independent of CO_2 production

(C)   is not dependent on dead space ventilation

(D)   varies directly with CO_2 production and inversely with alveolar ventilation

(E)   decreases when dead space ventilation increases

167.   A healthy 26-year-old man underwent open herniorrhaphy. He had a Class I preoperative airway examination and the medical student intubated him on her first attempt. When deciding when to extubate him, you should consider that

(A)   laryngospasm is of no concern, as it only occurs during induction

(B)   laryngospasm should be managed with positive pressure ventilation, oxygen, suctioning of oropharyngeal secretions, and, in severe cases, a small dose of IV succinylcholine

(C)   airway obstruction only occurs in the first 4 to 6 min after extubation

(D)   extubation during deep anesthesia carries the risk of a profound cardiovascular response

(E)   in patients who were difficult to intubate, extubation should be carried out during deep anesthesia

168.   A 70-year-old man underwent left carotid endarterectomy two years ago and is about to have the same operation on his right side. Following this right-sided surgery, he will

(A)   have no respiratory changes

(B)   show no change in arterial carbon dioxide

(C)   respond to hypoxia with hyperventilation

(D)   be more susceptible to hypoxemia

(E)   always develop hypertension

169.   Mechanisms that may cause hypoxemia under anesthesia include all of the following EXCEPT

(A)   hypoventilation

(B)   hyperventilation

(C)   increase in functional residual capacity (FRC)

(D)   supine position

(E)   increased airway pressure

170.   A healthy 44-year-old woman underwent ablation of a dysrhythmia focus. The procedure required two hours, and the cardiologist requested apnea during periods of image acquisition. You hyperventilated her throughout the procedure. Now that she is extubated and breathing room air, she will

(A)   return to normal parameters within 30 min

(B)   remain hypocarbic for 2 h

(C)   possibly become hypoxemic if not treated with oxygen

(D)   become hypoxemic and hypercarbic

(E)   be well oxygenated if the air exchange is unimpaired by drugs

171.   All of the following lead to decreases in lung compliance, EXCEPT

(A)   pneumothorax

(B)   emphysema

(C)   pulmonary fibrosis

(D)   pneumonectomy

(E)   hyperinflation

172. The ventilatory response to $Paco_2$

    (A) is independent of hypoxemia
    (B) has a major peripheral component
    (C) is depressed by metabolic acidemia
    (D) is unaffected by opioid antagonists
    (E) is augmented by norepinephrine

173. When considering oxygen transport in the lung, the LEAST important cause of hypoxemia is

    (A) ventilation/perfusion mismatch
    (B) diffusion barrier
    (C) venous admixture
    (D) bronchial artery blood flow
    (E) altitude

174. In pulmonary function testing, carbon monoxide diffusing capacity (DLCO)

    (A) is greater than functional residual capacity (FRC)
    (B) is unchanged in anemia
    (C) is increased in pulmonary fibrosis
    (D) estimates the gas transfer ability of the lung
    (E) estimates the dead space ratio (V_D/V_T) of the lung

175. All of the following lead to decreases in chest wall compliance, EXCEPT

    (A) chest wall edema
    (B) thoracic deformities
    (C) flail chest
    (D) ventilator dyssynchrony
    (E) abdominal distension

176. The oxyhemoglobin dissociation curve describes the relationship of oxygen saturation to oxygen tension. All of the following are true EXCEPT that

    (A) at an oxygen tension of 60 mm Hg, the saturation is approximately 90%
    (B) the curve is shifted to the left with a more acidic pH
    (C) the curve is shifted to the right with an increase in carbon dioxide tension

    (D) the curve is shifted to the left with a decrease in temperature
    (E) the curve is shifted to the right with increased levels of 2,3-DPG

177. The definitive test of adequacy of ventilation is

    (A) listening to the esophageal stethoscope
    (B) watching the rise and fall of the chest
    (C) analyzing arterial blood gases
    (D) measuring tidal volume with a spirometer
    (E) using an apnea monitor

178. Pulmonary vascular resistance

    (A) is entirely dependent on the cardiac output
    (B) is entirely dependent on the pressure in the pulmonary artery
    (C) is equal to pressure divided by radius of the artery
    (D) depends on the state of vasomotor tone, flow, and pressure
    (E) is not affected by cardiac output

179. The work of breathing

    (A) can be excessively high during SIMV (spontaneous intermittent mandatory ventilation)
    (B) is solely due to airway resistance
    (C) is solely due to elastic forces
    (D) is at its lowest at a respiratory rate of 25 breaths per minute
    (E) is increased in the patient with restrictive disease if the respiratory rate is increased

180. Anatomic dead space

    (A) is independent of lung size
    (B) is about 1 mL/kg body weight
    (C) is not affected by equipment
    (D) combined with alveolar dead space constitutes physiologic dead space
    (E) is of less importance in the newborn than the adult

181. The term P_{50} in reference to the oxyhemoglobin dissociation curve

    (A) refers to the position on the curve at which the P_{O_2} is 50 mm Hg

    (B) normally has a value of 27 mm Hg

    (C) describes an enzyme system in hemoglobin

    (D) is constant

    (E) is affected only by type of hemoglobin

182. All of the following are frequently found in carbon monoxide poisoning EXCEPT

    (A) seizures and coma

    (B) lactic acidosis

    (C) desaturation by pulse oximetry

    (D) carboxyhemoglobin

    (E) normal Pa_{O_2}

183. The carotid bodies primarily

    (A) respond to elevated P_{CO_2}

    (B) respond to Sv_{O_2}

    (C) respond to Pa_{O_2}

    (D) signal the medulla via the vagus nerve

    (E) respond to hydrogen ions

184. Hypercapnia under anesthesia may be a result of

    (A) hyperventilation

    (B) decreased dead space ventilation

    (C) decreased carbon dioxide production

    (D) use of an Ayre T-piece at less than peak inspiratory flow rate

    (E) increased pulmonary artery flow

185. All of the following statements about the diaphragm are true EXCEPT

    (A) it is innervated via the vagus nerve

    (B) it has no fixed insertion

    (C) it is mainly active in inspiration

    (D) it has an equal mix of slow twitch and fast twitch fibers

    (E) it is deficient in stretch receptors

DIRECTIONS: Use the following figure to answer Questions 186-189:

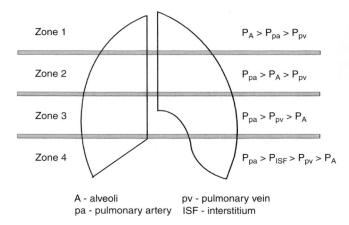

Zone 1 $P_A > P_{pa} > P_{pv}$

Zone 2 $P_{pa} > P_A > P_{pv}$

Zone 3 $P_{pa} > P_{pv} > P_A$

Zone 4 $P_{pa} > P_{ISF} > P_{pv} > P_A$

A - alveoli   pv - pulmonary vein
pa - pulmonary artery   ISF - interstitium

186. In Zone 1 of the lung

    (A) no air is moving

    (B) circulation is highest

    (C) venous pressure is high

    (D) dead space is high

    (E) shunting is high

187. In Zone 2 of the lung

    (A) there is good blood flow regardless of ventilation

    (B) venous pressure is high

    (C) dead space is high

    (D) the pulmonary vessels are collapsed

    (E) the blood flow is determined primarily by pulmonary artery pressure and alveolar pressure

188. In Zone 3 of the lung

    (A) blood flow is governed by the arteriovenous pressure difference

    (B) dead space is high

    (C) there is high alveolar pressure

    (D) venous pressure is very low

    (E) little blood flow occurs

189. All of the following are true EXCEPT

    (A) Zone 2 is the "waterfall" region of the lung

    (B) Zone 1 will increase in hypovolemic shock

    (C) Zone 4 will increase with lymphatic blockage

    (D) these zones would matter less if we could breathe in water

    (E) these zones are independent of gravitational effects

190. Hypoventilation in the recovery room

    (A) should always be treated with opioid reversal

    (B) is common after inhalation anesthesia

    (C) is uncommon after upper abdominal procedures

    (D) is best detected by pulse oximetry

    (E) is always accompanied by increases in blood pressure

191. All of the following statements about preoxygenation are true EXCEPT

    (A) 80% of the nitrogen in the functional residual capacity (FRC) is being replaced with oxygen during preoxygenation

    (B) during preoxygenation, nitrogen is eliminated rapidly, dependent on the volume of the breaths

    (C) preoxygenation preceding induction of general anesthesia can sustain vital organs for up to 15 min even without active ventilation

    (D) preoxygenation should always be considered before induction of general anesthesia

    (E) preoxygenation should be carried out over 2-3 min, or as a series of four vital capacity breaths

192. Which one of the following statements is true about Type II alveolar cells?

    (A) They produce surfactant.

    (B) They are the major component of gas exchange.

    (C) They line the capillary endothelium.

    (D) They can be replaced by Type I cells.

    (E) They are migratory and phagocytic.

193. A 56-year-old female patient is scheduled for emergent exploratory laparotomy for acute bowel obstruction. After rapid sequence induction of general anesthesia, the patient is noted to have regurgitation of gastric contents during direct laryngoscopy. Regarding perioperative aspiration of gastric content, all of the following are true, EXCEPT

    (A) the severity of symptoms depends on the type and volume of material aspirated

    (B) initial management comprises suctioning, administration of bronchodilators, supplemental O_2, and ICU transfer

    (C) bronchoscopy may be of benefit to remove particulate material

    (D) pulmonary lavage with large volumes of saline should be carried out repeatedly

    (E) administration of empirical antibiotic is not recommended

194. Regarding hypoxemia during the postoperative period, which one of the following is true?

    (A) Hypoxemia necessitates reintubation in most cases.

    (B) Hypoxemia is rarely caused by decreased ventilatory drive.

    (C) Opioid antagonists should be avoided, as they impede pain therapy.

    (D) The incidence of postoperative hypoxemia is relatively independent of surgical site.

    (E) Analgesics can enhance postoperative respiratory mechanics in some cases.

195. Comparing infant (<1 yr) and adult (>8 yr) airways,

    (A) the angle between trachea and right bronchus is smaller in infants

    (B) the narrowest position of the airway is glottis in infants and cricoid cartilage in adults

(C) only adults have a prominent protrusion of the corniculate and cuneiform tubercles into the laryngeal aditus

(D) the angle between trachea and left bronchus remains unchanged

(E) the epiglottic cross-section shape remains unchanged

196. If a patient is allowed to breathe 100% oxygen under anesthesia

(A) areas of atelectasis will disappear

(B) bowel distention will decrease

(C) the P_{O_2} will rise due to increased dead space

(D) lung units with low ventilation/perfusion (V/Q) ratios may become shunt units

(E) the oxygen tension will rise due to an increase in functional residual capacity (FRC)

197. All of the following statements are true about the esophageal-tracheal airway, Combitube, EXCEPT

(A) the combitube enters the trachea in approximately one third of cases

(B) the device has two lumens, one opening at the distal end, one at fenestrations between the balloons

(C) ventilation takes place using the more proximal lumen in the majority of cases

(D) the combitube does not need to be replaced even if it enters the trachea

(E) it is intended to establish emergency airway access if the operator is not able to perform face mask ventilation or conventional intubation

198. Independent risk factors for difficult mask ventilation include all of the following, EXCEPT

(A) sleep apnea

(B) limited mandibular protrusion

(C) body mass index <21 kg/m^2

(D) facial hair

(E) age >55 years

199. A 46-year-old woman with a history of scleroderma for more than twenty years is being evaluated in the preoperative clinic. She would be expected to have all of these pulmonary manifestations of scleroderma EXCEPT

(A) increased compliance

(B) diffuse fibrosis

(C) decreased vital capacity

(D) hypoxemia

(E) increased V_D/V_T ratio

200. All of the following statements are true about alveoli EXCEPT

(A) they are 100–300 microns in diameter

(B) they are mostly lined with Type I alveolar cells

(C) they are partially lined with Type II alveolar cells

(D) they are partially lined with Type III alveolar cells

(E) they are surrounded by capillaries

201. Auto-PEEP (positive end-expiratory pressure)

(A) decreases end-expiratory lung volume

(B) can be measured by applying an expiratory pause in mechanically ventilated patients

(C) promotes venous return

(D) decreases with increasing respiratory rate

(E) decreases with increasing minute ventilation

202. Chest wall compliance

(A) normally is 200 mL/cm H$_2$O

(B) decreases in the setting of a flail chest

(C) is increased in patients with kyphoscoliosis

(D) is increased in patients with abdominal distension

(E) is increased in morbidly obese patients

203. The work of breathing

(A) involves both resistive and elastic work
(B) is expended mostly in expiration
(C) to overcome elastic forces is decreased when breathing is deep and slow
(D) to overcome resistive forces is decreased when breathing is fast and shallow
(E) is expended mostly in inspiration

DIRECTIONS: Use the following figure to answer Questions 204-205:

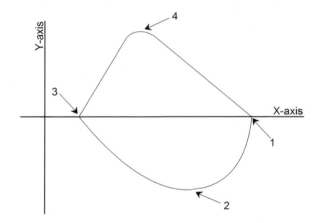

204. All of the following are TRUE of the flow-volume loop shown in the figure EXCEPT

(A) the X axis is volume
(B) the Y axis is pressure
(C) vital capacity is the distance from point 1 to point 3
(D) a breath proceeds through points 1, 2, 3, and 4, in that order
(E) there is no air leak

205. In this flow-volume loop

(A) there is evidence of tracheal stenosis
(B) point 2 is at maximum expiratory volume
(C) point 3 is at maximum inspiratory volume
(D) one can determine inspiratory reserve volume
(E) one can determine functional residual capacity (FRC)

206. Functional residual capacity (FRC) can be measured by

(A) use of an esophageal balloon
(B) computed tomography
(C) spirometry
(D) inert gas dilution technique
(E) bioimpedance

207. End-tidal CO_2 is increased by

(A) bicarbonate administration
(B) a circuit leak around the endotracheal tube cuff
(C) hypotension
(D) cardiac arrest
(E) intracardiac air embolism

208. Hypoxic pulmonary vasoconstriction

(A) leads to an increase in the shunt fraction
(B) is increased with increases in pulmonary artery pressure
(C) is increased with increases in central blood volume
(D) is decreased with the use of sodium nitroprusside
(E) is increased with the use of inhaled nitric oxide

209. Conditions aggravated by hypercapnia include all of the following EXCEPT

(A) elevated intracranial pressure
(B) right-to-left cardiac shunts
(C) pulmonary hypertension
(D) cardiac dysrhythmia
(E) ARDS

210. The patient who is hyperventilated to a P_{CO_2} of 20 mm Hg under anesthesia will have

(A) increased cerebral blood flow
(B) increased ionized calcium
(C) increased oxygen delivery to the tissues
(D) increased ventilation/perfusion (V/Q) mismatch due to inhibition of hypoxic pulmonary vasoconstriction
(E) increased respiratory drive

211. Specific effects of anesthesia on control of breathing include a decreased response to all of the following, EXCEPT

    (A) carbon dioxide
    (B) hypoxemia
    (C) metabolic acidemia
    (D) added airway resistance
    (E) external stimuli

212. Factors leading to pulmonary edema include all of the following, EXCEPT

    (A) increased capillary pressure
    (B) decreased oncotic pressure
    (C) lymphatic insufficiency
    (D) increased capillary permeability
    (E) hyperinflation during ventilation

213. The respiratory quotient

    (A) depends on the CO_2 output and O_2 uptake
    (B) is independent of the metabolic substrate
    (C) depends on the O_2 uptake and cardiac output
    (D) depends on the CO_2 output and metabolic equivalent
    (E) is always 0.8

214. Positive end-expiratory pressure (PEEP) usually

    (A) decreases functional residual capacity (FRC)
    (B) decreases compliance
    (C) decreases work of breathing
    (D) increases work of breathing
    (E) decreases lung volume

215. In comparing closing capacity (CC) and functional residual capacity (FRC),

    (A) obesity increases both CC and FRC
    (B) increasing FRC relative to CC results in areas of low ventilation/perfusion (V/Q)
    (C) anything that decreases CC below FRC results in areas of atelectasis

    (D) increasing CC above the tidal volume plus FRC results in areas of atelectasis
    (E) compared to adults, young children are less likely to suffer atelectasis from tidal breathing occurring from end-expiratory lung volumes close to closing capacity

216. During anesthesia, the diaphragm assumes a more cephalad position because of all of the following, EXCEPT

    (A) paralysis from muscle relaxants
    (B) increased end-expiratory tone of the abdominal wall
    (C) surgical retraction
    (D) second gas effect
    (E) pneumoperitoneum

217. Forced exhaled vital capacity (FVC)

    (A) may vary with patient cooperation
    (B) is measured in the first second
    (C) is a measure of inspiratory reserve volume
    (D) is affected by restrictive disease in the first second
    (E) can only be measured using body-plethysmography or the inert gas dilution technique

218. The medullary chemoreceptors are maximally stimulated by

    (A) low oxygen tension
    (B) reflex activity from the diaphragm
    (C) carbon dioxide
    (D) ondansetron
    (E) hydrogen ion

219. The composition of alveolar gases differs from that of inhaled gas. Concerning this, all of the following are true, EXCEPT

    (A) oxygen is being absorbed from the alveoli
    (B) carbon dioxide is being added to the alveoli
    (C) water vapor is being added
    (D) nitrogen is taken up by the alveolar capillaries
    (E) inhalational anesthetic agents are absorbed from or eliminated into the alveoli

220. The endotracheal tube position in a female adult patient is evaluated by the following: examining the patient, the numerical markings on the tube, and the chest x-ray. Which one of the following is consistent with the proper position?

(A) The left side is ventilated better than the right side.

(B) The tip of the tube is 30 cm from the upper front teeth.

(C) The tip of the tube overlies the 6th thoracic vertebra.

(D) Both sides ventilate equally.

(E) The ideal tube position is approximately 2 mm above the carina.

221. During mechanical ventilation inspiratory airway resistance

(A) cannot be estimated

(B) is decreased with the use of longer tubes

(C) is independent of endotracheal tube diameter

(D) is typically lower compared with expiratory airway resistance

(E) is independent of endotracheal tube length

222. A right shift in the oxyhemoglobin dissociation curve is caused by

(A) decreased temperature

(B) hypercarbia

(C) alkalosis

(D) the presence of fetal hemoglobin

(E) hypocarbia

223. Factors that increase the incidence of postoperative pulmonary complications include all of the following, EXCEPT

(A) upper vs. lower abdominal surgery

(B) chronic obstructive pulmonary disease

(C) heart failure

(D) asthma

(E) longer surgical duration

224. All of the following statements are true of closing capacity EXCEPT it is

(A) the lung volume at which the onset of airway closure is detected

(B) increased in smoking

(C) greater than residual volume

(D) greater than closing volume

(E) a smaller fraction of the total lung capacity in infants, compared to adults

225. Transpulmonary pressure

(A) measures intralung pressure

(B) is equal to intrapleural pressure at FRC

(C) is a gradient between the airway opening and the alveolar pressure

(D) increases with increasing lung volume

(E) is independent of tidal volume

226. All of the following statements are true in interpreting pulmonary function tests EXCEPT

(A) vital capacity measurement is not a timed measurement

(B) spirometry fails to detect early disease in small airways

(C) maximal breathing capacity is dependent on cooperation

(D) the FEV_1 will detect restrictive disease

(E) absolute lung volumes cannot be determined using standard spirometry

227. A patient who arrives in the recovery room after a general anesthetic should

(A) be sedated to prevent overt postoperative stress

(B) always be encouraged to lie on the back for easier access to the airway

(C) be closely observed for respiratory depression

(D) be given opioids at fixed intervals

(E) always be maintained on arterial blood pressure monitoring, using a radial artery catheter

228. A 14-gauge catheter is inserted through the cricothyroid membrane and attached to a wall oxygen source in such a way that oxygen can be delivered intermittently. With this technique

(A)   pneumothorax is inevitable

(B)   adequate oxygenation is possible

(C)   gastric dilatation is a hazard

(D)   larynx injury is impossible

(E)   prevention of hypercapnia is possible

229.   Patients with pneumoconiosis, e.g., asbestosis or silicosis, often require surgery on other organs. In the preoperative assessment, one must recognize that

(A)   the lung volumes will be increased

(B)   the x-ray abnormality fully reflect the functional changes

(C)   early airway closure is the hallmark

(D)   fibrosis usually is present

(E) FEV_1/FVC is regularly decreased in these patients

230.   Vital capacity includes all of the following, EXCEPT

(A)   tidal volume

(B)   inspiratory reserve volume

(C)   expiratory reserve volume

(D)   functional residual capacity (FRC)

(E)   closing volume

231.   Hypoxemia may occur under anesthesia because of all of the following, EXCEPT

(A)   blood loss

(B)   increased release of oxygen from hemo-globin to the tissues

(C)   depressed myocardial function

(D)   shunting

(E)   airway obstruction

232.   Diffusion hypoxia

(A)   is due to a large volume of nitrous oxide in the lungs

(B)   is due to a large volume of carbon mon-oxide in the bloodstream

(C)   is due to the second gas effect

(D)   can occur up to 48 h after surgery

(E)   does not respond to oxygen supplementation

233.   Pneumothorax may be due to all of the follow-ing EXCEPT

(A)   alveolar rupture

(B)   chest wall trauma

(C)   connection between the distal airway and the pleural space

(D)   extrathoracic tracheal puncture

(E)   a break in the parietal pleura

234.   When assessing the acutely hypoxemic patient, causes that may be important are all of the fol-lowing EXCEPT

(A)   hypoventilation

(B)   hypoperfusion

(C)   ventilation/perfusion (V/Q) mismatch

(D)   intracardiac shunts

(E)   abnormal diffusion

235.   Total pulmonary compliance

(A)   is measured by dividing pressure by volume

(B)   is usually decreased in elderly patients

(C)   involves the lung only

(D)   is independent of previous breaths

(E)   is increased by surfactant

Answers and Explanations

150. (E) At FRC, there is no pressure difference between the alveoli and atmosphere. Further ventilation is possible, since FRC is the volume that exists at the end of a normal tidal volume. Elastic forces of the lung and chest wall are balanced. The total pulmonary vascular resistance is at its lowest at FRC. The gradient between the alveoli and the intrapleural space will be non-zero, balancing the elastic tension of the lung. *(6:2087-8)*

151. (E) Dyspnea associated with obesity is likely due to multiple problems, including high cardiac output and decreased compliance of the chest wall. Chemoreceptors are activated by hypoxemia, acute hypercarbia and acidosis and are located in the medulla and carotid bodies. J-receptors are activated during the accumulation of pulmonary edema. Changes in the biochemical milieu of skeletal muscle can activate metaboreceptors that can contribute to the sensation on dyspnea. *(6:277-9)*

152. (C) In ventilated patients proximal airway pressure increases with increases in flow, higher tidal volumes, lower respiratory system compliance, higher airway resistance, higher inspiratory flow, higher PEEP, and presence of auto-PEEP. *(5:470)*

153. (B) Spirometry can only detect relative volume changes. In order to determine absolute volumes including residual volume and to calculate total lung capacity, other methods like inert gas dilution or body plethysmography have to be applied. *(6:2091)*

154. (B) Endobronchial intubation with a double-lumen tube allows selective lung ventilation and isolation of a bleeding lung segment. When one lung contains either blood or infectious secretions, isolation of the lungs should be applied in order to prevent spillage of blood or secretions into the unaffected lung. *(5:417, 963)*

155. (E) Carboxyhemoglobin is involved in the transport of carbon monoxide. Carbon dioxide exists as dissolved, bicarbonate and carbaminohemoglobin. *(5:461, 525, 1336)*

156. (C) The V/Q ratio is higher at the apex and thus P_{O_2} is higher in this location as well. Blood flow is greatest at the base. *(5:959)*

157. (B) Measures to improve oxygenation during one-lung ventilation include, among others, improving V/Q distribution and/or blood flow in the dependent lung (lung recruitment maneuver, PEEP, prostacyclin, nitric oxide), increasing Pa_{O_2} (through CPAP) or decreasing blood flow in the non-dependent lung (ligature). A ligature placed on the pulmonary artery of the dependent lung would result in massive shunting and profound hypoxemia. *(5:970)*

158. (B) As an air-fluid mixture, the lung tends to sag with gravity, causing a gravity-induced pleural pressure gradient. Pleural pressure increases by approximately 0.25 cm H_2O with every centimeter from apex to base. Thus, it is lowest at the apex and highest at the base. Pleural pressure is related to body position because in different positions, different areas of the lung will be dependent. Pleural pressure variation is caused by the hydrostatic pressure exerted by gravity. *(5:959)*

159. **(D)** The LaPlace law, P = 2T/R, states that the pressure within an elastic sphere is directly proportional to the tension of the wall and inversely proportional to the radius of the curvature. In this case, the sphere is the alveolus. Alveoli are lined with a film of surfactant that lends stability to the alveoli by decreasing the surface tension as the radius of the alveolus becomes smaller. Without this ability to vary surface tension, small alveoli, which have a smaller radius of curvature and thus a higher pressure, would empty into large alveoli and alveolar stability would be lost. *(6:2154)*

160. **(D)** Surfactant is a substance containing dipalmitoyl lecithin produced by the type II alveolar epithelial cells of the lung. The substance is important in adults as well as newborns, providing alveolar stability. It is 90% lipid and 10% protein. *(5:250; 6:2206)*

161. **(D)** The FRC is composed of expiratory reserve volume and residual volume. Tidal volume plus inspiratory reserve volume comprise the inspiratory capacity. The other options are not designated capacities. *(5:256)*

162. **(B)** In order to determine the FEV$_1$, the patient is asked to forcefully exhale from total lung capacity to residual volume. While the FEV$_1$ measures the volume exhaled after the first second of the maneuver, the patient is asked to complete the exhalation process. This allows among others for the calculation of the FEV$_1$/FCV ratio. *(5:131)*

163. **(C)** During high frequency jet ventilation (HFJV), gas is injected into the trachea under high pressure, creating a "jet drag" effect entraining (not preventing the entry of) secondary gases, thus providing ventilation to a non-sealed airway. It has been used successfully in surgeries where establishing a closed airway is not possible, e.g. upper airway surgery. Simple HFJV systems have been used to provide emergency ventilation by placing an injector through the cricothyroid membrane. An escape pathway for the injected gases must be present, however. *(5:1419)*

164. **(A)** Muscle paralysis will decrease chest and abdominal wall tone, improving compliance. The decrease in FRC and the supine position will move the patient to a less compliant region of the lung volume relationship. The endotracheal tube increases airway resistance, worsening dynamic compliance. Controlled ventilation changes the pressure gradient entirely; the airway pressure must be supra-atmospheric instead of sub-atmospheric. *(5:362, 471, 1406)*

165. **(B)** The dependent areas are better ventilated, since the alveoli in the dependent areas are smaller and more compliant. *(5:959)*

166. **(D)** Arterial CO_2 rises with CO_2 production and decreases with increases in alveolar ventilation. As dead space ventilation does not contribute to gas exchange, the larger the ratio of dead space ventilation to total ventilation becomes the higher Paco$_2$ rises. *(5:460)*

167. **(B)** Laryngospasm is common after extubation, especially in children. It should be treated as outlined in option B. Delayed airway obstruction can occur, for instance as a result of laryngeal edema. Extubation during deep anesthesia minimizes the cardiovascular response, but increases the risk of airway complications. It should not be attempted in patients who were difficult to intubate, as reintubation might become necessary. *(5:575)*

168. **(D)** After bilateral carotid endarterectomy, a patient will be more susceptible to hypoxemia because of bilateral denervation of the carotid bodies. The patient will not respond to hypoxemia with hyperventilation. In addition, the resting Pco$_2$ is elevated, and the response to small doses of opioids may be accentuated. Hypertension is not a constant finding in these patients. *(5:1021)*

169. **(C)** Anesthesia usually causes a decrease in FRC that leads to hypoxemia. All of the other options can lead to hypoxemia: hypoventilation

by decreased FRC and increased shunt, hyperventilation by shift of the oxyhemoglobin dissociation curve to the left and decreased cardiac output, supine position by decreased ventilation and decreased FRC, and increased airway pressure by change in the ventilation-perfusion relationships. *(5:363, 459, 550)*

170. **(C)** Patients who are hyperventilated for long periods of time have their carbon dioxide stores depleted. Postoperatively, these patients hypoventilate in an effort to restore their carbon dioxide and, in doing so, may become hypoxemic if not given supplemental oxygen. *(5:460)*

171. **(B)** Normal lung compliance is 100 mL/cm H_2O and is decreased by pulmonary edema (cardiogenic or noncardiogenic), pneumothorax, lung consolidation, atelectasis, pulmonary fibrosis, pneumonectomy or lung resection, bronchial intubation, and hyperinflation. Lung compliance is increased with emphysema and flail chest. *(5:471)*

172. **(E)** The CO_2 response curve is shifted to the left by norepinephrine, acidosis, and hypoxia. Naloxone will reverse opioid depression. Peripheral chemoreceptors contribute 15% of the control. *(5:324, 529, 612, 710)*

173. **(B)** Diffusion is rarely the limiting component of oxygen transport. High altitude lowers the Pa_{O_2}. The other factors contribute to shunt. *(6:287)*

174. **(D)** DLCO is a measure of the diffusing capacity of the lung. Increased hemoglobin and pulmonary blood volume will affect it. It is not a lung capacity in the same sense as FRC. *(5:953; 6:2093)*

175. **(C)** All conditions lead to decreased chest wall compliance through either increased muscular tone or mechanical impairment of elasticity, except flail chest that leads to increased chest wall compliance through instability *(5:471)*

176. **(B)** The curve is shifted to the right with acidosis. The other options are correct. *(5:459; 6:853)*

177. **(C)** All of the factors cited are presumptive evidence of ventilation. The only sure measure of demonstrating effective gas exchange is the analysis of blood gases, specifically carbon dioxide. *(5:459)*

178. **(D)** Pulmonary vascular resistance is the result of cardiac output, the state of vasomotor tone, and pressure. A change in cardiac output will normally be followed by changes in the radius of the vessels to allow maintenance of normal pressure. The resistance is equal to pressure divided by flow. *(6:1856)*

179. **(A)** As the mandatory ventilatory rate is reduced during SIMV, the work of breathing for both mandatory and spontaneous breaths increases. The optimum rate is about 15 breaths per minute in normal adults. In the patient with restrictive disease, short shallow breaths decrease the effort. In general, humans adjust their breathing pattern to minimize the work of breathing while maintaining adequate ventilation. *(5:1410)*

180. **(D)** Anatomic dead space increases with increased lung volume. The normal dead space is approximately 2 mL/kg. Equipment dead space may greatly increase the amount of dead space that can be disproportionately large in infants. *(5:460)*

181. **(B)** P_{50} is the P_{O_2} level on the oxyhemoglobin dissociation curve at which hemoglobin is 50% saturated. The normal value is 27 mm Hg and may change due to the influence of factors that cause a shift in the oxyhemoglobin dissociation curve. *(5:200, 274)*

182. **(C)** Carbon monoxide binds hemoglobin avidly, forming carboxyhemoglobin. Because oxyhemoglobin and carboxyhemoglobin absorb light at the same wavelength, it is not possible to detect carbon monoxide poisoning with pulse oximetry. *(5:1336)*

183. **(C)** The chemoreceptors of the carotid body sense Pa_{O_2} (less than 65 mm Hg) and send afferents via the glossopharyngeal nerve. *(5:251; 6:277)*

184. **(D)** Hypercapnia may result from rebreathing of CO_2 while using an Ayre T-piece at low fresh gas flow. The other options all cause decreased carbon dioxide tension. *(5:638)*

185. **(A)** The diaphragm is innervated by the phrenic nerve. *(5:952)*

186. **(D)** In Zone 1, the alveolar pressure is higher than the arterial or venous pressure; therefore, these areas act as dead space units. *(5:460, 960)*

187. **(E)** In Zone 2, the blood flow is dependent on arterial pressure and the alveolar pressure. These change with the status of ventilation. Venous pressure is still not a determinant of blood flow in this zone. *(5:414, 460, 960)*

188. **(A)** In Zone 3, blood flow is determined by the arteriovenous pressure difference. Dead space is low, since the units are being perfused, alveolar pressure is not high, and the venous pressure is lower than arterial but higher than alveolar pressure. *(5:414, 460, 960)*

189. **(D)** Gravity is the cause of the hydrostatic pressure gradient in the arterial and venous circulations. If the density of the alveolar gas were closer to blood, the pressure gradient in the alveoli would be closer to the vascular gradient. *(5:414, 460, 960)*

190. **(D)** Residual anesthetic, both inhaled and intravenous, inhibits hypoxic drive. It may or may not respond to opioid reversal, depending on the anesthesia technique employed. The patient with hypoventilation may be hypotensive. The best way to identify the hypoxia is a continuous convenient monitor: pulse oximetry. It is important to note that patients receiving a high concentration of supplemental oxygen might not display oxygen desaturation even in the setting of hypoventilation. *(5:1286)*

191. **(C)** All of the facts are true except C. Preoxygenation can sustain vital organs for up to approximately 8 min. *(5:551)*

192. **(A)** Type I alveolar cells form the majority of the alveolar gas exchange surface. When injured,

Type II cells create new Type I cells. Type II cells produce surfactant. Type III cells are alveolar macrophages. *(6:2206)*

193. **(D)** All of the options are appropriate, except pulmonary lavage with large volumes of saline that is believed to cause detrimental effects. *(5:1288)*

194. **(E)** Hypoxemia can be treated by supplementing the spontaneously breathing patient with O_2 in most cases. A major reason for postoperative hypoxemia is residual respiratory depression from hypnotics or analgesics, necessitating application of antagonists in some cases. However, improved pain control by administration of opioids might facilitate deep breathing and thus prevent hypoventilation and atelectasis. The surgical site, especially if thoracic or upper abdominal, is known to have a major influence on postoperative hypoxemia. *(5:1286)*

195. **(D)**

	Infant (<1 yr)	Adult (>8 yr)
Angle between trachea and right bronchus (deg)	30	20
Angle between trachea and left bronchus (deg)	45	45
Narrowest position of the airway	Cricoid cartilage	Glottis
Protrusion of corniculate and cuneiform tubercles into aditus	Prominent	Minimal
Shape of epiglottic cross-section	Omega-shaped	Crescent-shaped or flat

(5:549)

196. **(D)** When patients breathe an increased F_{IO_2}, there is an increased amount of shunt present due to absorption atelectasis. This occurs in all air spaces. The lung units with low V/Q ratios have a greater tendency to collapse. *(5:970)*

197. **(A)** The Combitube enters the trachea in about 4-6% of cases and can then still be used to ventilate the lungs, by using the distal rather than the more proximal lumen. All other facts are true. *(5:558)*

198. (C) Independent risk factors for difficult mask ventilation include age older than 55 years, body mass index greater than 30 kg/m², facial hair, limited mandibular protrusion, abnormal neck anatomy, sleep apnea, and a history of snoring. *(5:549)*

199. (A) The pulmonary involvement in scleroderma results in restrictive disease. The chest wall and the lung itself both contribute to the restriction. There is fibrosis and a decreased vital capacity leading to decreased arterial saturation. The V_D/V_T ratio increases. *(6:2757)*

200. (D) Type III alveolar cells are macrophages that are not stationary elements of the alveolar lining. *(6:2206)*

201. (B) Auto-PEEP occurs if the expiratory phase is terminated prematurely. When this occurs, alveolar pressure does not equilibrate with proximal airway pressure at end-exhalation and gas trapping results. It increases end-expiratory lung volume and can be measured by applying an expiratory pause in mechanically ventilated patients. The pressure measured at the end of this maneuver that is in excess of the PEEP set on the ventilator is auto-PEEP. Auto-PEEP may reduce venous return and increases with increasing respiratory rate and minute ventilation. *(5:470)*

202. (A) Chest wall compliance is calculated from the change in esophageal pressure (pleural pressure) during passive inflation. Chest wall compliance normally is 200 mL/cm H₂O, and can be decreased by abdominal distension, chest wall edema, chest wall burns, thoracic deformities (e.g., kyphoscoliosis), in obese patients, and through an increase in muscle tone (e.g., a patient who is dyssynchronous with the ventilator). Chest wall compliance is increased with flail chest and paralysis. *(5:471)*

203. (A) The work of breathing involves both elastic and resistive work. If breathing is deep and slow, more effort is expended in overcoming elastic work. Most of the breathing effort is expended in inspiration. *(6:2089)*

204. (B) A flow-volume loop has flow on the y-axis and volume on the x-axis. An air leak would be manifest by an open curve. *(5:997)*

205. (C) Dynamic tracheal stenosis would be seen with inspiratory or expiratory flattening, depending on whether the affected area was extrathoracic or intrathoracic, respectively. Point 2 is the point of peak inspiratory flow, while maximum expiration is at point 1. Point 3 is at maximum inspiration, and point 4 at peak expiratory flow. Since a flow-volume loop is done from maximum expiration to maximum inspiration and back, the point at rest, FRC, cannot be determined. Without knowing the residual volume, FRC, or tidal volume, none of the classical lung volumes can be determined. Vital capacity, the sum of inspiratory reserve, expiratory reserve, and tidal volumes can be determined, but it is a capacity, not a volume. *(5:997; 6:2086)*

206. (D) The FRC measurement is possible through the use of body plethysmography or a trace gas (such as helium) dilution. The residual volume component of the FRC cannot, by definition, be measured with spirometry. An esophageal balloon is used to estimate pleural pressure, and is not relevant to this measurement. *(6:2084)*

207. (A) The breakdown of bicarbonate will lead to CO₂ production and thus increased ETCO₂ levels. Any decrease in sampling, reduced production or delivery of CO₂ to the lungs will decrease ETCO₂. *(5:466)*

208. (D) Vasodilators attenuate the hypoxemic pulmonary vasoconstrictive response. Anything that increases pressure in the pulmonary circulation will decrease hypoxic pulmonary vasoconstriction, including increases in pulmonary pressure, central blood volume, and arterial pressure. *(5:969)*

209. (E) All of the conditions mentioned are aggravated by hypercapnia, partly through increased catecholamines, respiratory acidosis, and increased plasma potassium, except ARDS, where a certain degree of permissive hypercapnia can augment unloading of oxygen to the tissues by virtue of a rightward shift of the oxygen-hemoglobin dissociation curve. *(5:532, 551)*

210. **(D)** Hypocapnia leads to decreased cerebral blood flow, decreased ionized calcium, and decreased oxygen delivery to the tissues. Respiratory drive is decreased. There is an inhibition of hypoxic pulmonary vasoconstriction leading to V/Q mismatch. *(5:970)*

211. **(D)** The anesthetized patient has decreased ability to respond to increased CO_2, low oxygen, metabolic acidemia, and external stimuli. The ability to respond to added airway resistance is not lost. *(5:612)*

212. **(E)** Surgery can cause capillary damage from rough handling and can interrupt lymphatic drainage. Injudicious fluid administration can add more fluid than the pulmonary circulation can handle. Hyperinflation may cause parenchymal lung damage, but usually not pulmonary edema. *(5:422; 6:2232)*

213. **(A)** The respiratory quotient is the rate of CO_2 output divided by the rate of O_2 uptake. It may vary with the metabolic substrate and, therefore, will not always be 0.8. *(5:1468)*

214. **(C)** PEEP increases FRC and decreases the work of breathing. Compliance is increased, and the lung volume is increased. *(5:470, 651)*

215. **(D)** The FRC/CC relationship is important in determining if the airway will remain open. If CC is below FRC, lung areas will stay open. If CC is above FRC, lung areas will collapse with each breath. If CC is above FRC plus tidal volume, lung areas will stay collapsed. In obesity, FRC is decreased, while CC stays constant. Younger children are more prone to experiencing airway closure and alveolar collapse with atelectasis because the end-expiratory lung volume from which tidal breathing occurs is close to closing capacity. *(5:253, 302)*

216. **(D)** When paralyzed, the diaphragm is pushed cephalad by abdominal contents in the supine and lateral positions. Under spontaneous, anesthetized breathing, active expiration with increased abdominal tone also pushes the diaphragm cephalad. Pneumoperitoneum, retraction, and packing in the abdomen can also decrease the diaphragm's descent. The second gas effect is the concentrating effect of the initial uptake of nitrous oxide on the other alveolar gases. *(5:605, 1041)*

217. **(A)** The forced vital capacity (FVC) is the volume of gas that can be exhaled from maximal inhalation. The results vary with patient cooperation. The FEV_1 is that portion of the procedure performed in the first second. The FEV_1 is greatly reduced in obstructive disease. Inspiratory reserve volume is only a portion of the FVC. Unlike residual volume, FVC can be determined using standard spirometry. *(6:2084)*

218. **(E)** The primary stimulus is pH. Carbon dioxide reacts with water to form hydrogen ions; thus, CO_2 is involved indirectly. Hypoxia acts peripherally at the level of the carotid bodies. Ondansetron is an antiemetic agent. *(5:528)*

219. **(D)** The composition of alveolar gas differs from that of the inhaled gas since there is active CO_2 production, O_2 consumption, uptake or elimination of inhalational anesthetic agents (depending on concentration on either side), and humidification. Nitrogen undergoes no metabolism and insignificant excretion, so at equilibrium, no net transfer occurs across the alveolar membrane. *(5:459, 596)*

220. **(D)** Equal ventilation of both sides is consistent with proper tube placement, although it does not guarantee it. Unequal ventilation obviously demonstrates poor tube placement, or lung pathology. The distance from the lips to the carina in an adult female is about 25 cm. Therefore, the tube distance of 30 cm from the upper teeth is excessive. The carina lies at the level of the 4th–5th thoracic vertebra. Therefore, the tube placement by chest x-ray also is incorrect. *(5:573)*

221. **(D)** Airway resistance is typically higher during exhalation than inhalation. Factors influencing resistance include the diameter

and length of the endotracheal tube. In mechanically ventilated patients the resistance can be estimated as the difference between peak and plateau pressure divided by inspiratory flow. *(5:472)*

222. **(B)** A right shift in the oxyhemoglobin dissociation curve is caused by hyperthermia, acidosis, hypercarbia, and increases in DPG. Fetal hemoglobin will shift this curve to the left. *(5:460)*

223. **(D)** The rate of pulmonary complications correlates strongly with all these factors, except asthma. The existence of chronic or acute pulmonary disease and the specific location of the incision can influence the level of postoperative pulmonary dysfunction. However, risk of complications is surprisingly low in well-controlled asthma and in patients treated preoperatively with corticosteroids. *(5:63)*

224. **(E)** All of the options regarding closing capacity are true, except E. Closing capacity is the sum of closing volume and residual volume. As a fractional part of the total lung capacity, it is decreased during infancy and childhood. *(5:255)*

225. **(D)** Transpulmonary pressure is the pressure gradient across the lung measured as the pressure difference between the airway opening and the pleural surface, and therefore is associated with tidal volume and lung volume. It is zero at FRC. *(5:1415)*

226. **(D)** Vital capacity is the full exhalation from total lung capacity without time limit for the maneuver. Closing capacity is the earliest test of small airway disease, but requires gas analysis. Maximal breathing capacity is effort dependent. FEV_1 is altered in obstructive disease. To determine absolute lung volumes as opposed to relative volume changes, body plethysmography or an inert gas dilution technique is required. *(6:2209)*

227. **(C)** Patients in the recovery room do not normally require sedation. Opioids should be used carefully in an amount that will treat the pain but still allow the patient to breathe deeply and mobilize secretions, rather than at fixed intervals. Positioning is dependent on the type of surgery performed; invasive arterial blood pressure monitoring is not indicated in low-risk patients after low-risk surgery. *(5:87)*

228. **(B)** This describes a method of emergency ventilation that can be used to oxygenate a patient adequately. If there is no obstruction above, pneumothorax is unlikely but one of the possible complications of the procedure. Gastric dilatation does not occur, since the air will be vented to the atmosphere. Injury to the surrounding structures (larynx, esophagus, trachea) are possible complications. Ventilation may be inadequate to prevent hypercapnia. *(5:572)*

229. **(D)** Pneumoconiosis is associated with fibrosis. Since a restrictive component is present, the diaphragm may move very little. The x-ray may look much worse than the functional state. Decreased FEV_1/FVC is a measure for obstructive lung disease. *(6:2121)*

230. **(D)** Vital capacity includes tidal volume, closing volume, and inspiratory and expiratory reserve volumes but not all of FRC. FRC includes residual volume. *(5:256; 6:2209)*

231. **(B)** All of the factors cited may be involved in causing hypoxemia, except B. Decreased release of oxygen from hemoglobin to the tissues is a cause of hypoxia. Blood loss, cardiac output, and shunting are involved in oxygen transport; airway obstruction is involved in ventilation. *(5:459)*

232. **(A)** Diffusion hypoxia is due to an outpouring of nitrous oxide from the circulation into the alveoli that displaces oxygen and leads to hypoxia. It can easily be treated and prevented through oxygen supplementation. It occurs only during the phase of nitrous oxide elimination, minutes after emergence from anesthesia. The second gas effect occurs during induction and refers to enhanced uptake of a second volatile anesthetic in the presence of nitrous oxide.

Carbon monoxide does not cause diffusion hypoxia. *(5:605, 612)*

233. **(D)** Pneumothorax is caused by a loss of the sealed, negative pressure in the pleural space. Gas tracking through fascial planes, a connection to the airways, a connection through the chest wall, or intrathoracic tracheobronchial injury can all cause pneumothorax. Chest wall trauma can either produce a penetrating injury to the chest wall, or airway rupture, or a rib fracture, that in turn can puncture the lung. *(5:857; 6:2181)*

234. **(E)** Hypoventilation, low cardiac output, V/Q mismatch, and intracardiac or pulmonary shunting are problems that are of the highest importance. Abnormal diffusion is rarely important in this situation, and is associated with chronic lung diseases, such as sarcoidosis. *(5:459)*

235. **(E)** Total pulmonary compliance is volume divided by pressure. Net pulmonary compliance remains relatively unchanged in elderly people due to a combination of loss of tissue elasticity and stiffening of costochondral joints, compared to younger individuals. Pulmonary compliance involves the lung and the chest wall. There is hysteresis in the alveolar expansion, so hypoventilation and atelectasis will decrease compliance. Compliance is increased by surfactant. *(5:280, 470)*

Nervous System
Questions

236. A 44-year-old woman is undergoing total pelvic exenteration for metastatic ovarian cancer. Several hours into the procedure her body temperature has dropped to 34.6°C despite measures to keep her warm. Core body temperature may decrease intraoperatively because of all the following factors EXCEPT

    (A) exposure of body surfaces to room temperature air
    (B) administration of room temperature intravenous fluids
    (C) administration of muscle relaxants
    (D) low humidity of inspired gases
    (E) high inspired oxygen concentration

237. Of the cranial contents contributing to intracranial pressure (ICP), which one has the smallest volume?

    (A) brain tissue
    (B) tissue water
    (C) venous blood
    (D) arterial blood
    (E) cerebrospinal fluid (CSF)

238. In the sympathetic nervous system

    (A) preganglionic fibers synapse only in paravertebral sympathetic ganglia
    (B) preganglionic cell bodies are located throughout the spinal cord

    (C) the preganglionic neurotransmitter is acetylcholine
    (D) target organ receptors are only adrenergic
    (E) effects are mediated entirely through cyclic AMP

239. A 22-year-old man has an unidentified parietal mass and presents for open brain biopsy. He has some symptoms associated with a mild increase in intracranial pressure. Which one of the following induction agents may increase his intracranial pressure even further?

    (A) thiopental
    (B) methohexital
    (C) ketamine
    (D) propofol
    (E) midazolam

DIRECTIONS: Use the following figure to answer Questions 240-243:

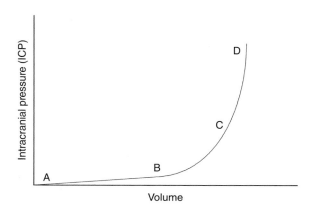

240. Between A and B on the curve

(A) there is a small ICP increase with increased intracranial volume

(B) a small ICP increase indicates poor compensatory effect

(C) pressure increases are compensated for by increased blood flow

(D) intracranial contents do not effect ICP

(E) compensatory mechanisms are not functional

241. Intracranial pressure measurements similar to those shown in the graph are obtained from a

(A) needle in the caudal canal

(B) needle in the cervical epidural space

(C) catheter positioned in the lateral ventricle

(D) catheter positioned in the carotid siphon

(E) catheter positioned in the jugular bulb

242. A patient at position B on the curve would be expected to

(A) have clinical manifestations of increased ICP

(B) move toward position C with hyperventilation

(C) have unilateral mydriasis

(D) move toward position A with administration of isoflurane

(E) may benefit from administration of intravenous hypertonic saline

243. At position C on the curve, a patient

(A) moves toward position D with hyperventilation

(B) moves toward position D with coughing

(C) will not benefit from intravenous mannitol

(D) will likely be hypotensive

(E) will likely be tachycardic

244. The ventilatory control centers

(A) contain no expiratory neurons

(B) receive no mechanical sensory input

(C) receive input from airway oxygen receptors

(D) are located in the medulla and pons

(E) are activated by peripheral CO_2 tension

245. Absorption of cerebrospinal fluid (CSF) takes place through

(A) ependymal cells

(B) arachnoid villi

(C) the pia mater

(D) the foramen of Monro

(E) the foramen of Magendie

246. The smallest nerve fiber, a postganglionic fiber associated with slow conduction, is the

(A) A-alpha fiber

(B) A-beta fiber

(C) A-gamma fiber

(D) B fiber

(E) C fiber

247. Integrity of all of the following structures can be monitored by sensory-evoked potentials EXCEPT the

(A) dorsal columns

(B) cerebellum

(C) thalamus

(D) vestibular-cochlear nerve

(E) inferior colliculus

248. A 61-year-old man has developed a resting tremor in his right hand. His neurologist believes it is consistent with early Parkinson disease. He is therefore likely to have dysfunction within the

(A) cerebellum

(B) lateral ventricle

(C) pons

(D) basal ganglia

(E) aqueduct of Sylvius

249. A nuclear group in the brain involved in transmission of sensory information to the cortex is the

(A) cerebellum

(B) caudate

(C) hypothalamus

(D)   thalamus

(E)   hippocampus

250.   All of the following cranial nerves contain parasympathetic efferent fibers EXCEPT the

(A)   oculomotor nerve (III)

(B)   trigeminal nerve (V)

(C)   facial nerve (VII)

(D)   glossopharyngeal nerve (IX)

(E)   vagus nerve (X)

251.   The electroencephalographic (EEG) waveform with a frequency range of 8 to 13 Hz is associated with

(A)   alpha activity

(B)   beta activity

(C)   gamma activity

(D)   delta activity

(E)   theta activity

252.   In face of a declining supply of nutrients

(A)   neuronal function deteriorates in an all-or-none fashion

(B)   there is no reserve below the normal level of cerebral blood flow

(C)   irreversible neuronal damage occurs with EEG evidence of ischemia

(D)   the actual CBF level at which neuronal function deteriorates varies with anesthetics

(E)   an isoelectric EEG indicates irreversible neuronal damage

253.   The substantia gelatinosa

(A)   has the highest concentration of opioid receptors in the spinal cord

(B)   is located in the lateral columns

(C)   is part of the dorsal column

(D)   is in the motor area of the brain

(E)   is in the ventral column

254.   The oculocardiac reflex involves all of the following structures EXCEPT

(A)   vagus nerve

(B)   trigeminal ganglion

(C)   ophthalmic division of cranial nerve V

(D)   oculomotor nerve

(E)   brain stem

255.   Hormonal products of the anterior pituitary include all of the following EXCEPT

(A)   growth hormone

(B)   luteinizing hormone

(C)   antidiuretic hormone

(D)   follicle-stimulating hormone

(E)   thyrotropin

256.   After bringing a traumatized patient to the emergency department, the paramedic team reports that his Glasgow Coma Score is 11. This assessment is based on

(A)   eye opening, verbal response, and motor response

(B)   assessment of knee jerk and other motor reflexes

(C)   assessment of pupil size and brain stem reflexes

(D)   assessment of respiration and autonomic brain stem functions

(E)   assessment of EEG

257.   An increase in Pa_{CO_2} from 40 to 50 mm Hg will increase cerebral blood flow

(A)   not at all

(B)   1 to 2 mL/100 g/min

(C)   5 to 10 mL/100 g/min

(D)   10 to 20 mL/100 g/min

(E)   25 to 50 mL/100 g/min

258.   The oxygen reserves of the brain are

(A)   infinite

(B)   capable of maintaining function for 25 min

(C)   greater under anesthesia

(D)   very low

(E)   carried primarily in the cerebral hemispheres

259. Cerebral perfusion pressure may be estimated by

(A) MAP + ICP
(B) SBP − ICP
(C) MAP − ICP
(D) MAP + CVP − ICP
(E) SBP − CVP

MAP: mean arterial blood pressure
ICP: intracranial pressure
SBP: systolic arterial blood pressure
CVP: mean central venous pressure

DIRECTIONS: Use the following case to answer Questions 260-262: A 47-year-old man is brought to the interventional radiology suite for insertion of a suprapubic catheter to provide long-term bladder drainage. He sustained a C6 fracture with transection of the cervical cord at age 23 in a motor vehicle accident. He takes no medications but has had several urinary tract infections treated with antibiotics. He has no motor function or sensation below the shoulders. He is sedated with 2 mg midazolam and 50 mcg fentanyl.

260. In the patient with an injury at the C 6-7 level, one would expect

(A) a major loss of diaphragmatic power
(B) no effective ventilation and ventilator dependency
(C) difficulty swallowing and pulmonary aspiration
(D) impaired alveolar ventilation
(E) profound bradycardia

261. On instillation of the bladder with saline, the blood pressure rises from 128/75 to 221/120 mm Hg and the heart rate falls from 87 to 45 bpm. What is the likely cause of these changes to blood pressure and heart rate?

(A) response to pain
(B) autonomic hyperreflexia
(C) micturition reflex
(D) response to cold solution in the bladder
(E) anxiety

262. This event could have been prevented by

(A) pretreatment with beta blockers
(B) lithotomy position
(C) instillation of body temperature fluid
(D) light general anesthesia
(E) spinal anesthesia

263. A 38-year-old woman is in the neurological intensive care unit following rupture of an aneurysm of the right middle cerebral artery. A CT scan shows extensive subarachnoid hemorrhage. Which one of the following findings would be considered to be LEAST likely?

(A) hyponatremia
(B) dysrhythmias
(C) normal ICP
(D) cerebral vasospasm
(E) ECG abnormalities consistent with ischemia

264. The basilar artery is formed by the merger of

(A) the vertebral arteries
(B) branches of the internal carotid artery
(C) branches of the external carotid artery
(D) the anterior and posterior communicating arteries
(E) the anterior and posterior spinal arteries

265. The celiac plexus

(A) contains visceral and somatic afferent and efferent fibers
(B) receives efferents from both sympathetic and parasympathetic ganglia
(C) innervates abdominal viscera
(D) is formed from nerve roots from T7 through T10
(E) may be blocked to relieve intractable angina pain

266. Cerebrospinal fluid (CSF)

(A) is formed in the choroid plexus by a passive process
(B) functions as a cushion for the brain
(C) is produced at a rate of about 100-200 mL/h

(D)   production is affected to the least extent by enflurane of all of the volatile agents

(E)   normally contains protein at about one-tenth the plasma concentration

267.   Neurotransmitters in the central nervous system that exert an inhibitory action on post-synaptic neurons include

(A)   dopamine, glycine, serotonin, γ-aminobutyric acid (GABA)

(B)   acetylcholine, dopamine, histamine

(C)   dopamine, epinephrine, glutamate

(D)   acetylcholine, γ-aminobutyric acid (GABA), glutamate

(E)   dopamine, serotonin, epinephrine, histamine

268.   Low cerebral blood flow (CBF) may disrupt adequate brain perfusion, and one of the main determinants of CBF is the cerebral metabolic rate for oxygen ($CMRO_2$). Which one of the following statements regarding $CMRO_2$ and CBF is TRUE?

(A)   In adults, the normal rate of neuronal oxygen utilization is 30-40 mL/100 g/min.

(B)   Blood flow in the brain is independent of $CMRO_2$.

(C) $CMRO_2$ reflects the amount of oxygen utilization in neurons to produce ATP.

(D)   Oxygen utilization is higher in the white matter as compared to the gray matter.

(E)   Blood flow in the brain is coupled to $CMRO_2$ in a ratio of 5:1.

269.   A typical neuron has

(A)   numerous branching dendrites

(B)   three or four axons to conduct impulses

(C)   no nucleus in the cell body

(D)   a dendritic zone devoid of receptors

(E)   a myelin sheath that covers the entire cell

270.   Propofol

(A)   has little effect on SSEP or MEP

(B)   can decrease $CMRO_2$, CBF, and ICP

(C)   does not cross the blood brain barrier

(D)   increases the frequency of EEG

(E)   has little effect on seizure activity

271.   All of the following are true concerning hyperthermia EXCEPT that it

(A)   increases ICP

(B)   increases cerebral metabolic demand

(C)   worsens outcome from cerebral ischemia

(D)   decreases cerebral blood flow

(E)   increases cardiac output

272.   A typical reflex arc includes all of the following EXCEPT a

(A)   sense organ

(B)   afferent neuron

(C)   efferent neuron

(D)   synapse on a peripheral effector

(E)   ascending axon within the ventral column

273.   The electroencephalogram (EEG)

(A)   alone is sufficient for the diagnosis of brain death, because a flat line is synonymous with death

(B)   shows decreased cortical activity with hypercapnia

(C)   is unaffected by hysterical seizures

(D)   is unaffected by hypothermia

(E)   is not useful in the diagnosis of a convulsive disorder

274.   A 15-year-old girl is undergoing surgery to correct scoliosis. Intraoperative monitoring includes motor evoked potentials. These potentials

(A)   test integrity of the descending corticospinal tracts

(B)   are unaffected by muscle relaxants

(C)   cannot be performed under anesthesia with a volatile agent

(D)   are increased during hypothermia

(E)   are produced by electrical stimulation within the cerebellum

275. When the cranium is open, the ICP is

(A) increased by volatile anesthetic agents

(B) reduced by hyperventilation

(C) dependent upon the position of the head relative to the heart

(D) equal to ambient pressure

(E) cannot be measured by a ventricular catheter

276. The act of vomiting is an integrated activity that includes

(A) activation of the vomiting center in the cerebral cortex

(B) opening of the glottis

(C) closing of the esophageal and gastric cardiac sphincters

(D) activity mediated by cranial nerves VIII and XI

(E) activation of the chemoreceptor trigger zone in the area postrema

277. The compressed spectral array (CSA) recording of the electroencephalogram (EEG)

(A) is more accurate than a standard EEG tracing

(B) presents data in a format of amplitude, time, and frequency

(C) is more accurate for determination of sudden events

(D) requires no training for interpretation

(E) should be in use for all neurosurgical procedures

278. Which one of the following is NOT involved in sensory transmission?

(A) dorsal root ganglion

(B) spinothalamic tract

(C) parietal cortex

(D) ventral posterior and ventral lateral nuclei of the thalamus

(E) precentral gyrus

279. In the adult, the spinal cord ends

(A) at the lower border of the second sacral vertebra

(B) at the lower border of the first lumbar vertebra

(C) at a segment in the lower lumbar region depending upon the patient's height

(D) midway between the 3rd and 4th lumbar vertebra

(E) at the lumbosacral junction

280. The normal brain

(A) has a constant metabolic rate

(B) maintains nearly constant blood flow between mean arterial blood pressures of 80 to 120 mm Hg

(C) requires only glucose and oxygen to maintain function

(D) couples regional blood flow to metabolic demand

(E) requires fructose for energy

281. The blood–brain barrier

(A) permits free passage of bicarbonate ion

(B) does not include the brainstem

(C) is impermeable to carbon dioxide

(D) is permeable to mannitol

(E) is composed of tight junctions in the vascular endothelium

282. Hyperventilation may lead to

(A) cerebral vasodilatation

(B) reduced Pa_{CO_2} in CSF

(C) shift of the oxyhemoglobin dissociation curve to the right

(D) increased cardiac output

(E) metabolic alkalosis

283. In administration of anesthesia to a patient with Arnold–Chiari malformation, all of the following considerations are important EXCEPT

(A) coughing on the endotracheal tube should be prevented

(B) a moderate increase in mean arterial pressure may lead to subarachnoid hemorrhage

(C) postoperative respiratory depression may be encountered

(D) a coexistent syrix in the spinal cord is common

(E) extreme flexion-extension of the neck should be avoided

284. In the patient with amyotrophic lateral sclerosis, the anesthetic plan should include

(A) succinylcholine but not non-depolarizing muscle relaxants

(B) non-depolarizing muscle relaxants but not succinylcholine

(C) awareness of the patient's respiratory limitation

(D) avoidance of respiratory depressants

(E) avoidance of isoflurane

285. Loss of cerebral autoregulation

(A) will cause the cerebral blood pressure to fall with systemic hypertension

(B) affects the entire brain at the same time

(C) may be focal

(D) only affects the lower end of the blood pressure range

(E) has no clinical significance

286. A 15-year-old girl with a history of myotonic dystrophy is scheduled for tonsillectomy and adenoidectomy under general anesthesia. Considerations regarding her anesthesia management include

(A) postoperative hyperthermia may precipitate a myotonic response

(B) myotonia can be relieved by nondepolarizing relaxants

(C) mechanical ventilation is contraindicated

(D) myotonia can be precipitated by succinylcholine

(E) neostigmine prevents myotonia

287. A 26-year-old man is scheduled to undergo elective resection of an arteriovenous malformation. In planning the anesthesia, the anesthesiologist should be prepared to manage

(A) blood pressure during induction within a very narrow range

(B) malignant brain swelling

(C) barbiturate-induced coma to decrease oxygen demand prior to resection

(D) vasospasm during surgery treated with deliberate hypertension

(E) elevated ICP treated with the head-up position

288. Brain tumors affect intracranial pressure by all of the following processes EXCEPT

(A) increasing intracranial tissue content

(B) increasing cerebral metabolic rate

(C) altering cerebral blood volume

(D) obstructing CSF flow

(E) increasing interstitial fluid volume

289. Which is the most profound chemical stimulus for regulation of cerebral blood flow?

(A) metabolic alkalosis

(B) hypothermia

(C) hyperthermia

(D) carbon dioxide

(E) hypercalcemia

Answers and Explanations

236. **(E)** Oxygen concentration does not influence body temperature. Exposure to low ambient temperature may cause hypothermia. This is a problem especially in small children because of their large body surface to mass ratio. Cold intravenous fluids and dry inspired gases are sources of heat loss and cause a fall in body temperature. Muscle relaxants prevent shivering, a principal means by which the body maintains a normal temperature. *(1:528; 5:1507-9; 6:165-6)*

237. **(D)** Under normal conditions, intracranial arterial blood volume is about 7 to 8 mL and constitutes about 15% of the 50 mL of total intracranial blood volume. Conceptually, brain tissue can be divided into solid material (about 168 g or 12% of intracranial contents) and tissue water (about 1092 g or 78% of intracranial contents). Intracranial CSF volume is about 75 mL. Although occupying the smallest volume within the cranium, cerebral blood volume is altered rapidly by physiological and pharmacological intervention. *(5:871-3; 6:2254)*

238. **(C)** Preganglionic neurons are located in the thoracic and lumbar spinal cord (T1 through L3) and synapse upon postganglionic nerves either in paravertebral sympathetic ganglia or in plexi adjacent to organs of innervation. Except for sweat glands that are cholinergic, target organ receptors are adrenergic. β-adrenergic receptors mediate their effects through cyclic AMP; α-adrenergic receptors act via a more complex second messenger system involving G proteins. All preganglionic neurons are cholinergic. *(1:171-4; 5:1574; 6:3351)*

239. **(C)** Ketamine causes increases in intracranial pressure, cerebral metabolism, and cerebral blood flow. It is relatively contraindicated in patients with an intracranial mass or increased intracranial pressure. The other induction agents will decrease intracranial pressure. *(1:538-9; 5:699-700)*

240. **(A)** On the flat part of the compliance curve, there is a small rise in pressure for increases in volume. In this area of the curve, there is good compensation. As one moves to the right, there is a sudden increase in pressure with small changes in volume. *(5:873, 880; 6:2256-7)*

241. **(C)** ICP is measured typically with a ventriculostomy catheter positioned in the lateral ventricle or from a fiberotic intraparenchymal ICP monitor. ICP only can be determined accurately within the cranium; measurements from the spine may not accurately reflect intracranial events. Pressure determined within vascular structures will not reflect ICP. *(5:875, 880; 6:2255)*

242. **(E)** Although this patient is approaching the steep portion of the intracranial compliance curve, they may not manifest signs of increased ICP. Unilateral mydriasis often occurs with brain distortion from extremely high ICP or herniation. Hyperventilation reduces intracranial blood volume and pressure by vasoconstriction of cerebral arteries. Isoflurane, in contrast, increases cerebral blood flow by causing cerebral vasodilation and raises ICP. Hypertonic saline reduces ICP by reducing brain water content. *(5: 537-8, 880; 6:2255-7)*

243. (B) This patient is on the steep portion of the intracranial compliance curve. Since compensatory mechanisms have been exhausted, small increases in the volume of intracranial contents (such as an increase in blood volume due to coughing) will produce large increases in intracranial pressure. Reduction in brain volume by decreasing brain water content will move the patient toward position A. The Cushing's response to elevated ICP is hypertension, and sometimes bradycardia. *(5:880, 893; 6:1868, 2256-7)*

244. (D) The ventilatory control centers, located in the pons and medulla, integrates information from peripheral mechanical receptors and peripheral and central chemosensors. The apneustic center contains both inspiratory and expiratory neurons. Peripheral oxygen sensors are located in the carotid body (not the airway). Receptors for hydrogen ion are centrally located; when the hydrogen ion concentration increases, ventilation is stimulated. *(5:528-9; 6:277, 288)*

245. (B) The absorption of CSF takes place through the arachnoid villi. The ependymal cells and the pia mater are not involved. The foramina of Monro and Magendie are conduits for CSF flow. *(5:871-3)*

246. (E) A very small postganglionic fiber with slow conduction is the C fiber. *(5:1520; 6:93, 3352)*

247. (B) The cerebellum is not monitored by sensory-evoked potentials. The dorsal columns of the spinal cord transmit proprioception and are assessed by somatosensory-evoked potentials. The vestibular-cochlear nerve (cranial nerve VIII) and the inferior colliculus are assessed by brainstem auditory-evoked potentials. Peaks corresponding to thalamic nuclei are detected with both. *(5:484-6)*

248. (D) Parkinson disease is due to loss of dopaminergic cells in the basal ganglia of the brain. A non-intention tremor may be a symptom. *(5:149; 6:3317)*

249. (D) The thalamus is located at the base of the brain and contains many distinct nuclear groups. Sensory information is processed here before conduction to the cortex. Distinct peaks corresponding to the thalamus are found in somatosensory and brain stem auditory-evoked potentials. *(5:484-8; 6:187)*

250. (B) The trigeminal nerve contains somatic afferent fibers from the face and supplies motor innervation to the muscle of mastication. The oculomotor nerve contains parasympathetic efferents that control pupillary constriction; the facial nerve contains parasympathetic fibers supplying the submandibular gland; the glossopharyngeal nerve supplies the parotid gland; and the vagus nerve supplies the heart, respiratory system, and gut. *(5:1208; 6:224, 243, 3352)*

251. (A) Alpha activity has a frequency range of 8 to 13 Hz. Beta activity has a frequency of greater than 13 Hz. Theta rhythm has an activity of 4 to 7 Hz. Delta rhythm has an activity of less than 4 Hz. There are no gamma waves in the EEG. *(5:475-7)*

252. (D) In humans undergoing carotid endarterectomy, volatile anesthetics have been shown to alter the cortical blood flow level at which EEG evidence of ischemia first develops; halothane had the least effect, isoflurane reduced the threshold most, and enflurane was intermediate between the two. Although neuronal function deteriorates progressively with decreasing blood flow, not until CBF is less than half the normal level (22 mL/100 g/min) does EEG evidence of ischemia manifest. The EEG is isoelectric at 15 mL/100 g/min, but irreversible damage does not occur until flow falls below 6 mL/100 g/min. *(5:478-9, 1019; 6:2255)*

253. (A) The substantia gelatinosa has the highest concentration of opioid receptors in the spinal cord. This area is in the dorsal horn of the spinal cord. *(5:798, 1306-8, 1520-1, 1603-4)*

254. (D) The oculocardiac reflex is chacterized by bradycardia (even to the point of asystole) produced by pressure or traction on the eye.

The afferent limb of the reflex is composed of fibers from the ophthalmic division of the trigeminal nerve that synapse upon brain stem neurons and ultimately increase vagal efferent activity. Activation of the reflex can occur from manipulation of any of the structures that carry afferent impulses, including the trigeminal ganglion and the long ciliary nerves that innervate the globe. The oculomotor nerve is not involved in the reflex. *(5:866, 1220; 6:3351-2)*

255. **(C)** Antidiuretic hormone (ADH) and oxytocin are secreted by the posterior pituitary. Growth hormone, leutenizing hormone, follicle-stimulating hormone, thyrotropin, prolactin, and adrenocorticotropin are all secreted by the anterior pituitary. *(5:1127-31; 6:2876-7)*

256. **(A)** The Glasgow Coma Score is based on the ability to open the eyes and verbal and motor responses. Responses to knee jerk, pupil size, respiration, and EEG are assessed as part of a general neurologic examination but are not part of the Glasgow Coma Score. *(5:1328, 1355; 6:3381)*

257. **(D)** Cerebral blood flow increases 1 to 2 mL/ 100 g/min with each 1 mm Hg rise in Pa_{CO_2} in the normal physiologic range of Pa_{CO_2}. For this reason it is important to have good airway control at all times when dealing with patients with increased intracranial pressure. *(5:874; 6:2255-6)*

258. **(D)** The oxygen reserves are very low. The reserves are not changed under anesthesia, but oxygen use is decreased. Since oxygen reserves are so low, the brain is subject to hypoxia with any bout of ischemia. *(5:1464-6; 6:2257)*

259. **(C)** Cerebral perfusion pressure is the fundamental concept underlying the autoregulation curve. It represents the blood pressure available for global perfusion of the brain. Because the brain is enclosed in the cranium, which functions as a noncompliant container, CPP is defined as the pressure of the blood entering the cranium (MAP) minus the pressure exerted within the cranium (ICP). This assumes that central venous pressure is less than intracranial pressure, as is the case when the head is elevated and there is no resistance to venous outflow from the cranium. *(5:871; 6:2255)*

260. **(D)** The phrenic nerve arises from cervical segments C3–C5 and supplies motor innervation to the diaphragm. The intercostal muscles receive motor innervation from nerves originating in the thoracic cord. Although disruption of the cervical cord between C6 and C7 would compromise ventilation, some diaphragmatic function would remain intact. Sympathetic supply to the heart is from the sympathetic ganglia that receive afferents from the thoracic cord below the injury; parasympathetic innervation is from the vagus and is unaffected by the injury. In the absence of hypoxia, no disturbance in heart rate is expected. Cranial nerves IX and X supply motor and sensation to the pharynx and glottis. *(5:828; 6:2182-5)*

261. **(B)** Autonomic hyperreflexia occurs with spinal lesions above T5. Any noxious stimulation (e.g., urinary catheter insertion or bladder distention) may lead to hypertension accompanied by sweating and bradycardia. Anxiety or pain would produce hypertension and tachycardia. *(5:1138-9; 6:3356)*

262. **(E)** Disruption of noxious afferent signals emanating from the bladder to the intact lower spinal cord can prevent the autonomic hyperreflexic response. This can be accomplished with deep general anesthesia or regional anesthesia. *(5:1138-9; 6:3356)*

263. **(C)** After subarachnoid hemorrhage, rhythm disturbances and ischemic ECG changes are common. Spasm of the cerebral arteries can result in decreased cerebral blood flow with resulting cerebral ischemia. Hyponatremia can occur from SIADH (syndrome of inappropriate secretion of antidiuretic hormone). The mass effect of hematoma in the subarachnoid space as well as obstruction of CSF egress commonly leads to hydrocephalous. *(5:85-7; 6:2261-5)*

264. **(A)** The left and right vertebral arteries merge to form the basilar artery. *(5:870)*

265. (C) The celiac plexus is a major abdominal plexus composed of a number of ganglia and innervates most of the abdominal contents. Sympathetic nerve fibers are derived from T5 through T12 and convey only visceral afferent and efferent information with no somatic inputs. *(5:1134, 1574; 6:3352)*

266. (B) The majority of CSF is formed in the choroid plexus by filtration and by active transport, the latter responsible for about two-thirds of the total amount. The active transport process requires energy. Transependymal diffusion from the brain interstitium also contributes to total volume. Continuous production at a rate of 30-40 mL/h results in a complete turnover three times daily. The brain and spinal cord essentially float in this fluid. Enflurane acts to increase production and decrease absorption. The normal protein concentration in CSF is about one-hundredth the plasma concentration. *(5:873; 6:3435, 3600)*

267. (A) The major inhibitory transmitter in the central nervous system is GABA, but other transmitters may have inhibitory effects as well. Acetylcholine, glutamate, histamine, and epinephrine are excitatory. *(5:323, 474-5, 585-7; 6:3523)*

268. (C) In adults, the normal rate of neuronal oxygen utilization is 3.0 to 3.8 mL/100 g/min that is coupled to blood flow of 50 mL/100 g/min, resulting in a ratio of 15:1. This coupling of $CMRO_2$ to CBF causes an increase in CBF during neuronal activity. Oxygen utilization is higher in the gray matter as compared to the white matter. *(5:873-4)*

269. (A) The typical neuron has numerous dendrites that branch out and a dendritic zone that is rich in receptors. The neuron has a single cell body with an active nucleus and only one axon. The myelin sheath covers the axon only in myelinated neurons. *(5:474-5, 1518-21; 6:95)*

270. (B) Propofol decreases the frequency of EEG and diminishes both the SSEP and MEP. It decreases cerebral metabolism, blood flow, and ICP. It is an effective anticonvulsant. *(5:875-6)*

271. (D) The consequences of hyperthermia include increased cerebral blood flow and ICP. Metabolic demand is increased and cerebral ischemia has been shown to have a worse outcome during hyperthermia. Cardiac output is increased to meet metabolic demand. *(5:1469-71; 6:143-5)*

272. (E) A reflex arc includes a sense organ, an afferent neuron and efferent neuron that form a synapse on a peripheral effector such as a muscle. Reflexes can be mediated by descending inputs from higher centers within the CNS. The ventral column contains descending fibers of the corticospinal tract. *(1:261, 265, 5:489-90)*

273. (C) The EEG is not sufficient for the diagnosis of brain death. Brain death requires a careful history and patient assessment. Patients who are hypothermic or deeply anesthetized with barbiturates, volatile agents, or propofol may display a flat EEG. Cortical activity increases with hypercapnia. Hysterical seizures do not produce a seizure spike pattern on EEG. *(6:2252-3)*

274. (A) Motor evoked potentials are produced by direct transcranial electrical stimulation of the motor cortex; action potentials in contracting muscles are measured peripherally. They test integrity of the ventral spinal cord that contains the corticospinal tracts. MEPs are depressed by hypothermia, muscle relaxants, and high concentrations of volatile anesthetics. *(5:484-8)*

275. (D) ICP is produced within a closed cranium. Opening of the cranium at surgery relieves intracranial pressure and ICP equals ambient pressure or zero. While positioning of the head and anesthetic agents impact upon brain relaxation, they do not alter ICP. *(5:880)*

276. (E) The act of vomiting requires the activation of the vomiting center located in the reticular formation of the lower medulla near the area postrema. It requires the opening of the esophageal and gastric cardiac sphincters. The process is mediated by cranial nerves IX and X.

It may be initiated by stimulation of the chemoreceptor trigger zone. *(5:711; 6:301)*

277. **(B)** The compressed spectral array presents data from the EEG in a format of amplitude, time, and frequency. Although this format is more convenient, some specificity and accuracy are lost. The CSA is not as accurate for sudden events. In spite of its convenience, a certain amount of training and familiarity are needed to interpret the tracing accurately. CSA is not necessary for every anesthetic. *(5:1019)*

278. **(E)** The precentral gyrus is primarily involved with motor functions. Sensation involves the dorsal root ganglion cell, the lateral spinothalamic tract, the thalamic nuclei, and the postcentral gyrus. *(5:1520-21; 6:187-8)*

279. **(B)** The spinal cord ends at the lower border of the first lumbar vertebra in the adult. The subarachnoid space continues further caudally and ends at S2. Although in children the cord ends in the lower lumbar region and moves rostral as the child reaches adulthood, the position of the end of the cord is not dependent upon patient height. *(5:786)*

280. **(D)** In the normal brain, metabolic rate and blood flow are relatively constant. The autoregulatory range in which constant blood flow is maintained occurs between a mean arterial blood pressure of approximately 50 to 150 mm Hg. Fructose is not a required energy source of the brain. While the brain requires only glucose and oxygen to maintain energy supply, this is insufficient to maintain the structural and functional integrity. *(5:871-4; 6:2255-7)*

281. **(E)** The blood-brain barrier is present in all regions of the brain and spinal cord and is formed by tight junctions between vascular endothelial cells and foot processes of the glia. Carbon dioxide freely crosses the blood-brain barrier; bicarbonate is charged and crosses the blood-brain barrier more slowly. Mannitol is excluded from normal brain. *(5:538, 874-5, 880; 6:2254-6)*

282. **(B)** Hyperventilation reduces the Pa_{CO_2} in CSF. It decreases cardiac output and constricts cerebral vasculature. The oxyhemoglobin curve is shifted to the left. The reduction in Pa_{CO_2} produces respiratory alkalosis; prolonged hyperventilation produces loss of bicarbonate ion and metabolic acidosis. *(5:528-9)*

283. **(B)** The Arnold–Chiari malformation is characterized by brain stem compression from herniation of the cerebellar tonsils through the foramen magnum and caudal displacement of the brain stem. Hydrocephalus is common from obliteration of the foramina of Lushka and Magendie that drain the fourth ventricle. Increases in intracranial pressure may be encountered. Extreme flexion-extension of the neck may increase brain stem compression. Postoperative respiratory and hemodynamic patterns should be monitored closely because of possible brain stem compression. The syndrome is commonly associated with syrinx. *(5:251, 1180, 1193; 6:127)*

284. **(C)** The patient with amyotrophic lateral sclerosis is chronically weak and has muscle wasting from loss of descending input in the spinal cord. Succinylcholine should be avoided. Nondepolarizing muscle relaxants may have profound impact; if required, they should be used in low doses. If the patient has any respiratory compromise postoperatively, mechanical ventilation is indicated. Although these patients may exhibit exaggerated changes in hemodynamics in response to inhalational anesthetics, there is no specific recommendation to avoid these agents. *(5:139, 500-1; 6:3345-7)*

285. **(C)** Loss of cerebral autoregulation will cause cerebral blood flow to vary directly with blood pressure. This may be focal and only affect part of the brain. Loss of autoregulation has great clinical significance with respect to blood pressure and cerebral ischemia. *(5:873-4; 6:2255)*

286. **(D)** The patient with myotonic dystrophy presents an anesthetic problem with regard to muscle relaxation. While succinylcholine may cause myotonia, myotonic episodes are not necessarily reversed by nondepolarizing

muscle relaxants. Furthermore, neostigmine may aggravate myotonia. Postoperative shivering in the recovery room may induce myotonia. At the end of the procedure, mechanical ventilation is preferable to reversal of muscle relaxants. *(5:144-5; 6:3487-9)*

287. **(B)** Arteriovenous malformations are high-flow, low-pressure lesions, and hypertension-induced hemorrhage is rare, if not nonexistent. Vasospasm is also rare. Intraoperative hemorrhage can be severe if rupture occurs. In addition, reperfusion breakthrough (development of severe brain swelling as a result of the sudden alteration in blood flow and perfusion pressure in the brain parenchyma surrounding the malformation) during resection can result in severe intraoperative problems. Treatment may include induced hypotension and high-dose barbiturates. *(5:887-8; 6:3298)*

288. **(B)** Because intracranial contents are not compressible, any increase in the mass of intracranial material will result in a rise in intracranial pressure unless the volume of another compartment decreases. Edema in tissue surrounding the tumor increases interstitial fluid volume and contributes to the rise in ICP. Cerebral blood volume may be either increased or decreased by tumor growth. Hydrocephalus can result from tumor obstruction of CSF outflow from the brain. *(5:80-3; 6:2254-7)*

289. **(D)** The most profound chemical stimulus affecting cerebral blood flow is carbon dioxide. Changes in electrolytes and acid-base balance may have an effect, but the predominant effect is from Pa_{CO_2}. Hypothermia decreases cerebral blood flow by decreasing cerebral metabolic rate. *(5:873-4; 6:2255-7)*

CHAPTER 6

Renal, Hepatic, Endocrine, Hematologic, and Metabolic Systems
Questions

DIRECTIONS (Questions 290-365): Each of the numbered items or incomplete statements in this section is followed by answers or by completions of the statement. Select the ONE lettered answer or completion that is BEST in each case.

290. A 50-year-old patient underwent a thyroidectomy that finished at 1000, and at 2200 he complained to the nurse of difficulty in breathing. She took his blood pressure that was moderately elevated above previous determinations, but she also noticed that his wrist flexed when the blood pressure cuff remained inflated. The cause of the stridor is probably

    (A) vocal cord paralysis
    (B) partial vocal cord paralysis
    (C) laryngeal edema
    (D) cervical hematoma
    (E) hypocalcemia

291. A 62-year-old man with chronic renal failure who is receiving dialysis three times weekly suffers a fracture of the humerus in a fall. He is brought to the operating room for an open reduction of the fracture on the evening of a day on which he missed his dialysis due to the injury. Expected abnormalities in this patient include all of the following EXCEPT

    (A) metabolic acidosis
    (B) hyperkalemia
    (C) uremia
    (D) thrombocytopenia
    (E) hypervolemia

292. A previously healthy 25-year-old man suffers a ruptured spleen during a rugby game. During the emergency splenectomy, he is given ten units of packed red blood cells. After achieving hemostasis, an acceptable hematocrit value of 27%, and euvolemia via the administration of normal saline, the most likely electrolyte abnormality is

    (A) hypercalcemia
    (B) hypermagnesemia
    (C) hypophosphatemia
    (D) hypokalemia
    (E) hyperkalemia

293. A 50-year-old alcoholic man with a long history of tobacco abuse and who is chronically dyspneic at rest is in the recovery room after an emergency appendectomy. He is receiving supplemental oxygen by mask and appears to be hypoventilating. An arterial blood gas is obtained that shows pH = 7.19, P_{O_2} = 85 mm Hg, and P_{CO_2} = 90 mm Hg. This state can best be described as

    (A) pure respiratory acidosis
    (B) combined respiratory acidosis and metabolic acidosis
    (C) respiratory acidosis with compensating metabolic alkalosis
    (D) metabolic acidosis with compensating respiratory alkalosis
    (E) pure metabolic acidosis

294. A hypotensive, comatose 47-year-old man is brought to the operating room after being struck by a bus. He is emaciated and has a long history of alcoholism. It is important to administer thiamine to this patient because thiamine deficiency may

(A) be the cause of the observed coma
(B) be the cause of the observed hypotension
(C) be precipitated by the administration of glucose-containing solutions
(D) cause rhabdomyolysis if succinylcholine is given
(E) potentiate the cardiovascular depressant effects of volatile anesthetics

295. A 59-year-old woman requires treatment for non-Hodgkin's lymphoma. Antineoplastic chemotherapy with which one of the following agents may cause a peripheral neuropathy?

(A) methotrexate
(B) doxorubicin
(C) busulfan
(D) bleomycin
(E) vincristine

296. A 20-year-old college student is found dead in his dormitory room after consuming a large amount of alcohol. When a lethal amount of ethanol is ingested, the toxic effect of ethanol usually leading to death is

(A) hypotension due to vasodilation
(B) hypotension due to decreased cardiac output
(C) seizure
(D) apnea
(E) ventricular arrhythmia

297. A 73-year-old patient is undergoing implantation of a hip prosthesis under general anesthesia. She has been taking prednisone for rheumatoid arthritis for 6 months. During the procedure, there is a sudden drop in blood pressure. The first step to be taken is to

(A) administer hydrocortisone 100 mg intravenously
(B) establish the cause of the hypotension

(C) cancel the procedure
(D) begin an infusion of phenylephrine
(E) discontinue all anesthetic agents

298. A 72-year-old man with esophageal carcinoma has been receiving total parenteral nutrition with a solution containing 20% glucose and 4% amino acids for several weeks prior to surgery through a central venous catheter in the left subclavian vein. The patient is undergoing a left thoracotomy for resection, and during the procedure the medical student holding the rib retractor accidentally removes the subclavian catheter. Regarding the infusion of total parenteral nutrition, the most appropriate maneuver to perform during the surgical procedure would be to

(A) do nothing
(B) position the patient supine, insert a right subclavian catheter, and restart the infusion of parenteral nutrition
(C) restart the parenteral nutrition solution via a peripheral intravenous catheter
(D) administer 5 units of regular insulin intravenously and measure the serum glucose concentration in 15 min
(E) begin an infusion of 10% glucose via a peripheral vein

299. A 36-year-old nurse in good health is stuck with a used needle during the unsuccessful resuscitation of a homeless man with an unknown medical history. She is at potential risk of all of these diseases from exposure to a needle contaminated with blood or tissue from an infected patient EXCEPT

(A) Creutzfeldt–Jakob disease
(B) hepatitis A
(C) hepatitis C
(D) cytomegalovirus
(E) syphilis

300. A 29-year-old anesthesia resident is found dead of an overdose in his call room one morning. The following statements are true concerning substance abuse among anesthesiologists EXCEPT

(A) alcohol and fentanyl are the drugs most likely to be abused

(B) a proper drug accountability system will prevent misuse

(C) an individual confrontation with the drug user is not recommended

(D) the relapse rate of anesthesiology residents allowed to reenter a program is about 66%

(E) it is the policy of the ASA to treat substance abuse disorders as a disease

301. A 37 year-old-woman with a history of scleroderma is brought to the hospital after a motor vehicle accident and requires an emergency laparotomy for management of intraabdominal bleeding. Problems that may be encountered in scleroderma include all of the following EXCEPT

(A) limited mouth opening

(B) arterial dilatation

(C) pulmonary fibrosis

(D) contractures

(E) pericardial effusion

302. A 2-year-old child with Hurler syndrome (gargoylism), a disturbance of mucopolysaccharide metabolism, needs anesthesia for an umbilical hernia repair. Anesthesia for such patients is complicated by all of the following EXCEPT

(A) dwarfism

(B) macroglossia

(C) hypertelorism

(D) hepatosplenomegaly

(E) short neck

303. An 80-year-old patient has a normal value of 1.0 mg/dL for serum creatinine. Compared with a 20-year-old patient of the same weight and with the same serum creatinine value, the 80-year-old patient has approximately what fractional value of creatinine clearance?

(A) 0.1

(B) 0.2

(C) 0.5

(D) 0.7

(E) 0.9

304. A 40-year-old alcoholic man with a massive gastrointestinal bleed is treated with a variety of blood components. The blood component with the least risk of transmitting hepatitis C is

(A) cryoprecipitate

(B) fresh frozen plasma

(C) packed red blood cells

(D) frozen washed red blood cells

(E) 5% albumin

305. A 64-year-old man with a history of stable exertional angina for 3 years presents for preoperative evaluation before an elective hip replacement for severe degenerative arthritis. In terms of his preoperative medications or his need for additional evaluations prior to surgery, he

(A) needs a cardiac catheterization

(B) needs a dobutamine stress echocardiogram

(C) needs a myocardial perfusion scan

(D) should be taking a beta-blocker unless there is a specific contraindication

(E) should discontinue his statin preoperatively

306. You are the anesthesiologist assigned to the preoperative testing area for the day. All of the following statements regarding stopping or continuing medications are true EXCEPT

(A) patients with coronary artery disease should ideally never stop aspirin because of a rebound phenomenon resulting in an increased risk of perioperative cardiac complications; risk of bleeding versus thrombosis need to be assessed

(B) statins should be continued and may even exert a protective effect in patients undergoing vascular surgery

(C) metformin should be stopped 2 weeks preoperatively because of the risk of metabolic acidosis

(D) it is advisable to stop furosemide a day before surgery because of an increased risk of hypovolemia

(E) birth control pills should be continued on the day of surgery

307. A 79-year-old man with coronary artery disease develops acute kidney injury after a carotid endarterectomy. The circulation to the kidney is

(A) autoregulated over a mean arterial pressure range of about 80 to 160 mm Hg

(B) not regulated by neural factors

(C) innervated by sympathetic nerves originating in T2-T3

(D) not affected by epinephrine

(E) constricted by prostaglandin E_2

308. A 33-year-old woman takes clarithromycin chronically for sinusitis. After falling on ice, she suffers a complex fracture of her ankle. In the emergency department, her ankle is too swollen to permit immediate operative repair so it is casted and she is scheduled for surgery in a week. She is given a fentanyl patch, 25 mcg/h, for pain. The following morning, she is found dead in bed. The most likely mechanism for her death is

(A) excessive fentanyl effect due to excessive dose

(B) excessive fentanyl effect due to impaired metabolism

(C) myocardial infarction

(D) pulmonary embolus of clot originating in injured leg

(E) bone marrow embolus

309. A morbidly obese 42-year-old woman is scheduled for bariatric surgery. Which one of the following statements is true about the perioperative management of a morbidly obese patient?

(A) Obese patients have different fasting guidelines compared to non-obese patients.

(B) Neck circumference is the single best predictor of problematic intubations in obese patients.

(C) Postoperative continuous positive airway pressure increases the incidence of major anastomotic leakage after gastric bypass surgery.

(D) Patients with obesity-hypoventilation syndrome have a decreased sensitivity to the respiratory depressant effects of general anesthetics.

(E) Succinylcholine should be dosed based on lean body weight in obese patients.

310. A 59-year-old man with moderate chronic obstructive pulmonary disease (COPD) is scheduled for a nephrectomy for renal cell carcinoma. All of the following statements about patients with chronic pulmonary disease are correct EXCEPT

(A) a patient with severe but stable COPD should routinely have preoperative pulmonary function tests before major abdominal or pelvic surgery

(B) to prevent intraoperative bronchospasm in patients with asthma, pretreatment with a β_2-adrenoceptor agonist and/or an anticholinergic agent is indicated

(C) in patients with severe asthma, propofol and ketamine are the induction agents of choice

(D) ketamine has little effect on ventilatory drive in patients with COPD

(E) in patients with COPD, longer-acting neuromuscular blockade is associated with a greater risk of postoperative pulmonary complications than use of shorter acting neuromuscular blockers

311. The liver affects glucose metabolism by all of the following mechanisms EXCEPT

(A) glycogen storage

(B) gluconeogenesis

(C) glycogenolysis

(D) insulin production

(E) conversion of galactose to glucose

312. A 55-year-old woman with recurrent nephrolithiasis is treated with extracorporeal shock wave lithotripsy. The shock wave during extracorporeal shock wave lithotripsy is timed to coincide with a particular point in the ECG, and occurs

(A) at the peak of the P-wave.

(B) 100 msec after the peak of the P wave

(C)   20 msec after the peak of the R wave

(D)   200 msec after the peak of the R wave

(E)   at the peak of the T wave

313.   A 60-year-old man with a history of well-controlled type 2 diabetes and a myocardial infarction 7 years ago with no recent cardiac symptoms presents for preoperative evaluation prior to prostatectomy. All of the following statements about perioperative cardiac risk assessment are true EXCEPT

(A)   most ischemic events occur postoperatively rather than intraoperatively

(B)   in terms of cardiac risk stratification for noncardiac surgery, intrathoracic and intraperitoneal surgeries are deemed intermediate risk

(C)   according to the American College of Cardiology/American Heart Association (ACC/AHA) guidelines, patients with asymptomatic type 2 diabetes have the same risk of perioperative cardiac complications (PCC) as a patient with a previous MI

(D)   cardiomegaly by itself is not a risk factor for PCC

(E)   renal insufficiency is one of the five perioperative risk factors in the ACC/AHA guidelines

314.   A 40-year-old alcoholic man is found to have massive ascites. Ascites

(A)   follows chronic decreased portal vein pressure

(B)   follows periods of hyperalbuminemia

(C)   is usually accompanied by hypernatremia

(D)   may have an adverse cardiopulmonary effect

(E)   should be removed rapidly to avoid reaccumulation

315.   An elderly woman is brought into the hospital after being found on the floor of her apartment. She is found to have prerenal failure and her urine will

(A)   be positive for nitrites

(B)   be concentrated

(C)   have a specific gravity of approximately 1.010

(D)   be excreted in large amounts

(E)   have a reddish tinge due to presence of red blood cells

DIRECTIONS: use the following scenario to answer Questions 316-317: A 46-year-old woman with myxedema is scheduled for emergency intraabdominal surgery.

316.   A finding consistent with the myxedematous state is

(A)   fine, soft hair

(B)   moist skin

(C)   bradycardia

(D)   heat intolerance

(E)   pitting edema of the eyelids

317.   Fluid and blood replacement in this patient

(A)   should be guided by blood pressure

(B)   should be guided by electrocardiographic voltage

(C)   does not differ from that in normal patients

(D)   should be guided by invasive arterial and central venous pressure monitoring

(E)   should be accompanied by rapid restoration of the euthyroid state

318.   A 75-year-old woman with aortic stenosis and depression treated with fluoxetine presents for aortic valve replacement surgery. All of the following statements about depression are correct EXCEPT

(A)   St. John's wort is an herbal remedy often taken by patients to treat depression

(B)   successful treatment of depression has been shown to correlate with a reduced risk of postoperative death

(C)   it is estimated that more than 75% of hospitalized elderly patients suffer from depression

(D)   depression may be a symptom of hypocalcemia

(E)   depression may be a symptom of Cushing syndrome

319. A 60-year-old woman presents with episodic hypertension to 180/105 associated with headache and profuse sweating. A diagnosis of pheochromocytoma is made. She

    (A) requires immediate surgery
    (B) should be treated for 10 to 14 days with an α-adrenoceptor antagonist
    (C) can be anesthetized regardless of the level of blood pressure readings
    (D) is usually hypervolemic
    (E) should have a Swan-Ganz catheter in place preoperatively

DIRECTIONS: use the following scenario to answer Questions 320-321: A 52-year-old woman with a one-year history of type 2 diabetes controlled on metformin is scheduled for a partial colectomy for recurrent diverticulitis.

320. The most important goal in the treatment of a middle-aged diabetic patient undergoing anesthesia is to

    (A) keep blood sugar in the normal range
    (B) prevent glycosuria
    (C) prevent hypoglycemia
    (D) prevent ketoacidosis
    (E) prevent acetonuria

321. Hypoglycemia in the awake patient

    (A) is identical to that in the anesthetized patient
    (B) is characterized by bradycardia
    (C) is characterized by hypertension
    (D) is due to ketoacidosis
    (E) is characterized by a marked parasympathetic response

322. You are called to see a patient on the medical service in need of a cholecystectomy for acute cholecystitis. The patient was admitted with abdominal pain and hyperosmolar coma. Hyperosmolar coma

    (A) usually occurs in young people
    (B) occurs at osmolar levels of 150 to 175 mOsm/L

    (C) occurs in the absence of ketonemia
    (D) is usually accompanied by oliguria
    (E) requires treatment with large doses of insulin

323. A 33-year-old woman with type 1 diabetes who uses an insulin pump presents for surgical drainage of a pilonidal abscess. She has been fasting since the night before surgery. All of the following statements regarding perioperative management of this patient are correct EXCEPT

    (A) in general, it is best to maintain the basal infusion rate of insulin
    (B) scheduled preprandial insulin boluses should be omitted
    (C) glucose levels should be monitored at frequent intervals
    (D) she should resume her usual diet and insulin therapy regimen as soon as possible postoperatively
    (E) uptake of insulin from the pump is not affected by alterations in tissue perfusion

324. A 26-year-old otherwise healthy female trauma patient is brought to the operating room with massive injuries and requires multiple units of blood to attempt to maintain euvolemia. Which one of the following statements about blood transfusions in her is correct?

    (A) Cross-matching is necessary for fresh frozen plasma (FFP).
    (B) Most platelet transfusions are given to treat dilutional thrombocytopenia after massive transfusion.
    (C) Human error is the root cause of most fatal hemolytic transfusion reactions.
    (D) A unit of packed red blood cells should increase the hemoglobin level by 3 g/dL.
    (E) FFP transfusion should be guided by the INR value.

325. A 47-year-old patient is to be operated on for a tumor of the small bowel. In the preoperative interview, a history of flushing, diarrhea, and joint pain is elicited. There are also symptoms compatible with congestive heart failure. A likely diagnosis is

   (A) Zollinger-Ellison syndrome
   (B) carcinoid syndrome
   (C) pheochromocytoma
   (D) Peutz-Jeghers syndrome
   (E) adrenal tumor with metastasis

326. A 59-year-old man with cirrhosis needs hip replacement surgery for severe osteoarthritis. Which one of the following statements regarding cirrhotic patients is correct?

   (A) The serum albumin level will be elevated.
   (B) Excessive sodium is lost in the urine.
   (C) Pancuronium is more effective.
   (D) Serum gamma globulin level will be low.
   (E) Less thiopental is required for induction.

327. The optimal anesthetic regimen for a 50-year-old patient with fulminant hepatic failure from hepatitis C undergoing liver transplantation

   (A) will avoid fentanyl
   (B) will avoid nondepolarizing relaxants
   (C) is a balanced technique
   (D) will avoid halogenated hydrocarbons
   (E) will depend on the cause of the liver failure and the patient's status

328. A 35-year-old woman with hyperparathyroidism undergoes a parathyroidectomy. Features of hypocalcemia relevant to the perioperative period include all of the following EXCEPT

   (A) hypocalcemia predisposes to laryngospasm
   (B) hypocalcemia can present as change in mental status
   (C) hypocalcemia can lead to difficult to treat hypertension in the postoperative setting

   (D) one gram of calcium chloride solution provides three times the amount of elemental calcium present in one gram of calcium gluconate
   (E) concentrated calcium solutions may be caustic to peripheral veins

329. A 43-year-old male patient who has had a transsphenoidal hypophysectomy for acromegaly several years ago presents for cholecystectomy. Which one of the following hormones should be given in the perioperative period?

   (A) ACTH
   (B) TSH
   (C) vasopressin
   (D) cortisol
   (E) insulin

330. A 39-year-old diabetic man is scheduled for a podiatric procedure. Which one of the following statements is TRUE regarding the effects of medications on blood sugar?

   (A) Propranolol potentiates the hyperglycemic response to stress.
   (B) Lisinopril increases insulin requirements in the diabetic.
   (C) Hydrochlorothiazide potentiates the hypoglycemia produced by glyburide.
   (D) Atenolol decreases insulin release from the pancreas.
   (E) Prednisone increases the blood glucose concentration.

331. Cryoprecipitate contains all of the following clotting factors EXCEPT

   (A) factor VIII
   (B) factor IX
   (C) factor XIII
   (D) von Willebrand factor
   (E) fibrinogen

332. The treatment of a hemolytic transfusion reaction in a middle-aged female patient who received blood during a surgical procedure may involve the immediate administration of all of the following EXCEPT

(A) crystalloid intravenous fluids
(B) furosemide
(C) hydrocortisone
(D) sodium bicarbonate
(E) mannitol

333. An elderly man with urosepsis develops disseminated intravascular coagulation (DIC). Which one of the following statements is FALSE regarding DIC?

(A) DIC is usually due to the abnormal consumption of clotting factors.
(B) DIC may be treated with heparin.
(C) Gram-negative endotoxemia is a common cause of DIC.
(D) Abnormalities in laboratory tests include a prolonged prothrombin time and decreased values for platelet count and plasma fibrinogen.
(E) Regardless of the etiology, therapy of DIC is directed toward replacement of clotting factors and inhibition of the clotting cascade.

334. A middle-aged man with long-standing hypertension and chronic renal insufficiency on a beta-blocker and simvastatin requires an intraoperative angiogram while undergoing a vascular procedure. What should be done to decrease his risk of developing contrast-induced acute tubular necrosis?

(A) Administer a fluid bolus of normal saline prior to the procedure.
(B) Stop his statin a week before surgery.
(C) Start a diuretic on the morning of surgery.
(D) Start a calcium channel blocker immediately after the procedure.
(E) Start a beta-blocker at a low dose one week before surgery.

335. Which one of the following patients requires stress doses of steroids on the day of surgery to drain a postoperative wound infection a week after a partial colectomy for recurrent diverticulitis?

(A) A patient who uses topical steroids daily for eczema on both elbows as needed.
(B) A patient who uses inhaled budesonide daily in the spring and fall for allergy-related asthmatic symptoms.
(C) A patient who took oral prednisone for three weeks to treat her severe poison ivy 9 months ago.
(D) A patient who was treated with one dose of dexamethasone last week for postoperative nausea.
(E) A patient treated with steroids for lymphoma 3 years ago.

336. Perioperative management of a 47-year-old man with carcinoid syndrome undergoing a prostatectomy should include

(A) infusion of epinephrine to treat bronchospasm
(B) avoiding the use of vasopressin to treat intraoperative hypotension
(C) the preferential use of muscle relaxants in the benzylisoquinoline class as opposed to those in the steroid class
(D) administration of octreotide preoperatively
(E) starting a calcium channel blocker one week before surgery

337. All of the following facts about antidiuretic hormone (ADH) are true EXCEPT

(A) release is under control of osmoreceptors in the hypothalamus
(B) release is from the posterior pituitary
(C) release is inhibited by increased stretch of the atrial baroreceptors
(D) acts on the proximal convoluted tubule
(E) causes increased reabsorption of free water from the kidney

338. A 50-year-old man with long-standing obstructive sleep apnea who uses a CPAP machine intermittently at home and needs a cholecystectomy

(A) would benefit from a short-acting benzodiazepine given at bedtime for the week before surgery

(B) should be kept intubated and mechanically ventilated for the night following surgery

(C) is at high risk for developing postoperative hypoxemia

(D) would usually require large doses of opioids to treat postoperative pain

(E) should completely stop using CPAP for a week prior to surgery

339. The perioperative management of a middle-aged man with gout undergoing knee replacement should include the avoidance of

(A) local anesthetics in the amide class

(B) succinylcholine

(C) β-adrenergic antagonists

(D) hypovolemia

(E) etomidate

340. Which one of the following abnormalities does not cause a hypercoagulable state?

(A) Factor V Leiden

(B) Protein S deficiency

(C) Protein C deficiency

(D) Antithrombin III deficiency

(E) Von Willebrand disease

341. You are called to see a 57-year-old patient in the recovery room with a serum potassium concentration of 5.9 mEq/L after a colonic resection for colon cancer. Treatment of hyperkalemia includes all of the following EXCEPT

(A) elimination of exogenous sources

(B) correction of cause of endogenous sources

(C) administration of glucose with insulin

(D) administration of acidifying solutions

(E) administration of calcium gluconate

342. Regarding a young adult with Duchenne muscular dystrophy who is to undergo general anesthesia, all of the following are true EXCEPT

(A) the patient often has delayed gastric emptying

(B) the patient has an increased risk of malignant hyperthermia

(C) the patient can safely receive nondepolarizing muscle relaxants

(D) the patient is usually a difficult intubation

(E) ineffective cough from diminished respiratory muscle strength can cause retention of secretions post-operatively

343. Relatively rare diseases that are much more common in patients with the acquired immunodeficiency syndrome include all of the following EXCEPT

(A) pneumonia due to *Pneumocystis carinii*

(B) Addison disease

(C) infection due to *Mycobacterium avium* complex

(D) B-cell lymphoma

(E) Kaposi's sarcoma

344. A 56-year-old woman with a diagnosis of the syndrome of inappropriate secretion of antidiuretic hormone (SIADH) requires a mastectomy for recently diagnosed breast cancer. Findings seen in patients with SIADH includes all of the following EXCEPT

(A) hypernatremia

(B) low serum osmolality

(C) excessive renal secretion of sodium

(D) normal renal function

(E) absence of edema

345. A 26-year-old man with severe inflammatory bowel disease is being treated with complete bowel rest for several weeks. A nutritionist recommends parenteral nutrition. All of the following facts about parenteral nutrition administered via a peripheral vein are true EXCEPT that peripheral nutrition

(A) IV catheters should be changed every three days

(B) has a low incidence of phlebitis if the dextrose concentration is kept below 10%

(C) uses lipid as a source of calories

(D) uses protein as a source of calories

(E) can be stopped during patient transport if it will be restarted within an hour

346. The blood supply to the liver is by two vessels, the hepatic artery and the hepatic portal vein. Which one of the following statements regarding hepatic circulation is correct?

(A) 60% of the blood supply comes from the hepatic artery.

(B) The portal vein provides 90% of the oxygen supply.

(C) Portal vein blood has a higher oxygen saturation than the hepatic artery.

(D) The portal vein supplies the bulk of the nutrients to the liver.

(E) The hepatic artery is more important than the portal vein in transporting orally administered medications to the liver.

347. A 61-year-old woman who had a cadaveric kidney transplant seven years ago now presents for knee replacement surgery. All of the following statements about immunosuppression are correct EXCEPT

(A) immunosuppression may occur with protein–calorie malnutrition

(B) renal transplant recipients have a higher incidence of acute rejection and immunologic graft loss than recipients of any other solid organ

(C) opioids induce immunosuppression in part by decreasing natural killer cell activity and antibody production

(D) cyclosporine use after renal transplantation may cause hypertension, hyperlipidemia, and accelerated atherosclerosis in renal transplant patients

(E) the most common cause of invasive fungal infections in immunocompromised patients is *Candida* species

348. A 59-year-old man with recent cholangitis undergoing an open cholecystectomy under general anesthesia develops intraoperative hypotension unresponsive to vasopressors and fluids. There is no sign of hemorrhage. What drug should you administer at this point?

(A) hydrocortisone 100 mg intravenously

(B) regular insulin 5 units intravenously

(C) glucagon 1 mg intravenously

(D) levothyroxine 100 mcg intravenously

(E) 50 mL of 50% glucose intravenously

349. When evaluating renal function in a 75-year-old healthy man undergoing preoperative assessment for an elective orthopedic procedure, one must consider that

(A) proteinuria is always pathological

(B) a specific gravity of 1.023 or greater demonstrates good concentrating function

(C) BUN elevation is always indicative of renal dysfunction

(D) less creatinine is produced by muscular persons

(E) by the eighth decade of life, GFR is reduced by 85% in otherwise healthy adults

350. A 40-year-old woman with no history of diabetes develops hyperglycemia during abdominal surgery. Mechanisms by which blood glucose can increase during surgery include all of the following EXCEPT

(A) intravenous administration

(B) secretion from the liver secondary to catecholamine-stimulated glycogenolysis

(C) increased catecholamine output inhibiting glucose uptake by insulin-dependent tissues

(D) increased catecholamine output stimulating pancreatic insulin secretion

(E) stress-induced cortisol release from the adrenal cortex

351. All of the following statements about a 47-year-old male patient with diabetes insipidus (DI) are correct EXCEPT

(A) the serum sodium is high

(B) the osmolality of the serum is high

(C) the urine is concentrated

(D) thirst need not be present

(E) pituitary DI is treated with desmopressin

352. A 39-year-old man has been diagnosed with primary hyperaldosteronism. He is expected to have all of the following manifestations EXCEPT

(A) excess secretion of hormone from the adrenal medulla

(B) hypertension

(C) metabolic alkalosis

(D) hypokalemia

(E) inability to concentrate urine

353. A 49-year-old woman with hyperthyroidism due to Graves disease is having a thyroidectomy. She

(A) is likely to have an increased MAC

(B) is likely to have a palpable nodule

(C) should be heavily sedated in the preoperative period

(D) should not be treated with beta blockers perioperatively

(E) should be pretreated with iodide one hour before surgery

354. A 56-year-old man with Gilbert syndrome is scheduled for a bone marrow harvest for donation to his sister. Important considerations in the perioperative period for this patient should include

(A) avoidance of preoperative sedation

(B) preoperative transfusion of fresh frozen plasma

(C) preoperative administration of multiple antiemetic medications

(D) recognition of the benign etiology of the laboratory abnormality

(E) liver biopsy for confirmation of the diagnosis

355. A 52-year-old woman undergoes a total thyroidectomy for a toxic goiter. Upon arrival to the PACU her temperature is 38°C; all other vital signs are normal. Thirty minutes later you are called by the patient's nurse who tells you the patient is now in atrial fibrillation with a heart rate of 140. What medication should you order first?

(A) metoprolol

(B) amiodarone

(C) furosemide

(D) nitroglycerin

(E) diltiazem

356. A 20-year-old African-American woman with sickle cell disease develops severe knee pain after pelvic surgery for a tubal pregnancy. She tells you this pain is typical of her sickle cell crises and usually responds well to opioids. The sickling of red blood cells in this patient

(A) is a reversible process

(B) occurs when oxygenated hemoglobin molecules precipitate

(C) impairs the clotting cascade

(D) may cause infarction in tissues with a high oxygen extraction ratio

(E) may be related to acute splenic infarction given her age

357. A 57-year-old man with cirrhosis develops hepatorenal syndrome. Regarding the hepatorenal syndrome, all of the following are true EXCEPT

(A) it is associated with kidneys that are normal on biopsy

(B) type I is an indication for urgent liver transplantation

(C) it is associated with oliguria

(D) it may be readily diagnosed by the abnormalities in urinary sediment analysis

(E) the prognosis is poor

358. A 19-year-old male patient arrives at the hospital with a gunshot wound through the liver and is brought immediately to the operating room hypotensive and still bleeding heavily. He remains hypotensive following fluid resuscitation with 3 L of lactated Ringer solution. Fluid resuscitation should continue using

(A) uncrossmatched O-negative packed red blood cells

(B) platelets

(C) 5% albumin

(D) fresh frozen plasma

(E) cryoprecipitate

359. A 36-year-old woman with polycythemia vera (PV) presents for a diagnostic laparoscopy as part of an infertility work-up. All of the following statements about PV are correct EXCEPT

(A) PV is the most common of the chronic myeloproliferative disorders

(B) PV is most often diagnosed by the incidental finding of a high hemoglobin and hematocrit

(C) chemotherapy is the usual first line treatment for this condition

(D) if untreated, erythrocytosis causes hyperviscosity that can lead to thrombosis

(E) the goal of treatment in female patients is to maintain the hemoglobin level <12 g/dL

360. A 32-year-old female patient with Sipple syndrome (multiple endocrine neoplasia type IIa) is scheduled for a thyroidectomy. Soon after induction, hypertension of 210/130 is recorded. A likely cause for this is

(A) light anesthesia

(B) pheochromocytoma

(C) inadvertent injection of a pressor agent

(D) hypercarbia

(E) allergic response to an anesthetic agent

361. A middle-aged woman is found to have a plasma calcium concentration of 11 mg/dL while undergoing a preoperative evaluation for an elective cholecystectomy. All of the following are true about hypercalcemia in this patient EXCEPT

(A) mild hypercalcemia as seen in this patient is usually asymptomatic

(B) hypercalcemia decreases renal concentrating ability that can cause polyuria and polydipsia

(C) hypercalcemia can result in bradycardia and shortened QT intervals on ECG

(D) primary hyperparathyroidism is an unlikely cause of her hypercalcemia

(E) if her parathyroid hormone level is suppressed, she is likely to have an underlying malignancy as the cause of her hypercalcemia

362. Which one of the following statements is true regarding anion gap?

(A) An anion gap of 12 mEq/L is considered abnormal.

(B) Diabetic ketoacidosis is associated with a low anion gap.

(C) Metabolic acidosis accompanying diarrhea has a normal anion gap.

(D) Anion gap may be estimated by subtracting the serum chloride concentration from the serum sodium concentration.

(E) Acetazolamide therapy causes increased anion gap metabolic acidosis.

363. Factors released in response to hypovolemia include all of the following EXCEPT

(A) atrial natriuretic peptide

(B) renin

(C) antidiuretic hormone

(D) aldosterone

(E) arginine vasopressin

364. Physiologic compensation for anemia includes all of the following EXCEPT

(A) increased plasma volume

(B) increased cardiac output

(C) increased levels of 2,3-diphosphoglycerate

(D) bradycardia

(E) increased minute alveolar ventilation

365. A few months into her anesthesiology residency, a previously healthy 27-year-old woman is diagnosed with herpetic whitlow. This infectious disease

(A) is caused by the varicella zoster virus

(B) may be effectively prevented by wearing gloves

(C) usually affects the CNS causing encephalitis

(D) is usually acquired from a needle stick

(E) is initially treated with intravenous antiviral agents

Answers and Explanations

290. (E) Stridor occurring twelve hours after thyroidectomy and accompanied by signs of tetany is most likely due to hypocalcemia due to iatrogenic hypoparathyroidism. This patient has an airway problem, and that should be given priority in management. The patient should be observed and intubated if necessary to protect the airway. *(5:172, 1122)*

291. (D) The patient with chronic renal failure who has missed a scheduled dialysis is expected to have uremia, hyperkalemia, hypervolemia, and metabolic acidosis. Platelet function is abnormal due to the uremia, which inhibits platelet aggregation, and a decrease in platelet factor III. The platelet count should not be abnormal unless there is another coexisting problem causing decreased platelet production or increased utilization. *(6:2307, 2310-11)*

292. (D) Stored, cold red cells leak potassium ion, however, the cells avidly take up potassium once they are warmed. The primary electrolyte abnormalities associated with massive transfusion are those associated with citrate intoxication such as hypocalcemia and hypomagnesemia. In addition, since citrate is metabolized to bicarbonate ion, the resulting metabolic alkalosis may lead to hypokalemia. Judicious administration of potassium may be required following massive transfusion assuming preserved hepatic and renal function. *(5:1452)*

293. (C) By the Henderson–Hasselbalch equation, $pH = pK + \log [HCO_3^-]/[H_2CO_3]$. $[H_2CO_3]$ may be replaced by $Pa_{CO_2} \times 0.03$. With the values given, a bicarbonate concentration of 33.2 mEq/L is calculated. Therefore, it appears that this patient has, at baseline, a metabolic alkalosis as a compensatory mechanism for chronic respiratory acidosis. In the postoperative period, the respiratory acidosis has become worse, possibly as a result of medications that depress ventilation or the supplemental oxygen that has diminished this patient's hypoxic ventilatory drive. *(6:364, 369-71)*

294. (C) Thiamine deficiency is common in malnourished persons, especially in those who rely on alcohol as a source of calories. The administration of glucose to such a person may cause symptoms of acute thiamine deficiency. *(6:595)*

295. (E) Vincristine is commonly associated with the development of a peripheral neuropathy. *(6:699, 703-4)*

296. (D) At very high blood levels of ethanol, approximately 400 mg/dL in the nontolerant person, apnea is likely. The resulting hypoxemia may cause seizures and/or ventricular arrhythmias. Ethanol causes dose-dependent vasodilation; however, blood pressure is usually maintained (until hypoventilation leads to hypoxemia) because of reflexive increases in heart rate and cardiac output. *(5:320)*

297. (B) A possible cause of hypotension is acute adrenal insufficiency in a patient with suppression of the pituitary-adrenal axis. However, more likely causes of hypotension during hip arthroplasty include hypovolemia due to blood loss, marrow or fat embolus, methyl methacrylate-induced vasodilation, excessive anesthetic depth, or an allergic reaction to an antibiotic or other medication. The appropriate therapy is dependent upon the etiology. (*5:157, 424, 1280*)

298. **(E)** This patient's parenteral nutrition solution is too concentrated to administer via a peripheral vein. The immediate concern is hypoglycemia resulting from the high circulating insulin level that accompanies infusions of solutions high in glucose. The administration of a 10% glucose solution (the highest concentration recommended by peripheral vein) with concurrent regular monitoring of the blood glucose concentration would be the most appropriate temporary measure to take during the operation. (*5:1331*)

299. **(B)** Hepatitis C, cytomegalovirus, and syphilis infections can be transmitted by blood transfusions, and infected patients should be considered able to transmit disease to health care workers who receive parenteral injuries with needle or surgical instruments contaminated with blood. Similarly, the prion of Creutzfeldt–Jakob disease is thought to be present in neural (and perhaps other) tissue in infected patients, and a parenteral injury with a contaminated instrument may be a method of transmission. The virus of hepatitis A is shed in feces, thus a possible mode of transmission to a health care worker is by the hand-to-mouth route after handling fecal-contaminated material. (*5:189-90, 1448-50*)

300. **(B)** There is no practical system for drug use accountability that can prevent the diversion of drugs by an anesthesia care provider. The other statements listed are correct. (*5:1621-31*)

301. **(B)** Scleroderma is associated with many problems, but arterial dilatation is not one of them. The arterial problem is usually arterial constriction. Raynau's phenomenon is frequently seen. (*6:2762-6*)

302. **(C)** Hurler syndrome is associated with all of the options listed. Hypertelorism may be present, but it should not be a factor complicating the anesthetic. (*6:3192*)

303. **(C)** Creatinine clearance may be estimated according to the following equation:

$$Cl_{Cr} \approx [(140 - age) \times weight]/(Cr \times 72),$$

where age is in years, weight is in kg, and Cr is in mg/dL. The values obtained at 20 and 80 years of age are approximately 117 and 58 mL/min, respectively, for patients weighing 70 kg. (*6:334-5*)

304. **(E)** Albumin is thought to have no risk of transmitting viral diseases such as hepatitis. There is a theoretical concern, not proven, that prion diseases (such as Creutzfeldt-Jakob disease) may be transmitted via transfusion of albumin. (*5:539, 1448*)

305. **(D)** The presence of preexisting coronary artery disease does not automatically indicate a need for preoperative invasive interventions. Rather the risks to the patient should be assessed and minimized. Orthopedic surgery is considered intermediate risk. The patient has stable cardiac disease and no history of diabetes or congestive heart failure, two important risk factors for perioperative cardiac complications (PCC). Beta-blockers reduce long-term PCC. His statin should be continued. (*5:104, 109, 112-5*)

306. **(C)** In the past metformin was stopped up to one week preoperatively because of concerns about metabolic acidosis. Recent analyses have not shown this to be a problem and metformin likely has a role in improving endothelial function. It is not necessary to stop this drug preoperatively. The other statements are true. (*5:114-7*)

307. **(A)** Renal circulation is autoregulated over a wide range of blood pressures. There are many neural factors that control the vessel diameter and the renal blood flow, including the renin-angiotensin system. Innervation comes from T4 to T12, the vagus, and the splanchnic nerves. Epinephrine also has an influence. Prostaglandin E_2 causes vasodilatation. (*6:2281, 2294-5*)

308. **(B)** In an opioid-naïve person, fentanyl administered at a rate of 25 mcg/h should not cause apnea. However, if fentanyl metabolism by CYP3A4 is inhibited, as by clarithromycin, then the possibility of apnea becomes likely. Although the other mechanisms of death are plausible in a person with an acute fracture of the ankle, all would be considered quite rare. *(1:505, 1534)*

309. **(B)** Obese patients should follow the same fasting guidelines as non-obese patients. Postoperative continuous positive airway pressure does not increase the risk of major anastomotic leakage after gastric bypass surgery. Patients with obesity-hypoventilation syndrome have an increased sensitivity to the respiratory depressant effects of general anesthetics. Succinylcholine dosing should be based on total body weight. *(5:301-9)*

310. **(A)** Preoperative evaluation of pulmonary patients is meant to gather information to allow optimization of the patient's pulmonary status. A detailed history and physical examination is the single most useful tool in the preoperative assessment of these patients and should be the basis for deciding on the necessity for further testing. Recent data suggest that spirometry is not an independent predictor of postoperative pulmonary complications. *(5:135, 687)*

311. **(D)** Insulin production occurs in the pancreas and not in the liver. Glycogen storage, gluconeogenesis, glycogenolysis, and the conversion of galactose to glucose all take place in the liver and are important to glucose metabolism. *(6:2520, 2972, 3004)*

312. **(C)** The shock wave is timed to occur 20 msec after the peak of the R wave that corresponds to a point during the absolute refractory period. Shock wave-induced dysrhythmias are therefore minimized. *(5:1141)*

313. **(D)** The American College of Cardiology/American Hospital Association guidelines list five risk factors associated with an increased risk of perioperative cardiac complications. These are a history of ischemic heart disease, diabetes, congestive heart failure and/or cardiomegaly, renal insufficiency, and cerebrovascular disease. *(5:99, 104-7)*

314. **(D)** Ascites may be associated with severe cardiorespiratory symptoms. Ascites follows chronic increased portal vein pressure. It is usually accompanied by hyponatremia. Ascitic fluid should be removed slowly to avoid hypotension. *(6:331-3)*

315. **(B)** When trying to diagnose the cause of renal failure, one should obtain a urine specimen before treatment is begun. The urine will be concentrated in the patient with prerenal failure and will have a higher specific gravity. The urine need not be blood-tinged. Oliguria is present. *(6:336-7)*

316. **(C)** Patients with myxedema have coarse hair and dry skin. Cold intolerance and bradycardia are present. The edema is nonpitting. *(5:152; 6:2919-20)*

317. **(D)** Such patients should be well monitored. Too rapid replacement of thyroid hormone may cause myocardial ischemia. The electrocardiogram and blood pressure are not sufficient to monitor fluid status. *(5:153)*

318. **(C)** It is estimated that more than a third of hospitalized elderly patients suffer from depression. Depression may be related to disturbances in other systems such as the hypothalamic-pituitary-adrenal axis. *(5:81, 109, 156, 172, 286)*

319. **(B)** The patient with pheochromocytoma should be well prepared preoperatively. This may take two weeks of α-adrenoceptor blockade. These patients are usually hypovolemic. While the level of monitoring varies with the amount of concurrent illness in the patient, a pulmonary artery catheter is not mandatory in all cases. *(5:158)*

320. **(C)** The most important goal is to prevent hypoglycemia. One can monitor glucose levels and try to keep them in the normal range, but

this should not be done at the risk of hypoglycemia. Many regimens can be used for perioperative glucose control. (*5:163*)

321. **(C)** Hypoglycemia may be manifest as sympathetic discharge, including hypertension and tachycardia. The skin is cold and clammy. Ketoacidosis is more likely to occur with insulin deficiency. (*6:3005*)

322. **(C)** Hyperosmolar coma may occur in the absence of ketosis. The osmolarity is over 320 mOsm (normal is about 285 mOsm). The condition is seen more often in the elderly and is accompanied by polyuria. Treatment is with rehydration and small doses of insulin. (*5:1114-5*)

323. **(E)** Insulin pumps deliver insulin subcutaneously and so uptake of the drug may be affected by alterations (usually reductions) in tissue perfusion that are commonly encountered during the perioperative period. In certain cases, it may be beneficial to substitute intravenous infusions of insulin. (*5:1115; 6:2976, 2979*)

324. **(C)** One unit of packed red cells should increase the hemoglobin concentration by about 1 g/dL. Unfortunately, most hemolytic transfusion reactions are the result of human error. FFP should be ABO-type compatible but does not usually need to be Rh (D) compatible and a crossmatch is unnecessary. Transfusion of FFP should be guided by improvements in the PT, and aPTT values; the INR value is used solely to guide warfarin therapy. Most transfusions of platelets are to treat thrombocytopenia associated with malignancies. (*5:1439, 1442-6*)

325. **(B)** The symptoms are compatible with carcinoid syndrome. The Zollinger-Ellison syndrome is associated with hypersecretion of gastric acid. Pheochromocytoma is associated with hypertension and a catecholamine-secreting tumor. Peutz-Jeghers syndrome is associated with multiple polyps of the gastrointestinal tract. (*5:1035*)

326. **(E)** Decreased plasma albumin levels decrease the bound fraction of thiopental and result in a greater fraction of free thiopental. Serum gamma globulin is higher in cirrhosis. Pancuronium has a larger volume of distribution; therefore, it is less effective for a given dose. Patients with cirrhosis excrete sodium-poor or sodium-free urine. (*5:695-6*)

327. **(E)** There is no ideal anesthetic technique for liver transplantation, although no class of anesthetic drugs is contraindicated. The effects of the agents should be titrated against the patient's responses. (*5:1068-72*)

328. **(C)** Hypotension is a feature of hypocalcemia. Particularly when symptomatic, hypocalcemia should be treated if total calcium is less than 7.5 g/dL. (*5:1123*)

329. **(D)** A patient who has had a transsphenoidal hypophysectomy for acromegaly is likely to be lacking all of the hormones of the anterior pituitary (GH, ACTH, TSH, FSH, LH, prolactin). The patient probably has been maintained on a glucocorticoid and thyroxine, both of which should be given in the perioperative period. The posterior pituitary is usually not removed during a transsphenoidal hypophysectomy; therefore, the patient is unlikely to require vasopressin therapy. (*5:1129, 1133*)

330. **(E)** Glucocorticoids, such as prednisone, have a hyperglycemic effect. Nonspecific β-adrenergic antagonists, such as propranolol, antagonize the hyperglycemic response to stress. Hydrochlorothiazide also causes hyperglycemia, and antagonizes the hypoglycemic effect of glyburide. Insulin release from the pancreas is stimulated by $β_2$-adrenergic agonists, and would not be affected by atenolol that is specific for the $β_1$-adrenoceptor. Inhibitors of angiotensin converting enzyme, such as lisinopril, have no effect on glucose homeostasis. (*5:1116*)

331. **(B)** Factor IX is not present in cryoprecipitate. Treatment of factor IX deficiency (hemophilia B) involves transfusion of prothrombin complex that contains factors II, VII, IX, and X. (*5:1333*)

332. **(C)** In a hemolytic transfusion reaction, the immediate goals include maintenance of intravascular volume and increasing urine flow with diuretics to prevent acute tubular necrosis from hemoglobinemia. Alkalinizing the urine may decrease the likelihood of hemoglobin precipitation in the renal tubules. There is no indication for the immediate use of cortisol. (*5:1441*)

333. **(E)** DIC has many causes and the most effective therapy is to treat the underlying cause, if possible. (*5:215*)

334. **(A)** Radiocontrast dye can cause acute kidney injury. Hydration before administration of contrast lowers the rate of contrast-induced renal failure. (*5:1373-4*)

335. **(C)** Using glucocorticoids at doses exceeding 5 to 7.5 mg of prednisone or the equivalent for three weeks or longer within the last year is considered a risk factor for perioperative adrenal insufficiency. In most cases, topical or inhaled glucocorticoids do not suppress the pituitary-adrenal axis. (*5:1126*)

336. **(D)** Measures should be taken to decrease the likelihood of a carcinoid crisis. These include giving octreotide to prevent or decrease the release of factors by the carcinoid tumor, and avoiding medications that increase release of such factors such as catecholamines and benzylisoquinoline muscle relaxants such as mivacurium and cisatracurium. Vasopressin is the preferred drug for treating hypotension. (*5:1035*)

337. **(D)** ADH release is in response to decreased plasma osmolarity detected by osmoreceptors in the hypothalamus. It is also released in response to decreased tension in the stretch receptors in the atrium. ADH is secreted from the posterior pituitary. The principal effect is on the collecting tubules. (*5:1127; 6:342, 1903*)

338. **(C)** The patient with obstructive sleep apnea is at high risk for developing postoperative hypoxemia and for this reason usually warrants a longer period of postoperative observation. This is not however an indication for routine postoperative intubation and ventilation. Apneic episodes are more likely in the patient who uses nighttime sedatives or alcohol. Patients with obstructive sleep apnea are also at increased risk for opioid-induced hypoventilation or apnea. (*5:64, 68, 134*)

339. **(D)** Hypovolemia may decrease renal excretion of uric acid and increase the risk of an acute attack. Although aspirin increases uric acid levels, other COX inhibitors, especially indomethacin, are effective in preventing or treating an attack. There is no reason to avoid succinylcholine or β-adrenoceptor antagonists. (*6:2820-1, 2838*)

340. **(E)** Protein C, protein S, and antithrombin III are endogenous anticoagulants. Their deficiencies make patients hypercoagulable, as does the presence of the abnormal form of factor V designated as factor V Leiden. Von Willebrand disease (vWD) is an autosomal dominant congenital disorder of platelet function caused by a deficiency of normally functioning von Willebrand factor and results in a hypocoagulable state that manifests as bleeding episodes. (*5:209, 214*)

341. **(D)** Hyperkalemia may be treated by the administration of insulin and glucose solutions, eliminating exogenous sources (one of the major causes), and correcting causes of endogenous sources. Treatment includes alkalinizing the blood, not acidifying it. (*5:517-8*)

342. **(D)** Duchenne muscular dystrophy is often accompanied by delayed gastric emptying and susceptibility to malignant hyperthermia. Nondepolarizing muscle relaxants may be used if needed. There is no definite association with airway difficulties. (*5:143-4*)

343. **(B)** The two listed infections and the two listed malignancies are all much more common in patients with AIDS. (*6:1507, 1531, 1535, 1547-8*)

344. **(A)** Inappropriate secretion of ADH is sometimes seen after surgery. The syndrome includes hyponatremia and low serum osmolality. The kidneys excrete an excessive amount of sodium under the influence of ADH. Underlying renal function is normal and peripheral edema is not part of the syndrome. (5:159-60; 6:2908-11)

345. **(E)** Parenteral nutrition is very important in the pre- and postoperative care of patients, however there may be problems associated with its use. It can be administered through a peripheral vein, and the problem with phlebitis is less if the glucose concentration is limited. Both lipids and proteins are used as sources of calories. Sudden cessation of parenteral nutrition can lead to hypoglycemia. (5:1393; 6:617-8)

346. **(D)** The liver has a dual blood supply. The hepatic artery supplies only 25% of the blood. The oxygen supply is evenly divided by the two vessels, even though the portal vein blood is less saturated. Most of the nutrients come from the portal vein. (6:2520)

347. **(B)** Pancreas transplant recipients have the highest incidence of acute rejection and immunologic graft loss of all solid organ transplant recipients. (5:243, 713, 1099, 1103)

348. **(A)** Relative adrenal insufficiency occurs when the pituitary-adrenal axis fails to mount a sufficient response to an acute and severe stressor like surgery or infection, despite adequate output when the patient is healthy. In such cases, the patient may benefit from exogenous administration of corticosteroids. (5:1320, 1366, 1396)

349. **(B)** Proteinuria may be normal with exercise or stress, and BUN elevation may occur with a high-protein diet or when there is blood present in the gastrointestinal tract. Creatinine load is reduced by atrophy of skeletal muscle mass. By the eighth decade of life, GFR is reduced by one-third to one-half. (5:168-9, 282)

350. **(D)** Blood sugar rises during surgery by many mechanisms, including administration of intravenous fluids, secretion from the liver due to increased circulating levels of catecholamines, and insulin suppression. Uptake into the tissues leads to a decrease in blood sugar. (5:163)

351. **(C)** In diabetes insipidus, the serum sodium is high and the serum osmolality is high. The urine is dilute. In spite of polyuria, thirst need not be present. (6:2904-7)

352. **(A)** The patient with hyperaldosteronism has hypertension and hypokalemia. The excess secretion comes from the adrenal cortex. Alkalosis is present. (5:157; 6:2949-50)

353. **(B)** The patient with hyperthyroidism does not have an increased MAC. Iodide is given for one to two weeks preoperatively to decrease thyroid hormone release and to decrease the vascularity of the gland. Propranolol may also be needed pre- or intraoperatively to manage tachycardia. In contrast to the usual practice of many years ago, heavy preoperative sedation is no longer necessary. In fact, many patients scheduled for thyroidectomy are admitted on the day of surgery. (5:151-2, 1117-9)

354. **(D)** Gilbert syndrome is a common and entirely benign cause of unconjugated hyperbilirubinemia. Although serum bilirubin levels may rise in response to fasting or stress, they are not elevated to hazardous levels. The most important measure in the perioperative period is to elicit the history of Gilbert syndrome from the patient so that the isolated abnormality of hyperbilirubinemia is not investigated further. (6:2534-5)

355. **(A)** In the setting of thyroid-induced atrial fibrillation, the initial drug administered should be a beta-blocker. (5:1118)

356. **(D)** In sickle cell anemia, the abnormal hemoglobin molecule precipitates when deoxygenated. When a significant fraction of the hemoglobin molecules in a red cell precipitate, the cell irreversibly assumes the sickle shape. This alteration in red cell shape increases blood viscosity, decreases microcirculatory flow, and causes platelet aggregation and fibrin deposition. Tissues with a high oxygen extraction ratio are at increased risk for infarction because

hemoglobin molecules are more likely to become deoxygenated. The spleen is generally lost within the first three years of life due to repeated microinfarctions. (*6:855-7*)

357. (D) Hepatorenal syndrome, which is accompanied by oliguric renal failure, carries a very poor prognosis. Urinary sediment and renal biopsy are normal. (*5:177, 194, 323*)

358. (A) If there is inadequate time to crossmatch packed red blood cells, then uncrossmatched O-negative red cells should be given to expand circulating volume and increase oxygen carrying capacity. The patient might very well require FFP and platelets if blood loss exceeds approximately one blood volume. There is little support in the literature for the use of albumin in the management of hypovolemic shock from trauma. (*5:1160*)

359. (C) Polycythemia vera is a clonal disorder in which phenotypically normal red cells, granulocytes, and platelets accumulate in the absence of a physiologic stimulus. It is a generally indolent disorder and first line therapy is periodic phlebotomy. (*6:898-900*)

360. (B) The patient with Sipple syndrome who develops hypertension must be suspected of having a pheochromocytoma. Light anesthesia and hypercarbia should be quickly ruled out. Allergic reactions are not usually associated with hypertension. The inadvertent injection of a vasopressor agent may occur but should be easy to rule out. (*5:157-9*)

361. (D) Chronic hypercalcemia is most commonly caused by primary hyperparathyroidism. The second most common etiology is an underlying malignancy. (*6:360-1*)

362. (C) Anion gap may be estimated by subtracting the sum of the serum chloride and bicarbonate concentrations from the serum sodium concentration. A normal value is 10 to 12 mEq/L. The acidosis that occurs due to

gastrointestinal loss of bicarbonate ion with diarrhea has a normal anion gap because it is accompanied by hyperchloremia. Diabetic ketoacidosis has a high anion gap because of the presence of increased levels of unmeasured anions such as acetoacetate and β-hydroxybutyrate. Acetazolamide causes metabolic acidosis with a normal anion gap. (*5:171, 461*)

363. (A) Renin is released by the kidney in response to sympathetic stimulation or hypotension. Renin generates angiotensin I that is converted to angiotensin II, a stimulator of aldosterone release. Hypovolemia leads to ADH release while hypervolemia releases atrial natriuretic peptide. Arginine vasopressin is another name for ADH. (*6:331, 336, 344*)

364. (D) Heart rate and minute alveolar ventilation initially increase after hemorrhage in the absence of volume replacement. Hyperventilation and tachycardia serve to increase cardiac output that in turn increases blood flow to tissues. Acute hemorrhage is also associated with redistribution of water from the extravascular space into the intravascular space. Another compensatory mechanism for acute anemia occurs within the erythrocyte; red blood cells can increase their intracellular concentration of 2,3-diphosphoglycerate (2,3-DPG). Increased levels of 2,3-DPG reduce the affinity of hemoglobin for oxygen and result in increased tissue oxygen delivery. (*5:198-9*)

365. (B) Herpetic whitlow is a painful infection of a finger caused by the herpes simplex virus. It is most commonly acquired from contact with herpetic lesions or respiratory secretions containing virus. The wearing of gloves is highly protective. Edema, erythema and tenderness of the infected finger, as well as fever and lymphadenitis are common. Oral antiviral medications are used as first-line therapy. (*6:1064, 1457, 1461*)

Pharmacology
Questions

DIRECTIONS (Questions 366-523): Each of the numbered items or incomplete statements in this section is followed by answers or by completions of the statement. Select the ONE lettered answer or completion that is BEST in each case.

366. A 72-year-old female with a past medical history of osteoporosis underwent open reduction and internal fixation of her left hip. She was previously diagnosed with heparin induced thrombocytopenia type II and has a platelet count of 56,000. Which one of the following agents can be administered for immediate postoperative prophylaxis of deep vein thrombosis?

    (A) low-molecular-weight heparin
    (B) warfarin
    (C) tirofiban
    (D) unfractionated heparin
    (E) fondaparinux

367. Drug elimination from the body

    (A) is most efficient for substances with high lipid solubility
    (B) may occur by metabolism
    (C) is usually complete after 2 half-lives
    (D) is usually not modifiable with pharmacologic interventions
    (E) is independent of drug binding to blood and tissues

368. Sevoflurane

    (A) can cause hepatotoxicity
    (B) is flammable at a concentration of 6%
    (C) gives poor muscle relaxation

    (D) undergoes hepatic metabolism
    (E) causes myocardial irritability

369. In an 80-kg patient with severe pain, administration of thiopental 80 mg will

    (A) produce sleep
    (B) will have analgesic effects
    (C) will have no effect
    (D) will sedate the patient but not induce sleep
    (E) will blunt the hemodynamic response to painful stimuli

370. Administration of ketamine causes

    (A) decreased heart rate
    (B) increased heart rate
    (C) decreased cardiac output
    (D) no change in cardiac output
    (E) no change in heart rate

371. Atracurium 0.5 mg/kg is administered for induction of paralysis in a hemodynamically stable, anesthetized patient as an intravenous bolus. Shortly after drug administration, the patient becomes hypotensive. This is most likely due to

    (A) adrenoceptor mediated effects
    (B) ganglionic blockade
    (C) histamine release
    (D) negative inotropic effects
    (E) hemodynamic effects of laudanosine

372. Rocuronium

    (A) is a ganglionic blocker
    (B) at 4 × ED95 causes significant histamine release
    (C) may be administered intramuscularly
    (D) is eliminated by the kidney
    (E) is not suitable for continuous infusion

373. With regard to drug metabolism reactions

    (A) the phase I reactions usually involve conjugation
    (B) the phase II reactions generally result in the loss of pharmacological activity
    (C) they typically lead to an increased rate of renal tubular reabsorption of the drug
    (D) they usually result in an increase in the duration of action of the drug
    (E) they can be differentiated into three distinct phases

374. Transdermal scopolamine

    (A) will not produce behavioral side effects
    (B) is safe for emesis prophylaxis in children
    (C) is a muscarinic agonist
    (D) does not cross the blood–brain barrier
    (E) can prevent postoperative nausea in adult patients

375. A drug that is a pure opioid antagonist is

    (A) butorphanol
    (B) levallorphan
    (C) naloxone
    (D) neostigmine
    (E) edrophonium

376. Milrinone

    (A) decreases cyclic-AMP levels
    (B) is metabolized by monoamine oxidase
    (C) inhibits phosphodiesterase
    (D) is a β-adrenergic agonist
    (E) increases peripheral vascular resistance

377. Bupivacaine

    (A) is an ester local anesthetic with a short duration
    (B) should be used in a concentration of 0.75% for epidural anesthesia during labor
    (C) is associated with cardiac toxicity due to its effect on sodium channels
    (D) toxicity is not a problem unless it is injected intravenously
    (E) cardiotoxicity is noted by the onset of tachycardia

378. A 23-year-old male is scheduled to undergo repair of an elbow fracture under ultrasound guided brachial plexus blockade. With regard to choice of local anesthetic, which one of the following statements is most accurate?

    (A) Tetracaine is less cardiotoxic than chloroprocaine.
    (B) The extent of blockade of cardiac sodium channels by bupivacaine is predicted by its local anesthetic potency.
    (C) Chloroprocaine is a suitable choice due to its long duration of action.
    (D) The maximum recommended local anesthetic dosage for ropivacaine is 3 mg/kg.
    (E) Lidocaine has a longer duration of action as compared to mepivacaine.

379. Etomidate

    (A) has anticonvulsant activity
    (B) releases histamine
    (C) has analgesic properties
    (D) has an antiemetic effect
    (E) increases intraocular pressure

380. Glucuronide metabolites of medications will be excreted in the urine more rapidly than the parent compounds by which one of the following processes?

    (A) tubular secretion
    (B) glomerular filtration
    (C) facilitated diffusion
    (D) passive nonionic diffusion
    (E) tubular reabsorption

381. The correct ranking of the potencies of the volatile anesthetics, from most potent to least potent, is

(A) sevoflurane > desflurane > isoflurane > halothane

(B) desflurane > sevoflurane > isoflurane > halothane

(C) isoflurane > halothane > desflurane > sevoflurane

(D) halothane > isoflurane > sevoflurane > desflurane

(E) halothane > sevoflurane > desflurane > isoflurane

DIRECTIONS: Use the following figure to answer Questions 382-383:

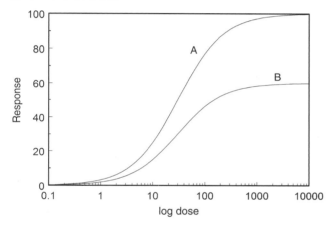

382. If A and B are two different medications producing the same effect, then the figure shows that

(A) A has higher efficacy than B

(B) A has lower efficacy than B

(C) A and B must act via different receptors to produce their effects

(D) A is more potent than B

(E) A has a higher ED_{50} than B

383. If A depicts the dose-response relationship of drug X acting alone, and B depicts the dose-response relationship of drug X in the presence of drug Y, then it can be said that drug Y

(A) is a competitive antagonist of drug X

(B) is a noncompetitive antagonist of drug X

(C) must act via a different receptor than drug X

(D) increases the efficacy of drug X

(E) decreases the potency of drug X

384. A 63-kg patient with a history of glaucoma who suffered a second degree burn of 10% of the total body surface area in a motor vehicle accident is undergoing surgery for intramedullary nailing of an open tibia fracture 18 h after the accident under general endotracheal anesthesia. Induction of anesthesia was accomplished by administration of fentanyl 2 mcg/kg, propofol 2.5 mg/kg, and succinylcholine 1 mg/kg intravenously. Antibiotic prophylaxis consisted of gentamicin 5 mg/kg intravenously prior to incision. Prolonged duration of neuromuscular blockade after succinylcholine in this patient would be most likely due to

(A) potentiation of the neuromuscular blocking effects by gentamicin

(B) the burn suffered in the motor vehicle crash

(C) chronic treatment of glaucoma with topical isofluorophate

(D) prolonged immobilization

385. Desflurane

(A) is highly lipid soluble

(B) has a MAC of 6% when administered with O_2

(C) is highly water soluble

(D) is not irritating to the airway

(E) metabolism releases significant quantities of fluoride ion

386. A patient scheduled for an emergency procedure gives a history of heroin abuse. A problem that must be anticipated in the perioperative period is

(A) delayed gastric emptying

(B) presence of left ventricular hypertrophy

(C) progressive sensory-motor polyneuropathy

(D) decreased need for anesthetics

(E) increased sensitivity to catecholamines

387. Local anesthetics have their effect at the

(A) presynaptic nerve terminal

(B) postsynaptic nerve terminal

(C) GABA receptor

(D) membrane

(E) calcium channel

388. The action of propofol after injection is terminated by

(A) its elimination unchanged by the kidneys

(B) its biotransformation by the liver

(C) its being bound to proteins

(D) its redistribution

(E) being taken up in fatty tissues

389. Methohexital

(A) is metabolized to a greater extent than thiopental

(B) is converted to active metabolites

(C) has a longer terminal half-life than thiopental

(D) causes histamine release from mast cells

(E) is contraindicated in asthma

390. The first-pass effect refers to

(A) the biotransformation of a drug in its vehicle of administration

(B) the change of a drug by enzymes in muscle

(C) biotransformation of a drug as it passes through the intestinal mucosa and liver

(D) the drug lost by urinary excretion

(E) the drug lost by fecal excretion

391. An expected cardiovascular change after ketamine administration is

(A) elevated diastolic pressure, normal systolic pressure

(B) elevated diastolic and systolic pressure

(C) decreased diastolic and systolic pressure

(D) decreased diastolic pressure, increased systolic pressure

(E) no change in blood pressure

392. A small dose of a nondepolarizing muscle relaxant given 3 min before an intubating dose of succinylcholine

(A) increases the dose of succinylcholine required

(B) will not prevent the rise in intracranial pressure

(C) is useful in preventing arrhythmias

(D) doubles the time to recovery from neuromuscular blockade

(E) permits faster intubation

393. A drug is administered by bolus intravenous injection. Approximately what percentage of the drug remains after four half-lives have elapsed?

(A) 1%

(B) 4%

(C) 6%

(D) 10%

(E) 12%

394. Flecainide is

(A) an antiarrhythmic drug in Class IC

(B) a lidocaine analog

(C) a muscle relaxant

(D) the drug of choice for local anesthesia reactions

(E) administered only orally

395. The administration of anticholinesterase drugs will

(A) prolong all neuromuscular blockade

(B) always reverse nondepolarizing agents

(C) shorten the block of a depolarizing agent

(D) reverse nondepolarizing agents if the plasma concentration of the drug is low enough

(E) reverse the action of a depolarizing agent if only partial paralysis is present

396. A patient is admitted for emergency orthopedic surgery. Preliminary data show a BUN value of 85 mg/dL and serum potassium of

6.0 mEq/L. The least desirable drug for intubation would be

(A) rocuronium
(B) vecuronium
(C) cisatracurium
(D) mivacurium
(E) pancuronium

397. The most sensitive test to determine adequate recovery from neuromuscular blockade is

(A) five-second head lift
(B) five-second hand grip
(C) inspiratory force
(D) tactile response to double-burst stimulation
(E) tactile response to train-of-four

398. A patient who had been given vecuronium received neostigmine, 3 mg, at the termination of the surgical procedure. Six minutes later, a large amount of white, frothy secretions was noted in the endotracheal tube. Vigorous suctioning was required to remove these secretions in order to ventilate the patient. The treatment of choice for such secretions is

(A) atropine
(B) digoxin
(C) more neostigmine
(D) readministration of vecuronium
(E) use of a ventilator

399. Heparin inhibits blood coagulation

(A) by binding calcium ions
(B) through interactions with protamine
(C) by activating antithrombin III
(D) by activating plasmin
(E) by activating von Willebrand factor

400. The patient with myasthenia gravis

(A) has normal reactions to muscle relaxants
(B) reacts abnormally to relaxants only when the condition is not well controlled
(C) has decreased sensitivity to nondepolarizing relaxants

(D) has an increased sensitivity to nondepolarizing relaxants
(E) has an increased sensitivity to depolarizing relaxants

401. Labetalol

(A) is a nonselective α-adrenergic receptor blocker
(B) has intrinsic sympathomimetic activity at β_2-adrenergic receptors
(C) undergoes significant placental transfer and should not be used in pregnancy
(D) has a potency ratio of $\beta-$ to $\alpha-$adrenergic blockade of approximately 10:1
(E) is a short acting, selective β_1-adrenergic receptor blocker

402. Physostigmine

(A) may be used for the treatment of central anticholinergic syndrome
(B) does not cross the blood–brain barrier
(C) is less effective than neostigmine in treating emergence delirium
(D) is the drug of choice for reversal of the sedative effect of benzodiazepines
(E) often produces an uncomfortably dry mouth

DIRECTIONS: Use the following scenario to answer Questions 403-408. Many patients are unaware of the reasons for which they are taking their medications. When provided with a list of medications by a patient, an anesthesiologist must be able to recognize the medications and know the likely pathological states for which the medications are indicated. For Questions 403-408, a medication is followed by five diseases or pathological states. Choose the ONE disease for which the medication may be indicated.

403. Lisinopril

(A) panic disorder
(B) hypertension
(C) paroxysmal supraventricular tachycardia
(D) premature ventricular contractions
(E) hyperthyroidism

404. Amiodarone

    (A) Wolff-Parkinson-White syndrome
    (B) hyperthyroidism
    (C) angina pectoris
    (D) pulseless electrical activity
    (E) ventricular tachycardia

405. Fexofenadine

    (A) hay fever
    (B) insomnia
    (C) schizophrenia
    (D) chronic pain
    (E) inflammatory bowel disease

406. Budesonide

    (A) deep venous thrombosis
    (B) control of asthma
    (C) claudication
    (D) angina pectoris
    (E) atrial fibrillation

407. Dofetilide

    (A) muscle spasticity
    (B) trigeminal neuralgia
    (C) atrial fibrillation
    (D) peripheral edema
    (E) insomnia

408. Allopurinol

    (A) systemic lupus erythematosus
    (B) gout
    (C) osteoarthritis
    (D) rheumatoid arthritis
    (E) psoriatic arthritis

409. A 42-year-old female with a BMI of 32 and a history of severe postoperative nausea and vomiting (PONV) is scheduled for a laparoscopic cholecystectomy for symptomatic cholelithiasis. Your anesthetic plan includes the administration of a 5-HT$_3$ receptor antagonist and droperidol for the prevention of PONV. If you were to add a third agent, the most useful drug would be

    (A) metoclopramide
    (B) prochlorperazine
    (C) famotidine
    (D) dexamethasone
    (E) ephedrine

DIRECTIONS: Use the following figure to answer Questions 410-411:

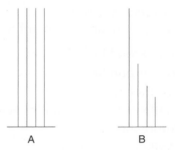

410. The train-of-four stimulus is depicted in the figure. Stimulation is at 2 Hz. The response in A is normal. By looking at B, you know that

    (A) a depolarizing block is present
    (B) the patient is partially paralyzed
    (C) the patient is partially paralyzed, but one would need a baseline recording to know how much
    (D) the train-of-four ratio is 50%
    (E) the patient could sustain a head lift

411. The train-of-four ratio for a depolarizing block is

    (A) variable
    (B) 50%
    (C) 60%
    (D) 75%
    (E) 100%

412. Propofol as compared to thiopental

    (A) is less likely to provoke bronchospasm
    (B) if administered in equipotent doses for induction of anesthesia causes less reduction in systemic blood pressure
    (C) causes adrenal suppression after prolonged infusion
    (D) has no effect on cerebral metabolic rate
    (E) does not cause excitatory motor activity

413. Verapamil

(A) increases myocardial contractility

(B) is a β-adrenergic antagonist

(C) is poorly bound to plasma protein

(D) may produce AV-block when combined with volatile anesthetics

(E) belongs to the class of dihydropyridines

414. Lepirudin and argatroban exert their anticoagulant effect by

(A) vitamin K antagonism

(B) inhibition of platelet aggregation

(C) glycoprotein IIb/IIIa inhibition

(D) increasing the rate of the thrombin-antithrombin reaction

(E) direct thrombin inhibition

415. If a patient is taking a monoamine oxidase (MAO) inhibitor, which one of the following should be avoided?

(A) local anesthetics

(B) halothane

(C) vecuronium

(D) meperidine

(E) aspirin

416. The most common electrolyte alteration caused by the thiazide diuretics is

(A) hypokalemia

(B) hypoglycemia

(C) hyperchloremia

(D) hypernatremia

(E) hyperuricemia

417. Nifedipine

(A) is quite effective in supraventricular tachycardia

(B) is used for the treatment of ischemic heart disease

(C) has a half-life of 30 min

(D) is a peripheral vasoconstrictor

(E) is an effective drug for ventricular tachycardia

418. The interaction of protamine and heparin to terminate anticoagulation is of

(A) competition for binding sites

(B) a chemical interaction leading to an inactive compound

(C) pH change

(D) a conformational change

(E) platelet stimulation

419. Epinephrine causes a prolongation of activity of local anesthetics by

(A) chemical interaction

(B) decreasing absorption

(C) altered protein binding

(D) competition for binding sites

(E) altered metabolism

420. The combination of nitrous oxide at 0.5 MAC plus isoflurane 0.5 MAC is one of

(A) antagonism

(B) potentiation

(C) additive effect

(D) synergism

(E) no effect

421. Glycopyrrolate

(A) is a quaternary amine

(B) crosses the blood–brain barrier with ease

(C) is associated with the central cholinergic syndrome

(D) is a cholinergic agonist

(E) is a naturally occurring belladonna alkaloid

422. Lidocaine

(A) is eliminated chiefly by the liver

(B) is effective orally

(C) is toxic at levels over 1 mcg/mL

(D) toxicity is noted by the appearance of hematuria

(E) is useful in supraventricular tachycardia

423. The interaction of phenobarbital and phenytoin can be described as one of

    (A) chemical interaction
    (B) interaction at site of absorption
    (C) altered protein binding
    (D) competition for binding sites
    (E) altered metabolism

424. Midazolam

    (A) is contraindicated in the child
    (B) is shorter-acting than thiopental
    (C) is associated with less frequent venous irritation than diazepam
    (D) suppresses adrenal cortical function
    (E) has a high incidence of histamine release

425. The patient who has recently abused cocaine

    (A) will be calm and sedated
    (B) may be treated with propranolol
    (C) exhibits signs of sympathetic blockade
    (D) will have bradycardia
    (E) will have hypotension

426. The methylxanthine group of drugs

    (A) includes caffeine
    (B) have a strong β_1-adrenergic mimetic effect
    (C) stimulates production of phosphodiesterase
    (D) causes bronchoconstriction
    (E) leads to a decrease in cyclic AMP

427. Sublingual drug administration

    (A) leads to lower drug levels compared to oral administration
    (B) is more effective for ionized drugs
    (C) circumvents the first-pass effect
    (D) leads to rapid liver breakdown of the drug
    (E) requires a much larger dose for effectiveness

428. Metoclopramide

    (A) is a dopaminergic agonist
    (B) decreases gastric acid secretion
    (C) stimulates motility of the upper gastro-intestinal tract
    (D) may lead to vomiting
    (E) leads to an ileus and increased small intestinal transit time

429. A patient is scheduled for surgery who is a Jehovah's Witness. She adamantly refuses to receive blood products. The procedure may require volume replacement. A product that may be used is

    (A) 5% albumin
    (B) washed red cells
    (C) autologous blood
    (D) hetastarch
    (E) platelets to decrease bleeding, thus making transfusion unnecessary

430. A 21-year-old female is emergently taken to the operating room for exploratory laparotomy after sustaining multiple injuries including a grade 4 splenic rupture in a high-speed motor vehicle accident. Upon transfer to the operating room table, the patient is noted to have pulseless ventricular fibrillation, and cardiopulmonary resuscitation according to ACLS guidelines is initiated. Despite resuscitation according to protocol including the administration of epinephrine intravenously, the patient remains in ventricular fibrillation. Which one of the following drugs or procedures is recommended as an alternative to epinephrine in this setting?

    (A) phenylephrine 80 mcg IV push
    (B) adenosine 6-12 mg IV push
    (C) vasopressin 40 U IV push
    (D) sodium bicarbonate 50 mEq IV push
    (E) overdrive pacing with isoproterenol

431. Edrophonium, in a dose of 1 mg/kg

    (A) has a slower onset time than neostigmine
    (B) has a much shorter duration than neostigmine

(C) has greater muscarinic side effects than neostigmine

(D) has a faster onset and decreased duration than neostigmine

(E) should be preceded by atropine

432. Sodium nitroprusside is to be used for treatment of intraoperative hypertension. This drug

(A) causes venous dilatation only

(B) will be needed in increased doses if the patient has been previously treated with propranolol

(C) may cause cyanide toxicity in high doses, evidenced by alkalosis and increasing drug dosage needed to achieve the same result

(D) may cause acidosis as a sign of toxicity

(E) may cause a toxicity that is evidenced by an acidosis that is responsive to sodium bicarbonate

433. Postoperative pain control with methadone

(A) is limited by its short half-life

(B) is more effective with oral administration

(C) is used on an every-2-h regimen

(D) may take 48 h to obtain a stable effect

(E) does not depress respiration

434. Dopamine

(A) is a transmitter confined to the central nervous system

(B) stimulates dopaminergic receptors only at an infusion rate of 10 mcg/kg/min

(C) decreases renal blood flow

(D) increases cardiac output by stimulating β_1-adrenergic receptors

(E) decreases pulmonary artery pressure

435. A patient has undergone a laparotomy for a bowel obstruction. A rapid sequence induction was performed using succinylcholine for muscle relaxation, and pancuronium was subsequently given. Neuromuscular blockade was reversed with neostigmine. A few minutes after extubation, the surgical dressing is stained with blood and the surgeon decides that the wound must be reexplored. If another rapid sequence induction is to be performed,

(A) succinylcholine will be ineffective

(B) succinylcholine will lead to severe hyperkalemia

(C) succinylcholine will be effective, however the time of onset will be delayed

(D) succinylcholine will be effective, however its duration will be prolonged

(E) succinylcholine will behave as it did during the first rapid sequence induction in this patient

436. Drug clearance

(A) is solely a function of volume of distribution

(B) is a function of age

(C) is independent of protein binding of a drug

(D) is dependent on drug concentration

(E) may be due to elimination of an unchanged drug

437. Pharmacotherapy with cimetidine may impair the metabolism of which one of the following drugs?

(A) atracurium

(B) dopamine

(C) remifentanil

(D) lidocaine

(E) succinylcholine

438. Glucagon produces all of the following effects EXCEPT

(A) increased insulin secretion

(B) inotropic cardiac effects

(C) relaxation of gastrointestinal smooth muscle

(D) increased hepatic gluconeogenesis

(E) increased lipolysis in adipose tissue

439. Which one of the following statements regarding injectable benzodiazepines is most accurate?

(A) They significantly induce the synthesis of hepatic CYP isozymes.

(B) Administration of benzodiazepines is safe in patients with acute intermittent porphyria.

(C) They should be avoided in patients with a history of MH.

(D) They exert their therapeutic effect by increasing chloride conductance and hyperpolarizing membranes.

(E) Excessive sedation following IV administration of benzodiazepines should be antagonized with IV naloxone.

DIRECTIONS: Use the following figure to answer Questions 440-442:

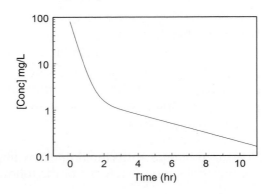

440. The figure shows the blood concentration of a drug as a function of time after an intravenous bolus of 400 mg. The volume of distribution of this medication in the central compartment is

(A) 5 L

(B) 8 L

(C) 10 L

(D) 12 L

(E) 15 L

441. The redistribution half-life for this drug is

(A) 5 min

(B) 10 min

(C) 15 min

(D) 20 min

(E) 30 min

442. The terminal half-life for this drug is

(A) 1 h

(B) 2 h

(C) 3 h

(D) 4 h

(E) 5 h

443. A patient who has had surgical ablation of the pituitary gland is scheduled for surgery. She is on desmopressin twice daily. The drug

(A) may be given intravenously during the procedure

(B) may lead to hypotension

(C) has a half-life of a few minutes in the circulation

(D) is equally effective in nephrogenic diabetes insipidus

(E) may increase blood loss at the time of surgery

444. Hydralazine

(A) is a vasodilator due to its catecholamine inhibitor properties

(B) may cause bradycardia

(C) may lead to a lupus-like syndrome

(D) leads to diuresis and sodium loss

(E) has beneficial effects in patients with angina

445. An age-related difference in drug response in the elderly is

(A) increase in MAC

(B) decreased rate of hepatic glucuronidation of morphine

(C) lower required induction dose of thiopental

(D) shorter recovery time to normal ventilatory response after fentanyl

(E) lower intubating dose of vecuronium

446. Nonparticulate antacid administration

(A) should be given 3 h before surgery

(B) decreases gastric volume

(C) may lead to pulmonary distress if aspiration occurs

(D) has a lag time of 1 hour for effectiveness

(E) is aimed at raising the pH to at least 2.5

447. A drug that is a mixed opioid agonist–antagonist is

(A) butorphanol

(B) naloxone

(C) bleomycin

(D) methohexital

(E) midazolam

448. Patients with alcohol abuse

(A) will have increased anesthetic requirements in the acute state of intoxication

(B) will have reduced anesthetic requirements in the chronic abuse state

(C) will develop tolerance to its CNS effects with chronic usage

(D) will develop tolerance to its respiratory effects with chronic usage

(E) are more resistant to the toxic effects of local anesthetics

449. A 24-year-old patient is undergoing brachial plexus blockade for open reduction and internal fixation of a forearm fracture. After injection of 30 mL of local anesthetic, blood is aspirated through the injection needle. Assuming significant inadvertent intravascular injection, which one of the following agents is least likely to cause Local Anesthetic Systemic Toxicity (LAST)?

(A) tetracaine

(B) chloroprocaine

(C) ropivacaine

(D) lidocaine

(E) mepivacaine

450. The pKa of mepivacaine is 7.6. At physiologic pH (7.4), what percentage of mepivacaine molecules are in the uncharged form?

(A) 3.9%

(B) 6.1%

(C) 39%

(D) 61%

(E) 100%

451. If a patient presenting for emergent craniotomy has increased intracranial pressure, which one of the following techniques is most likely to result in a net decrease in intracranial pressure by virtue of reducing cerebral blood flow?

(A) A combination of halogenated inhalational anesthetics with nitrous oxide

(B) Hyperventilation combined with a balanced anesthetic technique including the use of opioids

(C) Ketamine bolus for induction followed by continuous infusion, combined with a halogenated inhalational anesthetic

(D) Administration of a dobutamine

(E) Administration of phenylephrine

452. In the distribution phase of an intravenous drug,

(A) the delivery of the drug to tissues is independent of blood flow

(B) highly charged, lipid-insoluble drugs distribute to the vessel-rich group of tissues because of poor uptake by fat

(C) distribution to the vessel-poor group of tissues is facilitated by binding to plasma proteins

(D) the interstitial concentration of the drug is affected by the pH of the interstitial fluid

453. The loading dose of a drug

(A) is calculated based on the central volume of distribution (Vc)

(B) is designed to achieve immediate steady-state plasma concentration

(C) is not affected by the bioavailability (F) of the drug

(D) may lead to undesirable effects

454. Which one of the following statements about amiodarone is true?

(A) It is the drug of choice for the treatment of Wolff-Parkinson-White (WPW) syndrome.

(B) It is considered the most effective of the antiarrhythmic drugs for the prevention of recurrences of atrial fibrillation.

(C) Hypotension does not occur with intravenous administration.

(D) It should be avoided in the patient with refractory ventricular fibrillation and tachycardia.

(E) Drug toxicity during oral loading regimes is common, and mostly affects the kidneys.

455. A 78-year-old patient with past medical history of chronic renal insufficiency and congestive heart failure is admitted to the intensive care unit with symptoms of nausea, visual disturbances, confusion, and sinus bradycardia. The patient is unable to give a reliable history including medication regimen. Based on the patients' presentation, the drug most likely to cause these symptoms is

(A) amiodarone
(B) quinidine
(C) triazolam
(D) carvedilol
(E) digoxin

456. The decrease in cerebral metabolic rate caused by inhaled anesthetics is

(A) more pronounced with isoflurane as compared to sevoflurane

(B) independent of dose

(C) associated with a decrease in cerebral electrical activity

(D) present during seizure activity

(E) due to vasoconstriction and resulting decreased cerebral blood flow

457. A patient has been on oral steroid therapy for a dermatologic problem for two years. She is to undergo a cholecystectomy. In order to prevent secondary adrenal insufficiency, the most appropriate approach to perioperative steroid coverage would include which one of the following?

(A) hydrocortisone 100 mg PO at the time of oral benzodiazepine premedication

(B) 50-75 mg hydrocortisone IV at the time of induction

(C) 50-75 mg hydrocortisone IV at the time of induction, followed by a rapid taper back to the usual dose

(D) 25 mg hydrocortisone IV at the time of induction

(E) 100-150 mg hydrocortisone IV at the time of induction, followed by a rapid taper back to the usual dose

458. A 78-kg, 36-year-old patient is undergoing saphenous vein stripping of her left lower extremity. After uneventful induction of general anesthesia with placement of LMA, cefazolin 2 gm IV is being administered, when there is a sudden increase in airway pressure, wheezing, tachycardia, and decreased blood pressure. In addition to stopping infusion of cefazolin, an IV fluid bolus, and administration of 100% oxygen, which one of the following actions is most appropriate?

(A) administration of IV glucocorticoid and phenylephrine

(B) administration of subcutaneous epinephrine and IV glucocorticoid

(C) administration of diphenhydramine and ephedrine

(D) administration of IV epinephrine and IV glucocorticoid

(E) administration of IV dopamine and IV glucocorticoid

459. A 37-year-old patient with a history of chronic alcohol abuse is admitted to the hospital for palpitations. On examination, the patient appears weak and malnourished, and is complaining about muscle cramps. An ECG obtained is significant for polymorphic ventricular tachycardia with QT prolongation. An electrolyte panel obtained from a venous blood draw will most likely show which one of the following electrolyte abnormalities?

(A) hypochloremia

(B) hypocalcemia

(C) hyponatremia

(D) hyperkalemia

(E) hypomagnesemia

460. Opioid agonists produce

(A) dilated pupils

(B) nausea and vomiting mediated through the gastrointestinal tract

(C) good amnesia

(D) unconsciousness at high doses

461. A drug suitable for the patient with hyperthyroidism is

(A) amiodarone

(B) propranolol

(C) levothyroxine

(D) aspirin

462. Inhalational anesthetic-mediated coronary "steal"

(A) results in a higher incidence of perioperative ischemia when isoflurane is used in patients with coronary artery disease

(B) involves the diversion of blood flow away from areas of fixed stenotic lesions

(C) is a common problem under desflurane anesthesia

(D) is associated with increased postoperative mortality

(E) is a common problem under sevoflurane anesthesia

463. Corticosteroids given for the treatment of asthma

(A) have an immediate onset of action

(B) are best given by the inhalation route to decrease onset time

(C) have no use in the anesthetized patient

(D) should involve only those drugs with little mineralocorticoid effect

(E) are less effective in controlling inflammation as compared to inhaled β_2-agonists

464. An anesthetic agent with a prolonged duration of action in patients with renal failure is

(A) pancuronium for intubation

(B) fentanyl for analgesia

(C) maintenance of anesthesia with isoflurane

(D) propofol for induction

(E) etomidate for induction

465. Ionization of a drug

(A) is affected by volume of distribution

(B) is independent of the pKa of the drug

(C) is described by the Michaelis-Menten equation

(D) does not affect the ability of the drug to cross membranes

(E) is a function of pH of the fluid in which it is dissolved

466. A pharmacologic difference in the obese patient as compared to the lean patient is a(n)

(A) decreased degree of metabolism of isoflurane

(B) decreased terminal half-life of thiopental

(C) increased volume of distribution of midazolam

(D) prolonged duration of action of succinylcholine

(E) increased volume of distribution of digoxin

467. Granisetron exerts its therapeutic effect via which one of the following mechanisms?

(A) blockade of 5-HT$_3$ receptors in the chemoreceptor trigger zone

(B) histamine H$_2$-receptor antagonism

(C) blockade of dopaminergic receptors in the chemoreceptor trigger zone

(D) histamine H$_1$-receptor antagonism

(E) neurokinin receptor antagonism

468. A patient with acute intermittent porphyria

(A) voids urine containing uroporphyrins that are pathognomonic for the disease

(B) will likely suffer a cardiac arrest if administered thiopental for induction of anesthesia

(C) will have urine negative for porphobilinogen

(D) may be given morphine safely

469. A patient who has been treated in the past with high doses of cisplatin may have which one of the following permanent problems?

(A) pulmonary fibrosis

(B) chronic pancreatitis

(C) peripheral neuropathy

(D) congestive heart failure

(E) hepatic cirrhosis

470. A comparison of dissociative and inhalational anesthesia shows that

(A) the relaxed, nonresponding state is present in each

(B) there is decreased muscle tone in each

(C) the presence of movement is a sign of insufficient dosage in each

(D) the eyes may remain open during dissociative anesthesia

(E) complete unconsciousness is a hallmark feature of dissociative anesthesia

471. A patient is suspected to have had an allergic reaction to an injection of lidocaine obtained from a multiple dose vial. Which one of the following statements is most accurate?

(A) The patient will probably have a reaction if a second injection is made with lidocaine from a fresh, single-dose vial.

(B) The patient may be exhibiting a reaction to methylparaben.

(C) The risk of an allergic reaction to procaine in the same individual is low.

(D) The patient is probably reacting to a bacterial contaminant previously introduced into the vial.

(E) The reaction may be avoided by addition of a vasoconstrictor.

472. Captopril

(A) activates angiotensin-converting enzyme

(B) increases levels of angiotensin II

(C) decreases venous capacitance

(D) decreases arteriolar resistance

(E) increases cardiac contractility

473. Drug antagonism

(A) may occur when two drugs chemically combine in the body

(B) occurs when two drugs affect a physiologic system in a similar way

(C) is considered competitive when a drug with affinity for a receptor, and intrinsic efficacy competes with the agonist for the primary binding site

(D) may occur when two drugs displace the dose-response curve in the same direction

(E) when competitive, will decrease the maximal response of the agonist on the dose-response curve

DIRECTIONS: Use the following scenario to answer Questions 474–476: A 46-year-old, 63-kg woman enters the hospital for correction of strabismus. She has been using echothiophate iodide drops for 2 years. She undergoes induction of anesthesia with propofol 2.5 mg/kg and succinylcholine 1 mg/kg is given to facilitate intubation. Anesthesia is maintained with 70% N_2O in O_2 and fentanyl 1 mcg/kg. During the procedure she is mechanically ventilated, and no untoward effects occur during the case. At the end of the surgery, the patient does not awaken and does not move or breathe.

474. The most likely cause of the apparent prolonged anesthesia is

(A) fentanyl overdose

(B) prior use of echothiophate iodide

(C) effects of succinylmonocholine

(D) effect of nitrous oxide

(E) propofol overdose

475. A maneuver that can be done to ascertain the cause of the prolongation is

(A) use of a nerve stimulator

(B) inhalation of carbon dioxide

(C) administration of flumazenil

(D) administration of another dose of succinylcholine

476. Application of a nerve stimulator reveals that the patient has no twitch or tetanic response to nerve stimulation. Opioid antagonism with naloxone is attempted without response. The appropriate intervention is

(A) administration of pralidoxime

(B) administration of a stimulant (e.g., epinephrine)

(C) administration of neostigmine

(D) continued ventilation

(E) administration of physostigmine

477. Intramuscular injection

(A) into the gluteus maximus permits a more rapid onset than if the drug were injected into the deltoid muscle

(B) permits a more rapid onset than after subcutaneous injection

(C) results in the same rate of drug absorption between males and females

(D) cannot be used for nonaqueous solutions

(E) avoids first-pass elimination in the lung prior to distribution to the rest of the body

478. When reversing nondepolarizing neuromuscular blockade,

(A) atropine should be given at the same time as neostigmine

(B) glycopyrrolate should be given at the same time as edrophonium

(C) neostigmine should be titrated until reversal is complete, up to a maximum dose of 200 mcg/kg

(D) lack of fade during double-burst stimulation is a good indicator of sufficient muscular function to permit endotracheal extubation

(E) a TOF ratio = 0.7 indicates complete recovery of pharyngeal function

479. A 24-year-old female, G1 P0, with a history of CHF is presenting for cesarean section at 36 weeks gestation. Rapid sequence intubation facilitated by fentanyl, propofol, and succinylcholine is performed. Shortly after successful intubation of the trachea, the patient suffers cardiac arrest. The underlying disease most likely implied as the cause of the cardiac arrest is

(A) myasthenia gravis

(B) Duchenne muscular dystrophy

(C) hypokalemic periodic paralysis

(D) Charcot-Marie-Tooth disease

(E) myotonic dystrophy

480. The neuroleptic state is characterized by

(A) amnesia

(B) increased motor activity

(C) indifference to the environment

(D) analgesia

(E) loss of consciousness

481. Which one of the following agents has the highest propensity for producing carbon monoxide during inhalational anesthesia?

(A) isoflurane

(B) halothane

(C) sevoflurane

(D) desflurane

(E) enflurane

482. Two drugs are said to have an additive effect when

(A) one drug will accelerate the speed of onset of the other

(B) one drug will prolong the action of the other

(C) both drugs are of the same chemical family

(D) the combined effect of the two drugs is the algebraic sum of the individual actions

(E) the combined effect of the two drugs exceeds the sum of each drug given alone

DIRECTIONS: Use the following figure to answer Question 483:

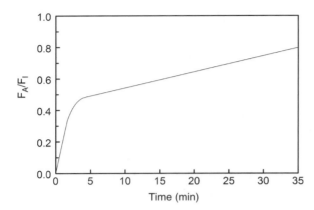

483. The figure shows the ratio of the concentrations of sevoflurane in alveolar gas to inspired gas as a function of time. A factor that will increase the initial slope is

(A) presence of nitrous oxide in inspired gas
(B) decreased inspired sevoflurane concentration
(C) decreased minute ventilation
(D) increased cardiac output
(E) pulmonary right-to-left shunting

484. Eaton–Lambert syndrome is characterized by

(A) decreased production of acetylcholine by the nerve cell
(B) decreased release of acetylcholine at the neuromuscular junction
(C) nondepolarizing neuromuscular blockade that is readily reversed by neostigmine
(D) decreased sensitivity to depolarizing muscle relaxants
(E) increased susceptibility to malignant hyperthermia

485. A patient is infected with *Clostridium perfringens* and has gas gangrene. Which one of the following drug regimens is considered first line for the treatment of this organism?

(A) parenteral penicillin G and parenteral clindamycin
(B) parenteral cefoxitin and parenteral imipenem

(C) oral levofloxacin and oral cephalexin
(D) parenteral gentamicin and parenteral vancomycin
(E) oral penicillin V and parenteral amikacin

486. A 56-year-old, 85-kg patient with a history of gastroduodenal ulcers is presenting for elective resection of the sigmoid colon for chronic diverticulitis. The patient is premedicated with 10 mg diazepam orally, and undergoes placement of an epidural catheter in the midthoracic area for postoperative pain control. Induction of anesthesia is performed with propofol 2 mg/kg, fentanyl 2 mcg/kg, and rocuronium 0.6 mg/kg. Anesthesia is maintained with desflurane in nitrous oxide and oxygen. At the conclusion of an uncomplicated case, the patient is noted to have prolonged emergence from anesthesia, and appears oversedated after tracheal extubation, despite full recovery from neuromuscular blockade. Which one of the following is the most likely cause?

(A) administration of desflurane
(B) chronic therapy with cimetidine
(C) chronic ingestion of ethanol
(D) fentanyl overdose
(E) diazepam overdose

487. The metabolism of nitrous oxide in humans

(A) yields nitric oxide as the main product
(B) occurs in the liver
(C) is a reductive process
(D) is increased by phenobarbital pretreatment
(E) occurs in the lungs

488. When methylmethacrylate (MMA) cement is used to secure the femoral component of a hip prosthesis in the femoral canal,

(A) hypertension is a common occurrence
(B) acute vasodilation and cardiac collapse can occur due to hypersensitivity reaction to MMA
(C) cardiovascular collapse and bronchoconstriction may occur due to embolization of fat particles and debris from the intramedullary canal

(D) the patient should have a central venous catheter for the removal of an air embolus

(E) the technique of venting the canal can reliably prevent cardiovascular compromise during the procedure

489. Ondansetron

(A) facilitates gastric emptying

(B) decreases gastroesophageal reflux

(C) is sedating at higher doses

(D) has antiemetic effects

(E) acts on dopaminergic receptors in the area postrema

DIRECTIONS: Use the following figure to answer Question 490:

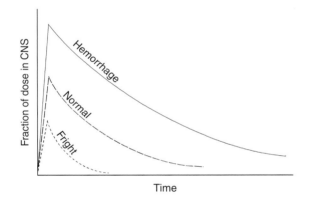

490. The figure depicts the relative effect of propofol in three physiologic states. From this we can say that

(A) the potency of propofol in the anxious patient is increased

(B) the anxious patient will require a larger dose

(C) a patient in shock will have a decreased effect from propofol

(D) the bleeding patient has a faster decrease in brain concentration as a result of the propofol being lost with the blood

(E) the anxious patient will have loss of consciousness sooner after IV bolus, as compared to the bleeding patient

491. A recommended single-agent perioperative prophylaxis regimen against a surgical site infection for patient populations with low incidence of methicillin-resistant *Staphylococcus aureus* (MRSA) is

(A) penicillin G

(B) vancomycin

(C) cefazolin

(D) ampicillin

(E) levofloxacin

492. Carbon monoxide

(A) when bound to hemoglobin can be differentiated from oxyhemoglobin by standard pulse oximetry

(B) causes oxygen to be released less efficiently from hemoglobin in tissues

(C) does not produce toxicity in the presence of an increased FIO_2

(D) combines and dissociates from hemoglobin at a rate equal to that of oxygen

(E) leads to a right-shift of the oxygen-hemoglobin dissociation curve

493. An active transmembrane transport mechanism is

(A) transport via filtration

(B) channel mediated diffusion

(C) passive nonionic diffusion

(D) transport of solute by carrier protein down an electrochemical gradient

(E) saturable

494. An active metabolite of heroin is

(A) thebaine

(B) morphine

(C) hydromorphone

(D) codeine

(E) apomorphine

495. Low-molecular-weight heparins

    (A) are pentasaccharides
    (B) cause a lower incidence of heparin-induced thrombocytopenia than unfractionated heparin
    (C) are administered intravenously
    (D) all have equivalent antithrombotic effects
    (E) are able to bridge antithrombin to thrombin to the same extent as unfractionated heparin

496. A 42-year-old female is admitted to the hospital approximately 18 h after supposedly ingesting a large quantity of an unknown drug in tablet form. The patient appears confused, tachypneic, complains about nausea and tinnitus, and is febrile at 39°C. Pupils are equal bilaterally at 3 mm and reactive. Shortly after arrival, the patient starts to vomit. Blood gas analysis is significant for a mixed picture consisting of respiratory alkalosis and metabolic acidosis. The patients' symptoms are most consistent with drug overdose from

    (A) acetaminophen
    (B) aspirin
    (C) oxycodone
    (D) diphenhydramine
    (E) lithium

497. Of the following metabolic reactions, which one is most likely to be catalyzed by cytochrome P450?

    (A) acetylation of hydralazine
    (B) demethylation of ketamine
    (C) conjugation of morphine to glucuronide
    (D) oxidative deamination of norepinephrine
    (E) conjugation of acetaminophen to sulfate

498. In a patient who is physically dependent on morphine, which one of the following is a symptom of the abstinence syndrome that begins within 12 h of the last dose of morphine?

    (A) bradycardia
    (B) lacrimation
    (C) seizures
    (D) pilomotor activity ("gooseflesh")
    (E) coma

499. A 72-year-old man with a history of congestive heart failure presents for evaluation of acute renal insufficiency. On evaluation, the patient also complains about a loss of sense of taste and a chronic cough. Urinalysis is significant for proteinuria. He was started on a new antihypertensive medication a few months ago. The drug most likely implied in his symptoms is

    (A) carvedilol
    (B) hydralazine
    (C) labetalol
    (D) nifedipine
    (E) captopril

500. The rapidly perfused (vessel-rich) tissues

    (A) include the kidneys
    (B) receive an increasing proportion of cardiac output with increasing age
    (C) receive the same proportion of cardiac output in the neonate as the vessel-poor group
    (D) include muscle
    (E) account for 30% of total body weight in adults

501. Ketorolac 60 mg and morphine 10 mg produce approximately equivalent magnitudes of which one of the following effects after intramuscular injection?

    (A) nausea
    (B) sedation
    (C) ventilatory depression
    (D) analgesia
    (E) abdominal pain

502. The CNS response to an induction dose of propofol would be most altered by which one of the following conditions?

(A) obesity

(B) hypoalbuminemia

(C) advanced age

(D) renal failure

(E) hypovolemia due to blood loss

503. Which one of the following statements regarding the CNS effects of halogenated volatile anesthetics is most accurate?

(A) Isoflurane, in contrast to halothane, abolishes autoregulation

(B) Halothane can produce an isoelectric EEG at clinically relevant doses

(C) Isoflurane lowers the ischemic threshold for EEG changes

(D) Isoflurane decreases cerebral blood flow

(E) Sevoflurane decreases epileptic brain activity

504. Lamotrigine

(A) is an atypical antipsychotic drug

(B) has a prolonged half-life when pentobarbital, carbamazepine, or phenytoin are administered concomitantly

(C) is not effective in absence epilepsy

(D) is effective against a broader spectrum of seizures than phenytoin and carbamazepine

(E) is not metabolized in humans

505. A 42-year-old patient with alcohol induced liver cirrhosis, Child-Pugh class B, underwent operative repair of a femur fracture sustained in a motor vehicle accident under general anesthesia. There were no other associated injuries. Induction of anesthesia was performed with propofol, fentanyl, and cisatracurium, and the anesthesia was maintained with sevoflurane in oxygen and nitrous oxide. After uneventful postoperative extubation and recovery, the patient is transferred to the floor. Three days later, the orthopedics team consults you to evaluate the patient for jaundice, lethargy, and signs of encephalopathy. The patient most likely suffered intraoperative hepatocellular injury due to

(A) immune reaction associated with sevoflurane administration

(B) sevoflurane-mediated decreased hepatic blood flow

(C) hepatotoxic effects of propofol

(D) hepatotoxic effects of nitrous oxide

(E) hepatotoxic effects of sevoflurane

506. A drugs that may suppress the symptoms of opioid withdrawal is

(A) butorphanol

(B) chlorpromazine

(C) nalbuphine

(D) clonidine

(E) flumazenil

507. Emergence sequelae with ketamine include delirium and dreaming that

(A) are always of an unpleasant nature

(B) are caused by $GABA_A$ antagonism of ketamine

(C) are not remembered because of the amnestic effects of ketamine

(D) can be minimized by giving a benzodiazepine

(E) occur equally across all age groups

508. Omeprazole

(A) in typical doses diminishes the daily acid production by approximately 70%

(B) inhibits the metabolism of some medications by cytochrome P450

(C) facilitates gastric emptying

(D) decreases the volume of gastric juice

(E) is a histamine H_2-receptor antagonist

509. A 42-year-old schoolteacher underwent trans-abdominal hysterectomy for endometrial carcinoma. Her past medical history is significant for vitamin B_{12} deficiency diagnosed three years ago and is otherwise unremarkable. According to the patient, she is in excellent health because of her strictly vegan diet. The case was conducted under general anesthesia with propofol, fentanyl, and vecuronium for induction, followed by isoflurane, nitrous oxide, and oxygen for maintenance of anesthesia. After four hours of surgery, the patient was extubated and transferred to the PACU. On the third postoperative day, you are called to evaluate the patient on the floor because she has developed signs of lower extremity paresthesias and has an unsteady gait. Which one of the anesthetics used for induction and/or maintenance of anesthesia could have a role in this patient's symptoms?

(A) propofol
(B) isoflurane
(C) vecuronium
(D) nitrous oxide
(E) fentanyl

510. Histamine H_2 antagonists administered in the immediate preoperative period

(A) facilitate gastric emptying
(B) should be used in all patients
(C) increase the pH of fluid in the stomach at the time of administration
(D) protect against aspiration of gastric juice
(E) do not change the need for a cuffed tube

511. Which one of the following drugs is considered unsafe for the patient known to be susceptible to malignant hyperthermia?

(A) nitrous oxide
(B) succinylcholine
(C) xenon
(D) ketamine
(E) atracurium

512. An antihypertensive that interacts with the renin-angiotensin system is

(A) losartan
(B) prazosin
(C) nesiritide
(D) minoxidil
(E) hydralazine

DIRECTIONS: Use the following figure to answer Questions 513-514:

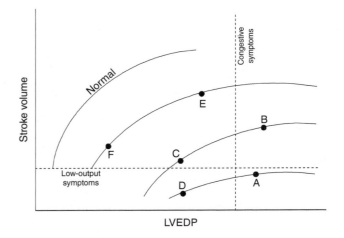

513. The position on the ventricular function (Frank-Starling) curve for a patient with systolic heart failure is depicted as point A in the figure. Administration of nicardipine would move the patient's ventricular function

(A) from A to C
(B) from A to B
(C) from A to normal
(D) from A to D
(E) from A to E

514. Administration of which one of the following drugs, or drug combinations, is most likely to move this patient's ventricular function from point A to point F?

(A) dobutamine
(B) dobutamine and furosemide
(C) nitroprusside
(D) dobutamine and losartan
(E) dobutamine, losartan, and furosemide

515. Fospropofol

(A) has a rapid onset of action after IV administration

(B) is a prodrug

(C) has a high volume of distribution

(D) is associated with pain on injection

(E) is administered as a bolus of 2 mg/kg for procedural sedation

516. Which one of the following agents will lead to a decrease in pulmonary vascular resistance through interaction with the endothelin-A receptor (ET_A) on vascular smooth muscle?

(A) inhaled nitric oxide

(B) epoprostenol

(C) sildenafil

(D) treprostinil

(E) bosentan

DIRECTIONS (Questions 517-520): Each group of items below consists of lettered headings followed by a list of numbered phrases or statements. For each numbered phrase or statement, select the ONE lettered heading or component that is most closely associated with it and fill in the circle containing the corresponding letter on the answer sheet. Each lettered heading or component may be selected once, more than once, or not at all.

(A) α_1-adrenoceptor

(B) α_2-adrenoceptor

(C) β_1-adrenoceptor

(D) β_2-adrenoceptor

(E) Na,K-ATPase

(F) PDE3

(G) PDE4

(H) PDE5

(I) AT_1

(J) AT_2

(K) V_1

For each medication, select the receptor or enzyme most responsible for its pharmacological effect.

517. antidiuretic hormone

518. inamrinone

519. sildenafil

520. valsartan

DIRECTIONS (Questions 521-523): Each group of items below consists of lettered headings followed by a list of numbered phrases or statements. For each numbered phrase or statement, select the ONE lettered heading or component that is most closely associated with it and fill in the circle containing the corresponding letter on the answer sheet. Each lettered heading or component may be selected once, more than once, or not at all.

(A) glomerulus

(B) proximal tubule

(C) descending limb of loop of Henle

(D) thin ascending limb of loop of Henle

(E) thick ascending limb of loop of Henle

(F) distal convoluted tubule

(G) collecting duct

For each diuretic, select the portion of the nephron most responsible for its pharmacological effect.

521. spironolactone

522. acetazolamide

523. furosemide

Answers and Explanations

366. **(E)** Use of heparin in a patient with heparin induced thrombocytopenia type II can lead to life-threatening thrombotic complications and is therefore not indicated. Low-molecular-weight heparins can cross-react with heparin and should also be avoided. Warfarin should not be used until the thrombocytopenia has resolved because it can cause venous limb gangrene or multicentric skin necrosis. Tirofiban is an antiplatelet drug that acts by inhibition of the glycoprotein IIb/IIIa receptor. Fondaparinux is a synthetic five-saccharide analog of a natural pentasaccharide sequence that is found in heparin and LMWHs and mediates their interaction with antithrombin. It has no intrinsic anticoagulant activity and instead it binds to antithrombin and accelerates the rate at which it inhibits various coagulation proteases. Its potency is assessed with an anti Xa assay. Other suitable alternatives would be lepirudin, bivalirudin, or argatroban. (*1:854, 859*)

367. **(B)** Drug elimination may occur by metabolism or excretion and is usually complete after five half-lives. Polar compounds are usually excreted more efficiently than substances with high lipid solubility. An example on how pharmacologic intervention can influence the rate of elimination from the body is alkalinization or acidification of the urine to hasten the excretion of some drugs in the treatment of drug poisoning. Protein binding of a drug to blood and tissues will affect the rate of elimination from the body. (*1:26-30*)

368. **(D)** Sevoflurane is not known to cause hepatotoxicity and it is not flammable. The agent produces good muscle relaxation, does not produce tachycardia and may be a preferable agent in patients prone to myocardial ischemia. Sevoflurane is metabolized in the liver by the cytochrome P450 system. (*1:546*)

369. **(D)** Barbiturates do not have a clinically relevant analgesic effect. Thiopental produces a dose-dependent effect on the EEG. If given in small doses for sedation, median EEG frequency increases because the predominant EEG activity changes from α to β waves. High doses of the drug can cause burst suppression, characterized by δ waves alternating with electrical inactivity. Methohexital may cause abnormal spiking activity of the EEG, and may elicit seizures in patients with seizure disorder. Thiopental injection is followed by decreased blood pressure and increased heart rate. Coronary blood flow is increased. Stroke volume is decreased, as is cardiac output. (*5:694*)

370. **(B)** Ketamine administration is associated with changes in cardiovascular parameters similar to those seen with sympathetic stimulation. Therefore, the heart rate is increased, and there is an increase in cardiac output. (*1:539*)

371. **(C)** The hypotension that may be seen after atracurium administration is due to histamine release, and may be exaggerated in a patient with hypovolemia. The extent of histamine release is dependent on the dose and the speed of injection. Atracurium does not cause clinically significant ganglionic blockade. Laudanosine, a metabolite of atracurium, can cause cerebral excitation and seizure activity in animal models; however, this has not been a clinical problem in humans. (*5:503*)

372. **(C)** Rocuronium is metabolized and eliminated by the liver. It can be administered intramuscularly and by continuous infusion and does not cause significant histamine release or ganglionic blockade. (*1:262; 5:504*)

373. **(C)** Drug metabolism is separated into two distinct phases, and usually results in a decreased duration of action because the drug is rendered inactive, more water soluble, more readily excreted by tubular secretion, and less likely to undergo tubular reabsorption. Reactions in phase I are most likely to consist of oxidation, reduction, or hydrolysis reactions, and generally result in the loss of pharmacological activity. Phase II reactions include conjugation reactions, aimed at facilitating the excretion of inactive drug metabolites. (*1:27-8*)

374. **(E)** Transdermal scopolamine is a muscarinic antagonist that can cross the blood–brain barrier. It is not recommended for the prophylaxis of emesis in children and can produce behavioral side effects. It has, however, been shown to be useful in adults if applied on the evening before, or 4 hours before the end of the operative procedure. (*1:230; 5:1256*)

375. **(C)** Naloxone is a pure opioid antagonist, meaning that the drug has no opioid effect of its own. Butorphanol and levallorphan are both mixed opioid agonist–antagonists. Neostigmine and edrophonium are cholinesterase inhibitors. (*1:483-4*)

376. **(C)** Milrinone is a vasodilating and inotropic agent thought to function through inhibiting phosphodiesterase and thereby elevating cyclic-AMP levels. It is not a catecholamine. (*1:795*)

377. **(C)** The toxicity associated with bupivacaine is due to blockade of sodium channels. The drug is an amide of long duration. It should not be used in concentrations above 0.5% for epidural anesthesia in pregnant patients. Toxicity may occur after injection other than intravenously. (*1:573; 5:1149*)

378. **(D)** Tetracaine is rarely used in peripheral nerve blocks because of the large doses that are typically required, its slow onset, and its potential for toxicity that is greater than chloroprocaine. Bupivacaine is more cardiotoxic than equieffective doses of lidocaine. Clinical manifestations of toxicity include severe ventricular arrhythmias and myocardial depression after inadvertent intravascular injection. The block of cardiac sodium channels is cumulative, and substantially more than would be predicted by its local anesthetic potency. Chloroprocaine is very short-acting, and probably not a good choice for the patient described in this vignette where postoperative analgesia from the brachial plexus blockade would be desirable. The duration of action of mepivacaine is about 20% longer than that of lidocaine. (*1:573-4; 5:824*)

379. **(A)** Etomidate has anticonvulsant activity, and it decreases intraocular pressure. There is no histamine release and it does not have any analgesic effects. Etomidate produces a higher incidence of postoperative nausea and vomiting than other intravenous induction agents. (*5:696-7*)

380. **(A)** The renal tubule has active transport processes for the tubular secretion of organic acids, such as glucuronides, and organic bases. Since the glucuronide derivative is likely to be much more polar than the parent compound, the rate of tubular reabsorption (which usually occurs by passive nonionic diffusion) will be less. (*1:26*)

381. **(D)** The correct ranking of the potencies of the volatile anesthetics, from most potent to least potent, is halothane > isoflurane > sevoflurane > desflurane. (*5:598*)

382. **(A)** A has higher efficacy than B because the maximum response produced by A is greater than the maximum response produced by B. Because A and B are located at the same place along the X-axis, A and B are said to have the same potency. The dose at which the half-maximal response occurs, the ED_{50}, is the same for both A and B. It is likely that A and B act via the same receptor. (*1:48-9*)

383. **(B)** The effect of drug Y is to decrease the efficacy of X without shifting the dose-response relationship of X. This is the definition of a noncompetitive antagonist. It is likely that X and Y act via the same receptor. (*1:46-7*)

384. **(C)** Administering succinylcholine to a patient with a massive burn may result in an exaggerated hyperkalemic response that can cause cardiac arrest. The recommendation is to avoid succinylcholine in these patients starting about 24 h after the burn. The pharmacokinetics of succinylcholine however will not be altered. Patients treated with inhibitors of cholinesterase (neostigmine, pyridostigmine, isofluorophate) or who have atypical cholinesterase will experience a prolonged succinylcholine effect. Aminoglycosides can produce neuromuscular blockade by inhibition of acetylcholine release from the preganglionic terminal, and to a lesser extent, by noncompetitively blocking the receptor. This effect however would be more likely in the patient described in the vignette had the patient received a nondepolarizing muscle relaxant during the case. In addition, the combination of a muscle relaxant with an aminoglycoside increases the incidence of myopathies in critically ill patients. (*1:267; 5:1345, 1392*)

385. **(B)** The MAC for desflurane is about 6% and it is irritating to airways. It is insoluble in water and lipids and is metabolized to a lesser extent than other halogenated anesthetics. (*1:545; 5:598*)

386. **(A)** The known heroin abuser may have a full stomach due to the slower emptying time of the gastrointestinal tract, and may be highly tolerant to opioids, necessitating higher doses of anesthetics to achieve adequate analgesia and sedation/hypnosis. Left ventricular hypertrophy can be expected in abusers of hallucinogens such as phencyclidine or LSD. Recent cocaine abuse can increase sensitivity to catecholamines. The so called "glue-sniffer's neuropathy" can be caused by inhalation of hexane-containing adhesives. (*5:326-7*)

387. **(D)** Local anesthetics act at the nerve membrane. The local anesthetics block sodium channels so that the membrane cannot conduct nerve impulses. (*1:565-7*)

388. **(D)** The action of propofol is terminated by redistribution. The drug is bound to protein, and various concomitant drugs may interfere with binding. It is taken up in fatty tissues, but that is not the mechanism of terminating its effect. (*5:691*)

389. **(A)** Methohexital is metabolized to a greater extent than thiopental. The drug is metabolized to hydroxymethohexital that is inactive. The terminal half-life is shorter than that of thiopental. Methohexital does not release histamine from mast cells and is not contraindicated in asthma. (*1:533-5; 5:731*)

390. **(C)** The first-pass effect is the biotransformation of a drug as it passes through the intestinal mucosa and liver. In some cases, much of the pharmacological activity is lost at this point, leaving little of the drug to have its desired effect. (*1:20*)

391. **(B)** Ketamine administration is associated with increases in both systolic and diastolic blood pressures. The mechanism for the increases is direct central nervous system stimulation as well as the liberation of catecholamines. (*1:539*)

392. **(A)** The small blocking dose of a nondepolarizing muscle relaxant given before an intubating dose of succinylcholine increases both the dose of succinylcholine required as well as the time to the onset of muscle paralysis. The rise in intracranial pressure is attenuated, but there is no effect on succinylcholine-induced arrhythmias. The time to recovery is not affected. (*1:261; 5:501*)

393. **(C)** After one half-life has elapsed, 50% of the drug remains; after two half-lives, 25%; after three half-lives, 12.5%; after four half-lives, 6.25%; and after five half-lives, 3.125%. (*6:35*)

394. **(A)** Flecainide is an antiarrhythmic drug in Class IC. The drug is not a muscle relaxant and can be administered orally or parenterally. It is not the drug of choice for local anesthetic reactions. *(1:840)*

395. **(D)** Administration of anticholinesterase drugs will reverse the block of a nondepolarizing agent only if the latter drug is in low enough concentration. Administration of an anticholinesterase will prolong the block of succinylcholine by inhibiting its metabolism. *(1:266-7)*

396. **(E)** Of the nondepolarizing muscle relaxants mentioned, the least desirable agent would be pancuronium due to its prolonged terminal half-life in renal failure. The intermediate–acting muscle relaxants have a shorter duration of action even in the presence of renal failure. *(5:504)*

397. **(D)** While all of the options are indicators of recovery, an objective measurement of recovery from neuromuscular block is better than a clinical assessment. Double-burst stimulation (DBS) with mechano-, electro-, or accelero-myography is the method of choice. If this is unavailable, tactile response to double-burst stimulation (DBS) is preferable to tactile estimation of the train-of-four ratio because it is easier to appreciate fade with DBS. Normal tidal volume is not sufficient to protect the airway; there must be enough force to generate a cough, and about 15 mL/kg are needed. Handgrip is a clinical assessment and must be sustained to correlate with recovery. Inspiratory force is a good measurement and should be at least 25 cm H_2O negative pressure. The advantage of inspiratory force is that it can be assessed in the patient who is still asleep and unable to respond. *(5:494-6)*

398. **(A)** Anticholinesterase drugs have potent muscarinic stimulating effects. These may be exhibited in the heart, bronchioles, or gut. It is important to consider each of these areas in the particular patient whose relaxants are being

reversed. Atropine or glycopyrrolate should be used with the reversal drug. Although the muscarinic manifestations are not common, their occurrence may be quite troublesome, such as the production of copious respiratory secretions. *(1:246-7)*

399. **(C)** The antithrombin III–heparin complex inactivates thrombin and the other proteases of the intrinsic clotting pathway. *(1:854)*

400. **(D)** The patient with myasthenia gravis has an altered sensitivity to relaxants. These patients are more sensitive to nondepolarizing agents. This sensitivity is present with or without control of the disease. These patients may also be resistant to depolarizing relaxants, particularly those treated with pyridostigmine. *(5:143)*

401. **(B)** Labetalol is a competitive antagonist at both, α_1-, and β-adrenoceptors. In addition, the drug has partial agonist activity at β_2-adrenoceptors, and inhibits neuronal uptake of norepinephrine (a cocaine-like effect). The potency for β-blockade is 5-10 fold greater than for α_1-blockade. Labetalol is suitable for the treatment of hypertensive emergencies, and maintains cardiac output, while maintaining, or slightly lowering, heart rate. Due to the poor lipid solubility of labetalol there is very little placental transfer, and the drug is safe for use in the setting of pregnancy-induced hypertensive crisis. *(1:328-9)*

402. **(A)** Flumazenil is the drug of choice for the reversal of high doses of benzodiazepines. While physostigmine may be effective in reversing the sedative effects of benzodiazepines, it is not considered the first-line agent. The drug crosses the blood–brain barrier well since it is a tertiary amine. It is used in the treatment of central anticholinergic syndrome and can cause hypersalivation. *(1:245-6, 461; 5:699, 1461)*

403. **(B)** Lisinopril is an inhibitor of angiotensin-converting enzyme used in the therapy of hypertension. *(1:731-2)*

404. (E) Amiodarone is a recommended pharmacologic treatment for mono- or polymorphic ventricular tachycardia in patients with structural heart disease. Sotalol is considered another first-line agent. The nonpharmacologic treatment of choice would be synchronized cardioversion. Amiodarone is also effective against most supraventricular arrhythmias, but has a number of serious toxicities, some of which are due to the drug's structural similarity to thyroid hormone. (*1:43; 6:1893, 1911*)

405. (A) Fexofenadine is a second-generation histamine H_1-receptor antagonist used to treat allergic conditions such as hay fever. It does not appreciably cross the blood-brain barrier and therefore lacks sedative effects. (*1:920*)

406. (B) Budesonide is an inhaled corticosteroid (ICS) used for the management and control of asthma. ICS are the most effective anti-inflammatory agents used in asthma therapy, reducing inflammatory cell numbers and their activation in the airways. (*1:1051; 6:2111*)

407. (C) Dofetilide is a class III antiarrhythmic agent that is an action potential-prolonging drug. It is effective in maintaining sinus rhythm in patients with atrial fibrillation. (*6:1883*)

408. (B) Allopurinol is an inhibitor of xanthine oxidase that decreases uric acid formation. It is used in the therapy of gout. (*1:996*)

409. (D) The most useful drug to add to this regimen is dexamethasone that has been shown to be effective either as a first-line agent, or in combination with 5-HT$_3$ receptor antagonists and/or droperidol. Metoclopramide is a short-acting prokinetic agent mainly used to ameliorate nausea and vomiting that accompany gastrointestinal dysmotility syndromes. Prochlorperazine should not be administered since the patient has already received a D_2 receptor blocker (droperidol). Famotidine is an H_2-receptor antagonist and not indicated for the prevention or treatment of PONV. Ephedrine is a non-catecholamine α- and β-adrenergic agonist and is a potent CNS stimulant; it is not recommended for the prevention or treatment of PONV. Additional considerations may include TIVA, as well as administration of a preoperative transdermal scopolamine patch, as well as oral aprepitant for the highest risk patients. (*1:233-4; 5:77-8*)

410. (B) The patient is partially paralyzed. The block that is present is not a depolarizing block. The train-of-four ratio is 75% and therefore the patient could not sustain a head lift. The advantage of the train-of-four is that it is not necessary to have a control tracing, since it serves as its own control. (*5:495-6*)

411. (E) The train-of-four ratio for a depolarizing block is 100%, since there is no fade. The fourth twitch will be as high as the first. (*5:500*)

412. (A) Excitatory phenomena after propofol induction occur more frequently than with thiopental, however, bronchospasm appears to occur less frequently. In equipotent doses, propofol produces a dose dependent decrease in blood pressure that is more pronounced than with thiopental administration. Propofol and thiopental cause a similar decrease in cerebral metabolic rate. Adrenal suppression occurs after the administration of etomidate. (*1:537; 5:689-90, 697*)

413. (D) Verapamil is a calcium channel blocker. All drugs in this class are highly bound to protein. Calcium channel blockers increase coronary blood flow, and decrease myocardial contractility. Verapamil, in combination with inhalational agents may produce varying degrees of AV-block. Structurally, it is a phenylalkylamine compound; representatives of the dihydropyridines include nifedipine, amlodipine, nimodipine, and nicardipine. (*1:755-7; 5:757*)

414. (E) Lepirudin and argatroban are direct thrombin inhibitors. (*1:874*)

415. (D) When meperidine is given to a patient on a monoamine oxidase inhibitor, hyperpyrexia and CNS excitation, which may be fatal, may result. Local anesthetics, halothane, vecuronium, and aspirin should not cause problems. (*1:504*)

416. **(A)** Hypokalemic, hypochloremic metabolic alkalosis is one of the most common problems in the patient being treated with thiazides. Hyperuricemia may occur, but it is not as common as hypokalemia. Hyponatremia and hyperglycemia also may occur. *(1:689)*

417. **(B)** Nifedipine is effective for coronary vasospasm due to its vasodilating activity. It has no antiarrhythmic effect. Its half-life is about 4 h. *(1:757-8)*

418. **(B)** The binding of protamine, a basic protein, and heparin, an acidic protein, results in a compound with no anticoagulation effect. There is no other mechanism involved. *(1:858)*

419. **(B)** Epinephrine causes vasoconstriction, which leads to decreased absorption of the local anesthetic, thus prolonging its effect. This action may also delay metabolism. Protein binding, chemical interaction, and binding site competition are not involved. *(5:776)*

420. **(C)** The combination of nitrous oxide in 0.5 MAC concentration and isoflurane in 0.5 MAC concentration will lead to an anesthetic effect of 1 MAC. For all practical purposes, nitrous oxide and a halogenated agent are the only agents that are administered together, but if 2 halogenated agents could be used together, their effect would be additive. *(1:50; 5:598)*

421. **(A)** Glycopyrrolate is a quaternary amine that is an anticholinergic agent. It is a synthetic alkaloid, and not naturally-occurring like atropine and scopolamine. Since it is a quaternary amine, it does not cross the blood–brain barrier and is not associated with the central cholinergic syndrome. *(1:233; 5:976)*

422. **(A)** Although well absorbed from the gastrointestinal tract, lidocaine is extensively metabolized on its first pass through the liver. The symptoms of toxicity are usually CNS stimulation, and usually occur at blood levels greater than 5 mcg/mL. Lidocaine is useful in ventricular arrhythmias. *(1:572-3; 5:781)*

423. **(E)** The interaction of phenytoin and phenobarbital is one of altered metabolism due to enzyme induction. If a patient has a stable drug level, it can be changed by starting another drug that may induce the enzyme system that metabolizes the first drug. *(1:592)*

424. **(C)** Midazolam is associated with fewer cases of venous irritation than diazepam. The drug is not contraindicated in children; in fact, it is very useful in children. The duration is longer than that of thiopental. There is no adrenal cortical depression and no histamine release. *(1:466; 5:698-9)*

425. **(B)** The patient showing signs of cocaine toxicity may be excited, anxious, and restless, and have hypertension and tachycardia. *(1:662; 5:324-5)*

426. **(A)** The methylxanthine group of drugs includes caffeine. This group has strong β_2-adrenergic-like effects such as bronchodilation but does not act via β_2-adrenergic receptors. The mechanism of action is by phosphodiesterase inhibition that leads to an increase in cyclic AMP. *(1:663)*

427. **(C)** Sublingual administration avoids the first-pass effect and bypasses the liver. This route is not useful with all drugs, only those that are unionized (e.g., nitroglycerin). This route leads to higher blood levels compared to oral administration. *(1:22)*

428. **(C)** Metoclopramide stimulates upper gastrointestinal motility. It is an antiemetic and has no effect on acid secretion in the stomach. Transit time is shorter and there is no ileus, since motility is stimulated. *(1:1325)*

429. **(D)** Hetastarch is a synthetic colloid. The other options all include administration of blood products. Some people of this belief will accept blood that is autologous while others will require that the blood be in the circuit continuously (e.g., in a cell saver). It is important to understand the particular patient's requirements before undertaking the procedure. *(5:46)*

430. **(C)** Vasopressin is recommended in the ACLS guidelines as an alternative agent to epinephrine in cases of refractory ventricular fibrillation and pulseless ventricular tachycardia. Because of its potential adverse effects, sodium bicarbonate should not be routinely administered during CPR. Phenylephrine, adenosine, and isoproterenol are not recommended for the treatment of refractory ventricular fibrillation. (*5:1433-4*)

431. **(E)** Edrophonium should be given with, or preceded by, atropine. The drug has a fast onset but, in the dose cited, a duration as long as neostigmine. The muscarinic effects are fewer than with neostigmine. (*1:239-243, 549*)

432. **(D)** Sodium nitroprusside may lead to cyanide toxicity that may be manifested as acidosis and a tolerance to the drug's effects. This drug affects both venous and arterial vessels. The acidosis that is seen is treated by stopping the drug and should not be treated with sodium bicarbonate. The hypotensive effect of sodium nitroprusside is potentiated by prior treatment with β-adrenergic antagonists. (*1:782-3; 5:746*)

433. **(D)** Postoperative pain control with methadone requires some time to obtain stable levels. While single small doses (< 10 mg) may have a duration of action less than an hour due to redistribution, larger doses are much longer-acting. Methadone is usually given in twice daily dosage, and does depress respiration. The oral dose is about 80-90% as effective as the same parenteral dose. (*5:718*)

434. **(D)** Dopamine has different actions depending on the dosage: at infusion rates greater than 10 mcg/kg/min, there is stimulation of α-adrenergic receptors. At lower infusion rates (approximately 1–3 mcg/kg/min), dopaminergic receptors are stimulated that leads to an increase in renal blood flow. Dopamine causes an increase in pulmonary artery pressure, making it a poor choice in the patient with right heart failure. Dopamine is a transmitter in both the central and peripheral nervous systems. (*1:355; 5:175*)

435. **(D)** The sequence that is proposed may result in a prolonged duration of succinylcholine action because the prior administration of neostigmine will result in pseudocholinesterase inhibition and decreased succinylcholine metabolism. (*5:500*)

436. **(E)** Drug clearance may occur by metabolism to inactive or less active products or by elimination of the unchanged drug. Clearance is independent of drug concentration, and is not a function of age; rather it is affected by volume of distribution that often is decreasing with increasing age. Similarly, the degree of protein binding is an important determinant of the rate of drug clearance. (*1:33*)

437. **(D)** Cimetidine may decrease the metabolism of lidocaine via inhibition of cytochrome P450. The other drugs listed are not metabolized by cytochrome P450. (*1:1314; 5:1033*)

438. **(A)** Glucagon inhibits insulin secretion and increases plasma glucose levels. (*1:1237, 1240*)

439. **(D)** Injectable benzodiazepines such as diazepam, lorazepam and midazolam do not induce the synthesis of hepatic CYP isozymes. They are safe to administer in patients with a history of MH, however, should be avoided in patients with acute intermittent porphyria because they have been shown to induce ALA synthase in animal models. They exert their effect through activation of the GABA$_A$ receptor as described in option D, and can be antagonized with flumazenil. Naloxone is a competitive opioid antagonist indicated only for ventilatory depression due to opioid overdose. (*1:1059; 5:697-9*)

440. **(A)** At zero time, the blood concentration is 80 mg/L. Volume of distribution is the dose of the drug divided by the concentration. Thus, the volume of distribution in the central compartment immediately after the injection of the drug is 400 mg/80 mg/L or 5 L. (*1:30-3*)

441. **(C)** To obtain the redistribution half-life, the initial straight portion of the curve is extrapolated. At zero time, the blood concentration is

80 mg/L. At 1 h, the extrapolated line gives a blood concentration of 5 mg/L. The time required for the blood concentration to drop from 80 mg/L to 5 mg/L is 4 half-lives: after one half-life, the blood concentration will be 40 mg/L; after two half-lives, 20 mg/L; after three half-lives, 10 mg/L; and after four half-lives, 5 mg/L. Since four half-lives occurred in 1 h, then the redistribution half-life must be 0.25 h or 15 min. (*1:33*)

442. **(C)** To obtain the terminal half-life, the final straight portion of the curve is extrapolated. At 10 h, the blood concentration is 1 mg/L. The blood concentration is 2 mg/L at 7 h, and 4 mg/L at 4 h. It is apparent that the blood concentration is declining by half every 3 h, thus the terminal half-life must be 3 h. (*1:33*)

443. **(A)** Desmopressin is usually taken twice daily by intranasal administration. In contrast to vasopressin that is rapidly inactivated, the duration of the effect of desmopressin is several hours. Desmopressin may increase blood pressure, but it does so to a much lesser degree than vasopressin. Desmopressin increases the circulating concentrations of factor VIII and von Willebrand factor, and has no effect in patients with nephrogenic diabetes insipidus. While there is not likely to be a need for intraoperative administration of desmopressin if the patient was given a dose by inhalation preoperatively, it may be given by intravenous infusion to decrease serum osmolality and increase water retention. (*1:708, 710*)

444. **(C)** Hydralazine may be associated with a lupus-like syndrome. It is a direct vasodilator and may cause reflex tachycardia that limits its usefulness in the patient with angina. There may be retention of sodium and water that may require diuretics. (*1:779-780*)

445. **(C)** The elderly generally require a lower dose of thiopental to induce anesthesia. With increasing age, MAC for inhalational anesthetics decreases, and recovery of normal ventilatory drive after fentanyl administration is delayed. In contrast, with increasing age there is no alteration in the intubating dose of vecuronium. The rate of hepatic synthetic reactions, such as the glucuronidation of morphine, is also unchanged in the elderly, while the rate of hepatic oxidative and reductive reactions declines with increasing age. (*5:607, 680-1*)

446. **(E)** The aim of antacid administration is to raise the pH. It should be given 15-30 min before surgery. Antacids will not decrease gastric volume but may actually increase it. Nonparticulate antacids should not cause any problem if aspirated. There is no lag time. (*1:1315; 5:1159, 1657*)

447. **(A)** Butorphanol is a mixed opioid agonist–antagonist. Naloxone is a pure opioid antagonist, methohexital a short-acting barbiturate, midazolam a benzodiazepine, and bleomycin a drug used in cancer chemotherapy. (*1:509-11*)

448. **(C)** Patients who abuse alcohol manifest tolerance to its CNS effects but not to its ventilatory effects. The acutely intoxicated person requires less anesthesia, whereas the chronic alcoholic who is not acutely intoxicated requires more. Because alcoholic liver disease may lead to a decreased capacity to metabolize local anesthetics, local anesthetic toxicity may be more likely in the alcoholic. (*5:321-3*)

449. **(B)** Chloroprocaine is the least toxic local anesthetic by virtue of its rapid hydrolysis after accidental intravenous injection. (*1:573-4; 5:781*)

450. **(C)** The Henderson–Hasselbalch equation states that pH = pK + log [proton acceptor/proton donor]. With a weak base like mepivacaine, the uncharged form is the proton acceptor, and 39% is present in this form at physiologic pH. Even without a calculator, an approximation is possible. If the pH were equal to the pK of the drug, equivalent amounts of the charged and uncharged moieties would be present. In this case, the pH is slightly lower than the pK, favoring slightly less than half of the drug to be in the uncharged form. (*5:769*)

451. (B) At levels below 1.5 MAC, the net effect of halogenated hydrocarbons is a decrease in cerebral blood flow. Opioids, ideally as a continuous infusion, should be administered concomitantly (balanced anesthetic), to decrease the amount of volatile anesthetic required. Nitrous oxide and ketamine are both likely to cause an increase in CBF. The administration of both phenylephrine and dobutamine can increase CBF. (*5:873-4*)

452. (D) A weak base is less ionized at higher pH values, thus rendering it more lipid-soluble and more likely to distribute to the interstitial fluid. The converse is true of weak acids. Increased blood flow to a tissue increases the distribution of drugs to that tissue. Distribution is decreased by binding to plasma protein and by decreased lipid solubility. (*1:30-3*)

453. (D) The loading dose of a drug is the dose given to achieve a faster blood concentration, and is calculated based on the volume of distribution at steady state (Vss), the desired plasma concentration (Cp), and the drugs bioavailability (F). While the loading dose decreases the time needed to achieve a steady state concentration, the drug concentration is initially higher because drug distribution after initial bolus is limited to the smaller, central compartment. With some drugs, the larger dose can have detrimental effects, e.g., a larger dose of relaxant may lead to a longer time of paralysis or cardiovascular effects. (*1:37*)

454. (B) Amiodarone is a structural analogue of thyroid hormone and exerts a variety of pharmacological effects. Hypotension after intravenous administration of the drug is due to vasodilation and depression of myocardial performance. Adenosine, verapamil, and procainamide are some of the drugs used for the treatment of cardiac dysrhythmias associated with the WPW syndrome; amiodarone is not indicated. Drug toxicity during oral loading regimens is uncommon, and may include nausea. Long-term therapy can cause significant pulmonary fibrosis. The adverse effects of amiodarone are thought to be attributable to the drugs interaction with

nuclear thyroid hormone receptors. (*1:834; 5:764; 6:1839, 1911*)

455. (E) Digoxin is an inotrope and may cause bradycardia. The mechanism involves inhibition of Na,K-ATPase. Calcium will potentiate the effects of digoxin. Digoxin toxicity can present as described in the vignette, including a variety of severe conduction disturbances. Side effects of carvedilol include bradyarrhythmias, but the drug is unlikely to cause visual disturbances. Quinidine can prolong the QT-interval and cause polymorphic ventricular tachycardia. The adverse effects of amiodarone include pulmonary fibrosis, and an overdose of benzodiazepines would cause respiratory depression. (*1:803-4; 5:749, 753*)

456. (C) All halogenated volatile anesthetics decrease cerebral metabolic rate in a dose-dependent manner, and are associated with a decrease in cerebral electrical activity. They differ, however, in their potential to cause cerebral vasodilation that could raise ICP in patients with poor compliance. Sevoflurane causes less vasodilation than either isoflurane or desflurane. Cerebral metabolic rate rises dramatically during seizure activity. (*1:542-6; 5:874*)

457. (C) Coverage of steroid therapy at the time of surgery is important to avoid stress reactions and acute adrenal insufficiency. Replacement doses are based on the anticipated stress of the operative procedure. Cholecystectomy is considered moderately invasive, and the most appropriate regimen is the one outlined in option C. Option D is appropriate for minor procedures, while option E would be the recommended regimen for cases such as cardiac, or major abdominal surgery. (*5:157*)

458. (D) A patient with the presented symptoms may be having an anaphylactic reaction. In addition to the interventions outlined in the vignette, blood pressure should be supported with epinephrine in 100-mcg increments that is the cornerstone of initial therapy. In addition, glucocorticoids and diphenhydramine should be administered as secondary treatment. The most common causes of anaphylactic reactions during anesthesia care include muscle relaxants and antibiotics. *(5:1484)*

459. **(E)** The patient is most likely suffering from magnesium deficiency that is common in malnourished alcoholic patients and often accompanied by hypokalemia. The arrhythmia described is consistent with torsades des pointes, while other findings might include Trousseau and Chvostek signs that are also found in states of hypocalcemia. *(5:520-1; 6:1891)*

460. **(D)** The opioids usually produce unconsciousness at high dosage, but it is important to recognize that unconsciousness is not absolute. The pupils are constricted. Opioids do not produce reliable amnesia, and the nausea and vomiting seen are mediated through the central nervous system in the chemoreceptor trigger zone. *(1:488-490)*

461. **(B)** The patient with hyperthyroidism should be adequately prepared preoperatively. This usually involves the preoperative administration of β-adrenergic antagonists to decrease the heart rate. Aspirin is usually avoided because it may displace thyroid hormone from its plasma protein binding sites. Administration of exogenous thyroid hormone should be avoided, as should administration of amiodarone that is a structural analogue of thyroid hormone and can trigger thyroid storm. *(1:834; 5:151-2)*

462. **(B)** For coronary "steal" to occur, there must be a stenosed vessel supplying an area of myocardium that is dependent upon flow through collateral vessels. Isoflurane may then cause vasodilation that diverts blood away from these collaterals, leading to ischemia in the collateral-dependent area of myocardium. In spite of this theory, and the fact that many persons have "steal-prone" coronary anatomy, there is no evidence that the use of isoflurane is associated with an increase in perioperative ischemia or mortality. The phenomenon of

"steal" does not occur with either desflurane or sevoflurane. *(1:543; 5:612)*

463. **(D)** Corticorticoids used for the treatment of asthma should be of the glucocorticoid type since no mineralocorticoid effect is desired. The onset time is measured in hours. Giving the drug by inhalation does not decrease the onset time but it decreases systemic toxicity because lower doses may be used. Inhaled corticosteroids are the most effective anti-inflammatory agents used in asthma therapy. *(5:131-2; 6:2110-1)*

464. **(A)** The patient with renal failure usually does not need an altered dose of medications whose effects are terminated by redistribution. Pancuronium is primarily eliminated unchanged by the kidney. *(1:274, 501)*

465. **(E)** Ionization of a drug is important in the drug's function, since charged particles do not cross membranes well. The degree of ionization is a function of the pH of the solution and the pKa of the drug as given by the Henderson–Hasselbalch equation. The Michaelis-Menten equation describes transporter-mediated processes across biological membranes. *(1:18-9, 95)*

466. **(C)** Obese patients have an increased volume of distribution and an increased terminal half-life for highly lipid soluble agents such as midazolam and thiopental. The degree of isoflurane metabolism is not significantly changed. Obese subjects have higher levels of pseudocholinesterase activity; when a larger dose of succinylcholine is given to an obese patient, the duration of action is similar to that seen when a similar dose (in mg/kg) is given to a lean patient. Even though digoxin is a highly lipophilic drug, it has a comparable volume of distribution in obese and lean individuals. *(5:308-10)*

467. **(A)** All of the options listed are targets for different classes of antiemetic agents. Granisetron is a 5-HT$_3$ receptor antagonist. *(1:1342)*

468. **(D)** Acute intermittent porphyria is an inborn error of metabolism in which porphobilinogen cannot be converted to uroporphyrin. Therefore, the urinalysis is positive for porphobilinogen, which is pathognomonic, and negative for uroporphyrins. Thiopental induces the enzyme δ-aminolevulinic acid synthetase that results in increased synthesis of porphobilinogen and therefore will worsen acute intermittent porphyria. This disease is associated with a constellation of symptoms and signs, the worst of which are neurologic; however, cardiac arrest with thiopental is not among them. Morphine may be safely administered. (*5:141-2, 695*)

469. **(C)** Both renal insufficiency and peripheral neuropathy may persist after courses of therapy with cisplatin. Congestive heart failure has been reported after high doses of doxorubicin. Pulmonary fibrosis is a serious complication of bleomycin therapy, and hepatic cirrhosis may occur after long-term therapy with methotrexate, for example in patients with psoriasis. (*1:1689, 1694, 1714, 1718*)

470. **(D)** Dissociative anesthesia is noted by the presence of open eyes and occasional muscle movements that are not signs of inadequate anesthesia. Muscle tone may be increased in dissociative anesthesia, and the patient is not necessarily unconscious. (*1:538; 5:1265*)

471. **(B)** This patient is most likely having a reaction to the methylparaben preservative present in multiple-dose vials of lidocaine. Persons allergic to methylparaben are also likely to be allergic to local anesthetics of the ester type, such as procaine. Since true allergy to lidocaine is extremely rare, a second dose of preservative-free lidocaine is very unlikely to cause a reaction. Bacterial contamination of a preservative-containing solution is also unlikely. Local anesthetic preparations containing a vasoconstrictor may also elicit allergic reactions due to sulfite added as an antioxidant. (*1:571-2; 5:777*)

472. **(D)** Captopril inhibits conversion of angiotensin I to angiotensin II and thus decreases arteriolar and venous tone. (*1:732-4*)

473. **(A)** Drug antagonism occurs when two drugs have effects that tend to counteract one another. This may occur by combination, as in the case of heparin–protamine interaction, or they may compete for the same receptor site, as with muscle relaxants and acetylcholine. The hallmark feature of competitive antagonism is the lack of intrinsic efficacy of the antagonist. The dose response curve of the agonist will be shifted to the right, with no change in the maximal response. (*1:46-8*)

474. **(B)** Succinylcholine will have a prolonged effect in a person deficient in pseudocholinesterase, either on the basis of a genetic defect or because they have taken a cholinesterase inhibitor such as echothiophate that is readily absorbed from the eye. Succinylmonocholine is a metabolite of succinylcholine with minimal potency and unlikely to be the cause of prolonged paralysis. While opioid overdose can cause apnea and unresponsiveness, the dose of fentanyl administered to the patient in the vignette is too small to explain her symptoms, and the same is true for the short-acting hypnotic propofol. Since 70% N_2O does not cause apnea, it is not likely to be associated with this patient's current signs. (*1:250; 5:500*)

475. **(A)** In trying to determine the cause, a nerve stimulator should be used to assess the level of muscle relaxation. If no twitches are elicited, a prolonged effect of succinylcholine is demonstrated. Administration of the benzodiazepine antagonist flumazenil is not indicated, since there is no mention of benzodiazepine administration in the vignette. Administration of carbon dioxide by inhalation is technically difficult in most settings and will not provide a definitive answer. There is no reason to administer another dose of succinylcholine. (*1:459; 5:500-1*)

476. **(D)** Once it has been established that there is no twitch, the only course to take is to ventilate the patient as long as is necessary. Even with no measurable pseudocholinesterase activity, paralysis due to an intubating dose of succinylcholine should wear off within an hour or two due to renal elimination of unmetabolized succinylcholine. Neostigmine will not reverse the paralysis if pseudocholinesterase deficiency is the cause. Pralidoxime is unlikely to be effective in reactivating cholinesterase that is chronically inhibited by echothiophate, and physostigmine is occasionally used in the treatment of central anticholinergic syndrome. (*1:86, 268; 5:500-1, 1461*)

477. **(B)** The intramuscular route may be used for aqueous or nonaqueous solutions and permits more rapid onset than after subcutaneous injection. Irritating substances that may cause pain if injected subcutaneously may be tolerated by the intramuscular route. Absorption from the deltoid or vastus lateralis muscles is more rapid than from the gluteus maximus. The rate of absorption following intramuscular administration can differ significantly between males and females, particularly with injections into the gluteus maximus that has been attributed to different distributions of subcutaneous fat. Drugs injected into the muscle are subject to first-pass metabolism in the lung; the only exception is the intra-arterial route. (*1:22-3*)

478. **(D)** Because of their rapid onset times, atropine should be given at the same time as edrophonium in order to minimize side effects. Similarly, glycopyrrolate should be given at the same time as neostigmine. The maximum recommended dose of neostigmine is 75 mcg/kg; this will produce maximal inhibition of acetylcholinesterase and a larger dose may actually cause depolarizing neuromuscular blockade. The disappearance of fade during double-burst stimulation indicates sufficient recovery of muscular function to permit endotracheal extubation. A TOF ratio of 0.7 does not guarantee complete recovery of pharyngeal function; even at TOF ratio of 0.9 some patients may have incomplete recovery of pharyngeal muscles. (*1:247, 267; 5:507*)

479. **(E)** Myotonic dystrophy is a member of a diverse group of hereditary skeletal muscle disorders. It is usually exacerbated during pregnancy, and is associated with CHF and restrictive lung disease. Administration of succinylcholine in these patients can lead to hyperkalemic cardiac arrest and to muscle spasm so severe that ventilation may be impossible. Nondepolarizing neuromuscular blocking agents would not prevent or treat the muscle spasms in myotonia because the pathologic lesion is at the muscle membrane level. Patients with myasthenia gravis are resistant to the effects of succinylcholine due to the decreased number of acetylcholine receptors. Duchenne type is the most common muscular dystrophy. It is recessive sex-linked, and will affect males; however, females may exhibit subclinical symptoms. Patients with hypokalemic periodic paralysis may have increased serum potassium levels after administration of succinylcholine, however, cardiac arrest is far less likely. Charcot-Marie-Tooth disease is the most frequent peripheral neuropathy. Avoidance of depolarizing NMB drugs is advisable but again, unlikely to cause cardiac arrest. (*5:140-5*)

480. **(C)** The neuroleptic state is characterized by reduced motor activity and indifference to the surroundings. Neither amnesia nor analgesia are produced when a neuroleptic agent is administered by itself. (*1:417; 5:701*)

481. **(D)** All inhalational anesthetics can produce CO due to their interaction with strong bases in carbon dioxide absorbents, particularly when the absorbent is dry (such as when it has been flushed with dry gas during an entire weekend). The relative propensity for producing carbon monoxide is desflurane > enflurane > isoflurane > sevoflurane > halothane. Recommendations to decrease the risk of carbon monoxide production include low fresh gas flows, use of fresh absorbent, and the use of soda lime instead of baralyme. (*5:614*)

482. **(D)** Additive effect refers to a combined effect that is the algebraic sum of the individual actions. The effect described in option E would be synergistic. (*1:77*)

483. (A) An increased initial slope of the curve indicates an increased rate of sevoflurane uptake. An increased rate of uptake will occur if the inspired concentration of sevoflurane is increased, if nitrous oxide is added to the inspired gas mixture (the second gas effect), or if minute ventilation is increased. An increased cardiac output will cause a decreased rate of anesthetic uptake. Pulmonary right-to-left shunting will lead to a decrease in alveolar uptake. (*5:603-5*)

484. (B) Patients with the Eaton–Lambert syndrome have increased sensitivity to both depolarizing and nondepolarizing muscle relaxants because of decreased release of acetylcholine at the neuromuscular junction. The syndrome does not respond to acetylcholinesterase inhibitors, and nondepolarizing neuromuscular blockade is difficult to reverse. As opposed to some patients with muscular dystrophies, the myasthenic syndrome is not associated with an increased risk of MH. (*5:143-4*)

485. (A) *Clostridium perfrigens* is a gram-positive rod. The drug of choice for gas gangrene is penicillin G that is often combined with clindamycin due to its ability to reduce toxin expression. Pharmacologic therapy always has to be combined with adequate debridement of infected areas. Gas gangrene has to be treated with intravenous antibiotics; none of the other combinations listed would be considered first-line regimens. (*5:1485, 1535*)

486. (B) Cimetidine inhibits the oxidative metabolism of many drugs, including diazepam, by inhibiting cytochrome P450. While oral diazepam is an excellent oral preoperative sedative for patients undergoing inpatient surgery, the dose may need to be reduced in the setting of chronic cimetidine therapy. Chronic ingestion of ethanol increases cytochrome P450 levels. There is no inhibitory effect of nitrous oxide on cytochrome P450. (*5:699*)

487. (C) Human enzymes are not thought to be able to metabolize nitrous oxide. The reduction of nitrous oxide to nitrogen occurs to a small degree in the gut and is catalyzed by bacterial enzymes. Nitrous oxide is almost completely eliminated, but not metabolized, by the lungs. (*1:546-7*)

488. (C) While methylmethacrylate can act as a direct vasodilator in vitro, plasma concentrations achieved during cementing of joint replacements are 10-20 fold below those required to cause hypotension. The mechanism of *bone implantation syndrome* is described in option C, and can lead to acute pulmonary hypertension and right heart failure. An air embolus of hemodynamic consequence is much less likely, and cannot be effectively treated via aspiration of blood through the central venous catheter. Venting of the long bone does not reliably prevent cardiovascular compromise. (*5:1204*)

489. (D) Ondansetron is a 5-HT$_3$ receptor antagonist. It is an antiemetic and acts at the chemoreceptor trigger zone. It produces no sedation and has few, if any, adverse effects. It has no effect on gastrointestinal motility. (*1:1341*)

490. (B) The same dose of propofol is not appropriate for all patients. An understanding of the diagram is important for the proper use of intravenous medications. A patient in shock will have an increased effect of propofol because the fraction of the cardiac output reaching the brain is higher in shock. Furthermore, the rate of redistribution from the brain is slower because of decreased perfusion of other tissues. The patient who is anxious and has an increased cardiac output will have faster redistribution, and the effect will be shorter. Another important factor to consider in propofol dosing is patient age: the effect-site concentration of a given propofol dose will increase with increasing age. (*5:680-3*)

491. (C) Most strains of *Staphylococcus aureus* produce beta lactamase that will render penicillin G and ampicillin ineffective. Cefazolin and other first generation cephalosporins and vancomycin are both effective drugs for single-agent prophylaxis of such a wound infection;

however, the latter is usually reserved for selected patients at higher risk for MRSA-infection. Levofloxacin is currently not recommended as a first-line agent for surgical site infection prophylaxis. *(5:235-6)*

492. **(B)** Carbon monoxide shifts the oxygen–hemoglobin dissociation curve to the left; thus oxygen is bound more tightly and is less easily released in tissues. Carbon monoxide combines with hemoglobin at one-tenth the rate of oxygen, but dissociates from hemoglobin at only 1/2200 the rate of oxygen. The affinity of hemoglobin for carbon monoxide is therefore 220 times that of oxygen, and an increased F_{IO_2} provides no protection from carbon monoxide. The absorbance spectra of carboxyhemoglobin and oxyhemoglobin are similar, and standard pulse oximeters cannot distinguish between the two. Oxygen saturation readings can therefore be normal, even in the presence of lethal amounts of carboxyhemoglobin. *(5:1336)*

493. **(E)** Filtration occurs when drugs diffuse through aqueous pores in membranes. Passive nonionic diffusion is the process by which lipid-soluble compounds diffuse through the lipoidal portions of membranes. Active transport mechanisms use carrier molecules for certain ligands and are thus subject to saturability. Option D, while a mediated transport process, falls into the category of passive transmembrane transport. *(1:19, 674)*

494. **(B)** Heroin is diacetylmorphine. One or both of the acetyl groups may be removed via hydrolysis to yield acetylmorphine and morphine, respectively. *(1:499-501)*

495. **(B)** Low-molecular-weight heparins (LMWH) have a more predictable pharmacokinetic profile than standard heparin that allows weight-adjusted subcutaneous administration without routine laboratory monitoring. If monitoring is deemed necessary, anti-factor Xa activity can be determined. The incidence of heparin-induced thrombocytopenia is lower as compared to standard heparin. Even if similar anti-factor Xa activity is achieved with any of these agents, it cannot be assumed that they

produce equivalent antithrombotic effects. At least half of the LMWH chains are too short to bridge antithrombin to thrombin; the same is true for the pentasaccharide fondaparinux. *(1:853-6)*

496. **(B)** Aspirin overdose is a leading cause of overdose morbidity and mortality. Peak plasma concentration may not be reached for 4-35 h after intoxication with the enteric-coated form. The drug causes the uncoupling of oxidative phosphorylation resulting in increased carbon dioxide production with resulting hyperventilation and hyperthermia. CNS symptoms include confusion, dizziness, tinnitus, delirium, psychosis, and in some cases coma. Miosis and respiratory depression are characteristic of intoxication with opioids. While lithium overdose can cause severe CNS symptoms and coma, symptoms would likely become apparent sooner after ingestion. The symptoms of acute acetaminophen poisoning are more insidious, presenting as predominantly GI symptoms over the first two days, followed by acute hepatic failure in severe cases. *(1:75, 450, 981, 984)*

497. **(C)** Cytochrome P450 performs many oxidative reactions, including the oxidative demethylation of ketamine. While cytochrome P450 is capable of performing the oxidative deamination of norepinephrine in vitro, the reaction is performed by monoamine oxidase in vivo. The acetylation of hydralazine is catalyzed by *N*-acetyltransferase, the conjugation of morphine to glucuronide is catalyzed by glucuronyl transferase, and the conjugation of acetaminophen to sulfate is catalyzed by sulfate transferase. *(1:127-8, 202)*

498. **(B)** Sweating and lacrimation are two of the early signs of the abstinence syndrome. Chills and pilomotor activity are prominent effects a day or two after the last dose of morphine. Seizures and coma are not a part of the opioid withdrawal syndrome, but do occur with abrupt withdrawal of barbiturates and benzodiazepines. Bradycardia is one of the symptoms of withdrawal from cocaine. *(1:660-2)*

499. (E) All of these symptoms may occur with ACE-inhibitor therapy. Cough is a common side effect, whereas a loss of sense of taste is rare. Acute renal insufficiency is a risk in persons with renal artery stenosis or a history of CHF. Proteinuria is less common, but is more likely to occur in persons with underlying renal impairment. (*1:735-6*)

500. (A) The vessel-rich group includes those organs that receive the bulk of circulation. It includes the heart, brain, kidneys, and liver. Muscle is more poorly perfused. The vessel-rich group of tissues receives decreasing blood flow with increasing age, and represents about 10% of total body weight in adults, and approximately 22% in the neonate, compared to 13% in accounting for the vessel-poor group in that age group. (*5:254*)

501. (D) Ketorolac is a cyclooxygenase inhibitor that has high efficacy as an analgesic. Its major adverse effect is epigastric distress. It is much less likely than morphine to cause sedation, ventilatory depression, or nausea. (*1:973, 986; 5:1304*)

502. (E) The hypovolemic patient has a greater fraction of the cardiac output reaching the brain, and redistribution is less rapid due to the decreased blood flow to peripheral tissues. The impact of blood loss on the effects of propofol is dramatic, with an estimated 5-fold increase in duration of action, and a need for 80% dose reduction in severe blood loss to provide effect-site concentrations equivalent to a person with normal cardiovascular physiology. The CNS response may also be affected by the other factors listed, which alter the amount of drug reaching the brain in the time immediately following injection, but not to the extent as option E. The patient with renal failure is often hypoalbuminemic; such patients need a decreased dose of induction agent due to less protein binding that causes a higher unbound fraction to be available. Most, but not all elderly patients require lower induction doses of intravenous anesthetics, although the mechanism is unclear. Drug dosing in obese patients should take into consideration lean body mass

for the initial bolus to avoid excessive effect-site concentrations. (*5:676-83*)

503. (C) Unlike halothane, isoflurane produces burst suppression of the EEG at 2 MAC. During carotid endarterectomy performed under isoflurane anesthesia, the cortical blood flow level at which EEG manifestations of ischemia are detected is lower than that of halothane. Neither agent abolishes autoregulation of cerebral blood flow. Isoflurane, although producing less increase in CBF than halothane, is still a cerebral vasodilator. Sevoflurane and enflurane have been reported to augment epileptic brain activity. (*5:611*)

504. (D) Lamotrigine is an anticonvulsant agent useful in the treatment of partial and generalized tonic-clonic seizures. It is also effective for the treatment of absence seizures. Its half-life is reduced when pentobarbital, carbamazepine, or phenytoin is administered concomitantly. The drug is primarily metabolized by glucuronidation as opposed to gabapentin that is not metabolized by humans. Lamotrigine also has a role in the treatment of various neuropathic pain syndromes, but is considered second line due to significant side effects. (*1:584, 599-600; 5:1562*)

505. (B) Alterations in total hepatic blood flow during anesthesia and surgery can cause hepatocellular ischemic injury with resulting hepatic failure in patients with stable, underlying chronic liver disease. Volatile anesthetics decrease hepatic blood flow, halothane to a greater degree than sevoflurane and isoflurane. There is little effect of propofol or nitrous oxide on hepatic blood flow. Halothane hepatitis is thought to be caused by an immune response to hepatic proteins that become trifluoroacetylated as a consequence of halothane metabolism. (*1:537, 543; 5:193, 613-5*)

506. (D) Clonidine is a centrally acting sympathetic inhibitor and may suppress some withdrawal symptoms. Chlorpromazine is ineffective for this indication. Butorphanol and nalbuphine are both opioid agonist–antagonist medications that are likely to precipitate withdrawal.

Flumazenil is a benzodiazepine receptor antagonist. (*1:468, 497, 661*)

507. **(D)** The emergence reactions that are seen with ketamine, an NMDA receptor antagonist, include dreaming, hallucinations, and delirium. These effects are less common in children. While ketamine produces amnesia for intraoperative events, the amnesia, as opposed to profound analgesia, does not persist into the postoperative period, and many patients remember their dreams or hallucinations. The emergence reactions can be minimized by the concurrent administration of a benzodiazepine. (*1:539; 5:699-700*)

508. **(B)** Omeprazole is an inhibitor of the H^+,K^+-ATPase responsible for the synthesis of hydrochloric acid in the stomach. In typical doses, it decreases the daily acid production by about 80-95%. In contrast, ranitidine, as a representative of the H_2 antagonists, will decrease acid production by about 70%. Omeprazole has no effect on gastric emptying or on the volume of gastric juice. It is metabolized by cytochrome P450 and inhibits the metabolism of some other medications by this enzyme. (*1:1311-2*)

509. **(D)** In patients with preexisting vitamin B_{12} deficiency, even relatively short exposures to nitrous oxide can produce megaloblastic changes and a neuropathy. The neurologic findings characteristic of vitamin B_{12} deficiency are a bilateral peripheral neuropathy that affects predominantly the lower extremities as well as an unsteady gait and diminished deep tendon reflexes. Nitrous oxide has been shown to irreversibly inactivate the enzyme methionine synthase that ultimately leads to impaired synthesis of phospholipids, myelin, and thymidine that is an essential DNA-base. Megaloblastic hematopoiesis and subacute combined degeneration of the spinal cord can ensue. (*1:546-7; 5:613*)

510. **(E)** Pharmacologic preparation of the patient does not preclude good airway management. Histamine H_2-receptor antagonists do not protect against aspiration, do not facilitate gastric emptying, nor do they have any effect on fluid that is already present in the stomach. If administered 2-3 h before induction of anesthesia, they will increase gastric pH and by decreasing gastric acid secretion lead to lower residual gastric volumes. There is no need to use histamine H_2-receptor antagonists in all patients. (*1:1313; 5:1033-4*)

511. **(B)** All volatile anesthetics and depolarizing muscle relaxants (eg, succinylcholine) are known to be triggering agents in patients susceptible to malignant hyperthermia. All other medications are considered safe. (*5:615, 1497*)

512. **(A)** Losartan is a competitive antagonist of angiotensin II. Prazosin is an α-adrenergic antagonist, nesiritide a recombinant B-type natriuretic peptide, and minoxidil and hydralazine are arterial vasodilators. (*1:767; 5:747*)

513. **(A)** Administration of a vasodilator such as nicardipine would move the ventricular function curve from A to C, resulting in improved ventricular function while reducing cardiac filling pressures. An inotrope, such as dobutamine would result in a higher ventricular curve, from A to B, resulting in greater cardiac work at the same ventricular filling pressures. Diuretics improve CHF symptoms by moving filling pressures along the same ventricular function curve from A to D. The combination of inotropes and vasodilators would result in a shift of the Frank-Starling curve from A to E. (*1:792*)

514. **(E)** The combination of inotrope, diuretic, and vasodilator would result in a shift of the Frank-Starling curve from A to F. (*1:792*)

515. **(B)** Fospropofol is a water-soluble prodrug of propofol supplied as a 3.5% aqueous solution and is not associated with pain on injection. Unlike propofol the drug has a small volume of distribution, and has a significant lag time of approximately 3-4 min after intravenous administration before consciousness is lost. The recommended bolus dose is 6.5 mg/kg. (*1:536; 5:693*)

516. **(E)** All of the agents mentioned will lead to a decrease in pulmonary vascular resistance, each through a different mechanism. Inhaled nitric oxide is used for the treatment of acute pulmonary hypertension and acts through stimulation of soluble guanylate cyclase with resultant vascular smooth muscle relaxation. Intravenous prostacyclin (epoprostenol, PGI_2) induces relaxation of smooth muscle by stimulating the production of cyclic AMP and can also be administered via inhalation. Other drugs in this category are inhaled iloprost and subcutaneous treprostinil. Sildenafil is a phosphodiesterase type 5 inhibitor. These drugs have an acute pulmonary vasodilator effect that is due to enhancement of nitric oxide-mediated pulmonary vasodilation. Bosentan is an orally active endothelin antagonist used for the treatment of primary pulmonary hypertension. *(1:1059-60)*

517. **(K)** Antidiuretic hormone, or arginine vasopressin, is an agonist at the vasopressin V_1 receptor. *(1:704)*

518. **(F)** Inamrinone is an inhibitor of phosphodiesterase-3 (PDE3). *(1:805)*

519. **(H)** Sildenafil is an inhibitor of phosphodiesterase-5 (PDE5). *(1:50)*

520. **(I)** Valsartan is a competitive antagonist at the angiotensin-1 (AT_1) receptor. *(1:736)*

521. **(G)** Spironolactone is a competitive antagonist of aldosterone in the collecting duct. *(1:692-3)*

522. **(B)** Acetazolamide in an inhibitor of carbonic anhydrase in the proximal tubule. *(1:677-8)*

523. **(E)** Furosemide is an inhibitor of the Na^+-K^+-$2Cl^-$ symport in the thick ascending limb of the loop of Henle. *(1:682)*

CHAPTER 8

General Anesthesia
Questions

DIRECTIONS (Questions 524 through 558): Each of the numbered items or incomplete statements in this section is followed by answers or by completions of the statement. Select the ONE lettered answer or completion that is BEST in each case.

524. A patient with obstructive lung disease has an altered anesthetic induction with an insoluble agent because of

   (A) decreased cardiac output
   (B) increased perfusion
   (C) increased P_{CO_2}
   (D) uneven ventilation
   (E) decreased minute volume

525. The term MAC refers to

   (A) the median anesthetic concentration
   (B) the anesthetic concentration that prevents movement after skin incision in 50% of patients
   (C) a measurement that is not affected by age
   (D) a measurement that is pertinent only to volatile anesthetics
   (E) the mean alveolar concentration

526. Signs of inadequate general anesthesia include all of the following EXCEPT

   (A) eyelid movement
   (B) pupillary constriction
   (C) hyperventilation
   (D) sweating
   (E) limb movement

527. A patient has chronic obstructive pulmonary disease requiring the constant administration of oxygen. He is dyspneic at rest and can walk at most 20 feet before needing to rest. He is scheduled to undergo an exploratory laparotomy because of a small bowel obstruction. He would be classified by the American Society of Anesthesiologists as physical status

   (A) III
   (B) IIIE
   (C) IVE
   (D) V
   (E) VE

528. The person who performed the first public demonstration of diethyl ether as a general anesthetic was

   (A) Karl Koller
   (B) William Thomas Green Morton
   (C) Horace Wells
   (D) Charles Jackson
   (E) John Collins Warren

529. The most common postoperative visual complication following general anesthesia is

   (A) retinal detachment
   (B) retinal artery occlusion
   (C) ischemic optic neuropathy
   (D) vitreous hemorrhage
   (E) corneal abrasion

530. The correlation of anesthetic potency with lipid solubility is known as the rule of

   (A) Ferguson
   (B) Michaelis and Menten
   (C) Henderson and Hasselbalch
   (D) Singer and Nicholson
   (E) Meyer and Overton

531. One mL of desflurane liquid occupies what volume at 1 atm pressure and 37°C if all of the liquid is vaporized? The ideal gas constant is 0.082 L-atm-°K^{-1}-mole^{-1}, the specific gravity of desflurane is 1.45, and its molecular weight is 168.

    (A) 219 mL
    (B) 238 mL
    (C) 243 mL
    (D) 256 mL
    (E) 276 mL

532. The correct order of solubilities in blood, from greatest to least, among the volatile anesthetics is

    (A) halothane > isoflurane > sevoflurane > desflurane
    (B) sevoflurane > isoflurane > desflurane > halothane
    (C) desflurane > isoflurane > sevoflurane > halothane
    (D) desflurane > halothane > sevoflurane > isoflurane
    (E) sevoflurane > halothane > desflurane > isoflurane

533. The state of general anesthesia may be reversed by

    (A) the administration of a competitive antagonist
    (B) increasing the atmospheric pressure
    (C) increasing the ambient temperature
    (D) decreasing the ambient temperature
    (E) the administration of any medication that increases cerebral perfusion

534. A 30-year-old patient is to have a cholecystectomy. The anesthesiologist decides to use sevoflurane in oxygen as the sole anesthetic agent, with no other medications administered. Approximately what concentration of sevoflurane will be required to prevent hemodynamic changes in response to surgical incision?

    (A) 2.1%
    (B) 3.4%

    (C) 4.6%
    (D) 5.5%
    (E) 6.4%

535. If 2% isoflurane in oxygen, flowing at a rate of 3 L/min, is added to a circle system, what will the concentration of isoflurane be after 6 min? Assume complete mixing of gas in the system, and that excess gas is scavenged. The reservoir bag has a volume of 2 L, the carbon dioxide absorber has a volume of 3 L, and the connecting hose and valves have a volume of 1 L.

    (A) 1%
    (B) 1.26%
    (C) 1.73%
    (D) 1.90%
    (E) 1.96%

536. If the uptake of gaseous anesthetic in L/min is x, and the patient's cardiac output suddenly doubles, the rate of uptake

    (A) cannot be calculated without further information
    (B) will become x/2
    (C) will become 2x
    (D) will become 4x
    (E) will become x^2

537. The likelihood of intraoperative awareness under general anesthesia is highest with the use of

    (A) inadequate benzodiazepine doses
    (B) high-dose opioids
    (C) muscle relaxants
    (D) no premedication
    (E) nitrous oxide as the sole gaseous anesthetic

538. Stage 2 anesthesia can be characterized by all of the following signs EXCEPT

    (A) amnesia
    (B) purposeless movement
    (C) hypoventilation
    (D) disconjugate gaze
    (E) increased airway reflexes

539. Contraindications to the discharge to home of a patient who had a hernia repair under general anesthesia include all of the following EXCEPT

(A) nausea

(B) inability to drink liquids without vomiting

(C) heart rate 50% higher than the preoperative value

(D) inability to walk due to groin pain

(E) disorientation to person and place

540. You are given the honor of providing the first anesthetic in a new radiology room. The patient is a 38-year-old man with an arteriovenous malformation of the thoracic spine that is causing severe pain but no neurologic deficit. The radiologist plans to embolize the lesion, and estimates that the procedure will require ten hours. Which one of the following is the LEAST important requirement for the room in which this procedure will occur?

(A) Pipeline oxygen supply

(B) Pipeline nitrous oxide supply

(C) Adequate space to place an anesthesia machine in proximity to the patient

(D) Availability of suction

(E) Auxiliary lighting available to the anesthesiologist

541. A 22-year-old patient is brought to the operating room for repair of a fractured femur. He fell off a boat and remained in the water for a long time prior to rescue. He is hypothermic with a temperature of 33°C. Other vital signs and laboratory values are normal. It can be assumed that the MAC for isoflurane in this patient is approximately

(A) 1%

(B) 1.25%

(C) 1.5%

(D) 1.75%

(E) 2%

542. Which one of the following volatile agents undergoes the greatest degree of biotransformation?

(A) halothane

(B) isoflurane

(C) desflurane

(D) sevoflurane

(E) nitrous oxide

543. All of the following factors determine alveolar tension of an inhaled anesthetic EXCEPT

(A) minute ventilation

(B) blood:gas partition coefficient

(C) cardiac output

(D) inspired concentration

(E) body temperature

544. The second gas effect

(A) has its maximum effect early in an anesthetic

(B) applies only to anesthetic gases

(C) applies only to nitrous oxide

(D) involves two gases administered at similar concentrations

(E) may be responsible for diffusion hypoxia

545. At the anesthetic level associated with the alveolar concentration MAC-awake, patients

(A) do not respond to simple commands

(B) will not move in response to a surgical incision

(C) are likely to remember what is told to them

(D) may manifest signs of excitement

(E) will likely be apneic

546. During a surgical procedure to repair a traumatized liver in a patient who was in a motor vehicle accident, the patient required 100% O_2 in order to maintain an adequate value for oxygen saturation, and each time a volatile anesthetic was given, the blood pressure dropped to an unacceptable value. A medication that might prevent the occurrence of recall for intraoperative events in the absence of nitrous oxide and a volatile agent is

(A) morphine
(B) fentanyl
(C) scopolamine
(D) droperidol
(E) dexmedetomidine

547. During general anesthesia with isoflurane, nitrous oxide, and cisatracurium, expected ocular effects include

(A) mildly increased intraocular pressure in normal individuals
(B) ablation of the oculocardiac reflex
(C) mydriasis
(D) ocular akinesia
(E) angle closure glaucoma in susceptible patients

548. A patient has had a total laryngectomy in the distant past. The patient now presents for mastectomy and axillary node dissection for the management of breast cancer. A reasonable method of managing this patient's airway during general anesthesia is inserting a(n)

(A) low-pressure cuffed endotracheal tube via the mouth
(B) nasotracheal RAE tube
(C) oral airway to prevent obstruction
(D) laryngeal mask airway
(E) reinforced, cuffed endotracheal tube into the tracheostomy stoma

549. Nasotracheal intubation may be used safely in a patient who has

(A) fractures of the lower cervical spine and the ethmoid bone
(B) a LeFort I fracture of the maxilla

(C) a LeFort II fracture of the maxilla
(D) a LeFort III fracture of the maxilla
(E) a CSF leak requiring repair

550. A 24-year-old woman is to have diagnostic laparoscopy as an outpatient. Her medical history is significant only for symptomatic gastroesophageal reflux. She is 61 inches tall and weighs 185 pounds. Prior to the induction of general anesthesia, she should be premedicated with all of the following medications EXCEPT

(A) metoclopramide
(B) droperidol
(C) glycopyrrolate
(D) cimetidine
(E) ondansetron

551. Among all patients undergoing general anesthesia, the overall risk of awareness is approximately one case in how many anesthetics?

(A) 75
(B) 325
(C) 700
(D) 2,200
(E) 6,300

552. Moderate sedation is associated with all of the following characteristics EXCEPT the patient

(A) follows a simple command like making a fist
(B) may need a jaw thrust to relieve airway obstruction
(C) says "ouch" (or its equivalent) when pinched
(D) has a normal minute ventilation
(E) has a normal blood pressure

553. If nitrous oxide is administered at a constant concentration, the uptake into the bloodstream in milliliters per minute will

(A) be constant
(B) increase with time
(C) decrease with time
(D) depend on temperature
(E) be independent of concentration

554. An 85-kg patient was brought urgently to the operating room after sustaining multiple gunshot wounds to the abdomen. Exploratory laparotomy revealed multiple injuries to both large and small bowel that were repaired by resecting the damaged segments and performing anastomoses. There were no vascular injuries and the prolonged surgical procedure was associated with little blood loss. What is the most reasonable infusion rate of lactated Ringer solution intraoperatively in order to maintain adequate urine output in the absence of significant blood loss?

(A) 175 mL/h

(B) 400 mL/h

(C) 750 mL/h

(D) 1,400 mL/h

(E) 2,200 mL/h

555. Intraarterial injection of which one of these medications may lead to limb-threatening ischemia distal to the arterial catheter?

(A) sodium nitroprusside

(B) methohexital

(C) bupivacaine

(D) verapamil

(E) papaverine

556. Superficial thrombophlebitis may follow the intravenous injection of many medications. Which one of the following medications has the LOWEST incidence of thrombophlebitis?

(A) midazolam

(B) lorazepam

(C) diazepam

(D) etomidate

(E) dantrolene

557. Which one of the following medications is thought to be the safest during the first trimester of pregnancy?

(A) Prednisone

(B) Diazepam

(C) Warfarin

(D) Phenytoin

(E) Thalidomide

558. A young, previously healthy man suffered an extensive crush injury to his lower extremities at work. Before being brought to the operating room for debridement of devitalized tissue, he was given lactated Ringer solution in the emergency department and was considered euvolemic by the anesthesiologist at the beginning of the case. As the surgical procedure progressed, the surgeon requested that 5% albumin solution be given instead of additional lactated Ringer solution. Such use would be expected to cause

(A) an unequivocal decrease in mortality

(B) an unequivocal increase in mortality

(C) less of an impairment of coagulation than 10% dextran 40 solution

(D) less of an impairment of coagulation than 10% pentastarch solution

(E) a low incidence of allergic reaction as long as the blood types are matched

Answers and Explanations

524. **(D)** The patient with chronic obstructive lung disease has a prolonged induction due to ventilation/perfusion mismatching. The cardiac output is usually not decreased. The increased P_{CO_2} does not directly affect the uptake of the agent. Decreased minute volume is not a factor. *(5:604)*

525. **(B)** The term MAC refers to minimum alveolar concentration. It is defined as the alveolar anesthetic concentration sufficient to prevent movement in response to surgical incision in 50% of the subjects. It decreases with increasing age. MAC can be used to specify the potency of both volatile and gaseous anesthetics. It should be apparent to the reader that since MAC refers to a midpoint in a population, the word "minimum" is a misnomer and in fact "mean" or "median" would have been more accurate. *(5:598, 607)*

526. **(B)** Pupillary dilatation is one of the signs of light anesthesia, as are tachypnea, sweating, and somatic movement. Lack of eye movement and pupillary constriction are two determinants of adequate depth. *(5:608)*

527. **(C)** This patient would be classified as physical status IV because he has an incapacitating systemic illness. Because the patient is to undergo an emergency procedure, "E" is added to the physical status. *(5:54)*

528. **(B)** William Thomas Green Morton demonstrated the general anesthetic effect of diethyl ether at Massachusetts General Hospital on October 16, 1846. John Collins Warren was the surgeon. Charles Jackson was Morton's chemistry professor at Harvard Medical School and taught him about the chemical properties of ether. Horace Wells demonstrated the effects of nitrous oxide at MGH a year before Morton's demonstration; Wells' demonstration was considered a failure because the patient cried out when his tooth was extracted, although he later said that he felt no pain and remembered nothing. Karl Koller was the first person to use cocaine as a local anesthetic in surgery. *(5:2)*

529. **(E)** While all of the listed visual complications have been reported following general anesthesia, corneal abrasion is by far the most common. *(5:370)*

530. **(E)** The Meyer-Overton rule states that anesthetic potency is proportional to lipid solubility, and this rule is valid for the majority of gaseous anesthetics. Ferguson's rule states that anesthetic potency is proportional to thermodynamic activity (ideal solubility). Singer and Nicholson proposed the lipid bilayer hypothesis of membrane structure. *(5:600)*

531. **(A)** One mL of desflurane liquid is 1.45 g or 0.00863 mole (1.45 g/168 g/mole). Thus, by the ideal gas law, $V = nRT/P = (0.00863) \times (0.082) \times (273 + 37) = 0.219$ L = 219 mL. *(5:627)*

532. **(A)** The correct order of solubilities in blood, from greatest to least, among the volatile anesthetics is halothane > isoflurane > sevoflurane > desflurane. *(5:598)*

533. **(B)** The state of general anesthesia, produced by gaseous agents or barbiturates, may be reversed by increasing the atmospheric pressure. *(5:588)*

534. **(C)** MAC is defined in terms of the prevention of movement in response to skin incision in 50% of patients. It is therefore the value for the ED50 and is about 2.1% for sevoflurane. A more reasonable target for clinical anesthesia is the ED95 and that value is about 1.3-fold higher than the ED50. Blunting the autonomic response to skin incision requires about 1.7-fold higher a concentration than preventing movement in response to incision. Therefore, a reasonable target in this case is 2.1% $\times$ 1.3 $\times$ 1.7 = 4.6% sevoflurane. *(5:598, 607-8)*

535. **(D)** The time constant of the circuit is its total volume (6 L) divided by the fresh gas flow rate (3 L/min), or 2 min. The concentration at any point in time is given by the following exponential equation:

$$C = C_o(1 - e^{-(t/\tau)})$$

where C_o is the concentration in the fresh gas (2%), τ is the time constant (2 min), and t is the time in question (6 min). Thus, after one time constant has elapsed, the concentration in the system is 63.2% of the fresh gas concentration or 1.26% isoflurane; after two time constants, 86.5% or 1.73% isoflurane; after three time constants, 95% or 1.9% isoflurane; and after four time constants, 98.2% or 1.96% isoflurane. *(5:601)*

536. **(C)** Uptake by the blood of a gaseous anesthetic from the lung is proportional to cardiac output. Thus, if the cardiac output doubles, uptake will double. *(5:601-2)*

537. **(C)** The likelihood of recall is not correlated with the use, or the lack of use, of any anesthetic agent. However, the use of muscle relaxants, which may block the observation of movement as a sign of inadequate anesthesia, is the pharmacological risk factor of greatest importance for intraoperative awareness. *(5:609-10)*

538. **(C)** The second stage of anesthesia is characterized by excitement, somatic movement, increased airway reflexes, disconjugate gaze, hypertension, hyperventilation, loss of consciousness, and amnesia. *(5:606)*

539. **(A)** Nausea without vomiting is very common after general anesthesia and as an isolated symptom is not a contraindication to discharge to home. Patients should be oriented and their vital signs should be near their preoperative values. Their pain should be under reasonable control and they should be able to tolerate fluids without vomiting. *(5:1278-84)*

540. **(B)** This patient requires a general anesthetic because of his pain and because of the expected duration of the procedure. General anesthesia would most likely be provided by an anesthesia machine located near the patient. If the flow of nitrous oxide is set at 2 L/min, a single full cylinder would last for about 13 h. Conversely, the ventilator might require 10-20 L/min, meaning that an oxygen cylinder might last for only 30-60 min; a supply of wall oxygen is generally required whenever a ventilator is to be used. The anesthesiologist also must have the ability to suction the patient's airway and to see the patient and the anesthesia equipment, considering that much of the proposed procedure will take place with the room darkened. *(ASA Statement on Nonoperating Room Anesthetizing Locations, www.asahq.org/for-members/standards-guidelines-and-statements.aspx)*

541. **(A)** The effect of altered body temperature on MAC is to decrease MAC by approximately 5% for each 1°C decrease from normal body temperature. *(5:598, 607)*

542. **(A)** Nitrous oxide is not metabolized, and isoflurane and desflurane undergo minimal metabolism. Sevoflurane is about 5% metabolized while halothane is about 20% metabolized. *(5:598)*

543. **(E)** Minute ventilation, inspired concentration, blood:gas partition coefficient, and cardiac output all affect the alveolar tension of the anesthetic gas. Body temperature has no effect. *(5:600-2)*

544. **(A)** The second gas effect occurs when the administration of a high concentration of one gas increases the rise in alveolar concentration of another gas. This effect may apply to any

gas. The maximum effect in anesthesia is early in the course of the anesthetic, and one of the gases must be capable of being given in high concentration. Diffusion hypoxia may occur at the end of an anesthetic when the diffusion of large volumes of nitrous oxide from the pulmonary circulation to the alveoli dilutes the alveolar concentration of oxygen. *(5:605)*

545. **(D)** MAC-awake is the alveolar concentration of an inhalational anesthetic at which 50% of the patients respond to commands. This value may be applied to patients as general anesthesia is being induced, or as they are emerging from anesthesia, and is similar to the alveolar concentrations associated with the excitement stage. This concentration is lower than that which will prevent movement in response to incision (or MAC) or result in apnea. Patients are usually amnestic for events that occur at MAC-awake. *(5:607-8)*

546. **(C)** Scopolamine produces anterograde amnesia in most patients without adversely affecting blood pressure and cardiac output. Opioids (like morphine and fentanyl), butyrophenones (like droperidol), and α_2-adrenoceptor agonists (like dexmedetomidine) are not associated with amnesia. *(5:1374)*

547. **(D)** Isoflurane decreases intraocular pressure and cisatracurium renders the eye immobile. Deep general anesthesia does not prevent the oculocardiac reflex. Medications that cause mydriasis may precipitate an episode of angle closure glaucoma in susceptible patients. *(5:608, 1210, 1220)*

548. **(E)** A patient who has had a total laryngectomy usually has a permanent tracheostomy stoma in the neck. Such patients have no connection to the airway via the oral route, thus oral or nasal intubation or the placement of a laryngeal mask airway is impossible. The stoma may be intubated and a reinforced tube is a popular choice. An alternative is to supply supplemental oxygen via a tracheostomy mask while the patient breathes spontaneously during total intravenous anesthesia. *(5:127)*

549. **(B)** LeFort II and III fractures, fractures of the ethmoid bone, and a CSF leak all increase the risk of the endotracheal tube penetrating into the brain during nasotracheal intubation. This risk is not present if the patient has a LeFort I fracture. *(5:1243-4)*

550. **(C)** Patients with symptomatic reflux should be premedicated with a histamine H_2 antagonist (such as cimetidine) and a gastrointestinal prokinetic agent (such as metoclopramide) in order to decrease the volume and increase the pH of the gastric contents. This patient also has several risk factors for postoperative nausea and vomiting, including female gender, young age, obesity, and an emetogenic operative procedure. She should receive antiemetic prophylaxis such as with droperidol and ondansetron. She has no indication for preoperative glycopyrrolate. *(5:78, 80, 1034)*

551. **(C)** In a combination of studies including over 30,000 anesthetics, the incidence of awareness was found to be about 0.13%. *(5:608)*

552. **(B)** The patient under moderate sedation should maintain an unobstructed airway without assistance. Cardiorespiratory parameters should be normal or near normal, and the patient should respond appropriately to pain or a command. *(5:1261)*

553. **(C)** The uptake will decrease over time as equilibrium is reached. The uptake is dependent on concentration, being greater with a higher concentration. *(5:600-3)*

554. **(C)** This procedure would be considered a "major" surgical trauma in terms of intraoperative fluid replacement needs, and therefore intraoperative fluid replacement in the range of 6-12 mL/kg/h is likely to be appropriate for this patient. *(5:534)*

555. **(B)** The accidental intraarterial injection of a barbiturate solution is likely to lead to intense vasospasm that may put the limb at risk of loss unless there is timely treatment with a vasodilator such as papaverine, sodium nitroprusside, or verapamil, also injected intraarterially.

The accidental intraarterial injection of a local anesthetic into an artery above the diaphragm may result in retrograde flow of the local anesthetic and subsequent delivery to the brain by a carotid or vertebral artery resulting in a seizure. *(5:694)*

556. **(A)** Of the injectable benzodiazepines, midazolam has the lowest incidence of thrombophlebitis because it is the only one that does not contain propylene glycol in the vehicle. Etomidate solution also contains propylene glycol. Dantrolene solution is irritating because it has a high pH and is hyperosmolar. *(5:697, 699, 1500)*

557. **(B)** Older data suggested that diazepam might have teratogenic effects, but that is no longer thought to be the case. The other medications listed are likely or certain teratogens in humans. *(5:247, 298, 1150)*

558. **(C)** The use of albumin instead of crystalloid solution in the general patient population is associated with neither an increase, nor a decrease, in mortality, and somewhat controversial in the trauma population, particularly in those patients with traumatic brain injury. There is little effect on coagulation with albumin or with pentastarch, however dextran solutions do impair coagulation. Albumin solutions are not associated with a particular blood type. *(5:539-41)*

CHAPTER 9

Regional Anesthesia
Questions

DIRECTIONS (Questions 559-600): Each of the numbered items or incomplete statements in this section is followed by answers or by completions of the statement. Select the ONE lettered answer or completion that is BEST in each case.

559. As the supervising anesthesiologist you are assigned to four operating rooms staffed by CRNA's. Regional anesthesia is preferred in all cases; however, you are concerned about the use of regional anesthesia in the setting of anticoagulation. Of the following clinical scenarios, which patient is most likely to sustain a bleeding complication from regional anesthesia?

    (A) A 46-year-old male who takes a baby aspirin daily and undergoes a spinal anesthetic for a knee arthroscopy.

    (B) An elderly female with osteoporosis undergoing a total knee arthroplasty under epidural analgesia and receiving low-molecular-weight heparin once daily.

    (C) A 56-year-old female who discontinued clopidogrel ten days prior to having an epidural placed for postoperative pain control following a right hemicolectomy.

    (D) A 23-year-old healthy parturient who consumes daily garlic supplements undergoing an elective cesarean section.

560. As the chief of anesthesiology in your hospital, you are asked by the administration to discuss a process that is important in promoting a safe regional anesthesia practice. Which one of the following topics is the most important one to discuss?

    (A) Patient care team education and awareness of limb protection and neurologic evaluation.

    (B) Details regarding billing compliance.

    (C) Knowledge of when to change the bolus rate of a continuous intrathecal catheter.

    (D) Training of medical students and residents in appropriate use of liposomal local anesthetics.

561. A 71-year-old man with osteoarthritis of the right hip is undergoing a right total hip arthroplasty. You decide to perform a spinal anesthetic. While assessing the landmarks when choosing the interspace in which to perform the lumbar puncture, you must remember that the caudal termination of the adult spinal cord is typically at

    (A) T11-T12
    (B) L1-L2
    (C) L4-L5
    (D) L5-S1
    (E) S2-S3

562. A 92-year-old man is undergoing total knee arthroplasty for severe painful osteoarthritis. After struggling in the placement of a lumbar spinal anesthetic, you decide to use the Taylor approach. What best characterizes the Taylor approach to performing spinal anesthesia?

    (A) Uses image guidance to facilitate bony landmarks

    (B) Uses a midline and steep angled approach

    (C) Uses microcatheters to produce long-lasting blocks

    (D) Uses a loss of resistance technique with air

    (E) Uses a paramedian approach at L5-S1

563. You are discussing a labor epidural analgesia with a 25-year-old parturient. She also happens to be a physician who is curious on what is the most popular technique for confirming correct needle location when performing an epidural block. You respond that the most popular technique is

(A) loss of resistance to either saline or air
(B) ultrasound imaging
(C) radiographic confirmation
(D) patient response
(E) block quality

564. What is the primary barrier to drug absorption from the epidural space into the CSF?

(A) Arachnoid mater
(B) Dura mater
(C) Pia mater
(D) Spinous process
(E) Ligamentum flavum

565. A 68-year-old man with rheumatoid arthritis undergoes a left total knee arthroplasty. You prefer to use an isobaric solution over a hyperbaric or hypobaric solution because

(A) an isobaric solution will rise in the CSF when the patient is in the supine position
(B) a hyperbaric solution will sink in the CSF
(C) an isobaric solution will settle in the most dependent region of the thoracic spine in the supine position
(D) an isobaric solution will rise less than a hyperbaric solution and potentially lead to less hypotension
(E) an isobaric solution of 0.5% bupivacaine is approved by the FDA for spinal anesthesia

566. A 25-year-old football player presents for a right knee arthroscopy after sustaining a medial meniscus tear. He is frightened of general anesthesia and wants to remain awake throughout surgery. In your discussion of spinal anesthesia in the ambulatory setting, the topic of transient neurological symptoms

(TNS) arises. Which local anesthetic is associated with the highest risk of sustaining TNS?

(A) Tetracaine
(B) Bupivacaine
(C) Lidocaine
(D) Chloroprocaine
(E) Ropivacaine

567. A patient receives a lumbar epidural block with 2% lidocaine for a vaginal hysterectomy. Three hours after surgery the patient reports a dense motor block. An MRI demonstrates a lumbar epidural hematoma. For the best neurologic outcome, it is recommended that a surgical evacuation of the hematoma occurs within

(A) 2-4 h
(B) 4-6 h
(C) 6-8 h
(D) 10-12 h
(E) 16-24 h

568. A 54-year-old woman with rheumatoid arthritis is scheduled for total knee replacement. The anesthesiologist plans to use 0.5% plain bupivacaine to which 25 mcg of clonidine has been added for spinal anesthesia. Intrathecal clonidine

(A) will shorten the duration of the spinal block
(B) can prolong the spinal motor block
(C) is contraindicated in pregnant patients
(D) provides a reliable surgical block as a sole agent
(E) has not been approved by the FDA for epidural use

569. A 42-year-old man presents for ACL repair to your ambulatory surgery center. You decide to perform a spinal anesthetic because the patient asks to watch the surgery. You have a slow surgeon and contemplate adding 100 micrograms of epinephrine to your local anesthetic. What is the major drawback to adding epinephrine to a local anesthetic for spinal anesthesia in an ambulatory patient?

(A) Induces vomiting

(B) Does not add clinical benefit

(C) Delays gastric emptying

(D) Delays return of bladder function

(E) Causes itching

570. A 27-year-old healthy female presents for a triple arthrodesis of the ankle. She prefers to have a spinal anesthetic, but recalls feeling short of breath during a previous spinal anesthetic for cesarean section. You tell her that

(A) gross pulmonary function is maintained with spinal anesthesia in healthy adults

(B) spinal anesthesia never compromises pulmonary function

(C) spinal anesthesia results in severe pulmonary compromise and general anesthesia is her best choice

(D) spinal anesthesia routinely blocks the phrenic nerve and she probably had a phrenic nerve palsy during her previous cesarean section

(E) spinal anesthesia rarely impairs pulmonary function and is the anesthetic of choice in patients with severe cystic fibrosis

571. A 25-year-old parturient presents for an elective cesarean section. After performing a spinal anesthetic with 13.5 mg of hyperbaric bupivacaine, the patient reports "feeling sick to her stomach." Subsequently you notice the blood pressure is 62/30. The best description of the cardiovascular response to a spinal anesthetic is that

(A) no hemodynamic changes occur

(B) both arterial and venous vasodilation contribute to hypotension

(C) it exacerbates diastolic dysfunction

(D) hypotension only occurs in patients with stenotic valvular lesions

(E) it worsens regurgitant valvular lesions

572. A 33-year-old male undergoes a subgluteal sciatic nerve block for open repair of an ankle fracture. In preparing for the block, the primary drug therapy that the anesthesiologist must consider using for local anesthetic systemic toxicity is

(A) lidocaine

(B) epinephrine

(C) breytelium

(D) phenylephrine

(E) 20% lipid emulsion

573. What was the first drug used to produce local anesthesia?

(A) Lidocaine

(B) Procaine

(C) Cocaine

(D) Prilocaine

(E) Tetracaine

574. A 23-year-old parturient scheduled for an elective cesarean section undergoes a spinal anesthetic with 10.5 mg of hyperbaric bupivacaine. Ten minutes following the spinal anesthetic, she complains of nausea. Her vital signs are a BP of 75/52, pulse rate of 123 beats/min, and oxygen saturation of 98%. The best pharmacologic treatment for hypotension related to the spinal anesthetic is

(A) atropine

(B) epinephrine

(C) phenylephrine

(D) calcium

(E) labetalol

575. Twenty-four hours after performing a spinal anesthetic in a 27-year-old female for a vaginal hysterectomy, you are consulted to evaluate her for a presumed post-dural puncture headache. Regarding the symptoms of a post-dural puncture headache, you would expect the headache to

(A) be positional in nature with improvement when sitting

(B) be positional in nature with improvement lying down

(C) not be positional in nature

(D) localized to one eye

(E) be associated with delayed gastric emptying

576. A 72-year-old female presents for a right thoracotomy for a right lower lobe resection for lung cancer. She consents to a thoracic epidural catheter for postoperative analgesia. She understands the risks that may result and asks about the prognosis should she develop an epidural hematoma. The statement that best characterizes the prognosis of an epidural hematoma is

(A) a spinal epidural hematoma is universally fatal

(B) a spinal epidural hematoma always results in quadriplegia

(C) a spinal epidural hematoma always results in paraplegia or a chronic pain syndrome

(D) a spinal epidural hematoma is not diagnosable and thus has a very poor prognosis

(E) with prompt diagnosis, treatment strategies are effective

577. A 36-year-old otherwise healthy male with Crohn disease presents for open hemicolectomy. You place a thoracic epidural catheter for postoperative analgesia. What would be considered a positive heart rate response from a test dose of 15 mcg of epinephrine?

(A) Heart rate variability changes

(B) Systolic blood pressure drops

(C) Skin vasoconstriction noted

(D) Heart rate increases by 20 beats per minute

(E) Heart rate increases by 10 beats per minute

578. A 21-year-old male presents for ACL reconstruction of the left knee. The patient prefers to have a femoral nerve block but is worried because he has been told that he has an allergy to "Novacaine". Which statement best characterizes allergic reactions related to local anesthetics?

(A) Allergies do not occur related to local anesthetics.

(B) Reactions are usually limited to systemic hives and urticaria.

(C) Allergic reactions are more common after exposure to ester compounds than amides.

(D) Allergic reactions can be avoided by pre-treatment with diphenhydramine.

(E) Allergic reactions can effectively be treated with intravenous lipids.

579. A 50-year-old female is scheduled to undergo open repair of a distal right radius fracture. She prefers to have a supraclavicular nerve block but is concerned about nerve injury. Specifically, she is concerned about the risk of intraneural injection. Which statement best characterizes the risk of intraneural injection of local anesthetics?

(A) Ultrasound imaging suggests that it occurs frequently without leading to clinical injury.

(B) Nerve injuries do not occur by this mechanism.

(C) Intraneural injection must only be avoided in diabetics.

(D) Intraneural injections do not occur when ultrasound is used.

(E) Intraneural injections are only a concern in peripheral nerves and not in plexi.

580. A 28-year-old female is about to undergo left hand surgery and you discuss performing a supraclavicular nerve block. She appears concerned and asks about the incidence of pneumothorax. You respond that with traditional landmark techniques, the incidence of a pneumothorax when performing a supraclavicular block has been reported to be in the range of

(A) 0.1 - 0.3%

(B) 0.2 - 1%

(C) 0.5 - 5%

(D) 1 - 10%

(E) 5 - 30%

581. Maintaining the standards of care during regional anesthesia practice involves all of the following EXCEPT

    (A) offering regional anesthesia to all patients
    (B) informed consent
    (C) monitoring regional anesthesia practice
    (D) appropriate and timely postoperative follow up
    (E) monitoring vital signs

582. A 22-year-old parturient requests a labor epidural. During your evaluation of the patient she explains that she has an allergy to one local anesthetic but cannot remember which one. To which one of the following local anesthetics is a patient most likely to have an allergic reaction?

    (A) tetracaine
    (B) bupivacaine
    (C) lidocaine
    (D) ropivacaine
    (E) prilocaine

583. The rate of local anesthetic absorption from a particular injection site, from highest to lowest rate, is

    (A) epidural, intercostal, brachial plexus, subcutaneous tissue, lower extremity
    (B) epidural, intercostal, subcutaneous tissue, lower extremity, brachial plexus
    (C) brachial plexus, epidural, intercostal, subcutaneous tissue, lower extremity
    (D) intercostal, epidural, brachial plexus, lower extremity, subcutaneous tissue
    (E) subcutaneous tissue, intercostal, epidural, brachial plexus, lower extremity

584. You are providing informed consent to a patient about to undergo a popliteal sciatic block. She is concerned about the risk of long-term neurologic injury from a peripheral nerve block. You explain that the incidence of late neurologic deficits after peripheral nerve blocks is

    (A) 1/10,000
    (B) 4/10,000
    (C) 1/100,000
    (D) 4/100,000
    (E) 4/1,000,000

585. During the performance of a left femoral nerve block utilizing traditional landmark techniques and nerve stimulation, you obtain a patellar twitch at 2.5 mA current and proceed to decrease the current while still maintaining a patellar twitch. The highest stimulating current that reliably predict intraneural needle placement is

    (A) 0.2 mA
    (B) 0.5 mA
    (C) 1.0 mA
    (D) 1.5 mA
    (E) 2.0 mA

586. You are supervising a first-year anesthesia resident during her regional anesthesia rotation. You instruct the resident to use blunt-tip needles. Blunt-tip needles

    (A) are more likely to penetrate neural tissue
    (B) are less disruptive to neural tissue than sharp needles
    (C) are more disruptive to neural tissue than sharp needles
    (D) have a higher incidence of successful block
    (E) are only preferred when they are greater than 15 gauge

587. A 72-year-old female with painful osteoarthritis undergoes a right total knee arthroplasty. She receives an ultrasound-guided femoral nerve block. The following day, the patient reports inability to dorsiflex the right foot. The most likely reason would be

    (A) a persistent motor block to the right femoral nerve
    (B) neurologic injury to the right common peroneal nerve
    (C) a persistent motor block to the right saphenous nerve
    (D) neurologic injury to the right tibial nerve
    (E) neurologic injury to the superficial peroneal nerve

588. Twenty minutes after the performance of a lumbar plexus block with 40 mL of 0.5% bupivacaine for a total hip arthroplasty, the patient reports "ringing in the ears" and feeling "light headed." The patient's condition deteriorates and ECG monitoring shows progression to sinus bradycardia, ventricular fibrillation, and ultimately asystole. The most likely explanation for these symptoms is

(A) direct intravenous injection

(B) oversedation with midazolam

(C) direct intra-arterial injection

(D) profound vasodilatation

(E) vascular absorption of local anesthetic

589. Utilizing a transarterial axillary technique, a brachial plexus block is performed. After confirming negative aspiration of blood, 5 mL of 0.5% bupivacaine is administered. Suddenly the patient becomes unresponsive. Initial pharmacologic management should include the administration of

(A) 20% lipid emulsion

(B) epinephrine, 1 mg

(C) amiodarone, 150 mg

(D) atropine, 1 mg

(E) vasopressin, 40 units

590. A 54-year-old female with adenocarcinoma of the lung presents for right thoracotomy. You plan to place a thoracic epidural catheter for postoperative analgesia. In the process of providing informed consent, the patient becomes worried about the risk of an epidural hematoma. You explain that the incidence of an epidural hematoma following the administration of a neuraxial anesthetic is estimated to be less than

(A) 1 in 10,000

(B) 1 in 50,000

(C) 1 in 150,000

(D) 1 in 400,000

(E) 1 in 1,000,000

591. A 64-year-old female presents for a right total knee arthroplasty. A spinal anesthetic was performed in the L3-L4 interspace with 0.5% isobaric bupivacaine. Five minutes after the spinal anesthetic, the patient is insensate at the level of the umbilicus. This closely approximates which one of the following dermatome levels?

(A) T4

(B) T7

(C) T10

(D) L1

(E) L3

592. A 42-year-old previously healthy ASA I patient undergoes an awake fiberoptic intubation with topical anesthesia for a laparoscopic appendectomy. Upon extubation she was noticed to have a saturation of 93%. While in the PACU his oxygen saturation continued to drop to 85% despite being alert, taking large tidal volumes, having a normal chest x-ray, and not improving while breathing 100% oxygen via a non-rebreather mask. You suspect methemoglobinemia. Which one of the following topical anesthetics is most associated with methemoglobinemia?

(A) Cocaine

(B) Tetracaine

(C) Benzocaine

(D) Lidocaine

(E) Proparacaine

593. A 39-year-old female presents for carpal tunnel release surgery. You discuss performing an IV regional block (Bier block). All of the following are important to consider EXCEPT

(A) thorough exsanguination of the extremity should take place prior to the injection of local anesthetic

(B) preservative-free lidocaine is the most frequently used local anesthetic

(C) bupivacaine is the drug of choice because it provides a long duration block

(D) a double tourniquet permits longer surgical time than a single tourniquet

(E) a tourniquet is more reliable when placed proximal to the elbow than at a more distal location

594. A 51-year-old patient is scheduled to undergo a right lung lower lobectomy for lung cancer. You discuss the risks and benefits of thoracic epidural analgesia. You discuss that a common medical indication for performing regional anesthesia is

(A) increased professional billing

(B) less cardiac morbidity in the previously healthy patient

(C) reduction in postoperative wound infections

(D) reduction in the administration of opioids in the immediate perioperative period.

(E) less oxygen administration

DIRECTIONS: Use the following scenario to answer Questions 595-596: You have been following a 27-year-old former nurse in your chronic pain clinic for complex regional pain syndrome of the left hand. She initially sustained a work related injury to her hand a year ago and has since experienced ongoing chronic pain. After conservative treatment with neuropathic medications she has had little relief. You decide to offer her a regional nerve block as part of a multimodal approach to treating her pain.

595. Which one of the following nerve blocks would be most appropriate?

(A) Axillary brachial plexus block

(B) Stellate ganglion block

(C) Celiac plexus block

(D) A cervical transforaminal injection

(E) An infraclavicular brachial plexus block

596. After a successful nerve block, one would expect to see all of the following signs EXCEPT

(A) miosis

(B) nasal congestion

(C) anhidrosis

(D) a decrease in temperature of the blocked limb by at least 1°C

(E) ptosis

DIRECTIONS (Questions 597-598): Each group of items below consists of lettered headings followed by a list of numbered phrases or statements. For each numbered phrase or statement, select the ONE lettered heading or component that is most closely associated with it. Each lettered heading or component may be selected once, more than once, or not at all.

(A) Glossopharyngeal nerve

(B) Internal branch of the superior laryngeal nerve

(C) External branch of the superior laryngeal nerve

(D) Recurrent laryngeal nerve

(E) Trigeminal nerve

(F) Anterior ethmoidal nerve

(G) Greater palatine nerve

For each patient, select the appropriate airway block.

597. A 23-year-old obese female reports having a known difficult airway. She remembered having an awake intubation the last time she presented for surgery and anesthesia. Specifically she states having had a strong "gag reflex" when the fiberoptic scope made contact with her soft palate.

598. During your performance of an awake fiberoptic intubation, you are able to advance the fiberoptic scope just above the epiglottis. Just as you are about to advance the scope through the vocal cords, it makes contact with the posterior surface of the epiglottis and the vocal cords snap shut.

DIRECTIONS (Questions 599-600): Each group of items below consists of lettered headings followed by a list of numbered phrases or statements. For each numbered phrase or statement, select the ONE lettered heading or component that is most closely associated with it. Each lettered heading or component may be selected once, more than once, or not at all.

(A) C6
(B) C7
(C) T1
(D) T4
(E) T7
(F) T10
(G) L4

For each patient, select the vertebra described in the physical examination.

599. A 25-year-old female requests a labor epidural for analgesia. In assessing the appropriate landmarks, you palpate the anterior superior iliac spines and draw a line connecting both iliac crests.

600. A 25-year-old man presents for a right total shoulder replacement. You consent the patient for continuous cervical paravertebral blocks utilizing nerve stimulation. In assessing the appropriate topographical landmarks you palpate the most prominent spinous process in the neck.

Answers and Explanations

559. (B) Certain subsets of patients have been identified as high risk. This includes the scenario described in B. Such a patient has a 1 in 3600 risk of having an epidural hematoma in a ten-year Swedish observational study. *(5:784)*

560. (A) Extremities that have decreased sensation need to be protected from positional related injuries. Specific education and instructions to protect the extremities following regional anesthesia should be provided to care personnel and the patient. *(5:785)*

561. (B) The adult spinal cord typically terminates at L1-L2. The infant spinal cord terminates around L3. *(5:786)*

562. (E) The Taylor approach begins with identification of the posterior superior iliac spine (PSIS). The skin entrance site is 1 cm medial and 1 cm caudad to the PSIS. The needle is then directed approximately 45 degrees medial and cephalad to enter the L5-S1 interspace. *(5:792)*

563. (A) When the needle enters the epidural space, continuous or intermittent gentle pressure placed onto a syringe containing saline or air will result in the ability to inject into the epidural space. This is known as loss of resistance. *(5:793)*

564. (A) Local anesthetics and opioids must penetrate through the arachnoid mater to get to the CSF. The specifics of uptake of a drug by the CSF depend also on drug characteristics such as lipid solubility. *(5:794)*

565. (D) Isobaric means a baricity of 1.0, thus the drug will neither rise nor sink. *(5:795)*

566. (C) Lidocaine is the biggest risk factor for TNS. In particular, 5% lidocaine has the highest risk. *(5:796)*

567. (C) For the best neurologic outcome, decompression of an epidural hematoma must occur immediately and preferably within 6-8 h. Prognosis is worsened if decompression occurs after 8 h. *(5:860)*

568. (B) Intrathecal clonidine can prolong both the motor and sensory block associated with spinal anesthesia. Intrathecal clonidine cannot act as the sole anesthetic. *(5:798)*

569. (D) Intrathecal epinephrine can lead to urinary retention. Itching is thought to be a side effect of intrathecal opioids. *(5:799)*

570. (A) Although accessory muscles may be impacted by spinal anesthesia, as long as the phrenic nerve is not blocked, gross pulmonary function should be maintained. *(5:800)*

571. (B) Since both arterial and venous vasodilation occur, the recommended treatments for the hypotension accompanying spinal anesthesia are the administration of intravenous fluids and α_1-adrenoceptor agonists. *(5:801)*

572. (E) Lipid emulsion therapy has been documented to reverse local anesthetic systemic toxicity in both humans and animals. It is considered the treatment of choice and should be available wherever regional anesthesia is performed. *(5:780)*

573. (C) It has limited use in modern anesthesia practice because of its relatively high potential for systemic toxicity and addiction liabilities. Cocaine is an effective topical anesthetic agent, and it produces vasoconstriction at clinically useful concentrations. It is often used to anesthetize and constrict the nasal mucosa before nasotracheal intubation. It is the only local anesthetic that inhibits the reuptake of catecholamines in the central and peripheral nervous systems. *(5:781)*

574. (C) Most of the hypotension in a euvolemic patient is related to arterial and venous dilatation. Thus, administration of an α_1-adrenoceptor agonist like phenylephrine is the treatment of choice. Secondary treatment would be intravenous fluid administration. Atropine and/or epinephrine would be used in a situation of profound bradycardia. *(5:802)*

575. (B) The classic post-dural puncture headache (PDPH) is position-related in that recumbency helps to alleviate symptoms. Common symptoms are severe bi-frontal throbbing, nausea, vomiting, and malaise. Treatments include fluid, caffeine, theophylline, and epidural blood patch. *(5:802)*

576. (E) Although serious, prompt diagnosis with imaging studies and treatment with surgical decompression can result in full recovery. *(5:803)*

577. (D) A positive response should be concluded if any of the following occur: heart rate increase > 20 beats/min, systolic blood pressure increase > 15 mm Hg, T wave amplitude decrease by ≥ 25% on ECG. *(5:805)*

578. (C) The full spectrum of reactions from itching to anaphylaxis has been reported. Allergies are more common with ester compounds as compared to amides. *(5:786)*

579. (A) Ultrasound imaging has provided new information on the reality that conventional approaches to nerve localization often result in what appears to be intraneural injections. There is current debate as to what constitutes dangerous, versus safe, intraneural injections. *(5:855)*

580. (C) Traditionally the supraclavicular approach had been avoided due to a high incidence of pneumothorax. This high incidence of pneumothorax led to the popularity of the axillary approach. With ultrasound guidance, there has been renewed interest in the supraclavicular approach. *(5:833)*

581. (A) Practitioners should select appropriate patients for regional anesthesia considering absolute as well as relative contraindications. *(5:848)*

582. (A) Allergic reactions are more common after exposure to ester compounds than amide compounds. Tetracaine is the only ester compound listed. *(5:852)*

583. (D) A number of factors influence the absorption rate of local anesthetics from tissue. The most important factor is the site of injection. Absorption is more rapid in highly vascular tissue and less so in poorly perfused tissue. *(5:852)*

584. (B) A recent analysis of 7,000 peripheral nerve blocks reported an incidence of 0.04% of late neurologic deficits. *(5:855)*

585. (A) A recent study found that a stimulating current with 0.2 mA or less reliably predicts intraneural needle placement. However a threshold current greater than 0.2 mA does not reliably preclude intraneural needle placement. *(5:855)*

586. (C) Blunt tip needles are less likely to penetrate neural tissue and therefore are the preferred needle type. However, if they do penetrate neural tissue they are likely to be more disruptive to the neural tissue. *(5:855)*

587. (B) The motor innervation of the common peroneal is via the deep peroneal nerve that allows for dorsiflexion of the foot. Given its superficial nature, this nerve may be injured in the perioperative period after a total knee arthroplasty. The superficial peroneal nerve is a branch of the common peroneal nerve; however, it does not provide motor innervation. *(4:71-2)*

588. **(E)** The lumbar plexus block is associated with an increased risk of local anesthetic toxicity due to the high vascularity of the area and large volumes of local anesthetic required for the desired spread. This increases the vascular absorption of local anesthetic from the psoas muscle. With a direct intravascular injection, one would expect the manifestation of toxicity to be immediate upon injection. *(5:840)*

589. **(A)** With the administration of intravenous lipid emulsion, recent studies demonstrate improved hemodynamics and a survival benefit in animal models of bupivacaine toxicity. It has been suggested that lipid emulsion acts as a lipid sink binding local anesthetics and removing them from cardiac binding sites. Twenty percent lipid emulsion should be administered early as a bolus of 1.5 mL/kg over one minute and followed 0.25 mL/kg/min. *(5:853-4)*

590. **(C)** The true incidence is unknown but an epidural hematoma after neuraxial blockade is rare and estimated to occur in fewer than 1 in 150,000 cases. *(5:859)*

591. **(C)** The umbilicus closely approximates the T10 dermatome level. The nipple line closely approximates the T4 level. *(4:237)*

592. **(C)** Benzocaine is known to cause methemoglobinemia. The anesthesiologist must be cautious and vigilant to such an occurrence. *(5:970)*

593. **(C)** Bupivacaine is not recommended given the potential for cardiac toxicity. The duration of a Bier block is limited by tourniquet pain. When using a double tourniquet, the proximal tourniquet is inflated first. When the patient complains of tourniquet pain, the distal tourniquet (that is wrapped around an anesthetized area) is inflated followed by the proximal tourniquet being deflated. *(5:866)*

594. **(D)** Regional anesthesia is known to decrease the need for opioids and therefore decrease opioid related morbidity. *(5:785)*

595. **(B)** Complex regional pain syndrome (CRPS) is sympathetically-mediated pain. A sympathetic block of the upper extremity can be obtained by performing a stellate ganglion block. The stellate ganglion is also known as the cervicothoracic ganglion because it is a fusion of the seventh cervical and first thoracic ganglion. *(5:1579-81)*

596. **(D)** A sympathetic block would result in an increase in temperature to the block limb by at least 1°C. This is a result of the vasodilation that occurs to the extremity. Horner syndrome as well as nasal congestion would also occur. *(5:1579-81)*

597. **(A)** The glossopharyngeal nerve innervates the oropharynx, soft palate, posterior portion of the tongue, and the pharyngeal surface of the epiglottis. The pharyngeal nerve can be anesthetized by inhaling nebulized lidocaine, application of topical anesthesia, or direct glossopharyngeal nerve blocks. *(4:335)*

598. **(B)** The internal branch of the superior laryngeal nerve is a branch of the vagus nerve and provides sensory innervation to the base of the tongue, posterior surface of the epiglottis, aryepiglottic fold, and the arytenoids. The external branch of the superior laryngeal nerve provides motor innervation to the cricothyroid muscle. Besides topical administration, bilateral superior laryngeal nerve block can be performed by injecting local anesthetic at the level of the greater cornu of the hyoid bone. *(4:336)*

599. **(G)** The intercristal line reflects the spinous process of L4. *(5:810)*

600. **(B)** C7 is the most prominent and therefore easily palpated spinous process in the neck. *(5:809)*

CHAPTER 10

Practice Test
Questions

DIRECTIONS (Questions 1-150): Each of the numbered items or incomplete statements in this section is followed by answers or by completions of the statement. Select the ONE lettered answer or completion that is BEST in each case.

1. The interaction of rocuronium and acetylcholine at the myoneural junction is one of

    (A) synergism
    (B) competition for binding sites
    (C) chemical combination
    (D) alteration of metabolism
    (E) altered protein binding

2. As one moves from the apex of the lung to the dependent portions

    (A) the alveoli become larger
    (B) the caliber of the air passages becomes larger
    (C) pleural pressure decreases
    (D) compliance becomes greater
    (E) ventilation of the alveoli becomes less due to decreased compliance

3. A 70-year-old woman with long-standing type 2 diabetes mellitus presents for a preoperative assessment prior to femoral-popliteal bypass surgery. Her only medication is exenatide. Having never heard of this drug, the anesthesia resident looks it up and finds that it is

    (A) a glucagon-like peptide-1 receptor agonist
    (B) FDA approved for treatment of type 1 and type 2 diabetes mellitus
    (C) a member of the biguanide class of oral hypoglycemic agents like metformin
    (D) a thiazolidinedione like rosiglitazone
    (E) also used for prevention of heart disease in type 2 diabetics

4. The most important site of drug transformation is usually the

    (A) liver
    (B) spleen
    (C) kidney
    (D) lungs
    (E) bloodstream

5. Esmolol is chosen for a tachycardic patient with liver cirrhosis. The 9-minute half-life of the drug stems from

    (A) pseudocholinesterase
    (B) skeletal muscle esterase
    (C) red blood cell esterases
    (D) phosphodiesterase
    (E) alkaline phosphatase

6. A 49-year-old man with Addison disease presents for a herniorrhaphy. All of the following statements about Addison disease are true EXCEPT

(A) patient's with this condition undergoing even minor procedures require stress dose of steroids intraoperatively and a long postoperative taper

(B) typical laboratory abnormalities include hyponatremia and hyperkalemia

(C) Addison disease is a type of primary adrenal insufficiency caused by adrenal gland destruction

(D) both skin hyperpigmentation and vitiligo are signs of Addison disease

(E) common symptoms in untreated Addison disease are diarrhea and orthostatic hypotension

7. Bioavailability of a drug refers to the amount of drug that

(A) is administered intramuscularly

(B) is administered orally

(C) reaches the liver

(D) is excreted by the kidney

(E) reaches its site of action

8. A 21-year-old woman with a long history of anorexia nervosa typically has all of the following EXCEPT

(A) osteoporosis

(B) increased risk of intraoperative dysrhythmias

(C) delayed gastric emptying

(D) hypotension

(E) resting tachycardia

9. In cases of unequivocal intraoperative awareness, the incidence of posttraumatic stress disorder may be approximately

(A) 0.1%

(B) 1%

(C) 10%

(D) 50%

(E) 99%

10. A 40-year-old woman presents with a corrected QT interval (QTc) prolonged to 500 msec. She is

(A) at increased risk for perioperative morbidity and mortality related to cardiac arrhythmias

(B) recommended to receive amiodarone

(C) likely to be hypocalcemic

(D) at risk for Wolf-Parkinson-White syndrome

(E) at risk to require intraoperative pacemaker therapy

11. Renal clearance of a drug

(A) is usually of little importance

(B) has no relationship to creatinine clearance

(C) is constant for a given drug

(D) varies with pH, urine flow rate, and renal blood flow

(E) may exceed renal blood flow

12. A 50-year-old man planned for shoulder surgery is judged to be in New York Heart Association functional class III. He has

(A) marked limitation of physical activity

(B) symptoms at rest

(C) slight limitation of physical activity

(D) inability to comfortably carry out any physical activity

(E) no symptoms during ordinary activity

13. All of the following are true of closing volume EXCEPT that it is

(A) measured by a single-breath nitrogen technique

(B) useful in determining disease of small airways

(C) decreased at the extremes of age

(D) unchanged in obesity

(E) measured at phase IV on the nitrogen washout curve

14. A patient has been given an injection of ketamine in a dose calculated to be sufficient for anesthesia. His eyes remain open, and there is slight nystagmus and occasional purposeless movements. This is an indication that

   (A) the dose is inadequate
   (B) more ketamine should be given to stop the movements
   (C) the dose is excessive
   (D) the dose is adequate for anesthesia
   (E) the patient is having a seizure

15. Under normal physiologic conditions cerebral blood flow is

   (A) 1 mL/100 g/min
   (B) 10 mL/100 g/min
   (C) 25 mL/100 g/min
   (D) 50 mL/100 g/min
   (E) 100 mL/100 g/min

16. A 50-year-old man has a bicuspid aortic valve. Surgical repair of his ascending aorta is indicated at a diameter of

   (A) 4 cm
   (B) 4.5 cm
   (C) 5 cm
   (D) 5.5 cm
   (E) 6 cm

17. The peripheral chemoreceptors are

   (A) located in the medulla oblongata
   (B) poorly perfused and, therefore, respond slowly to changes in the oxygen content of the blood
   (C) responsible for the hypoxic drive to respiration
   (D) influenced by oxygen content rather than oxygen tension
   (E) not affected by increasing age

18. Which one of the following agents should be avoided in a patient with heparin-induced thrombocytopenia type II?

   (A) danaparoid
   (B) lepirudin
   (C) argatroban
   (D) warfarin
   (E) benzodiazepines

19. Possible ways to assure proper placement of the endotracheal tube include all of the following, EXCEPT

   (A) chest radiograph
   (B) bronchoscopic examination
   (C) auscultation of the thorax
   (D) continuous end-tidal carbon dioxide capnography
   (E) fogging within the endotracheal tube

20. Hypoxic pulmonary vasoconstriction

   (A) is not important in the intact human being
   (B) is active only at high altitude
   (C) causes more blood flow to the base of the lung
   (D) causes higher dead space/tidal volume ratio (V_D/V_T) than in the nonhypoxic lung
   (E) diverts blood flow from hypoxic to non-hypoxic lung areas

21. A 9-year-old boy sustained a 40% burn to the anterior portion of his body. On the twentieth day after the burn, he is brought to the operating room for a skin graft. Anesthesia is induced with thiopental, and succinylcholine is injected for relaxation. The ECG shows peaked T waves followed by asystole. The most likely cause of the arrhythmia is

   (A) an overdose of thiopental
   (B) hypoxia
   (C) hyperkalemia
   (D) electrocution
   (E) administration of the wrong drug

22. An anesthesia circuit is connected to a circle system and the combined volume of both is 5 L. The fresh gas flow is 1 L/min. After des-flurane 10% is turned on, how long will it take the concentration in the circuit to reach 8.5% desflurane?

    (A) 1 min
    (B) 5 min
    (C) 8.5 min
    (D) 10 min
    (E) 17 min

23. A 20-year-old patient with hemophilia B (Christmas disease) is planned for appendec-tomy. The coagulation deficit is that of clotting factor

    (A) II
    (B) VII
    (C) VIII
    (D) IX
    (E) XII

24. Propofol

    (A) increases cerebral blood flow
    (B) is very soluble in aqueous solutions
    (C) causes catecholamine release
    (D) has little analgesic activity
    (E) has a longer sleep time than thiopental

25. A 50-year-old woman with metabolic syn-drome presents for preoperative assessment prior to elective coronary artery bypass sur-gery. True statements about the metabolic syndrome include all of the following EXCEPT

    (A) patients with the metabolic syndrome are at increased risk for developing overt diabetes
    (B) to make the diagnosis, a patient must have 3 of the following 5 criteria: elevat-ed waist circumference, elevated triglyc-erides, reduced high-density lipoprotein cholesterol, elevated blood pressure, and elevated fasting blood sugar
    (C) patients with the metabolic syndrome are at increased risk of cerebrovascular disease

    (D) patients with the metabolic syndrome should be treated prophylactically with metformin
    (E) women with polycystic ovarian syndrome are at increased risk for developing metabolic syndrome

26. A discrepancy is noted in a patient bearing two arterial catheters. Normally the systolic blood pressure is highest in the

    (A) ascending aorta
    (B) descending aorta
    (C) femoral artery
    (D) dorsalis pedis artery
    (E) pulmonary artery

27. Recognition of hypoxemia in the recovery room

    (A) depends on the detection of cyanosis
    (B) depends on the detection of apnea
    (C) depends on the detection of circulatory responses
    (D) is best accomplished with pulse oximetry
    (E) is done better with a transcutaneous oxygen monitor than with a pulse oximeter

28. A 36-year-old male who recently suffered mul-tiple trauma including thermal injuries is to undergo general endotracheal anesthesia for elective orthopedic surgery. Which one of the following conditions would most likely explain resistance to non-depolarizing neuromuscular blockers during the operative procedure?

    (A) respiratory acidosis
    (B) recent large body surface area burn
    (C) administration of a volatile anesthetic
    (D) hypothermia
    (E) hypermagnesemia

29. The Hering–Breuer reflex

    (A) is accentuated in pre-term infants when compared to full-term infants
    (B) causes a deep inspiration after a total expiration in the laboratory animal

(C)   causes a deep inspiration after a cough

(D)   has a major role in the control of ventilation

(E)   is stimulated by barbiturates

30.   A 42-year-old African American woman with a multinodular goiter is diagnosed with hyperthyroidism. Clinical manifestations of hyperthyroidism include all of the following EXCEPT

(A)   sweating

(B)   fatigue

(C)   tachycardia

(D)   shivering

(E)   hypermotility and diarrhea

31.   A finding that may be used to distinguish deep sedation from general anesthesia is

(A)   ability to follow a simple command

(B)   adequate minute ventilation

(C)   response to a painful pinch

(D)   unobstructed airway

(E)   BIS value

DIRECTIONS: Use the following figure to answer Questions 32-33:

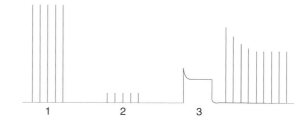

32.   The figure shows the evoked twitch response following an unknown drug. The segment (1) is the baseline before drug administration, and (2) is the response three minutes after drug administration. From these two segments, you can say that the drug

(A)   is not a muscle relaxant

(B)   is a depolarizing muscle relaxant

(C)   is a nondepolarizing muscle relaxant

(D)   caused complete paralysis

(E)   caused 90% depression

33.   At the time point (3), a tetanic stimulation was applied with the depicted result. Following this, one could state that

(A)   the drug is not a muscle relaxant

(B)   the drug is a depolarizing muscle relaxant

(C)   the drug is a nondepolarizing muscle relaxant

(D)   either the drug is a nondepolarizing muscle relaxant, or a dual block is present

(E)   the tracing shown is due to artifact

34.   A very fit amateur mountaineer wishes to climb without the use of supplemental oxygen or medications. He also wishes to avoid letting his arterial oxygen concentration decrease below 45 mm Hg. Using the table below, calculate the maximum height to which the mountaineer should ascend.

Altitude (ft)	7,000	10,000	12,000	15,000	18,000
P_{atm} (mm Hg)	595	534	496	443	395

(A)   7,000 ft

(B)   10,000 ft

(C)   12,000 ft

(D)   15,000 ft

(E)   18,000 ft

35.   The primary difference between cisatracurium and atracurium is that cisatracurium is

(A)   a different isomer than atracurium

(B)   optically active

(C)   substantially shorter-acting

(D)   less likely to result in histamine release

(E)   metabolized to a greater degree by nonspecific plasma esterases

36.   The second heart sound coincides with all of the following EXCEPT

(A)   closing of the aortic valve

(B)   isometric relaxation of myocardial fibers

(C)   closure of the mitral valve

(D)   the T wave of the electrocardiogram

(E)   closure of the pulmonic valve

37. In a carbon dioxide response curve, the minute ventilation is plotted against various concentrations of carbon dioxide. Which one of the following statements is TRUE about a carbon dioxide response curve?

   (A) The patient under anesthesia will show the same effects regardless of the agent.
   (B) The slope of the response may change, but the position of the curve remains the same.
   (C) The position and slope are the same in adults and infants.
   (D) Increased work of breathing leads to a steeper slope.
   (E) The slope of the line measures the patient's sensitivity to carbon dioxide.

38. The blood supply to the motor tracts of the spinal cord is primarily from the

   (A) posterior spinal artery
   (B) anterior spinal artery
   (C) penetrating branches of the radicular arteries
   (D) artery of Adamkiewicz
   (E) basilar artery

39. The inability to sustain contraction (fade) during tetanic contraction is due to

   (A) inability to transmit rapid electrical impulses
   (B) cellular loss of potassium
   (C) depletion of cellular DNA
   (D) inability of recording apparatus to show all contractions
   (E) the inability of the endplate to release sufficient acetylcholine

40. A 39-year-old woman being evaluated for cataract surgery has Von Willebrand disease. This disease

   (A) commonly first manifests as abnormal bleeding after tooth extraction or tonsillectomy in children
   (B) usually affects only females
   (C) is usually associated with a low platelet count

   (D) is caused by factor VIII deficiency
   (E) is one of the rarest of the congenital bleeding disorders

41. Calcium chloride is administered to a patient receiving citrated plasma transfusions. Calcium ion

   (A) decreases myocardial contractile force
   (B) decreases duration of systole
   (C) decreases vascular tone
   (D) decreases ventricular automaticity
   (E) enters the cardiac cell, causing excitation

42. Prolonged surgery on the spine in the prone position is occasionally followed by postoperative visual loss. The most common etiology of such visual loss is

   (A) central retinal artery occlusion
   (B) central retinal vein occlusion
   (C) cortical blindness
   (D) anterior ischemic optic neuropathy
   (E) posterior ischemic optic neuropathy

43. Transdermal scopolamine

   (A) is effective in the prevention of PONV if administered preoperatively
   (B) is effective in the treatment of PONV when administered postoperatively
   (C) patch should be applied to the deltoid muscle
   (D) is devoid of any side effects
   (E) in a multilayered adhesive unit has a duration of action of about 16 h

44. A pediatric patient weighing 14 kg is being ventilated with a traditional anesthesia machine ventilator using the following set parameters:

   Tidal volume = 50 mL

   Ventilatory rate = 20/min

   I:E ratio = 1:2

   Oxygen flow = 2.5 L/min

   Nitrous oxide flow = 3.5 L/min

The resulting minute ventilation is approximately

(A) 1 L/min
(B) 1.5 L/min
(C) 2 L/min
(D) 2.5 L/min
(E) 3 L/min

45. Compared to the young adult, the elderly patient

(A) has an unchanged venous admixture during general anesthesia
(B) has a decrease in true pulmonary shunting during general anesthesia
(C) has an increase in total lung capacity
(D) has an increase in closing capacity
(E) has a decrease in closing capacity

46. If succinylcholine is given to facilitate intubation, and the patient is allowed to recover fully from the depolarizing block, and then is given pancuronium, one would expect

(A) a lower than normal amount of pancuronium is needed to reestablish neuromuscular blockade
(B) the pancuronium to have a shorter duration of action as a result of the succinylcholine
(C) no change in the duration of action of pancuronium
(D) no change in the duration of action of pancuronium but less intensity of relaxation
(E) the development of a phase II block

47. A fourth-year medical student is on her anesthesia rotation. You are discussing local anesthetics for spinal anesthesia with her. The topic of baricity arises on which you explain that baricity is the

(A) milligram dose of an equipotent drug
(B) minimum concentration needed to reach clinical effect
(C) half-life of elimination

(D) context sensitive half-time
(E) ratio of the specific gravity of a drug to a reference specific gravity

48. When desflurane, but not sevoflurane, in a carrier gas of 100% oxygen is passed through very dry carbon dioxide absorbent, the patient may be exposed to a toxic concentration of

(A) ozone
(B) phosgene
(C) carbon dioxide
(D) carbon monoxide
(E) fluoride

49. Technical difficulties in treating patients with morbid obesity include all of the following EXCEPT

(A) spuriously low blood pressure cuff readings
(B) difficult venous access
(C) difficult intubation
(D) difficult airway maintenance with mask
(E) difficulty with nerve blocks

DIRECTIONS: Use the following scenario to answer Questions 50-52. Many patients are unaware of the reasons for which they are taking their medications. When provided with a list of medications by a patient, an anesthesiologist must be able to recognize the medications and know the likely pathological states for which the medications are indicated. For Questions 50-52, a medication is followed by five diseases or pathological states. Choose the ONE disease for which the medication may be indicated.

50. Omeprazole

(A) peptic ulcer disease
(B) diabetic gastroparesis
(C) vertigo
(D) urinary tract infection
(E) type II diabetes mellitus

51. Acetazolamide

(A) glaucoma

(B) asthma

(C) peptic ulcer disease

(D) deep venous thrombosis

(E) atrial fibrillation

52. Glyburide

(A) myasthenia gravis

(B) type II diabetes mellitus

(C) angina pectoris

(D) glaucoma

(E) hypercalcemia

53. Somatosensory-evoked potentials (SSEP)

(A) are extinguished by propofol

(B) are unaffected by deep levels of isoflurane anesthesia

(C) are evaluated from the standpoint of amplitude only

(D) are rendered unreadable by neuromuscular blocking agents

(E) are modestly affected by nitrous oxide

54. A team of anesthesiologists has traveled to a third-world country to provide anesthesia for their surgical colleagues who plan to perform plastic reconstructive procedures on children with cleft palate and similar craniofacial abnormalities. The anesthesiologists have brought an ample quantity of sevoflurane with them but find that there are no sevoflurane vaporizers at the hospital where they will work. In terms of the accuracy in delivering sevoflurane, the least difference between the set and delivered concentrations of sevoflurane will result if sevoflurane is delivered via which one of these vaporizers?

(A) Desflurane vaporizer

(B) Enflurane vaporizer

(C) Halothane vaporizer

(D) Isoflurane vaporizer

(E) Methoxyflurane vaporizer

55. An 18-year-old male presents for repair of a right shoulder rotator cuff tear. He agrees to an interscalene block for postoperative analgesia. You decide to avoid using the local anesthetic that is recognized as being the most cardiotoxic. You therefore decide to avoid

(A) bupivacaine

(B) ropivacaine

(C) chloroprocaine

(D) lidocaine

(E) mepivacaine

56. All of the following is true concerning the change in functional residual capacity (FRC) with body position, EXCEPT

(A) FRC is markedly reduced in the supine position

(B) in head-down, FRC is little different from supine

(C) FRC is reduced in sitting position when compared to supine position

(D) FRC is greater in lateral than in supine position

(E) FRC is greater in prone than in supine position

57. The inspired partial pressure of isoflurane is lower than the partial pressure of the anesthetic in the fresh gas because of all of the following processes EXCEPT

(A) absorption of the agent by rubber hoses

(B) dilution of fresh gas in the circle absorber

(C) metabolism of isoflurane

(D) adsorption of the agent by soda lime

(E) uptake of the agent by the patient

58. All of the following are factors that DECREASE the rate of onset of the effects of an inhalational anesthetic EXCEPT

(A) low (as opposed to high) fresh gas flow rate

(B) low (as opposed to high) minute ventilation

(C) low (as opposed to high) anesthetic concentration in inhaled gas mixture

(D) low (as opposed to high) blood:gas partition coefficient

(E) high (as opposed to low) cardiac output

59. Pulmonary edema in the recovery room

   (A) usually occurs as a late sign
   (B) is always associated with a rise of central venous pressure (CVP)
   (C) will be detected because of distended neck vessels
   (D) may be due to airway obstruction
   (E) usually occurs with normal breath sounds present

60. The number of calories required to raise the temperature of 1 g of a substance by 1°C is

   (A) the heat of vaporization
   (B) the specific heat
   (C) the critical temperature
   (D) thermal conductivity
   (E) equal for all substances

61. Your patient has dyspnea on mild exertion and peripheral edema. Mechanisms by which patients with failing hearts compensate for low cardiac output include all of the following EXCEPT

   (A) increased sympathetic drive to the heart
   (B) myocardial hypertrophy
   (C) renal loss of salt and decreased blood volume
   (D) secondary hyperaldosteronism
   (E) peripheral vasoconstriction

62. The pin index safety system (PISS)

   (A) prevents attachment of gas-administering equipment to the wrong type of gas
   (B) prevents incorrect yoke-tank connections
   (C) consists of quick-connectors typically mounted on the wall or hanging from the ceiling
   (D) is found on the wall end, but not the machine end, of gas hoses connected to anesthesia machines
   (E) is found on the machine end, but not the wall end, of gas hoses connected to anesthesia machines

DIRECTIONS: Use the following figure to answer Questions 63-64:

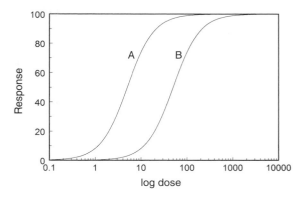

63. If A and B are two different medications producing the same effect, then the figure shows that

   (A) A has higher efficacy than B
   (B) A has lower efficacy than B
   (C) A and B must act via different receptors to produce their effects
   (D) A is more potent than B
   (E) A has a higher ED_{50} than B

64. If A depicts the dose-response relationship of a drug X acting alone, and B depicts the dose-response relationship of drug X in the presence of drug Y, then it can be said that drug Y

   (A) is a competitive antagonist of drug X
   (B) is a non-competitive antagonist of drug X
   (C) must act via a different receptor than drug X
   (D) decreases the efficacy of drug X
   (E) increases the potency of drug X

65. A 63-year-old male patient with end-stage renal disease from long-standing hypertension presents for preoperative assessment prior to elective repair of an abdominal aortic aneurysm. Laboratory abnormalities common in patients with end-stage renal disease include

   (A) anemia
   (B) thrombocytosis
   (C) hypokalemia
   (D) hypophosphatemia
   (E) leukocytosis

66. Four years after a heart transplant, a patient requires bowel resection. The transplanted heart

    (A) has an abnormal Frank–Starling mechanism
    (B) responds as does an innervated heart to atropine
    (C) bears functional α- and β-adrenoceptors
    (D) does not respond to isoproterenol
    (E) does not increase cardiac output with increased preload

67. Cerebrospinal fluid (CSF) flows through all of the following EXCEPT the

    (A) arachnoid villi
    (B) cerebral ventricle
    (C) lateral ventricle
    (D) subarachnoid space
    (E) epidural space

68. Verapamil

    (A) is useful in the treatment of supraventricular tachycardia
    (B) is contraindicated in patients with asthma
    (C) is useful when combined with propranolol
    (D) is a potent vasoconstrictor
    (E) has no effect on the pacemaker cells

69. A resident is carrying a Tec 5 vaporizer from the anesthesia workroom to the operating room and slips on the freshly washed floor. Although he did not drop it, he did tip it on its side when he fell. After properly mounting the vaporizer on the anesthesia machine, the proper procedure to flush the vaporizer is to

    (A) leave the vaporizer setting at "off" and press the oxygen flush valve for 10 min
    (B) leave the vaporizer setting at "off" and adjust the oxygen valve to deliver oxygen at 10 L/min for 10 min
    (C) turn the vaporizer setting to its maximum value and press the oxygen flush valve for 10 min

    (D) turn the vaporizer setting to its maximum value and adjust the oxygen valve to deliver oxygen at 10 L/min for 10 min
    (E) return the vaporizer to the manufacturer for service; do not mount it on the anesthesia machine

70. A 39-year-old female presents for a vaginal hysterectomy. Ten minutes after performing a spinal anesthetic with 15 milligrams of 0.5% hyperbaric bupivacaine, you notice a slowing of the heart rhythm on continuous EKG monitoring. A short period of asystole then develops at which time you administer 10 mcg of epinephrine and perform a brief period of chest compressions. The most important independent predictor of bradycardia following spinal anesthesia is

    (A) hypertension
    (B) hyperlipidemia
    (C) previous spinal anesthesia
    (D) preexisting bradycardia
    (E) ASA I status

71. A 45-year-old male with a history of hypertension that is controlled with a diuretic is scheduled for a hernia repair. He is completely asymptomatic, but his plasma potassium concentration is 3.0 mEq/L. The appropriate management is to

    (A) cancel the procedure
    (B) start a potassium infusion and proceed
    (C) proceed with the procedure but not administer potassium
    (D) give 40 mEq of potassium by mouth before starting
    (E) proceed with the procedure only if it can be done under regional anesthesia

72. Intracranial pressure (ICP) can be monitored with all of the following EXCEPT

    (A) a catheter implanted directly into brain parenchyma
    (B) by a pressure transducing bolt in the subarachnoid space

(C) by a pressure transducer in the epidural space

(D) a ventriculostomy catheter

(E) a catheter in the subdural space

73. In a mixture of gases (such as air)

(A) all vapors, but not all gases obey Dalton's law

(B) each gas contributes a partial pressure that is proportional to its solubility

(C) each gas contributes a partial pressure that is proportional to its molecular fraction

(D) the total pressure is equal to the sum of the gases multiplied by the number of gases

(E) the total pressure is equal to the sum of the gases divided by the number of gases

74. An effect of metoclopramide is

(A) dopamine receptor agonism

(B) β-adrenergic agonism

(C) antagonistic effects at 5-HT$_3$ receptors

(D) muscarinic cholinergic agonistic effects

(E) improvement of large bowel motility

75. A 22-year-old male gunshot victim requires urgent abdominal surgery. His record indicates that he has biopsy-proven hepatic cirrhosis but no history of drug or alcohol use, autoimmune disease, or hepatitis. Possible hereditary causes for cirrhosis in this patient include all of the following EXCEPT

(A) hemochromatosis

(B) α_1-antitrypsin deficiency

(C) Wilson disease

(D) antithrombin III deficiency

(E) cystic fibrosis

76. Hypovolemia is suspected in a septic patient in the ICU. All of the following may be seen in hypovolemia EXCEPT

(A) increased heart rate

(B) wide pulse pressure

(C) decreased urine volume

(D) flat neck veins

(E) pale mucous membranes

77. A 42-year-old man is scheduled for appendectomy for acute appendicitis. Four years ago, he had a myocardial infarction and was treated with the insertion of intracoronary stents. He underwent successful cardiac rehabilitation and now plays tennis regularly without angina or shortness of breath. He would be categorized as ASA Physical Status

(A) I

(B) II

(C) III

(D) IIIE

(E) IV

78. A 45-year-old male is to have a gallbladder procedure. He has heart disease and is on amiodarone. This drug

(A) should be stopped before surgery

(B) has a half-life of 4 h

(C) is used for ventricular arrhythmias

(D) is eliminated by the kidneys

(E) has no effects on β-adrenergic receptors

79. Spinal cord injury is feared in patients requiring thoracoabdominal aortic surgery. The arteria radicularis magna (of Adamkiewicz)

(A) is the largest of the radicular arteries supplying the spinal cord

(B) normally feeds the anteroposterior spinal artery system

(C) anastomoses with the splenic artery

(D) always originates from the suprarenal aorta

(E) may be ligated with impunity

80. The latent heat of vaporization

(A) is equal for all liquids

(B) is independent of the ambient temperature

(C) varies with the temperature of the liquid

(D) is very low for solids

(E) for water is 1 calorie/mL

81. Carbon monoxide diffusion capacity (DLCO) will decrease with

(A) smoking within 24 h of the test
(B) exercise
(C) pulmonary fibrosis
(D) increased hemoglobin
(E) congestive heart failure

82. A local anesthetic that inhibits the reuptake of norepinephrine is

(A) procaine
(B) cocaine
(C) bupivacaine
(D) mepivacaine
(E) lidocaine with epinephrine

83. A middle-aged man with a known pheochromocytoma is scheduled for elective abdominal surgery. Which one of the following statements about his preoperative pharmacologic management is correct?

(A) α-adrenergic blockade is instituted at the same time as β-adrenergic blockade
(B) diuretic antihypertensives are contraindicated
(C) preoperative drug therapy should be started 12 h before surgery
(D) dosage is adjusted according to the levels of urinary catecholamine metabolites
(E) calcium channel blockers are contraindicated in this condition

84. A patient with history of syncope is suspected of Wolff-Parkinson-White syndrome. In this condition, the

(A) heart rate is usually 60 to 80 beats/min during sinus rhythm
(B) PR interval is less than 0.12 sec during sinus rhythm
(C) QRS duration is usually longer than 0.12 sec
(D) the upstroke of the QRS complex is often slurred
(E) adenosine may increase heart rate

85. Atracurium

(A) has both prejunctional and postjunctional effects
(B) liberates histamine at all dose levels
(C) liberates histamine at all infusion rates
(D) breaks down into laudanosine that has caused seizures in humans
(E) causes increased blood pressure

86. A 70-year-old man is receiving anticoagulant drugs to inhibit platelet glycoprotein IIb/IIIa receptor. EXCEPT for the following, the receptor

(A) is activated by cyclic AMP
(B) participates in aggregation of platelets
(C) is inhibited by abciximab
(D) is inhibited by eptifibatide
(E) is activated by diverse stimuli

87. Cerebrospinal fluid pressure may be increased by

(A) coughing
(B) long expiratory time during positive pressure ventilation
(C) short inspiratory time during positive pressure ventilation
(D) low expiratory resistance
(E) negative expiratory phase

88. Isoflurane

(A) is a poor muscle relaxant compared with halothane
(B) has a vapor pressure of 175 mm Hg at 20°C
(C) stimulates ventilation
(D) has a MAC of approximately 1.2%
(E) should be delivered by spontaneous ventilation

89. When inhaling from functional residual capacity (FRC) to maximal inspiration, all of the following are true, EXCEPT

(A) pulmonary vascular resistance increases
(B) pleural pressure decreases
(C) residual volume stays constant

(D) basilar alveoli become larger than apical alveoli

(E) proximal airway pressure is greater than alveolar pressure

90. Propofol has all of the following pharmacological effects EXCEPT

(A) decreasing cerebral blood flow

(B) crossing the blood-brain barrier

(C) reducing ICP

(D) decreasing cerebral metabolic rate

(E) decreasing the latency of somatosensory evoked potentials

91. Which one of the following statements regarding heparin is most accurate?

(A) It inhibits several steps in the intrinsic pathway of blood clotting.

(B) Its dosage may be adjusted by estimating the patient's clotting ability via the bleeding time.

(C) It should not be injected subcutaneously.

(D) It interacts with drugs that inhibit the liver microsomal enzyme system.

(E) It should never be combined in therapy with an oral anticoagulant.

92. A patient undergoing a blood transfusion intraoperatively develops an acute hemolytic reaction. The diagnosis of such a reaction typically

(A) reveals ABO incompatibility to be an unlikely cause

(B) identifies incompatibility with a rare antigen after detailed testing

(C) first presents as hemoglobinuria if the patient is under general anesthesia

(D) shows that the severity of the hemolytic reaction is unrelated to the volume of transfused blood

(E) leads to shock-induced hepatic failure that is the etiology of most of the associated morbidity

93. A cyanotic child is suspected of tetralogy of Fallot. The condition includes all of the following EXCEPT

(A) atrial septal defect (ASD)

(B) ventricular septal defect (VSD)

(C) right ventricular hypertrophy

(D) pulmonary outflow obstruction

(E) overriding aorta

94. The pressure of oxygen delivered by the wall connectors in an operating room is approximately

(A) 1900 psi

(B) 750 psi

(C) 50 psi

(D) 1 atm

(E) 760 mm Hg

95. A 41-year-old patient with a history of drug abuse is admitted to the emergency department for acute onset, anterior chest pain that is radiating into the back between the shoulder blades. Vital signs on arrival include a HR of 107, and a BP of 172/98. The patient appears pale and diaphoretic. Emergent TEE findings include dilated cardiomyopathy and evidence of acute aortic dissection; the patient is referred for emergent cardiac surgery for aortic repair. When planning this patient's anesthetic, caution has to be exercised with the administration of which one of the following drugs?

(A) labetalol

(B) epinephrine

(C) midazolam

(D) ephedrine

(E) phenylephrine

96. An application of the Bernoulli theorem is the measurement of

(A) cardiac output with a thermodilution pulmonary artery catheter

(B) mean arterial pressure using an automated noninvasive blood pressure device

(C) minute ventilation using a spinning turbine

(D) the pressure gradient across a stenotic mitral valve using echocardiography

(E) airway resistance using a spirometer

97. A 45-year-old man with hypertension and a 60-pack-year smoking history is being evaluated in the preoperative clinic for an elective neurosurgical procedure to remove a benign spinal tumor. All of the following statements about exposure to tobacco in the perioperative period are correct EXCEPT

(A) nicotine replacement therapy should be started 1-2 weeks before an attempt at cessation

(B) smokers are more likely to experience wound infections

(C) patients presenting for surgery are more likely to quit smoking when so advised than smokers not having surgery

(D) varenicline for smoking cessation should be started 1-2 weeks before a quit attempt

(E) bupropion is effective pharmacotherapy to assist with smoking cessation in the perioperative period

98. Arterial oxygen tension can be improved by

(A) transferring an obese patient from the supine to the Trendelenburg

(B) decreasing inspired F_{IO_2}

(C) using calcium channel blockers in patients on one lung ventilation

(D) using PEEP in the presence of atelectasis

(E) increasing the concentration of the volatile agent

99. A 19-year-old patient presents for emergent craniotomy for evacuation of a subdural hematoma following a motor vehicle accident. Which one of the following anesthetics is most likely to increase cerebral blood flow?

(A) ketamine

(B) thiopental

(C) sevoflurane (1 MAC)

(D) midazolam

(E) propofol

100. A patient has an arterial catheter in place and the anesthesiologist can view the displayed value of pulse pressure variability. This value may be correlated with

(A) the probability of cardiac ischemia

(B) the depth of anesthesia

(C) the degree of hypovolemia

(D) the cardiac output

(E) the compliance of the lungs

101. A 37-year-old obese female with a known difficult airway presents for a laparoscopic cholecystectomy. You discuss performing an awake fiberoptic intubation with topical anesthesia. Which local anesthetic is used exclusively for topical purposes?

(A) Prilocaine

(B) Tetracaine

(C) Lidocaine

(D) Ropivacaine

(E) Benzocaine

102. A 40-year-old male patient with acromegaly presenting for prostate resection is likely to have all of the following EXCEPT

(A) a difficult airway

(B) glucose intolerance

(C) hypertension

(D) hyperthyroidism

(E) cardiomegaly

103. Calcium channel blockers

(A) should be stopped prior to elective surgery

(B) have a profound negative inotropic effect when administered to a patient who has been given a high dose opioid anesthetic

(C) may prolong atrioventricular conduction time when combined with volatile anesthetics

(D) may antagonize the effect of muscle relaxants

(E) can be used interchangeably due to identical effect sites and mechanisms of action

104. Which one of the following is true regarding the upper airway?

    (A) The hyoid bone suspends the sternothyroid muscle at the level of C7.
    (B) The anatomical structure referred to as "Adam's apple" is called cricoid cartilage.
    (C) The cricothyroid membrane is suitable for emergency airway access; it is located in the midline at the level of C6.
    (D) To each side of the larynx and inferior to the aryepiglottic folds is the rima glottidis, where the endotracheal tube should be placed during intubation.
    (E) The laryngoscope should be positioned in the piriform sinus during direct laryngoscopy.

105. The irrigating fluid for a 55-year-old otherwise healthy man undergoing transurethral prostatic resection

    (A) can cause hypotension and tachycardia in the anesthetized patient
    (B) should be water
    (C) should be isosmolar
    (D) should be hypertonic saline
    (E) should be a solution of a non-metabolized solute

106. Hypercarbia occurring under anesthesia may be due to all of the following, EXCEPT

    (A) increased dead space ventilation
    (B) exhaustion of soda lime
    (C) pulmonary embolism
    (D) hyperventilation
    (E) malignant hyperthermia

107. An anesthetic agent for which a specific antagonist exists is

    (A) etomidate
    (B) butorphanol
    (C) thiopental
    (D) propofol
    (E) succinylcholine

DIRECTIONS: Use the following scenario to answer Questions 108-109. A 55-year-old male is admitted with a history of hypertensive heart disease and evidence of acute myocardial infarction. Vital signs are: blood pressure 180/110, heart rate 124 per minute, body temperature 101°F, and respiratory rate 24 per minute.

108. Efforts to improve myocardial oxygenation should include the following EXCEPT

    (A) decreasing arterial blood pressure
    (B) decreasing body temperature
    (C) administration of intravenous fluid
    (D) slowing heart rate
    (E) administration of oxygen

109. Chest pain worsens as the heart rate and blood pressure are reduced with metoprolol and nitroglycerin. Additional measures might include

    (A) an inhibitor of cyclic-GMP phosphodiesterase
    (B) amiodarone
    (C) antifibrinolytics
    (D) anticoagulation
    (E) lidocaine

110. A contraindication to the discharge to home of a previously healthy, ASA I patient, who had a hernia repair under general anesthesia would be

    (A) heart rate 20% higher than baseline
    (B) systolic blood pressure 20% lower than baseline
    (C) inability to void
    (D) oxygen saturation of 93% on room air
    (E) requiring the assistance of another person to ambulate

111. Which one of the following factors introduces the greatest degree of error in the measurement of hemoglobin saturation by pulse oximetry?

    (A) High concentration of fetal hemoglobin
    (B) High concentration of sickle hemoglobin
    (C) High concentration of methemoglobin
    (D) High concentration of deoxyhemoglobin
    (E) Hyperbilirubinemia

DIRECTIONS: Use the following scenario to answer Questions 112-113: An operating room is protected by an isolated power system that is monitored by a line isolation monitor. During laparoscopic cholecystectomy surgery, the line isolation monitor alarms and the meter indicates 8 mA.

112. What action should initially be taken?

(A) Unplug the fluid warmer because it draws the most current.

(B) Unplug the surgeon's radio because it is unnecessary to the procedure.

(C) Turn off the fluorescent lights because they often interfere with the line isolation monitor.

(D) Unplug the last device that was connected to the circuit.

(E) Unplug the anesthesia monitors and operate them on battery power.

113. If none of the maneuvers taken by the OR staff removes the alarm condition, what action should be taken next?

(A) Relocate the patient to a different operating room while maintaining anesthesia.

(B) Convert to open cholecystectomy and avoid cautery.

(C) Continue the surgery because 8 mA is a harmless current that is flowing through the patient.

(D) Continue the surgery because a second, rare electrical fault will need to occur in order to cause electrical injury to the patient.

114. A 51-year-old patient is undergoing popliteal block under ultrasound guidance for postoperative pain control following ankle surgery. Midazolam 2 mg intravenously has been administered incrementally for procedural sedation. Shortly after injection of 30 mL of ropivacaine 0.5%, the patient starts to complain about visual disturbances that are quickly followed by loss of consciousness and respiratory arrest. Vital signs at the time are significant for new onset hypotension and cardiac arrhythmia. Assuming that the patient is experiencing symptoms of local anesthetic toxicity (LAST), which one of the following interventions is most appropriate?

(A) Ventilation with 100% O_2, propofol bolus, administration of lidocaine and phenylephrine

(B) Ventilation with 100% O_2, midazolam bolus, administration of lidocaine and vasopressin

(C) Ventilation with 100% O_2, administration of diazepam, a beta blocker, and epinephrine

(D) Ventilation with 100% O_2, administration of midazolam followed by continuous infusion of Intralipid 20%, administration of lidocaine and phenylephrine

(E) Ventilation with 100% O_2, administration of 1.5 mL/kg Intralipid 20% followed by continuous infusion, administration of phenylephrine

115. The principal disadvantage of methohexital is

(A) poor water solubility

(B) dose dependent decrease in blood pressure greater than that produced by propofol

(C) low pH of solution

(D) involuntary muscle movements

(E) increase in ictal activity

116. Assuming a constant rate of carbon dioxide formation, the relationship between alveolar ventilation (in a patient under general anesthesia) and carbon dioxide and hydrogen ion concentration is

(A) carbon dioxide is directly proportional to ventilation

(B) doubling ventilation will lead to respiratory alkalosis

(C) reducing ventilation to one fourth of normal will lead to metabolic acidosis

(D) interrupting ventilation for five minutes will cause, next to hypoxemia, profound respiratory alkalosis

(E) alveolar ventilation only responds to endogenous CO_2

117. Effects of fat embolism include all of the following, EXCEPT

(A) hypoxia
(B) tachypnea
(C) interstitial pulmonary edema
(D) neurological impairment
(E) left-axis deviation in the ECG

118. A 37-year-old woman presents for a brain biopsy under monitored anesthesia care. She has a family history of acute intermittent porphyria (AIP) and relates a history of several porphyric attacks over the last 20 years. All of the following statements about AIP are true EXCEPT

(A) propofol is safe in patients with AIP
(B) severe abdominal pain, mental status changes and peripheral neuropathy characterize acute porphyric attacks
(C) it is related to a specific enzyme deficiency in the biosynthesis of flavin-containing enzymes
(D) etomidate should be avoided in patients with AIP
(E) factors known to precipitate acute porphyric crisis include fasting, dehydration, and infection

119. The patient with myasthenia gravis

(A) has weakness of muscles innervated by cranial nerves
(B) usually has diaphragmatic weakness
(C) is very sensitive to succinylcholine
(D) has focal sensory deficits
(E) often has associated carcinomas

120. The brain stem is supplied with blood from the

(A) middle cerebral artery
(B) cingulate artery
(C) basilar artery
(D) posterior cerebral artery
(E) posterior communicating artery

121. When donated blood is initially collected, it is mixed with an anticoagulant and preservation solution containing glucose, citrate, phosphate, and adenine. It has a shelf life of five weeks.

If the unit of whole blood thus collected is fractionated into its components, the shelf life of the packed red cells may be extended to six weeks by adding additional glucose and

(A) ascorbic acid (Vitamin C)
(B) 2,3-DPG
(C) sodium bicarbonate
(D) α-tocopherol (Vitamin E)
(E) adenine

122. All of the following statements are true regarding smoking, EXCEPT

(A) smoking is the strongest modifiable risk factor for cardiovascular disease
(B) compared to non-smokers, FEV_1 tends to decrease more in smokers with increasing age
(C) smoking cessation before surgery may reduce airway hyperreactivity
(D) postoperative smoking cessation may improve wound healing
(E) risk of postoperative nausea and vomiting is higher in smokers

123. Ropivacaine

(A) is supplied as a racemic mixture
(B) is less likely than bupivacaine to cause ventricular arrhythmias after accidental intravenous injection
(C) produces motor blockade of longer duration than sensory blockade
(D) has a low degree of toxicity by virtue of its rapid intravascular metabolism
(E) is an aminoester agent

DIRECTIONS: Use the following case to answer Questions 124-126: A 67-year-old woman is brought to the operating room for an exploratory laparotomy for an intra-abdominal abscess. After induction of anesthesia, a hot air warmer is applied to the patient and but not initiated because the esophageal temperature is measured at 37.8°C. The skin is warm and wet to touch. Anesthesia is maintained with isoflurane in an air/oxygen mixture and muscle relaxation is provided by vecuronium. After opening the abdomen and washout of the abscess cavity, the temperature drops to 36.5°C.

124. The patient may sweat as a result of all of the following processes EXCEPT a

(A) thermal-regulating mechanism
(B) process mediated by β-adrenoceptors
(C) response to sepsis and hyperpyrexia
(D) response to emotional stimuli
(E) response to hypoglycemia

125. Core temperature in the patient under general anesthesia

(A) is closely regulated by the hypothalamus
(B) is elevated if the patient is peripherally vasodilated
(C) cannot be increased by increased metabolism
(D) is best assessed by skin temperature
(E) will tend to drift toward ambient temperature

126. Regulation of body core temperature involves all of the following EXCEPT

(A) heat production by muscle
(B) heat production by the liver
(C) heat dissipation by shivering
(D) heat dissipation by the lungs
(E) heat dissipation by the skin

127. The difference between the alveolar pressure and the ambient pressure is the sum of

(A) transpulmonary pressure and chest wall transmural pressure
(B) esophageal balloon pressure and chest wall transmural pressure
(C) chest wall transmural pressure and pulmonary artery occlusion pressure
(D) pulmonary artery occlusion pressure and esophageal balloon pressure
(E) esophageal balloon pressure and transpulmonary pressure

DIRECTIONS: Use the following figure to answer Questions 128–129:

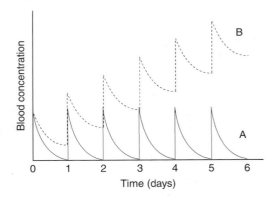

128. Drugs A and B were given by intravenous bolus every 24 h. From the graph, it can be concluded that

(A) drug A maintains persistent therapeutic levels when administered every 24 h
(B) drug B is cumulative when administered every 24 h
(C) drug A exhibits cumulative properties
(D) drug B is completely destroyed in less than 24 h
(E) drug B has reached steady state plasma concentration after 4 days

129. In addition, the graph shows that

(A) drug A has a long half-life in the body
(B) a large initial dose of both drugs was given
(C) different doses are given for initial doses and maintenance doses
(D) in the case of drug B, the body does not remove one dose before another is administered
(E) duration of action of the two drugs is identical

130. All of the following are true of airway resistance EXCEPT

(A) decreases with maximal inspiration
(B) increases with parasympathetic stimulation
(C) increases with sympathetic stimulation
(D) increases with acetylcholine inhalation
(E) increases with inhalation of smoke

131. Mannitol decreases cerebral edema because it

    (A) blocks reuptake of sodium in the collecting system
    (B) draws water across an intact blood brain barrier to dehydrate the brain
    (C) reduces red blood cell volume
    (D) is a peripheral vasodilator
    (E) can be given in kidney failure

132. Sickle cell formation is facilitated by all of the following EXCEPT

    (A) hypoxemia
    (B) sevoflurane
    (C) acidosis
    (D) fever
    (E) dehydration

133. A 33-year-old woman with a recent onset (3 weeks) of clinical hyperthyroidism is admitted for repair of a tendon laceration. She has not taken methimazole for 4 days. At this time the

    (A) patient should be essentially euthyroid
    (B) patient should have general anesthesia if at all possible
    (C) therapy with methimazole may have rendered the patient hypothyroid
    (D) patient would probably have bradycardia
    (E) patient should be considered as a high-risk hyperthyroid patient

134. Which one of the following is a characteristic of general anesthetic agents?

    (A) All inhaled anesthetics produce bronchodilation.
    (B) All general anesthetics are gases at body temperature.
    (C) All general anesthetic effects may be explained by their ability to disrupt membrane lipid-protein interactions.
    (D) General anesthetic effects may be reversed by decreasing the ambient pressure.
    (E) Nitrous oxide causes a dose-dependent inhibition of DNA synthesis.

135. Milrinone

    (A) inhibits Na,K-ATPase
    (B) causes vasodilation
    (C) is an endothelin receptor antagonist
    (D) stimulates phosphodiesterase
    (E) has inotropic effects via β_1-adrenoceptor stimulation

DIRECTIONS: Use the following figure to answer Questions 136-137:

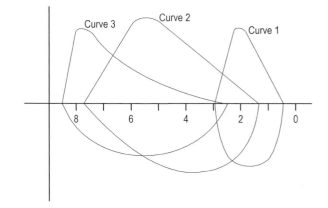

136. As compared to the normal Curve 2, all of the following are TRUE about Curve 3 EXCEPT

    (A) residual volume is elevated
    (B) late expiratory flow is reduced
    (C) vital capacity is relatively normal
    (D) total lung capacity is elevated
    (E) it is characteristic of restrictive lung disease

137. As compared to the normal Curve 2, all of the following are TRUE about Curve 1 EXCEPT

    (A) residual volume is reduced
    (B) late expiratory flow is reduced
    (C) vital capacity is reduced
    (D) total lung capacity is reduced
    (E) it is characteristic of restrictive lung disease

138. Thiopental is contraindicated in

    (A) porphyria congenita

    (B) porphyria cutanea tarda

    (C) acute intermittent porphyria

    (D) myotonia

    (E) chorea

139. Signs of hypoxemia include all of the following EXCEPT

    (A) decreased ventilatory effort due to chemoreceptor stimulation

    (B) increased heart rate due to sympathetic stimulation

    (C) cyanosis

    (D) decreased heart rate due to direct effect of hypoxemia on the heart

    (E) increased blood pressure due to sympathetic stimulation

140. Dopamine

    (A) in a low dose infusion can cause vasodilation and inhibit release of norepinephrine from sympathetic nerves

    (B) as a low dose infusion is selective for the α_2-adrenoceptor

    (C) as a high dose infusion is beneficial in patients with primary cardiac contractile dysfunction

    (D) acts via nicotinic receptors

    (E) is a β_1-selective inotrope

141. Agents in anesthetic practice that can cause bronchodilatation include all of the following, EXCEPT

    (A) ketamine

    (B) atropine

    (C) isoflurane

    (D) sevoflurane

    (E) thiopental

DIRECTIONS (Questions 142-143): Each group of items below consists of lettered headings followed by a list of numbered phrases or statements. For each numbered phrase or statement, select the ONE lettered heading or component that is most closely associated with it. Each lettered heading or component may be selected once, more than once, or not at all.

    (A) Pneumothorax

    (B) Myocardial infarction

    (C) Local anesthetic toxicity

    (D) Anaphylaxis

    (E) Hemidiaphragmatic paresis

    (F) Transient neurologic injury

    (G) Spinal stenosis

    (H) Total spinal anesthesia

For each patient reporting severe shortness of breath, select the most common reason for his or her symptoms

142. An 18-year-old cheerleader is scheduled to undergo open reduction and internal fixation of her wrist after sustaining a distal radial fracture. One hour before the scheduled surgical procedure she undergoes a supraclavicular brachial plexus block with 20 mL of 0.5% bupivacaine. One hour after returning to the PACU, she reports severe shortness of breath.

143. A 72-year-old patient with COPD undergoes a left interscalene brachial plexus block with 20 mL of 0.5% ropivacaine. Fifteen minutes after the local anesthetic injection, the patient reports severe shortness of breath. The monitor displays sinus tachycardia with a heart rate of 134.

DIRECTIONS (Questions 144-145): Each group of items below consists of lettered headings followed by a list of numbered phrases or statements. For each numbered phrase or statement, select the ONE lettered heading or component that is most closely associated with it. Each lettered heading or component may be selected once, more than once, or not at all.

(A) T2

(B) T4

(C) T6

(D) T7

(E) T10

(F) L1

For each patient, select the appropriate dermatome level corresponding to the height of the spinal anesthetic block.

144. A 21-year-old female presents for a cesarean section due to an arrest in labor. You perform a spinal anesthetic with 13.5 mg of hyperbaric bupivacaine. When assessing the level of block you determine that the patient is insensate to the level of the nipple line.

145. A 78-year-old man with a history of coronary artery disease presents for transurethral resection of the prostate. You decide to perform spinal anesthetic in order to be able to monitor the patient's neurologic status. Your goal is to achieve a level of blockade corresponding to the umbilicus.

DIRECTIONS (Questions 146-150): Each group of items below consists of lettered headings followed by a list of numbered phrases or statements. For each numbered phrase or statement, select the ONE lettered heading or component that is most closely associated with it. Each lettered heading or component may be selected once, more than once, or not at all.

(A) Acute pericarditis

(B) Chronic pulmonary hypertension

(C) Chronic constrictive pericardiopathy

(D) Myocarditis

(E) Pericardial tamponade

(F) Post-infarction ventriculoseptal defect (VSD)

(G) Pulmonary embolism

(H) Rheumatic fever

(I) Spontaneous pneumothorax

For each patient with a cardiac symptom or sign, select the most likely mechanism causing the symptoms or sign.

146. A 70-year-old man appears to be stabilizing well after a myocardial infarction. He suddenly develops profound hypotension and respiratory distress. An endotracheal tube is placed, and an intra-aortic balloon pump is initiated.

147. A 60-year-old woman with insidious dyspnea on mild exertion has a systolic heart murmur.

148. A young adult complains of recent onset of chest pain and breathlessness.

149. A 58-year-old man underwent uneventful coronary artery bypass grafting, and is transferred to the intensive care unit. After 4 h of hemodynamic stability, he suddenly develops profound hypotension, and equalization of invasive pressures is noted on initial evaluation.

150. A 60-year-old recipient of heart transplantation has poor cardiac output initially after the surgery but improves during treatment with inhaled nitric oxide and a phosphodiesterase inhibitor.

Answers and Explanations

1. **(B)** The interaction of rocuronium and acetylcholine at the myoneural junction is one of competition for binding sites. As the relaxant occupies the receptors, acetylcholine cannot bind and have an effect. *(1:60)*

2. **(D)** Compliance increases as one moves down the lung. Dependent alveoli are smaller due to the weight of the above tissue. However, this also means that they have a higher capacity for expansion. The shape of the thorax and diaphragm enhance this effect *(5:959)*

3. **(A)** *(1:1255, 1263)*

4. **(A)** The liver is the most important site of drug transformation. The kidney is responsible for the excretion of many drugs, and the metabolism of a few. There are some drug metabolism reactions that occur in the lung and a few that occur in the spleen. *(1:28)*

5. **(C)** Esmolol is inactivated by esterase activity in the cytosol of red cells. Pseudocholinesterase is a plasma protein attacking succinylcholine and ester local anesthetics. Remifentanil is degraded in skeletal muscle. Alkaline phosphatase activates water-soluble propofol. *(5:752-3)*

6. **(A)** The type of medical or surgical stress needs to be considered when ordering glucocorticoid supplementation in patients with adrenal insufficiency. Patients undergoing minor procedures such as herniorrhaphy or colonoscopy are supplemented with 25 mg of hydrocortisone or 5 mg of methylprednisolone IV for the procedure only. *(5:157)*

7. **(E)** Bioavailability is the amount of drug that reaches its site of action in active form. *(1:20)*

8. **(E)** Patients with anorexia nervosa may have profound electrolyte disturbances increasing the risk of dysrhythmias. Osteoporosis may result from malnutrition. Orthostatic hypotension, delayed gastric emptying and bradycardia are common. *(6:637)*

9. **(D)** In one small study, patients with unequivocal intraoperative awareness had a 50% incidence of developing posttraumatic stress disorder. *(5:609)*

10. **(A)** The congenital syndrome affects 1 in 5000 people and occurs because of cardiac ion channel mutations. The acquired syndrome is more common and is caused by medication side effects or electrolyte disturbances. A prolonged QT interval increases the likelihood of torsades de pointes and ventricular fibrillation. *(5:107-8)*

11. **(D)** Renal clearance of a drug in an individual with normal renal function may vary from patient to patient and from time to time, depending on such variables as urine pH and flow rate and renal blood flow. Excretion is correlated with renal blood flow. Renal elimination is correlated with creatinine clearance, and one may use changes in creatinine clearance to gauge how doses must be altered. *(1:28-30)*

12. **(A)** Class I is asymptomatic during ordinary exertion. Class II is slightly limited because ordinary activity is symptomatic. Class III is markedly limited but asymptomatic at rest. Class IV has symptoms at rest. *(6:1818)*

13. **(C)** Closing volume is the lung volume at which small airways collapse. Closing volume is related to lung elasticity. Factors that change FRC (general anesthesia, obesity, and supine position) can cause bronchioles to close during each breath, but do not change closing volume, per se. Closing capacity is measured by a single breath from maximal exhalation of a tracer gas, or by nitrogen washout after using 100% O_2 as the tracer gas. Measurement of closing volume will detect changes in the small airways before they become apparent by spirometry. *(5:133, 256)*

14. **(D)** Traditional signs of the anesthetic state are not seen with ketamine administration. Purposeless movements are seen, and these do not indicate the need for more anesthetic. *(5:699-701)*

15. **(D)** Global cerebral blood flow is 50 mL/100 g/min under normal physiological conditions. Cortical areas rich in gray matter receive more flow, 75 to 80 mL/100 g/min, whereas subcortical, white matter rich areas receive 20 mL/100 g/min. *(5:872; 6:171-2)*

16. **(B)** In Marfan syndrome, collagen vascular disease, familial aortic dissection, bicuspid aortic valve, ascending aortic repair is indicated at a diameter of 4.5 cm. For other patients the indication is a diameter of 5.5 cm, though 5.0 cm indicates ascending aortic replacement if the aortic valve requires surgery. *(5:915)*

17. **(C)** The peripheral chemoreceptors are primarily responsible for the hypoxic drive of respiration. They are disabled at very high oxygen tensions. The peripheral chemoreceptors respond to changes in oxygen tension, not content, and are located in the carotid arteries. In the elderly, dysfunction of the peripheral chemoreceptors can cause a 50-60% reduction in the ventilatory response to hypoxia and hypercapnia. *(5:134, 251; 6:277)*

18. **(D)** Warfarin should not be used until the thrombocytopenia has resolved because it can cause venous limb gangrene or multicentric skin necrosis. Danaparoid, lepirudin, and argatroban are anticoagulants that are approved for patients with heparin-induced thrombocytopenia. Benzodiazepines have no clinical effect on the coagulation system. *(5:214-5)*

19. **(E)** The presence of CO_2 can demonstrate respiratory gas exchange, but the correct position within the tracheo-bronchial tree can only be determined by bronchoscopy, X-ray, or (less reliably) auscultation. Fogging can appear during esophageal intubation. *(5:467, 573)*

20. **(E)** Hypoxic pulmonary vasoconstriction causes diversion of blood flow from hypoxic to non-hypoxic lung tissue. This causes a decrease in V_D/V_T and shunting. *(5:612)*

21. **(C)** Succinylcholine in the susceptible patient causes the release of potassium from inside the cell. The efflux of potassium, which is normal at the motor end plate, is seen over a much wider area of the membrane in the burned patient. This may result in a massive outpouring of potassium and cardiac arrest. *(5:1345)*

22. **(D)** The time constant of the system is the volume divided by the fresh gas flow, i.e., 5 L ÷ 1 L/min, or 5 min. Since $1 - e^{\frac{t}{\tau}} = 1 - e^{-1} = 0.63$, after one time constant the desflurane concentration will be 63% of the value set on the vaporizer. After two time constants, the percentage is 85%; after three time constants, 95%; after four time constants, 98%; and after five time constants, 99.3%. *(5:601)*

23. **(D)** Factor VIII is deficient in hemophilia A, while factor IX is the Hageman factor. *(5:208-9)*

24. **(D)** Propofol is an intravenous agent with a fast onset and short time to awakening. It is essentially insoluble in water and there is very little analgesic effect. When compared to thiopental, the sleep time is shorter. *(5:688)*

25. **(D)** Metabolic syndrome increases the risk of cardiovascular disease, cerebrovascular disease, and diabetes. Approximately one-half of patients with polycystic ovarian disease are obese and metabolic syndrome is common. There is no role for prophylactic medication. *(5:165-6; 6:387)*

26. **(D)** Pulse pressure widens in small distal vessels. *(5:406)*

27. **(D)** Analysis of arterial blood gases is the most reliable method of documenting hypoxemia, but pulse oximetry gives accurate, fast, and continuous results and thus is best as a monitor. Detection of cyanosis and circulatory responses are all subjective and may not be accurate. Residual anesthetics may blunt normal responses to hypoxia, and hypoxemia may be present without apnea. The pulse oximeter permits the detection of hypoxemia in less time than transcutaneous oxygen measurements. In a patient given supplemental oxygen, pulse oximetry is less sensitive in detecting hypoventilation. *(5:88)*

28. **(B)** Patients with burns over a large portion of their body surface area are resistant to nondepolarizing neuromuscular blockade. The other factors all potentiate such blockade. *(5:502-3)*

29. **(A)** The Hering-Breuer response is accentuated in preterm infants compared with full-term infants and leads to apnea with lung inflation in preterm infants. *(5:255)*

30. **(D)** Sweating and tachycardia are compensatory mechanisms to rid the body of the increased heat being produced in the patient with hyperthyroidism. Fatigue is common. Hyperthyroidism may produce hypermotility with resultant diarrhea. Shivering is not a heat-losing mechanism. *(6:314, 2923)*

31. **(C)** A patient who is deeply sedated should respond purposefully to a painful pinch while a patient under general anesthesia should not. The ability to follow a simple command, and maintain adequate minute ventilation and an unobstructed airway are all characteristics of moderate sedation. The BIS values associated with deep sedation and general anesthesia overlap substantially and therefore cannot be used to distinguish the two states. *(5:1261)*

32. **(E)** From the data presented in the two segments, the only statement that can be made is that there is a 90% block. The block could

represent either type of blockade. Complete relaxation is not present. *(5:494-6)*

33. **(D)** The drug is a muscle relaxant since tetanic stimulation produces fade. The drug may be either a depolarizing or nondepolarizing relaxant. If the cumulative dose of a depolarizing relaxant is sufficient to cause a phase II block, fade may be demonstrated. *(5:494-6, 500)*

34. **(B)** The mountaineer's alveolar oxygen concentration is estimated from the alveolar gas equation:

$$P_{AO_2} = F_{IO_2} \times (P_{atm} - P_{H_2O}) - P_{aCO_2}$$
$$\times (F_{IO_2} + (1 - F_{IO_2})/RQ))$$

Assuming a value of 0.8 for the respiratory quotient, the mountaineer's alveolar oxygen concentration would be approximately 54 mm Hg at an altitude of 10,000 feet. Because he is fit, his alveolar-arterial oxygen difference is probably less than 10 mm Hg, so he should avoid ascending above 10,000 feet to maintain his arterial oxygen concentration above 45 mm Hg. *(5:459)*

35. **(D)** Atracurium has four chiral centers and therefore there are 16 possible isomers. The marketed product contains a mixture of 10 isomers, each with different pharmacokinetic and pharmacodynamics properties. Cisatracurium is one of the isomers among the ten contained in atracurium. Even at very large doses, histamine release induced by cisatracurium is negligible. Atracurium is both more rapid in onset and shorter in duration than cisatracurium. *(5:498, 503-4)*

36. **(C)** At the time of the second heart sound, the mitral valve is opening. The closing of the aortic and pulmonic valves, isometric relaxation, and the T waves are coincident. *(6:1826)*

37. **(E)** The slope of the response curve is an index of the patient's sensitivity to carbon dioxide. The slope and position may change. Increased work leads to a flatter slope. Anesthetics differ in their effect on the curve. *(5:710)*

38. **(B)** The descending motor tracts are located in the ventral white matter in the spinal cord. The primary blood supply is from the anterior spinal artery. *(5:485; 6:3371)*

39. **(E)** When a nondepolarizing muscle relaxant is present, acetylcholine cannot be mobilized in sufficient quantities to sustain contraction. It is not a result of recording inabilities or potassium. Cellular DNA is not a factor. *(1:258-9)*

40. **(A)** Von Willebrand disease is one of the more common congenital bleeding disorders and is often diagnosed in children. The defect is in von Willebrand factor and has an autosomal-dominant transmission in most cases. There is an equal male-to-female distribution ratio. Von Willebrand factor participates in the process of platelet adhesiveness. Thus, affected patients usually have a prolonged bleeding time and a normal platelet count. *(5:209-10; 6:971-2)*

41. **(E)** Excitation of the cardiac cell membrane and depolarization are accompanied by calcium entering the cell. Calcium ions increase myocardial contractile force, prolong duration of systole, increase vascular tone, and increase ventricular automaticity. *(1:57-8, 755-6)*

42. **(D)** All of the listed causes of blindness have been associated with prolonged spine surgery in the prone position, but anterior ischemic optic neuropathy is the most common etiology. *(5:895-6)*

43. **(A)** The transdermal therapeutic system containing scopolamine should be applied to the postauricular mastoid region where drug absorption is especially efficient. The drug is much more effective in prevention of PONV than in treatment of nausea once it has occurred. The patch has a duration of action of about 72 h; side effects include dry mouth, drowsiness, and blurred vision. *(1:233-4, 923; 5:1288-9)*

44. **(E)** In a typical anesthesia ventilator, during inspiration, the pressure relief valve is closed so that the tidal volume delivered to the patient is the sum of the set tidal volume plus the fresh gas flow that occurs during inspiration. In this case, the total fresh gas flow is 6,000 mL/min or 100 mL/sec. With a ventilator rate of 20/min, each breath lasts for 3 sec. With an I:E ratio of 1:2, the inspiratory phase lasts for 1 sec. Therefore, the set tidal volume is augmented by fresh gas flowing for 1 sec, or 100 mL/ breath. The delivered tidal volume is therefore 150 mL and the minute ventilation is 3 L/min. *(5:650)*

45. **(D)** With increasing age closing capacity increases and total lung capacity decreases. While total venous admixture increases under general anesthesia more in the elderly due to increases in diffuse V/Q mismatch, the true intrapulmonary shunt increases only slightly with age. *(5:281)*

46. **(A)** After a patient has had and recovered from a dose of succinylcholine, it takes a smaller amount of nondepolarizing drug than normal to establish a neuromuscular block. This may be due to continued desensitization of the endplate. A longer duration of the nondepolarization block is also expected. *(1:267)*

47. **(E)** The baricity of a local anesthetic would be the specific gravity of the local anesthetic (numerator) divided by the specific gravity of CSF (denominator). A drug with baricity greater than 1 is considered hyperbaric. *(5:794)*

48. **(D)** Desflurane, but not sevoflurane, may react with dry soda lime to yield a potentially toxic concentration of carbon monoxide. The reaction of trichloroethylene, an obsolete anesthetic agent, yielded phosgene. *(5:614)*

49. **(A)** Blood pressure readings usually are falsely high due to the difficulty in obtaining a suitable cuff. The cuff bladder length should be at least 80%, and the width 40%, of the limb circumference. Venous and arterial access may be difficult. Intubation may be difficult. It may be impossible to get a suitable mask fit. Nerve blocks may be difficult because of the problem in finding landmarks. *(5:312)*

50. **(A)** Omeprazole is an inhibitor of the proton pump in the gastric mucosa and decreases gastric acid secretion. It is used to treat peptic ulcer disease. *(1:1311)*

51. **(A)** Acetazolamide is an inhibitor of carbonic anhydrase. It decreases the formation of aqueous humor and lowers intraocular pressure in glaucoma. *(1:677-8)*

52. **(B)** Glyburide is an oral hypoglycemic agent used to treat non-insulin-dependent (type II) diabetes mellitus. *(1:1255)*

53. **(E)** SSEPs are affected by nitrous oxide to a small extent and to a lesser degree than by volatile anesthetics. Deep levels of isoflurane will disrupt the tracings. They are not disrupted by lower doses of propofol. The tracings evaluate latency and amplitude. *(5:484-8)*

54. **(B)** The vapor pressure of sevoflurane at 20°C is 160 mm Hg and that of enflurane is 175 mm Hg. Therefore, the least error in the delivered concentration of sevoflurane would result by administering it with an enflurane vaporizer. The sevoflurane concentration would thus be slightly less than that set on the vaporizer dial. *(5:627, 629)*

55. **(A)** Of the options, bupivacaine is the most cardiotoxic. Chloroprocaine is the least cardiotoxic drug given its rapid metabolism by esterases in blood. This characteristic makes it an attractive drug to administer epidurally in obstetrical patients. *(5:779)*

56. **(C)** All of the options are true, if positioning is done properly, except C. This requires careful placement of rolls under the body in the prone position so that no pressure is placed on the abdomen. There is an overall increase in ventilation with increased vital capacity (VC) and FRC in the sitting position. *(5:362)*

57. **(C)** All of these effects act to increase the difference between the partial pressure of the agent in the fresh gas and the partial pressure in the inspired gas except metabolism since isoflurane is essentially not metabolized. *(5:598, 600-1)*

58. **(D)** Low fresh gas flow rate, low minute ventilation, low anesthetic concentration in the fresh gas, and high cardiac output all decrease the rate of onset of an inhaled anesthetic. A low blood:gas partition coefficient, indicative of a low-solubility agent, increases the rate of onset. *(5:600-2)*

59. **(D)** The patient who develops pulmonary edema in the recovery room usually does so within the first hour. Distended neck veins or increased CVP may be absent, but the patient is usually wheezing. An occluded endotracheal tube may be the problem. *(5:1288)*

60. **(B)** The number of calories required to raise the temperature of 1 g of a substance by 1°C is its specific heat. The specific heat varies for different substances. *(5:626)*

61. **(C)** The failing heart attempts to compensate by salt retention and increasing blood volume. Myocardial hypertrophy occurs, and there is an increased sympathetic outflow to improve output. Ventricular filling pressure increases as the heart decompensates. Vasoconstriction is part of the neurohumoral response to heart failure. *(5:176; 6:1906-7)*

62. **(B)** The pin index safety system consists of two pins located on the yoke of the anesthesia machine. The position of the pins is different for each medical gas. This system prevents the wrong medical gas tank from being hung on a particular yoke. Although it is found on the anesthesia machine, it is not at the site where gas hoses are connected. *(5:618)*

63. **(D)** A and B have the same efficacy because they produce the same maximum response. Because A is located to the left of B on the X-axis, A is said to be more potent than B; A will produce a particular magnitude of effect at a lower dose than will B. The dose at which the half-maximal response occurs, the ED_{50}, is lower for A than for B. It is likely that A and B act via the same receptor. *(1:44-5)*

64. **(A)** The effect of drug Y is to shift the dose–response relationship of X to the right with no effect on the maximum response to X. This is the definition of a competitive antagonist. It is likely that X and Y act via the same receptors. *(1:46-8)*

65. **(A)** Patients with end-stage renal disease are anemic because the kidney is the primary source of erythropoietin. They have an increased bleeding time due to platelet dysfunction, but the platelet count is not necessarily abnormal. Electrolyte abnormalities include hyperkalemia and hyperphosphatemia. *(6:2310-2)*

66. **(C)** The transplanted heart has intact α- and β-adrenoceptors. The Frank–Starling effect is intact. Atropine will not have any effect since there is neither autonomic innervation nor circulating cholinergic agonist. *(5:1093)*

67. **(E)** CSF flows through the cerebral ventricles and the subarachnoid space before absorption in the arachnoid villi. There is no CSF in the epidural space. *(5:871-3; 6:3435)*

68. **(A)** Verapamil is a calcium channel blocker that is useful in the treatment of supraventricular tachycardia. It is useful in the patient with asthma but should not be combined with propranolol, since it may cause profound bradycardia. The drug causes vasodilatation. It slows the rate in pacemaker cells. *(1:757-9)*

69. **(D)** When the dial on Tec 5 vaporizer is in the "off" position, no fresh gas flows through the vaporizer. When the oxygen flush valve is pressed, the delivered oxygen has not passed through the vaporizers. Therefore, when there is concern that liquid anesthetic has entered the gas delivery system, the vaporizer should be flushed with oxygen at 10 L/min for 10 min with the vaporizer dial set to its maximum value. *(5:629)*

70. **(D)** Although ASA I status is a predictor of bradycardia following spinal anesthesia, the most important predictor is preexisting bradycardia. *(5:801)*

71. **(C)** There is a growing consensus that the concern over hypokalemia is unfounded. If the likely cause of the hypokalemia is known and the patient is asymptomatic, there is no need to cancel the procedure in an otherwise healthy patient. Intraoperative infusions may cause hyperkalemia, and rapid administration of potassium may result in asystole. It is not possible to replenish the intracellular potassium over a short period of time. *(5:518)*

72. **(A)** Intracranial pressure is routinely monitored by transducing a small catheter introduced into the cerebral ventricle or subarachnoid space. Similarly, a hollow bolt with pressure transducer attached or a bolt-mounted transducer can be placed into the subdural space. Alternatively, ICP can be measured by placing a pressure transducer into the epidural space. A catheter implanted directly into brain parenchyma is not used; the Camino Bolt uses a fiberoptic cable placed on the brain parenchyma. *(5:875; 6:2256)*

73. **(C)** All gases and vapors obey Dalton's law. Each gas contributes to the total pressure in an amount that is proportional to its molecular fraction. Dalton's law states that each gas exerts the same pressure that it would if it alone occupied the container. Solubility plays a role in dissolved gases. *(5:626)*

74. **(C)** Metoclopramide has antagonistic effects on dopamine D_2 as well as 5-HT_3 receptors. Its main pharmacologic action is 5-HT_4 receptor activation. The main indication for metoclopramide is the amelioration of nausea and vomiting that often accompanies GI dysmotility syndromes. *(1:1325)*

75. **(D)** Hemochromatosis and Wilson disease result in cirrhosis due to the accumulation of excessive amounts of iron and copper, respectively, in the liver. $α_1$-antitrypsin deficiency causes bullous emphysema as well as cirrhosis. Cirrhosis can occur in patients with cystic fibrosis. Antithrombin III deficiency is a disorder of the clotting cascade that results in excessive thrombosis. *(6:2597)*

76. **(B)** In hypovolemic states, the pulse pressure is narrowed. Heart rate is increased to maintain cardiac output, and the neck veins are flat. Urine volume is decreased to preserve volume. The mucous membranes are pale, reflecting lower blood flow to peripheral areas. *(5:1398)*

77. **(D)** Most clinicians would classify a patient with a history of myocardial infarction as ASA physical status III at the minimum, regardless of the degree of recovery from the MI. In this case, "E" is added to the physical status because it is an urgent and unscheduled procedure. *(5:54)*

78. **(C)** Amiodarone is useful for both atrial and ventricular arrhythmias. Amiodarone has a half-life of many weeks, therefore stopping it before surgery would have little effect. It is eliminated through the liver. Autonomic effects of amiodarone include a noncompetitive β-adrenergic receptor blockade. *(1:834-7)*

79. **(A)** There are several radicular arteries that branch from intercostal and lumbar arteries to anastomose with the anteroposterior spinal artery system to supply the spinal cord with blood. The arteria radicularis magna (of Adamkiewicz) is the largest of these 4 to 10 radicular branches. Its origin may be either supra- or infrarenal. *(5:1573)*

80. **(C)** The latent heat of vaporization is the number of calories needed to convert 1 g of liquid into vapor at a constant temperature. This value is dependent on the ambient temperature. The colder the liquid, the more calories needed to vaporize a given amount of liquid. *(5:626)*

81. **(C)** DLCO depends on diffusion of CO across perfused alveoli to be avidly bound to hemoglobin. Smoking falsifies the test result through exogenous CO uptake. Exercise, congestive heart failure, and increased hemoglobin promote CO uptake, while fibrosis impedes diffusion and pulmonary embolism decreases effective gas transfer surface. *(5:953)*

82. **(B)** Cocaine is the only local anesthetic that blocks the reuptake of norepinephrine. The addition of epinephrine to a local anesthetic solution does not affect norepinephrine reuptake. *(1:278)*

83. **(B)** An α-adrenoceptor antagonist, such as phenoxybenzamine or prazosin, is begun one to two weeks prior to surgery. Once blood pressure control is achieved, if tachycardia persists, a β-adrenoceptor antagonist is added. Administration of a β-adrenoceptor antagonist prior to adequate α-adrenergic blockade may result in worsening of the hypertension. Because patients with pheochromocytoma are hypovolemic, diuretics are contraindicated in the control of the hypertension. The α- and β-adrenoceptor antagonists are titrated to blood pressure and heart rate control, and do not decrease the urinary excretion of catecholamine metabolites. *(5:158-9)*

84. **(D)** An accessory conduction pathway is evidenced by the wide QRS complex and its slurred upstroke (delta wave). The patients are prone to develop atrial fibrillation or paroxysmal supraventricular tachycardia. *(6: 1889)*

85. **(A)** Atracurium has both pre- and postjunctional effects. Histamine release is more likely only with higher doses (> 0.5 mg/kg) injected rapidly (in less than a minute). Laudanosine has caused seizures at high plasma levels in experimental animals, but this problem has not been observed in humans. The effect of atracurium on blood pressure is usually minor, but hypotension may occur if a large dose is given rapidly. *(5:503)*

86. **(A)** The glycoprotein is a receptor for fibrinogen or von Willebrand factor, proteins which, in turn, provide crosslinks to hold platelets together in an aggregate. Diverse platelet-activating stimuli operate via the glycoprotein. Abciximab is an inhibitory monoclonal antibody, and eptifibatide is an inhibitor peptide originally found in snake venom. *(6:991-2)*

87. **(A)** Cerebrospinal fluid pressure is increased with coughing. Coughing increases intrathoracic and intraabdominal pressure that is transmitted to the cranial vault. Maneuvers that decrease intrathoracic pressure will decrease intracranial pressure. *(5:880-3)*

88. **(D)** Isoflurane is a better muscle relaxant when compared to halothane. The vapor pressure is 238 mm Hg at 20°C. Isoflurane depresses ventilation and should be delivered by assisted or controlled ventilation. The value for MAC is correct. Cardiac output under isoflurane anesthesia in clinically relevant doses is well maintained. *(1:544; 5:598)*

89. **(D)** Basilar alveoli expand more than the apical ones, but in their end position are about the same size. Residual volume is independent of the state of inspiration. Pleural pressure decreases, balancing the increased elastic recoil of the lung. Pulmonary vascular resistance is lowest at FRC. Because of airway resistance, proximal airway pressure will always be greater than alveolar pressure during inspiration when flow is present. *(5:470; 6:2084)*

90. **(E)** Propofol is a potent metabolic suppressant. Since flow-metabolism coupling is maintained, there is a significant reduction in cerebral blood flow, blood volume, and ICP. Propofol, as do most anesthetic agents, increases the latency of SSEP's. *(5:688-92, 875)*

91. **(A)** Heparin increases the activity of antithrombin III that neutralizes the activated forms of factors II, IX, X, XI, XII, and XIII and of kallikrein. The effect of heparin is estimated by the activated partial thromboplastin time. It may be given subcutaneously and it may be given while waiting for the effect of an oral anticoagulant to occur. *(1:853-5)*

92. **(C)** Most hemolytic transfusion reactions are caused by clerical errors in which ABO-incompatible red cells are transfused. Many of the common signs of a hemolytic transfusion reaction (fever, chills, chest pain) may be masked by general anesthesia, and hemoglobinuria and coagulopathy are the signs most likely to be noted. The severity of the reaction is directly related to the volume of transfused cells, so immediate discontinuation of the transfusion is mandatory if a hemolytic reaction is suspected. Only a small percentage of hemolytic transfusion reactions are caused by the failure to detect incompatibility during serologic testing. Shock-induced renal failure and disseminated intravascular coagulation convey most of the morbidity and mortality. *(5:1441)*

93. **(A)** The tetralogy of Fallot includes a VSD, pulmonary outflow obstruction, overriding of the aorta, and right ventricular hypertrophy. An ASD is not part of the complex. *(6:1926-7)*

94. **(C)** The oxygen pressure at the wall connector is about 50 psi. The pressure in full E cylinders containing oxygen or nitrous oxide is about 1900 psi or 750 psi, respectively. *(5:619)*

95. **(B)** The patient described in this vignette most likely suffers from the consequences of chronic cocaine abuse. Cocaine causes the release of catecholamines and prevents their reuptake, thus raising the risk for hypertension, myocardial ischemia, and cardiomyopathy, as well as aortic dissection among many other complications. Exogenously administered catecholamines given intraoperatively can have an exaggerated effect. β-adrenergic antagonists are given for cocaine-induced arrhythmias, however in the acutely intoxicated patient, combined α-, and β-blockade with labetalol may be preferable to selective β-blockade, so as to avoid unopposed α-effects. There is no reason to withhold opioids for analgesia, or benzodiazepines for sedation. Ephedrine is an indirect vasoconstrictor, enhancing release of norepinephrine from sympathetic neurons. It may be ineffective in treating hypotension in the cocaine abuser due to catecholamine depletion; phenylephrine however will remain effective. *(1:300; 5:324-5)*

96. **(D)** The Bernoulli theorem may be used to estimate the pressure gradient across a stenotic valve:

$$\Delta P = 4(V_2^2 - V_1^2)$$

where ΔP is the pressure gradient, and V_1 and V_2 are the blood flow velocities on either side of the stenotic valve. *(5:432)*

97. **(A)** Exposure to tobacco either directly or through second-hand smoke increases the risk of many perioperative complications. Pharmacologic interventions to assist in smoking cessation such as varenicline and bupropion should be started one to two weeks before a quit attempt but nicotine replacement therapy is effective immediately. *(5:66-7)*

98. **(D)** The oxygen concentration in the blood is determined by the concentration in the alveoli, the efficiency of the lungs, and oxygen consumption. Decreasing shunting by using PEEP or reverse Trendelenburg positioning in the obese can reduce alveolar to arterial oxygen tension difference. Calcium channel blockers may decrease hypoxic vasoconstriction and thus increase shunting. *(5:312, 969)*

99. **(A)** Ketamine can lead to an increase in CBF by virtue of increasing $CRMO_2$. At levels below 1.5 MAC, the net effect of halogenated hydrocarbons is a decrease in cerebral blood flow. All other agents decrease CBF. *(5:873-4)*

100. **(C)** Pulse pressure variability is a function of the maximum and minimum values for pulse pressure during a positive pressure breath. The higher the value, the greater the degree of hypovolemia, and the greater the expected response to administered fluid. *(5:425)*

101. **(E)** Benzocaine is a local anesthetic commonly used as a topical analgesic, or in cough drops. Benzocaine is the ethyl ester of *p*-aminobenzoic acid (PABA); it can be prepared from PABA and ethanol. It is a common cause of methemoglobinemia. It is available only as a topical preparation. *(5:782)*

102. **(D)** Acromegaly is due to the hypersecretion of growth hormone. Hypertrophy of skeletal and connective tissue, especially of the face and head, may make intubation difficult. Diabetes mellitus and hypertension are also common. The pituitary adenomas usually responsible for acromegaly generally do not secrete TSH or cause hyperthyroidism. *(5:159)*

103. **(C)** Calcium channel antagonists should not be stopped in the preoperative period because of the possibility of worsening ischemia or hypertension. In patients undergoing inhalational anesthesia, they prolong atrioventricular conduction time, while in patients undergoing a high dose opioid anesthetic, they have little effect on cardiac output. Calcium channel blockers also potentiate neuromuscular blocking agents. Unlike the β-blockers, effect sites and mechanisms of action vary, and they cannot be used interchangeably. *(5:754-7)*

104. **(C)** The hyoid bone suspends the thyroid cartilage by the thyrohyoid membrane, at the level of C4. The Adams's apple is on the thyroid cartilage. The cricothyroid membrane at the level of C6 is an easily accessible, relatively avascular structure for cricothyrotomy or injection of local anesthetics for fiberoptic intubation. To each side of the larynx and inferior to the aryepiglottic folds is the piriform sinus. The endotracheal tube should be placed in the trachea, while the tip of the laryngoscope should be placed in the glossoepiglottic reflection. *(5:548, 563)*

105. **(C)** The irrigating fluids should be nonhemolytic and isosmolar. The composition should not be close to water, since water is hyposmotic. Electrolyte solutions should not be used because they conduct electricity and therefore interfere with the electrocautery. *(5:1140)*

106. **(D)** Increased dead space ventilation impedes CO_2 elimination. Exhausted soda lime is not capable of removing all CO_2 from the respiratory circuit. A pulmonary embolus or increased V_D/V_T will cause end-tidal CO_2 to fall while causing hypercarbia. The earliest signs of MH are hypercarbia, sinus tachycardia, and masseter muscle rigidity. Hyperventilation causes hypocarbia. *(5:460, 640, 1491)*

107. **(B)** Naloxone may reverse the effects of opioid agonists such as fentanyl and butorphanol,

and flumazenil may reverse the effects of a benzodiazepine such as midazolam. There is no specific antagonist for the hypnotic effects of propofol, thiopental, or etomidate. The only specific antagonist for steroidal muscle relaxants is sugammadex, a γ-cyclodextrin compound that encapsulates rocuronium and vecuronium, thus removing the drug from the neuromuscular junction. As of the end of 2012, it is not approved for use in the U.S. *(1:1059; 5:507)*

108. **(C)** This patient has the typical list of problems. A mainstay of therapy is to limit the mismatch of myocardial oxygen supply and demand by lowering the pressure, temperature, and heart rate. Administration of oxygen will increase the supply. *(5:902-3)*

109. **(D)** A cyclic-GMP phosphodiesterase inhibitor has a positive inotropic effect and would lower systemic vascular resistance. It would only be used in a patient with a low flow state due to low cardiac index or cardiogenic shock. A balloon pump is expected to reduce myocardial demand and improve supply. As a coronary thrombosis has probably occurred, fibrinolytics (not antifibrinolytics) and anticoagulants may help. *(5:97, 2015-20)*

110. **(C)** Inability to void is not always a contraindication to discharge to home, but since inguinal hernia repair has a high incidence of urinary retention, such patients should void before discharge. His heart rate, blood pressure, and oxygen saturation are within reasonable limits. It is not unusual for a person who has just undergone hernia repair to require assistance with ambulation. *(5:1278-84)*

111. **(C)** Pulse oximeters use dual-wavelength spectroscopy to measure the concentrations of oxyhemoglobin and deoxyhemoglobin. The presence of a significant concentration of methemoglobin introduces substantial error into the measurement. Interestingly, high concentrations of fetal or sickle hemoglobin or of bilirubin do not adversely affect the accuracy of the measurement. *(5:462)*

112. **(D)** An alarm of the line isolation monitor most commonly immediately follows the connection of a faulty electrical device. Disconnecting that device from the circuit is the initial step and most likely will resolve the alarm condition. *(5:376-8)*

113. **(D)** The meter on the line isolation monitor displays the maximum *potential* current that could flow through the patient *if* another fault were to occur. Since the likelihood of such an occurrence is rare in the short term, the operation should proceed. Of course the reason for the fault condition should be investigated more thoroughly after the operation is completed. *(5:376-8)*

114. **(E)** The presenting symptoms of LAST are isolated CNS symptoms in about 45% of cases, combined CNS and CV symptoms in about 44%, and isolated CV symptoms in 11% of cases; the latter occur by interference with sodium conductance. The cardiac toxicity with bupivacaine is of longer duration as compared to other local anesthetics and therefore harder to treat. Rapid recognition and immediate supportive care as described in E are paramount. In some instances, infusion of lipid emulsion may be beneficial by virtue of neutralizing circulating local anesthetic drug. It should be administered as a bolus, followed by continuous infusion. In cases of LAST, propofol should be avoided in patients with hypotension, as should vasopressin, β-blockers, calcium channel blockers, and local anesthetics. CNS symptoms such as seizure activity should be treated with injectable benzodiazepines. *(1:565, 571; 5:777-80)*

115. **(D)** The principal disadvantages of methohexital are pain on injection and involuntary muscle movements. The pH of the solution is high and it is water-soluble. Propofol has cardiodepressant effects far greater than those associated with administration of barbiturates. Because it lowers the seizure threshold, methohexital is a good choice for anesthesia in patients undergoing electroconvulsive therapy. *(1:535-7; 5:693-6)*

116. **(B)** Carbon dioxide is inversely proportional to ventilation, i.e., the higher the ventilation, the lower the CO_2. CO_2 will equilibrate with bicarbonate, acting as an acid. Reducing ventilation leads to respiratory acidosis, increasing ventilation leads to respiratory alkalosis. Ventilation will increase in response to endogenous or exogenous CO_2. *(5:461)*

117. **(E)** Fat emboli cause mechanical blockage, and then endothelial damage from free fatty acid breakdown products. The pulmonary and cerebral vascular beds can be involved. The ECG may show right-axis deviation or right bundle branch block. *(5:1203)*

118. **(C)** Porphyrias are a group of rare inherited disorders in which a specific enzyme deficiency leads to errors in the biosynthesis of heme. Drugs that induce cytochrome enzyme production may cause an acute porphyric attack and should be avoided. These include etomidate and thiopental. *(5:141-2, 695)*

119. **(A)** The patient with myasthenia gravis has weakness in the muscles innervated by cranial nerves and often experiences ophthalmoplegia and ptosis. Although the accessory muscles of respiration may also be weak, diaphragmatic weakness is uncommon. These patients are up to 100 times more sensitive to nondepolarizing muscle relaxants as compared to unaffected individuals, and resistant to the effects of succinylcholine. Myasthenia gravis is exclusively a motor disease. The myasthenic syndrome (Eaton-Lambert-syndrome), an acquired autoimmune disorder of the neuromuscular junction, is often associated with carcinomas. *(5:142-3)*

120. **(C)** The two vertebral arteries join to form the basilar artery. This unpaired midline structure gives rise to many branches and perforating arteries that supply the brain stem and the cerebellum. Transient ischemic attacks or strokes of the basilar arterial system result in unconsciousness from loss of reticular activating system function. In addition, motor function can be lost from ischemia of the cerebral pyramids that contain long motor tracts to the brain stem nuclei and spinal cord. *(5:872; 6:3286-7)*

121. **(E)** Packed red cells are mixed with an additive nutrient containing additional glucose and adenine in order to extend the storage period to 42 days. *(5:1439)*

122. **(E)** FEV_1 decreases with increasing age, in smokers even more than in non-smokers. A patient's risk for PONV is increased in non-smokers. *(5:113, 133, 1255)*

123. **(B)** Only the S-isomer of ropivacaine is present in solutions for clinical use, in contrast to other optically active local anesthetics that are supplied as racemic mixtures. The S-form appears to be less toxic, more potent, and longer acting that the R form, or the racemic mixture. Ropivacaine is much less toxic than bupivacaine and produces motor blockade that is of shorter duration than sensory blockade. Like other amide local anesthetics, ropivacaine is metabolized in the liver. *(5:768, 772, 779, 781)*

124. **(B)** Sweating is an important temperature-regulating mechanism that cools the body. It occurs in response to sympathetic nervous system-mediated stimulation of the sweat glands by cholinergic neurons and can result from a number of physiological perturbations that increase sympathetic activity, including hypoglycemia, emotional stress, and increased body temperature from infection. *(5:1506-8; 6:165, 2883)*

125. **(E)** In the patient under general anesthesia, core temperature will tend to drift toward ambient temperature. It is important to take steps to both prevent heat loss and to actively treat hypothermia. The problem is especially common during surgery involving open body cavities. Hypothalamic regulation and mechanisms to conserve and generate heat are obtunded by general anesthesia. Skin temperature unreliably reflects core temperature under general anesthesia *(5:1506-8)*

126. **(C)** Regulation of body temperature is a complex mechanism involving heat production by metabolism within muscles and liver and heat loss from skin and lungs. The conduct of anesthesia disrupts this system by vasodilation of the skin, preventing shivering with muscle relaxants, and general suppression of the hypothalamic function. *(5:1506-8; 6:165, 2883)*

127. **(A)** Transthoracic pressure is the sum of transpulmonary pressure and chest wall transmural pressure. Transpulmonary pressure is the gradient from alveoli to pleura, and transmural pressure is the gradient from pleura to ambient. Esophageal balloon pressure is a measure of pleural pressure. Pulmonary artery occlusion pressure (or wedge pressure) is a measure of left atrial pressure. *(5:470)*

128. **(B)** In the graph, the blood level of drug A decreases to nearly zero between doses. Drug B shows increasing levels over a period of time, i.e., it accumulates. Drug B never reaches steady state concentrations on this graph. *(5:32-5)*

129. **(D)** The graph shows that drug B is not completely eliminated before the next dose is given. The relative size of the dose cannot be determined from the diagram, but each of the doses is the same size. The half-life of drug A is not long, and its duration of action is shorter than B. *(5: 32-5)*

130. **(C)** Resistance decreases with inspiration because the airways dilate. Parasympathetic stimulation, acetylcholine, and smoke constrict the airway. *(5:470)*

131. **(B)** Mannitol is an osmotic diuretic in the kidney that does not cross the blood brain barrier and draws water out of brain tissue from which it is excluded. Rapid administration can produce transient peripheral vasodilation and hypotension. It reduces mean corpuscular volume similar in mechanism to reducing brain volume but this has no effect on cerebral edema. There is no diuretic effect in renal failure in which it is contraindicated. *(5:880; 6: 340-50)*

132. **(B)** Patients with sickle cell disease should be treated to prevent perioperative hypoxia, dehydration, acidosis, and hypothermia, all of which can result in a vasoocclusive crisis. General anesthesia per se does not overtly increase the risk of sickling. *(5:206)*

133. **(E)** The typical time it takes for methimazole to render a patient euthyroid is about 4-8 weeks. This patient would probably still have tachycardia. If a regional anesthetic is feasible, it might be safer for the inadequately treated hyperthyroid patient. *(5:151-2)*

134. **(E)** General anesthesia may be reversed by increasing the ambient pressure, regardless of the agent used to produce the anesthetic state. Some of the general anesthetics that are not gases at body temperature include halothane, isoflurane, and thiopental. While the perturbation of membrane lipid-protein interactions is an attractive hypothesis for general anesthetic action, most anesthetic agents have not been studied in terms of this action. While isoflurane, sevoflurane, and halothane are bronchodilators, nitrous oxide has little effect on airway resistance, and desflurane may cause bronchoconstriction. By irreversibly inhibiting methionine synthase, nitrous oxide inhibits many biochemical reactions, including DNA synthesis. *(5:588, 590-2, 598, 613)*

135. **(B)** The inotrope milrinone is a selective phosphodiesterase-3 inhibitor. It causes an increase in cyclic AMP and vasodilatation, and has no effect on β_1-receptors. Bosentan is an endothelin-antagonist used in the treatment of primary pulmonary hypertension. Inhibition of Na,K-ATPase is the principal effect of digoxin. *(1:801, 805, 1059)*

136. **(E)** This curve is characteristic of obstructive lung disease, with a higher residual volume and scooping of the expiratory limb from small airway closure. *(5: 997; 6:2089)*

137. **(B)** This curve is characteristic of restrictive lung disease, with smaller volumes and well preserved flows relative to volume. *(5: 997; 6:2089)*

138. (C) Thiopental is contraindicated in patients with acute intermittent porphyria. The other porphyrias listed as options are not associated with enzyme induction. *(5:697)*

139. (A) Chemoreceptor stimulation leads to an increased ventilatory effort. Cyanosis requires at least 5 g/dL deoxyhemoglobin in the blood to be apparent. Severe hypoxemia can cause bradycardia, in addition to a rapid fall in blood pressure and circulatory collapse. *(5:249-51)*

140. (A) Dopamine is not selective for any single adrenergic receptor; rather, the net effect of dopamine is dose-dependent. Dopaminergic receptors are activated by the lowest doses, while β-adrenergic, and then α-adrenergic, receptors are activated as the dose is increased. Dopamine in high doses is a poor choice for the patient with primary cardiac contractile dysfunction because of predominant vasoconstriction, increased afterload, and resulting worsening of left ventricular performance. *(1:804)*

141. (E) Ketamine has sympathomimetic activity that can reverse bronchospasm. Atropine causes bronchodilatation by its muscarinic antagonism, blocking the action of the vagus on bronchial smooth muscle. All potent inhalation agents block the bronchial response to mediators of bronchoconstriction, although in spontaneously ventilating patients, the respiratory depression will cause lower lung volumes. Therefore ventilation will occur at a less compliant range of the pressure–volume curve. Thiopental has no significant effect on bronchial tone. *(5:309, 612, 699, 977)*

142. (A) Traditionally supraclavicular blocks carried a relatively high risk of a pneumothorax, given the proximity of the lung to the brachial plexus. This risk has been reported to be as high as 5% in some studies. Hemidiaphragmatic paresis would be a less likely cause in an 18-year-old athlete with no prior pulmonary pathology. *(5:833)*

143. (E) Interscalene blocks have traditionally carried a 100% incidence of hemidiaphragmatic paresis from phrenic nerve blockade. Phrenic nerve blockade may reduce one's vital capacity by 40%. Depending on the severity of lung disease, patients with COPD may experience profound shortness of breath after an interscalene block. *(5:833)*

144. (B) The nipple line correlates to 4th thoracic dermatome (T4). *(4:198)*

145. (E) Bladder sensation is conducted by sympathetic afferent fibers of the hypogastric plexus that originate from T11-L2. Therefore a T10 sensory level is required to avoid the sensation resulting from bladder distension from irrigation fluid. The umbilicus correlates to a T10 level block. *(4:198; 5:1141)*

146. (F) Post-infarction VSD requires prompt surgery but can be stabilized with the aid of a balloon pump. The IABP supports diastolic perfusion pressure and reduces afterload. The latter action reduces the left-to-right shunt. *(6:2235-6)*

147. (H) Remote rheumatic fever can result in mitral stenosis. Antibiotic therapy of streptococcal infections has reduced the incidence. *(6:2752)*

148. (I) Spontaneous pneumothorax of idiopathic etiology rarely causes tension pneumothorax. *(5:979-80)*

149. (E) An arterial anastomosis suture line may be bleeding. A ligated branch of a vein graft may have opened. Sudden shock after cardiac surgery can prompt emergency opening of the chest. In event of tamponade, opening the chest may rapidly improve hemodynamics until control of bleeding is achieved. *(5:457-8)*

150. (B) Left heart failure before transplantation tends to increase pulmonary vascular resistance. A healthy transplanted heart may suffer right-sided failure in initially coping with the chronically insulted lung. *(5:1083-4)*

PART II

Advanced Topics in Anesthesiology

CHAPTER 11

Pharmacology
Questions

DIRECTIONS (Questions 1-63): Each of the numbered items or incomplete statements in this section is followed by answers or by completions of the statement. Select the ONE lettered answer or completion that is BEST in each case.

1. A child is brought to the emergency department for evaluation of his disoriented state. This began shortly after he ate some berries in the garden. He is noted to be very warm, flushed, and to have dilated pupils. The most appropriate action includes administration of

   (A) atropine
   (B) aspirin
   (C) diphenhydramine
   (D) physostigmine
   (E) phenylephrine

2. Fluoxetine is used for the treatment of

   (A) influenza
   (B) major depressive disorder
   (C) Graves disease
   (D) Parkinson disease
   (E) Hodgkin disease

3. A 52-kg patient undergoes anesthesia for removal of a bronchial carcinoma. His anesthesia consists of propofol, isoflurane, and N_2O/O_2, in addition to 50 mg of rocuronium after intubation. At the end of the procedure 3 h later, only one weak twitch is palpable on train-of-four stimulation, and the patient remains apneic. The most likely explanation for apnea in this patient is

   (A) rocuronium overdose
   (B) delayed pulmonary elimination of nitrous oxide after lung surgery
   (C) impaired release of acetylcholine from the nerve terminal
   (D) hypoxic pulmonary vasoconstriction
   (E) respiratory depression from residual effects of propofol

4. Dobutamine

   (A) is primarily an α-adrenoceptor agonist
   (B) has primarily β_1-adrenoceptor effects
   (C) causes decreased renal blood flow
   (D) is associated with severe increases in heart rate
   (E) is a naturally occurring catecholamine

5. A patient is scheduled for an elective cardioversion. A single intravenous injection of a short-acting agent is planned. Which one of the following agents is most likely to cause vomiting after the procedure when used in this patient?

   (A) Ketamine
   (B) Thiopental
   (C) Etomidate
   (D) Methohexital
   (E) Propofol

6. Esmolol is inactivated by

   (A) monoamine oxidase
   (B) catechol O-methyltransferase
   (C) erythrocyte esterase
   (D) plasma pseudocholinesterase
   (E) acetylcholinesterase

7. An 18-year-old patient with a history of asthma is brought to the operating room for emergent laparoscopic appendectomy for perforated appendix. Shortly after induction of general endotracheal anesthesia, the patient experiences severe bronchospasm. Which one of the following drugs, administered as monotherapy with a pressurized metered-dose inhaler via a spacer chamber through the ventilator circuit, is most likely to result in bronchodilation in the acute setting?

(A) Ipratropium bromide
(B) Albuterol
(C) Theophylline
(D) Terbutaline
(E) Salmeterol

8. A 55-year-old woman scheduled to undergo carotid endarterectomy has been smoking heavily for over 40 years and wishes to quit. Which one of the following medications is best at alleviating the symptoms of nicotine withdrawal?

(A) Buspirone
(B) Alprazolam
(C) Bupropion
(D) Zolpidem
(E) Citalopram

9. Botulinum toxin interferes with neuromuscular transmission by

(A) preventing synthesis of acetylcholine
(B) preventing breakdown of acetylcholine
(C) preventing storage of acetylcholine
(D) preventing release of acetylcholine
(E) blocking receptors for acetylcholine

10. A 62-year-old male with a history of diabetes mellitus, hypertension, and coronary artery disease is admitted to the hospital for unstable angina. He was recently diagnosed with heparin-induced thrombocytopenia type II and is now scheduled to undergo off-pump coronary artery bypass grafting for severe three-vessel coronary artery disease. A suitable agent for intraoperative anticoagulation would be

(A) heparin
(B) warfarin
(C) argatroban
(D) fondaparinux
(E) clopidogrel

DIRECTIONS: Use the following scenario to answer Questions 11-12: A 61-year-old male with a past medical history of diverticulosis is admitted to the intensive care unit after undergoing an emergent laparotomy with sigmoid colectomy and creation of Hartman's pouch for perforated diverticulitis. According to the surgeon, there was frank contamination of the peritoneal cavity. Despite broad-spectrum antibiotic coverage, the patient develops symptoms consistent with septic shock on the first postoperative day.

11. Despite aggressive fluid resuscitation and blood pressure support with norepinephrine, the patient remains hypotensive. A 2-D echocardiogram is obtained that shows no wall motion abnormalities, a hyperdynamic left ventricle, and a calculated cardiac index of 4.8 L/min/m². Which one of the following agents would be most useful in addition to the norepinephrine for the treatment of this patient's hypotension?

(A) Milrinone
(B) Ephedrine
(C) Phenylephrine
(D) Dobutamine
(E) Vasopressin

12. On the second postoperative day, the patient continues to require high-dose vasopressor support with two medications despite adequate fluid resuscitation. Low dose hydrocortisone therapy is started. Which one of the following statements is true?

    (A) In patients with septic shock, addition of low dose glucocorticoids may enhance the vascular reactivity to vasoactive substances.
    (B) Glucocorticoids in the setting of septic shock will enhance the bactericidal effect of broad-spectrum antibiotics.
    (C) Addition of glucocorticoids to the therapeutic regimen will improve glycemic control.
    (D) The major action of hydrocortisone in this setting is sodium retention with subsequent improvement of volume status.
    (E) Administration of glucocorticoids will most likely cause leukopenia in this patient.

13. A 51-year-old female with an anxiety disorder is admitted for elective surgery. Because the patient is extremely nervous, lorazepam is given IV in repeat, subhypnotic doses to manage her anxiety. Which one of the following statements is most accurate?

    (A) The patient's motor function is likely to be more impaired than her cognitive function.
    (B) Lorazepam is more rapid in onset as compared to midazolam.
    (C) The patient may experience extrapyramidal side effects.
    (D) To achieve anxiolysis, highly sedating doses of the drug have to be administered.
    (E) Administration of lorazepam will cause retrograde amnesia.

14. Milrinone

    (A) is a catecholamine used for treatment of congestive heart failure
    (B) is an antiarrhythmic drug
    (C) causes peripheral vasodilation
    (D) inhibits Na^+,K^+-ATPase
    (E) has a longer elimination half-life than inamrinone

15. A patient who is taking lithium for treatment of bipolar disorder is scheduled to have general anesthesia. The lithium

    (A) need not be considered in the anesthetic regimen
    (B) may affect both depolarizing and nondepolarizing muscle relaxants
    (C) decreases the duration of nondepolarizing muscle relaxants
    (D) should be stopped 2 weeks before surgery
    (E) may increase anesthetic requirements

16. A drug that is associated with pulmonary toxicity is

    (A) doxorubicin
    (B) bleomycin
    (C) vincristine
    (D) methotrexate
    (E) *l*-asparaginase

17. A 48-year-old woman takes a tricyclic antidepressant for depression. This patient

    (A) may have an increased number of arrhythmias
    (B) should have halothane and pancuronium as drugs of choice
    (C) should be cautioned to stop the medication before surgery
    (D) may become hypotensive with ketamine
    (E) may have short emergence with thiopental

18. A 66-year-old male with a history of diabetes mellitus, hypertension, and coronary artery disease is to undergo urgent surgery for an expanding 6.4 cm infrarenal abdominal aortic aneurysm. He had a myocardial infarction twelve months ago at which time he underwent percutaneous coronary angioplasty with placement of drug-eluting stents to the left anterior descending and right coronary arteries. Current medications include clopidogrel and aspirin that were started after the stent placement. With respect to the combination of these two drugs and the intraoperative risk of bleeding, it is true that

(A) both drugs exert their antiplatelet effect through the same mechanism

(B) clopidogrel does not add significantly to the risk of bleeding posed by aspirin

(C) if these drugs were stopped one day prior to surgery, the risk of bleeding would be minimized

(D) both drugs can be antagonized

(E) clopidogrel should be discontinued 5-10 days prior to surgery in elective cases were surgical hemostasis is needed

19. Gabapentin

(A) is approved for the monotherapy of partial seizures

(B) is a benzodiazepine

(C) is metabolized by the liver

(D) is useful for the treatment of migraine, chronic pain, and bipolar disorder

(E) increases the plasma concentrations of carbamazepine and phenobarbital when used concomitantly

20. A heroin addict injects six bags of heroin per day. After being involved in a motorcycle accident resulting in a fracture of the tibia, he is brought to the emergency department. Which one of the following analgesics is most likely to be effective and least likely to precipitate an acute withdrawal syndrome or cause significant toxicity?

(A) Meperidine

(B) Nalbuphine

(C) Buprenorphine

(D) Butorphanol

(E) Fentanyl

21. Which one of the following is a β-adrenoceptor antagonist?

(A) Isoproterenol

(B) Dobutamine

(C) Nadolol

(D) Albuterol

(E) Ritodrine

22. A 76-year-old male is undergoing CABG for severe three vessel coronary artery disease under cardiopulmonary bypass (CPB) with full anticoagulation with heparin. After uncomplicated weaning from CPB, the surgeon requests reversal of the anticoagulant with protamine. Shortly after administration of a ratio of 1 mg intravenous protamine to 1 mg heparin, the patient develops sudden onset of hemodynamic instability. Which one of the following statements regarding protamine is most accurate?

(A) Anaphylactic reactions occur in about 10% of diabetic patients on protamine-containing insulin (NPH insulin) who are administered intravenous protamine.

(B) Anaphylactic protamine reaction in the general population consisting of pulmonary hypertension, right ventricular dysfunction, and systemic hypotension is rare.

(C) The patient described in this vignette received a protamine overdose.

(D) Protamine is equally effective in reversing the anticoagulant activity of low molecular weight heparin as compared to unfractionated heparin.

(E) Protamine can be used as a specific antidote for fondaparinux.

23. Dantrolene

(A) has a half-life of about 36 h

(B) reduces concentrations of intracellular calcium

(C)   causes marked cardiac depression

(D)   in the setting of malignant hyperthermia is dosed at 1 mg/kg initial bolus

(E)   causes nephrotoxicity

24. A 76-year-old patient with a history of NYHA stage IV heart failure is admitted to the intensive care unit for the treatment of acute, decompensated heart failure. The patient is hypotensive, tachycardic, and in respiratory distress with increased work of breathing as well as hypoxemia documented on ABG. Which one of the following is the most appropriate therapeutic agent?

(A)   Losartan

(B)   Fenoldopam

(C)   Minoxidil

(D)   Nicardipine

(E)   Nesiritide

25. Nifedipine

(A)   may cause tachycardia as a compensatory effect

(B)   exerts its therapeutic effect by slowing AV-node conduction

(C)   achieves maximum plasma concentration more quickly when administered sublingual, as opposed to the oral route

(D)   is a coronary vasoconstrictor

(E)   has positive inotropic effects

26. Doxorubicin may produce a cardiomyopathy that

(A)   is present only during therapy

(B)   is independent of the dose administered

(C)   is not affected by radiation therapy

(D)   can be evaluated with echocardiography

27. A homeless person buys an inexpensive quart of denatured alcohol (90% ethanol, 10% methanol) at a hardware store. He mixes a pint of denatured alcohol with a half-gallon of orange juice and drinks the mixture over a period of an hour. A short while later, he is found unconscious and brought to the emergency department of a nearby hospital. All of the following statements about this patient are true EXCEPT

(A)   he is likely to have been drunk prior to drinking the denatured alcohol because he did not recognize the abnormal taste of the methanol present in it

(B)   he is likely to have a severe metabolic acidosis due to the effects of a metabolite of one of the alcohols he ingested

(C)   he is likely to be blind due to the effects of a metabolite of one of the alcohols he ingested

(D)   his decreased level of consciousness is likely due to the direct effects of one of the alcohols he ingested

(E)   he is likely to benefit from hemodialysis

28. Tachyphylaxis

(A)   can occur with administration of phenylephrine

(B)   describes the rapidly decreasing effectiveness of certain drugs with repeat administration

(C)   occurs with continuous administration of norepinephrine

(D)   is also known as "ceiling effect"

(E)   can occur due to induction of enzyme systems

29. A mechanism that accurately describes the effect of a drug used to produce deliberate hypotension is

(A)   sodium nitroprusside only dilates resistance vessels

(B)   nicardipine causes coronary and peripheral vasodilatation

(C)   isoflurane causes decreased cardiac output and peripheral vascular resistance

(D)   nitroglycerin primarily dilates resistance vessels

(E)   esmolol will attain a decrease in blood pressure faster than a decrease in heart rate

30. A patient with a history of type 1 diabetes mellitus, coronary artery disease, and COPD is to receive β-blocker therapy as part of an antihypertensive regimen. The most suitable agent for this indication is

(A) propranolol
(B) labetalol
(C) atenolol
(D) carvedilol
(E) pindolol

31. Which one of the following agents used as an adjunct in the therapy of chronic pain can cause rebound hypertension after abrupt cessation of therapy?

(A) Topiramate
(B) Clonidine
(C) Milnacipran
(D) Carbamazepine
(E) Gabapentin

32. Mannitol

(A) is effective at decreasing ICP in the absence of blood-brain barrier integrity
(B) is useful in the treatment of dialysis disequilibrium syndrome
(C) is a weak acid
(D) is almost completely reabsorbed from the renal tubule
(E) is effective at providing perioperative renal protection during high-risk urologic procedures

33. Based on the neurotransmitter aberrations that are thought to be responsible for the symptoms of Parkinson disease, which one of the following drug types would be therapeutic in a patient with Parkinson disease?

(A) Monoamine oxidase inhibitor
(B) Phenothiazine
(C) Butyrophenone
(D) Serotonin antagonist
(E) Serotonin reuptake inhibitor

34. The withdrawal syndrome in a person physically dependent on which one of the following drugs can be fatal?

(A) Amphetamine
(B) Phencyclidine
(C) Diazepam
(D) Heroin
(E) Eszopiclone

35. Fenoldopam

(A) activates α- and β-adrenoceptors
(B) causes a dose related decrease in renal blood flow and glomerular filtration rate
(C) is effective in preventing radiological contrast-induced nephropathy
(D) is a selective dopamine D_1 receptor agonist used to treat severe hypertension
(E) causes a dose-dependent increase in heart rate and cardiac contractility

36. Which one of the following agents may be administered via the intravenous route to treat postpartum hemorrhage?

(A) Oxytocin
(B) Prostaglandin $F_{2\alpha}$
(C) Methylergonovine
(D) Progesterone
(E) Prostaglandin E_2

37. A 34-year-old woman has a history of prolonged paralysis after a short, elective operation, and she was subsequently shown to be homozygous for the atypical form of the butyrylcholinesterase gene. Her 4-year-old son now needs anesthesia for bilateral myringotomy and ear tube placement. What is the probability that her son will have a prolonged response to succinylcholine?

(A) 25%
(B) 50%
(C) 100%
(D) Cannot be calculated without more information

38. A 22-year-old female college student is scheduled for placement of a tunneled IV catheter for total parenteral nutrition. She has a history of anorexia nervosa and is severely malnourished. It would be reasonable to avoid which one of the following medications in the perioperative period?

    (A) Cefazolin
    (B) Droperidol
    (C) Succinylcholine
    (D) Vancomycin
    (E) Sevoflurane

39. Each of the following characteristics applied to an anesthesiologist might be suggestive, but not diagnostic, of self-administration of intravenous opioids EXCEPT

    (A) wearing a long sleeve t-shirt underneath a scrub top
    (B) chronically showing up late for work
    (C) miosis in a dark room or mydriasis in a bright room
    (D) requesting more frequent breaks than other colleagues
    (E) avoiding changing into scrubs in the locker room

40. A 44-year-old woman with a significant history of prior postoperative nausea and vomiting is given aprepitant preoperatively before a diagnostic laparoscopy as part of a multidrug antiemetic regimen. Aprepitant interacts most strongly with which endogenous ligand?

    (A) β-endorphin
    (B) Dynorphin A
    (C) Substance P
    (D) Proopiomelanocortin
    (E) Leu-enkephalin

41. A person whose ancestors came from which one of the following geographical areas is most likely to need the lowest daily dose of warfarin to maintain a therapeutic value for INR?

    (A) Sub-Saharan Africa
    (B) China

    (C) Scandinavia
    (D) Southern Europe
    (E) Arabian peninsula

DIRECTIONS: Use the following table to answer Question 42:

	Chemical class	protein bound (%)
Diazepam	Weak base	98
Isopropanol	Nonionic	0
Aspirin	Weak acid	80
Pancuronium	Quaternary amine	10
Phenobarbital	Weak acid	50

42. The intravenous administration of sodium bicarbonate will increase the excretion rate of which one of the following drugs to the greatest degree?

    (A) Diazepam
    (B) Isopropanol
    (C) Aspirin
    (D) Pancuronium
    (E) Phenobarbital

43. An anesthesiologist is deployed in the desert of a Middle Eastern country. An artillery shell explodes in the midst of his base, and an alarm is sounded because a nerve gas has been detected. He is not wearing protective gear and should therefore immediately inject himself with

    (A) diazepam and atropine
    (B) physostigmine and diazepam
    (C) physostigmine and pralidoxime
    (D) pralidoxime and atropine
    (E) pralidoxime and diazepam

44. The benzodiazepine that is most appropriate as a bedtime sedative due to its pharmacokinetic properties is

    (A) oxazepam
    (B) nordazepam
    (C) diazepam
    (D) flurazepam
    (E) quazepam

45. Stereospecific binding of an agonist to the μ-opioid receptor produces all of the following effects EXCEPT

(A) euphoria
(B) cough suppression
(C) sedation
(D) constipation
(E) analgesia

46. Cyclooxygenase (COX) is associated with participating in numerous physiological functions. Which one of the following effects is primarily ascribable to COX-2 as opposed to COX-1?

(A) Platelet adhesiveness
(B) Inflammation
(C) Regulation of renal blood flow
(D) Pain perception
(E) Protection of GI mucosa against acid damage

47. Metoprolol exerts its therapeutic effect via

(A) β_1-adrenoceptor agonism
(B) β_1-adrenoceptor antagonism
(C) β_2-adrenoceptor antagonism
(D) α_2-adrenoceptor antagonism
(E) α_1-adrenoceptor antagonism

48. Both diazepam and buspirone

(A) lower seizure threshold
(B) cause sleepiness
(C) decrease abnormal behaviors in obsessive-compulsive disorder
(D) display cross-tolerance with ethanol
(E) decrease anxiety

49. A patient has been recently diagnosed with bipolar disorder. He is also on dialysis due to renal failure resulting from untreated ureteral reflux. His psychiatrist wishes to begin chronic therapy with a medication to prevent further manic episodes. Which one of the following is the BEST choice in this patient?

(A) Lithium carbonate
(B) Citalopram

(C) Carbamazepine
(D) Phenelzine
(E) Bupropion

50. Which one of the following opioids is ineffective as an analgesic in a significant fraction of the population due to a genetic polymorphism?

(A) Codeine
(B) Hydromorphone
(C) Meperidine
(D) Methadone
(E) Oxycodone

51. Soon after a patient is started on haloperidol he begins complaining of feeling stiff and having difficulty in performing rapid, fine motor movements like typing at his computer keyboard. Which one of the following medications will MOST likely help these new-onset symptoms?

(A) Fluoxetine
(B) Diazepam
(C) Aspirin
(D) Benztropine
(E) Lithium

52. Which one of the following characteristics of a substance make it less likely to be abused by humans?

(A) Tolerance develops to some of its effects.
(B) It potentiates dopamine neural activity.
(C) It is cheap and easy to obtain.
(D) It has a rapid onset.
(E) It has a long duration.

53. A 47-year-old man with long-standing type I diabetes mellitus has severe peripheral vascular disease and peripheral neuropathy. His feet are chronically cold and blue and are extremely painful. In commencing therapy for his painful feet, the least appropriate medication to try first is

(A) oxcarbazepine
(B) oxycodone

(C) gabapentin

(D) amitriptyline

(E) carbamazepine

DIRECTIONS (Questions 54-59): Each group of items below consists of lettered headings followed by a list of numbered phrases or statements. For each numbered phrase or statement, select the ONE lettered heading or component that is most closely associated with it. Each lettered heading or component may be selected once, more than once, or not at all.

(A) Agonists decrease the heart rate by inhibiting adenyl cyclase.

(B) Agonists cause vasoconstriction in arterioles by activating phospholipase C and increasing the intracellular concentration of calcium.

(C) Agonists relax bronchial smooth muscle by activating guanylyl cyclase.

(D) Agonists increase ganglionic transmission by activating phospholipase C and increasing the concentration of inositol triphosphate.

(E) Agonists cause vasodilation by inhibiting guanylyl cyclase.

(F) Agonists cause vasodilation by increasing endothelial nitric oxide synthase.

(G) Agonists relax bronchial smooth muscle by activating adenyl cyclase.

(H) Agonists inhibit transmission in sympathetic neurons by inhibiting adenyl cyclase.

For each autonomic receptor, select the corresponding mechanism of action:

54. Muscarinic M_1

55. Muscarinic M_2

56. Muscarinic M_3

57. Adrenergic α_{1A}

58. Adrenergic α_{2A}

59. Adrenergic β_2

DIRECTIONS (Questions 60-63): Each group of items below consists of lettered headings followed by a list of numbered phrases or statements. For each numbered phrase or statement, select the ONE lettered heading or component that is most closely associated with it. Each lettered heading or component may be selected once, more than once, or not at all.

(A) Increases numbers of adipocytes and increases uptake of fatty acids by adipocytes

(B) Blocks voltage-dependent calcium channels decreasing intracellular calcium in pancreatic β cells

(C) Stimulates tyrosine kinase associated with insulin receptors in hepatic cells

(D) Increases the activity of AMP-dependent protein kinase (AMPK) increasing fatty acid oxidation in hepatocytes

(E) Inhibits Na^+-K^+-ATPase thereby increasing intracellular potassium in adipocytes

(F) Inhibits phosphodiesterase (PDE) thereby increasing insulin release from pancreatic β cells

(G) Agonist at the GLP-1 (glucagon-like peptide) receptor

(H) Causes closure of K_{ATP} channels in pancreatic β cells increasing insulin release

For each medication used to treat diabetes mellitus, select the corresponding mechanism of action:

60. Exenatide

61. Rosiglitazone

62. Metformin

63. Repaglinide

Answers and Explanations

1. **(D)** The patient has all the symptoms of central anticholinergic syndrome that may follow the ingestion of jimson weed that contains atropine. The typical symptoms of "dry as a bone, blind as a bat, red as a beet, hot as a stove, and mad as a hatter" are due to the central and peripheral antimuscarinic effects of atropine. Physostigmine can cross the blood–brain barrier and will counteract both the central and peripheral effects. *(1:252)*

2. **(B)** Fluoxetine is an antidepressant used to treat persons with major depressive, obsessive-compulsive, and anxiety disorders. *(1:405)*

3. **(C)** The patient may be exhibiting the Eaton–Lambert syndrome, an acquired autoimmune disorder of the neuromuscular junction often associated with carcinomas. These patients are hypersensitive to the effects of both depolarizing and non-depolarizing muscle relaxants. Propofol should not be a factor in the apnea after a time period needed to complete a thoracotomy, and neither should be the fact that the patient received nitrous oxide. Hypoxic pulmonary vasoconstriction is a pulmonary vascular mechanism aimed at minimizing V/Q mismatch. *(5:143, 612)*

4. **(B)** Dobutamine is a synthetic catecholamine and contains a chiral center. The preparation used in clinical practice contains a racemic mixture of (+) and (−) enantiomers in equal amounts and the apparent effect of the combination of the two isomers is β_1-adrenoceptor stimulation. Dobutamine increases cardiac output and contractility. At higher doses, α-adrenoceptor agonist effects may be seen. It causes increased renal blood flow. *(1:290, 804-5)*

5. **(C)** Etomidate produces the highest incidence of postoperative vomiting after short procedures, propofol the lowest. *(5:697, 1255)*

6. **(C)** Catecholamines are inactivated by MAO and COMT. Pseudocholinesterase inactivates succinylcholine and mivacurium, while acetylcholinesterase inactivates acetylcholine. *(1:187, 200; 5:500-2)*

7. **(B)** Ipratropium bromide is an inhaled anticholinergic that causes bronchodilation. While anticholinergics are effective in severe acute asthma, they are less effective than β_2-adrenoceptor agonists and are often part of a combination therapy regimen. While terbutaline is an effective bronchodilator, it is only marketed in oral and subcutaneous forms in the US. Salmeterol is a long-acting β_2-adrenoceptor agonist with relatively slow onset, thus it is less suitable for therapy of the acute asthma attack. Theophylline is available in oral and parenteral preparations; however, it is less effective than nebulized β_2-adrenoceptor agonists and does not increase their bronchodilator response. *(1:291-3, 1043-5)*

8. **(C)** The antidepressant bupropion has efficacy in decreasing the symptoms of nicotine withdrawal and improving abstinence rates in smokers wishing to quit. *(1:407, 658)*

9. **(D)** Botulinum toxin leads to paralysis by preventing the release of acetylcholine from nerve terminals. *(1:186)*

10. **(C)** Use of heparin in a patient with heparin-induced thrombocytopenia type II can lead to life threatening thrombotic complications and is therefore not indicated. Warfarin is an oral anticoagulant. Fondaparinux is an activated factor X inhibitor approved for prophylaxis, and treatment of deep vein thrombosis and pulmonary embolus, and is administered subcutaneously. Clopidogrel is an inhibitor of ADP-induced platelet aggregation indicated for the secondary prevention of stroke and the reduction of cardiac events after percutaneous coronary intervention. It is administered orally. Argatroban is a direct thrombin inhibitor with a relatively short half-life of 1-2 h that can be continuously infused during CABG surgery. Other suitable alternatives would include lepirudin, bivalirudin, and danaparoid. *(1:855, 870; 5:211-2, 900)*

11. **(E)** Arginine vasopressin (AVP) concentrations in patients with septic shock are inappropriately low, and when administered exogenously, vasopressin can increase systolic blood pressure in this patient population. The proposed mechanism is twofold: first, endogenous AVP depletion may be the result of excessive baroreceptor-mediated release from sustained hypotension, and second, AVP appears to restore vascular sensitivity to norepinephrine. Another agent that could be added to restore blood pressure in septic shock is epinephrine instead of vasopressin. Milrinone and dobutamine are not indicated because this patient has good myocardial contractility. Ephedrine is a mixed-acting sympathomimetic drug that indirectly releases norepinephrine and has some direct effects on β_2-adrenoceptors. It is not indicated for continuous infusion in shock states. Phenylephrine is a selective α_1-adrenoceptor agonist and does not provide additional benefit. *(1:278, 708; 5:1321)*

12. **(A)** Administration of a low-dose glucocorticoid to patients in septic shock has been shown to decrease the time to discontinuation of vasopressor therapy in some clinical trials, and is recommended for patients with septic shock refractory to vasopressors and fluid therapy by the Surviving Sepsis Campaign Guidelines. One of the major actions of glucocorticoids on the cardiovascular system is to enhance the vascular reactivity to other vasoactive substances, for example norepinephrine or phenylephrine. Glucocorticoids do not improve the bactericidal activity of broad-spectrum antibiotics, they will increase blood glucose concentrations, and cause a leukocytosis due to increased release of polymorphonuclear leukocytes from the bone marrow. Sodium retention is much more pronounced with administration of mineralocorticoids; glucocorticoids play a permissive role in the renal excretion of free water. *(1:1224, 1231; 5:1321)*

13. **(A)** Lorazepam is a benzodiazepine and therefore does not cause extrapyramidal effects as are seen with the phenothiazines. Midazolam is more rapid in onset than lorazepam. Benzodiazepines usually produce a state of sedation accompanied by decreased anxiety and anterograde, not retrograde, amnesia. They can reduce anxiety at doses that are not highly sedating. Cognition tends to be less affected than motor performance, which is why most individuals who receive benzodiazepines underestimate their degree of impairment. *(1:465; 5:698)*

14. **(C)** Milrinone and inamrinone are phosphodiesterase inhibitors used for the short-term parenteral inotropic support in severe heart failure. They exhibit their therapeutic effect through inhibiting the breakdown of cyclic AMP and have no antiarrhythmic activity. Because milrinone has a shorter half-life and fewer side effects, it is a better choice than inamrinone for this indication. *(1:805)*

15. **(B)** Lithium may prolong the effect of both depolarizing and nondepolarizing relaxants. It is not necessary to stop the drug before induction, but it is necessary to consider the drug when planning the anesthesia. In addition to the effect on relaxants, the drug may lead to a reduction of anesthetic requirements. *(1:267)*

16. **(B)** Bleomycin is associated with pulmonary fibrosis, sometimes long after the drug has been stopped. Doxorubicin produces cardiac toxicity. Vincristine is associated with myelosuppression. Methotrexate toxicity is manifest as immunosuppression. *l*-asparaginase is associated with hepatic toxicity and allergic reactions. *(1:1717-8)*

17. **(A)** Arrhythmias are common in the patient on a tricyclic antidepressant and the combination of halothane, pancuronium, and a tricyclic antidepressant has been reported to be associated with severe intraoperative arrhythmias. The drug should not be stopped prior to surgery, but the anesthesiologist must be aware of its interactions with anesthetic agents. Ketamine and catecholamines may cause an exaggerated hypertensive response in these patients. *(1:411)*

18. **(E)** Aspirin irreversibly blocks the production of thromboxane A_2 in platelets, whereas clopidogrel exerts its antiplatelet effect by blocking the platelet ADP receptor. Because of their discrete mechanisms, the effect of these drugs is additive or even synergistic that results in a higher risk for excessive bleeding during surgical procedures. There are no antagonists available for these medications. Because of their long duration of action, stopping the drugs one day prior to surgery would not decrease the risk of bleeding. Current recommendations are to stop clopidogrel 5-10 d prior to surgery in elective cases where surgical hemostasis is needed. Aspirin in vascular surgical patients should be continued through the perioperative period *(5:115)*

19. **(D)** Gabapentin is approved for the treatment of partial seizures in adults when used in addition to other anticonvulsant drugs. It is not metabolized and is excreted unchanged in the urine. It is also used for the treatment of migraine, chronic pain, and bipolar disorder and concomitant use does not increase the plasma concentrations of carbamazepine or phenobarbital. *(1:599)*

20. **(E)** Of the medications listed, only fentanyl and meperidine are full agonists at the μ-opioid receptor. Because the patient is likely to have significant tolerance requiring a large dose of the agonist, meperidine would not be a good choice because it has an active metabolite that can cause CNS excitation resulting in seizures and inhibition of serotonin reuptake that can cause serotonin syndrome. Nalbuphine and butorphanol have μ-opioid antagonistic activity while buprenorphine is a μ-opioid partial agonist; each of these three medications may produce withdrawal if given to an opioid-tolerant person. *(5:715-6; 722-4)*

21. **(C)** Of the drugs listed, only nadolol is a β-adrenoceptor antagonist. Isoproterenol is a β-adrenoceptor agonist and dobutamine is a $β_1$-adrenoceptor agonist. Albuterol and ritodrine are $β_2$-adrenoceptor agonists. *(5:752)*

22. **(B)** Protamine is a naturally occurring protein salt (from salmon semen). It causes anaphylactic reactions in only about 1% of patients who have been sensitized to protamine (e.g., NPH insulin), while true anaphylactic reaction in the general population as described in option B is rare. Hypotension on administration is a frequent side effect that can be mitigated if injected slowly and into a peripheral vein. The patient in this vignette did not receive an overdose, as most protocols call for administration of protamine in slight excess of 1 mg per 1 mg (or 100 units) of heparin administered. Protamine only binds long heparin molecules, and therefore only partially reverses the effects of low molecular weight heparins, and has no effect on the very short molecules of fondaparinux. *(1:858-9; 5:900)*

23. **(B)** Dantrolene decreases intracellular calcium and causes generalized muscle weakness. The half-life is about 9 h. Hepatotoxicity is common after prolonged therapy. Cardiac toxicity is not usually seen. The initial dose of dantrolene in the setting of MH is 2.5 mg/kg, ideally administered into a large vein. It should be administered for at least 24 h after the MH episode until all signs of the hypermetabolic state are resolved and the concentration of creatinine kinase is decreasing. *(1:286, 626; 5:1499)*

24. **(E)** The major site of action for the human recombinant brain natriuretic peptide (nesiritide) is the inner medullary collecting duct (IMCD). It leads to an increase in urinary sodium excretion, decreases systemic and pulmonary resistances and left ventricular filling pressure, and results in a secondary increase in cardiac output. Nesiritide decreases dyspnea in patients with decompensated heart failure and pulmonary edema. The other drugs listed will decrease blood pressure, without increasing cardiac contractility. *(1:695-6, 5:746-8)*

25. **(A)** Nifedipine does not affect conduction through the AV-node at routine clinical doses and is used as a coronary vasodilator and antihypertensive. The drug has no positive inotropic effect. The arterial dilatation caused by nifedipine may cause a reflex tachycardia in some patients. Sublingual administration of the drug for control of acute hypertension has largely been abandoned, and sublingual administration will achieve target plasma concentrations no faster than oral administration. *(1:756-60, 777)*

26. **(D)** The cardiomyopathy seen with doxorubicin may be seen long after the chemotherapy has been discontinued. This side effect is dependent on the cumulative dose of doxorubicin and may be evaluated by echocardiography. Patients who have received radiation therapy to the mediastinum may have a greater likelihood of this effect. *(1:1714-5)*

27. **(A)** It is difficult to differentiate methanol from ethanol by taste. Methanol is converted to formic acid that is particularly toxic to the retina as well as being a major cause of the severe metabolic acidosis that occurs. Both methanol and ethanol are readily removed by hemodialysis. *(1:631-2)*

28. **(B)** Tachyphylaxis, or acute tolerance to a drug that develops rapidly, is seen with ephedrine because of depletion of norepinephrine stores. Tachyphylaxis also occurs due to desensitization of receptor systems because of repeat stimulation by agonists and is not due to induction of enzyme systems. Repeated or continuous administration of norepinephrine or phenylephrine does not reduce their effectiveness. A ceiling effect occurs when a patient does not exhibit an increasing effect with an increasing dose; an example of a ceiling effect is the analgesia produced by the opioid partial agonist buprenorphine. *(1:68)*

29. **(B)** Sodium nitroprusside dilatates both the resistance and capacitance vessels, whereas nitroglycerin primarily dilatates capacitance vessels. Nicardipine is a calcium channel blocker that causes coronary and peripheral vasodilatation. Isoflurane in clinically meaningful doses dilates the peripheral vasculature without any significant effect on cardiac output. The effects of esmolol on heart rate occur faster than those on blood pressure. *(1:543, 747-50, 757-8, 782-3; 5:753)*

30. **(C)** With the exception of atenolol, all agents listed are non-selective β-adrenoceptor antagonists. This class of drugs has the potential to delay recovery from hypoglycemia in patients with type 1 diabetes. Furthermore, there is a potential for life-threatening bronchoconstriction with nonselective β-adrenoceptor blockade, and selective agents such as atenolol are preferred. *(1:315)*

31. **(B)** Rebound hypertension can occur after abrupt cessation of β-adrenoceptor antagonists such as propranolol and centrally acting antihypertensives such as clonidine. Mechanisms of action for topiramate, an anticonvulsant, include sodium channel blockade, potentiation of GABA-mediated inhibition, and a decrease in glutamate neurotransmission. Milnacipran is a dual norepinephrine and serotonin reuptake inhibitor. Carbamazepine slows the recovery rate of sodium channels. Gabapentin increases GABA release. All of these agents are used as adjuncts in the therapy of chronic pain but as opposed to clonidine, do not cause potentially life-threatening hypertension upon acute cessation. *(5:1555, 1557, 1560-1)*

32. **(B)** Dialysis disequilibrium syndrome is caused by too rapid removal of solutes from the extracellular fluid by hemodialysis resulting in reduction of osmolality of extracellular fluid and associated CNS symptoms (headache, nausea, CNS depression, convulsions). Mannitol is filtered by the glomerulus and is negligibly reabsorbed. It is a nonelectrolyte that has almost no pharmacologic effects aside from its osmotic activity after intravenous injection. The drug's effectiveness at decreasing elevated ICP depends on preservation of the integrity of the blood-brain barrier in a significant portion of the brain. There is no evidence that administration of mannitol is of any benefit in surgical patients at high risk for renal damage. *(1:681-2; 5:1146, 1374)*

33. **(A)** The basal ganglia are thought to contain inhibitory dopaminergic neurons and excitatory cholinergic neurons. In Parkinson disease, there is a loss of dopaminergic neurons and relative excess in cholinergic neuronal activity. Dopamine agonists, acetylcholine antagonists, and monoamine oxidase inhibitors, by virtue of decreasing dopamine degradation and increasing dopaminergic activity, are therapeutic. Phenothiazines and butyrophenones have antidopaminergic effects and should be avoided in patients with Parkinson disease. Drugs affecting serotonin transmission have little positive or negative effect on the disease. *(5:149)*

34. **(C)** Withdrawal from barbiturates and benzodiazepines can result in grand mal seizures that may be fatal. Opioid and amphetamine withdrawal, while uncomfortable, are not considered to be life-threatening. Eszopiclone is a non-benzodiazepine sedative used for the long-term treatment of insomnia and sleep maintenance. Unlike the benzodiazepines, no signs of tolerance or serious withdrawal are associated with its use. Phencyclidine (PCP, "angel dust") is a psychedelic agent that is used intermittently by humans, therefore, tolerance and withdrawal syndromes have not been observed. *(1:411, 468, 665; 5:327; 6:3556)*

35. **(D)** Fenoldopam is a selective dopamine D_1 receptor agonist that is indicated for short term, rapid reduction of blood pressure in severe hypertension. The drug is devoid of α- and β-adrenoceptor and dopamine D_2 activity and causes a dose-related increase in renal blood flow and glomerular filtration rate. It does not increase heart rate or cardiac contractility. While fenoldopam has demonstrated nephroprotective properties in critically ill patients and those undergoing cardiac surgery, it has not been shown to mitigate the severity of contrast-induced nephropathy to date. *(5:747)*

36. **(A)** Methylergonovine and PGF_2 are administered intramuscularly, and PGE_2 is administered via the oral, rectal, or vaginal routes. Oxytocin is administered in slow intravenous increments; all of these drugs increase uterine contractions and may decrease postpartum hemorrhage. Progesterone usually relaxes the uterus. *(5:1157)*

37. **(D)** The mother has certainly passed onto her son one gene for the atypical form of butyrylcholinesterase, however without knowing the father's genotype, it is impossible to predict the son's phenotypic response to succinylcholine. He is, at least, a carrier for the atypical gene. If the father has no copies of the atypical gene, then the son will be phenotypically normal. If the father is a carrier and has one copy, the son has a 50% chance of being affected with a prolonged response to succinylcholine. If the father is homozygous and has two copies of the atypical gene, then the son has a 100% chance of being affected. *(5:79-80)*

38. **(B)** Persons with anorexia nervosa and resulting severe malnutrition are at increased risk for having prolonged QT and QTc intervals. Of the drugs listed, droperidol may increase the risk of torsades de pointes. *(5:108, 220)*

39. **(B)** The anesthesiologist who is dependent on opioids most typically arrives earlier to work than others so as to be able to obtain and divert opioid medication early in the day to avoid withdrawal and to request frequent breaks throughout the day to self-inject. They often take measures to hide cutaneous manifestations

of multiple injection sites from colleagues. Miosis in a dark room, indicating excessive opioid effect, or mydriasis in a bright room, indicating impending withdrawal, are also worrisome signs. *(5:1626-8)*

40. **(C)** Aprepitant is an antagonist of substance P at the neurokinin (NK$_1$) receptor. *(1:1344)*

41. **(B)** There is significant geographical heterogeneity in the VKORC1 phenotype that is responsible for the enzyme inhibited by warfarin. Persons of black African descent are most resistant to warfarin and require the highest daily maintenance doses, while persons of Chinese descent require the lowest daily doses. *(1:861-3)*

42. **(E)** The rate of the urinary excretion of weak acids is increased by increasing the pH of the urine with sodium bicarbonate. The greater the fraction of a drug bound to plasma protein, the less the renal clearance will be. *(1:19, 24-5)*

43. **(D)** The emergency management of poisoning with a nerve agent (an irreversible inhibitor of acetylcholinesterase) is the administration of atropine (to dry pulmonary secretions) and pralidoxime (an acetylcholinesterase reactivator). *(1:248-9)*

44. **(A)** A benzodiazepine used as a bedtime sedative should have a rapid onset after oral administration and a short duration that is not associated with excessive sedation the following day. That typically means that it has no active metabolites. Oxazepam meets these criteria. Diazepam is long-acting, with a half-life of about a day, and it has an active metabolite, nordazepam, with a half-life of about 4 d. Nordazepam is metabolized to oxazepam; flurazepam, and quazepam also have active metabolites with half-lives greater than a day. *(1:463-6)*

45. **(B)** Although all μ-opioid agonists used as analgesics have antitussive activity, this effect is not due to stereospecific binding to the μ-opioid receptor. All such μ-opioid agonists

are L-isomers. The D-isomers of these medications are devoid of analgesic effects and do not bind to the μ-opioid receptor, however they retain antitussive activity. Such a medication is dextromethorphan. *(1:491-5; 512-3)*

46. **(B)** Inflammation is mediated in part by prostaglandins synthesized by COX-2. Pain and GI mucosal integrity are associated with prostaglandins synthesized by both COX-1 and COX-2. Regulation of renal blood flow and platelet adhesiveness is due to prostaglandins or thromboxanes, respectively, synthesized by COX-1. *(1:849-51; 949-51)*

47. **(B)** Metoprolol is a selective β$_1$-adrenoceptor antagonist. Other members of this group are esmolol, atenolol, and acebutolol *(5:311)*

48. **(E)** Both diazepam and buspirone are antianxiety agents. Buspirone is neither a sedative nor an anticonvulsant. Buspirone has no efficacy in persons with obsessive compulsive disorder. *(1:343-4, 349, 412-3)*

49. **(C)** Of the medications listed, both lithium carbonate and carbamazepine have efficacy as mood stabilizers in persons with bipolar disorder. Lithium carbonate is contraindicated in persons with renal failure because of the increased risk of toxicity. *(1:447)*

50. **(A)** Codeine is a prodrug and requires metabolism by CYP2D6 to morphine for analgesic activity. About 10% of persons of western European descent are deficient in CYP2D6. *(5:42)*

51. **(D)** The symptoms are typical of the Parkinson-like rigidity the antidopaminergic antipsychotic agents may cause. Specific treatment is with a centrally-acting muscarinic cholinergic antagonist like benztropine. *(1:422, 437)*

52. **(E)** Factors that increase the likelihood that a substance will be abused include rapid onset and offset, easy availability, and low price, and that it potentiates dopaminergic reward pathways in the brain. *(1:650)*

53. **(B)** Some antidepressants and anticonvulsants, such as the ones listed, are effective in decreasing neuropathic pain. In contrast, opioids are less effective and their use in neuropathic pain is associated with significant toxicity as well as the development of tolerance requiring dose escalation. *(1:490, 518)*

54. **(D)** *(1:192)*

55. **(A)** *(1:220)*

56. **(F)** *(1:221)*

57. **(B)** *(1:203)*

58. **(H)** *(1:203)*

59. **(G)** *(1:204)*

60. **(G)** *(1:1261-3)*

61. **(A)** *(1:1260-1)*

62. **(D)** *(1:1258)*

63. **(H)** *(1:1257)*

DIRECTIONS (Questions 64-93): Each of the numbered items or incomplete statements in this section is followed by answers or by completions of the statement. Select the ONE lettered answer or completion that is BEST in each case.

64. A 73-year-old man undergoes a descending thoracic aortic aneurism repair. Following the surgical repair, the patient is unable to move his legs. Perfusion to the spinal cord appears to have been compromised during the repair. Which one of the following does NOT supply blood to the spinal cord?

   (A) Anterior spinal artery
   (B) Posterior spinal arteries
   (C) External carotid arteries
   (D) Anterior radicular arteries
   (E) Vertebral arteries

65. A 52-year-old female undergoes a right total knee arthroplasty. Her preference is to have an epidural catheter placed for postoperative analgesia. When threading a catheter into the epidural space, the anterior border of the epidural space may be encountered. The tissue creating the anterior border of the epidural space is

   (A) anterior longitudinal ligament
   (B) posterior longitudinal ligament
   (C) ligamentum flavum
   (D) dura
   (E) transverse process

66. A lumbar plexus block is performed in a 72-year-old man scheduled to undergo a total hip arthroplasty. Which nerve does NOT originate from the lumbar plexus?

   (A) Iliohypogastic
   (B) Ilioinguinal
   (C) Femoral
   (D) Genitofemoral
   (E) Sural

67. A 25-year-old female undergoing an elective cesarean section agrees to a spinal anesthetic. When performing a spinal anesthetic, the anesthesiologist must be knowledgeable of the fact that cerebral spinal fluid (CSF) is located between which two tissue layers?

   (A) Pia and arachnoid
   (B) Pia and dura
   (C) Pia and spinal cord
   (D) Dura and arachnoid
   (E) Dura and spinal cord

68. A 44-year-old female undergoes a right infraclavicular block for a right ulnar nerve transposition surgery at the elbow. The musculocutaneous nerve appears to have been missed. The musculocutaneous nerve usually emerges from the

   (A) lateral cord
   (B) inferior cord
   (C) C5 nerve root
   (D) posterior division
   (E) axillary nerve

69. A 22-year-old male presents for left hand reconstructive surgery. You discuss performing an axillary brachial plexus block. After performing an axillary brachial plexus block for forearm surgery, the nerve that will most likely need to be blocked by a separate injection is the

   (A) axillary nerve
   (B) suprascapular nerve
   (C) ulnar nerve
   (D) musculocutaneous nerve
   (E) median nerve

70. The normal bony vertebral column is made up of how many total vertebrae?

   (A) 27
   (B) 29
   (C) 31
   (D) 33
   (E) 35

71. A 72-year-old man presents for a total shoulder arthroplasty. He undergoes a continuous interscalene block utilizing a traditional landmark technique. Bone is contacted within 2 cm of the skin that likely represents the

   (A) first rib
   (B) clavicle
   (C) scapula
   (D) transverse process
   (E) vertebral body

DIRECTIONS: Use the following scenario to answer Questions 72-74: An 18-year-old male sustained an open right ulna forearm fracture after slipping on ice. He presented for open reduction and internal fixation. He undergoes a peripheral nerve block for surgical anesthesia with 20 mL of 0.5% bupivacaine. The following ultrasound image is obtained:

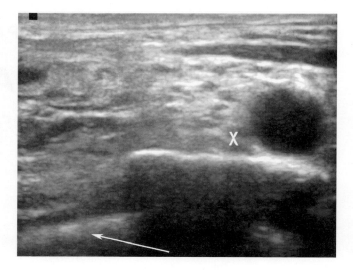

72. After successful completion of the block, all of the following are expected to occur on the ipsilateral side EXCEPT inability to

   (A) flex the wrist
   (B) shrug the shoulder
   (C) abduct the shoulder
   (D) flex the arm at the elbow
   (E) extend the arm at the elbow

73. The patient reports pain during skin incision on the ulnar side of his distal forearm. The most likely reason is the failure to

   (A) anesthetize the lateral antebrachial cutaneous nerve
   (B) advance the needle to the area represented by the "X"
   (C) anesthetize the ulnar nerve
   (D) anesthetize the medial brachial cutaneous nerve
   (E) advance the needle to the area represented by the arrow

74. If the needle is advanced to the area depicted by the arrow, which one of the following may occur?

   (A) Inability to further advance the needle
   (B) A complete and dense surgical block
   (C) A pneumothorax
   (D) An intravascular injection
   (E) Successful blockade of the inferior trunk of the brachial plexus

75. A 42-year-old male presents with neck pain of 1-year duration. He undergoes a cervical epidural steroid injection for what is presumed to be herniation of the inner contents of the intervertebral disk that resulted in inflammation. The inner contents of the intervertebral disk called is also called the

(A) annulus fibrosus
(B) ligamentum flavum
(C) nucleus pulposus
(D) posterior longitudinal ligament
(E) facet joint

76. A 41-year-old female undergoes right shoulder arthroscopy utilizing an interscalene block as the surgical anesthetic. Upon making a small skin incision on the cape of the shoulder, the patient reports feeling the painful incision. The skin on the top of the shoulder is innervated by which nerve?

(A) Radial
(B) Supraclavicular
(C) Axillary
(D) Median
(E) Ulnar

77. A 72-year-old male presents for repair of a distal humerus fracture. The patient prefers a regional anesthetic for surgery and a brachial plexus block is performed. The organization of the brachial plexus starting proximally in the neck and traveling distally to the axilla is

(A) trunks, divisions, roots, cords, branches
(B) divisions, trunks, roots, cords, branches
(C) branches, cords, divisions, trunks, roots
(D) roots, trunks, cords, divisions, branches
(E) roots, trunks, divisions, cords, branches

78. All of the following nerves provide exclusively cutaneous innervation to the foot EXCEPT the

(A) sural nerve
(B) saphenous nerve
(C) tibial nerve
(D) superficial peroneal nerve

79. An 18-year-old female sustained a closed right ankle fracture while skating. She presents five days later for open reduction and internal fixation of the ankle. She agrees to a regional anesthetic for surgical anesthesia as well for postoperative analgesia. Which nerve innervates the skin over the medial aspect of the lower leg?

(A) Saphenous
(B) Sciatic
(C) Sural
(D) Common peroneal
(E) Ilioinguinal

80. A 54-year-old male is scheduled to undergo a right total hip arthroplasty. You perform a lumbar plexus block as well as a gluteal sciatic block for postoperative analgesia. The sciatic nerve is composed of the ventral rami of

(A) L4 - S3
(B) T12 - L4
(C) T12 - S3
(D) S1-S3
(E) T10-S3

81. You are performing an ultrasound-guided supraclavicular block in a 15-year-old female for left hand surgery. You encounter bone with needle advancement. You suspect that the needle has most likely encountered the

(A) clavicle
(B) second rib
(C) transverse process of C6
(D) vertebral body of C6
(E) first rib

82. A 72-year-old female undergoes a transmetatarsal amputation of the left foot for peripheral vascular disease. All of the following are suitable regional anesthetics EXCEPT a(n)

(A) ankle block
(B) femoral and popliteal sciatic block
(C) saphenous and popliteal sciatic block
(D) femoral and saphenous nerve block
(E) spinal block

83. You are obtaining informed consent from 46-year-old lawyer for a femoral nerve block for a right ACL repair. You explain that you will be using ultrasound as the means of nerve localization. All of the following are true when using ultrasound in regional anesthesia EXCEPT that it

(A) decreases the incidence of unintentional vascular punctures

(B) decreases the number of needle passes

(C) decreases the volume of local anesthetic required

(D) decreases the onset time of a block

(E) has not been shown to facilitate the placement of epidural blocks in difficult patients

DIRECTIONS: Use the following scenario to answer Questions 84-85: A 25-year-old male undergoes ACL repair of the right knee utilizing a hamstring tendon. In the PACU, the patient reports intense pain and requests a peripheral nerve block. Utilizing ultrasound for the nerve block, 25 mL of 0.5% ropivacaine was administered and the following ultrasound-guided image was obtained:

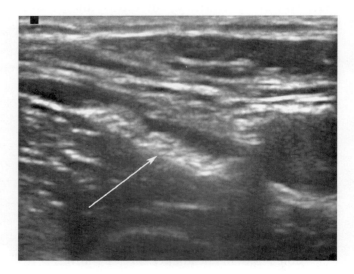

84. During the ultrasound-guided block shown above, anesthetizing the nerve depicted by the white arrow would result in inability to

(A) dorsiflex the foot

(B) plantarflex the foot

(C) extend the lower leg at the knee joint

(D) flex the lower leg at the knee joint

(E) flex the hip joint

85. After a successful block, the patient would be expected to have loss of sensation to the

(A) lateral aspect of the right thigh

(B) medial aspect of the right lower leg

(C) lateral aspect of the right lower leg

(D) posterior aspect of the thigh

(E) dorsum of the foot

86. A brachial plexus block is performed in a 26-year-old man for open reduction and internal fixation of the left elbow. A supraclavicular block is performed to anesthetize the entire brachial plexus. The brachial plexus is primarily derived from the nerve roots of

(A) C5-C8

(B) C5-T1

(C) C6-C8

(D) C6-T2

(E) C2-C4

87. A 66-year-old female with severe COPD presents for left upper extremity surgery. She prefers a regional anesthetic in order to avoid intraoperative intubation and wants to avoid the need for postoperative intubation. Which one of the following upper extremity blocks should be avoided because it typically results in phrenic nerve blockade with resulting ipsilateral diaphragm paralysis?

(A) Supraclavicular

(B) Interscalelene

(C) Infraclavicular

(D) Axillary

(E) Suprascapular

88. During a barroom fight, a man fractured his 5th metacarpal after throwing a punch. The following day he underwent a surgical repair of the 5th metacarpal. Which one of the following nerve(s) would need to be anesthetized to ensure adequate postoperative analgesia?

(A) Ulnar nerve

(B) Ulnar and radial nerves

(C) Median and radial nerves

(D) Median, radial, and ulnar nerves

(E) Musculocutaneous, median, radial, and ulnar nerves

89. A popliteal sciatic nerve block was performed for open reduction and internal fixation of the ankle. The patient reported feeling the painful surgical incision made on the medial aspect of the ankle. The nerve most likely missed was

(A) sural nerve

(B) saphenous nerve

(C) deep peroneal nerve

(D) superficial peroneal nerve

(E) tibial nerve

DIRECTIONS (Questions 90-91): Each group of items below consists of lettered headings followed by a list of numbered phrases or statements. For each numbered phrase or statement, select the ONE lettered heading or component that is most closely associated with it. Each lettered heading or component may be selected once, more than once, or not at all.

(A) Sciatic

(B) Femoral

(C) Supraclavicular

(D) Tibial

(E) Saphenous

(F) Infraclavicular

(G) Superficial Cervical Plexus

(H) Suprascapular

For each patient, select the best peripheral nerve block.

90. A 62-year-old morbidly obese patient sustained an open ankle fracture after falling. She undergoes general anesthesia for open reduction and internal fixation. In the PACU she reports intense pain not alleviated with opioids.

91. A 50-year-old gentleman is scheduled for elective rotator cuff repair of the left shoulder. You decide to perform an interscalene nerve block; however, you are unable to obtain an adequate ultrasound image. For complete surgical anesthesia, the most appropriate alternative technique is needed.

DIRECTIONS (Questions 92-93): Each group of items below consists of lettered headings followed by a list of numbered phrases or statements. For each numbered phrase or statement, select the ONE lettered heading or component that is most closely associated with it. Each lettered heading or component may be selected once, more than once, or not at all.

(A) Ulnar nerve block

(B) Musculocutaneous nerve block

(C) Median nerve block

(D) Radial nerve block

(E) Obturator nerve block

(F) Suprascapular nerve Block

(G) Medial brachial cutaneous nerve block

(H) Medial antebrachial cutaneous nerve block

For each patient, select the best rescue block.

92. A 26-year-old male sustained a left elbow fracture. After the performance of an infraclavicular block, you note that sensation is still intact on the ventral and lateral aspects of the forearm.

93. A supraclavicular nerve block is performed for surgical anesthesia of the hand. Upon testing the success of the block prior to surgery you notice that there is a lack of sensation on the volar and lateral aspect of the forearm but intact sensation on the medial side.

Answers and Explanations

64. **(C)** The only artery in the list that does not supply the spinal cord is the external carotid artery. *(5:780)*

65. **(B)** The posterior longitudinal ligament creates the anterior boarder of the epidural space. *(5:789)*

66. **(E)** The sural nerve originates from the common peroneal and tibial nerves. The common peroneal nerve and the tibial nerve originate from the sciatic nerve (sacral plexus). *(5:839)*

67. **(A)** The CSF is made by the choroid plexus and is found in the subarachnoid space. *(5:786)*

68. **(A)** The musculocutaneous nerve is a branch of the lateral cord. If the infraclavicular nerve block is performed in a more distal location with ultrasound guidance, the musculocutaneous nerve may be missed. The musculocutaneous nerve is more likely to be missed with an axillary approach and a separate injection is required. *(5:829)*

69. **(D)** The musculocutaneous nerve can be missed when an axillary block is performed because in many cases it has branched away from the neurovascular bundle more proximally. A separate injection is usually necessary. *(5:834)*

70. **(D)** There are 7 cervical, 12 thoracic, 5 lumbar, 5 sacral, and 4 coccygeal vertebrae. *(5:786)*

71. **(D)** The transverse process would represent the most superficial bony structure in the vicinity of a correctly performed landmark-based interscalene block. *(5:830)*

72. **(B)** This is an ultrasound image of a supraclavicular block. After a successful block, one would still be able to shrug the shoulders as the trapezius muscles are innervated by cranial nerve XI. *(5:831-3)*

73. **(B)** The medial aspect of the forearm is innervated by the medial antebrachial cutaneous nerve that is comprised of nerve fibers from the C8-T1 nerve roots or lower trunk of the brachial plexus. To consistently anesthetize these fibers the needle would need to be advanced closer to the area designated by the "X." This area has been termed the "corner pocket" that is formed by the subclavian artery and first rib. *(5:831-3)*

74. **(C)** The arrow depicts the pleura of the lung. Puncturing the pleura may result in a pneumothorax. *(5:831-3)*

75. **(C)** The nucleus pulposus represents the inner aspect of the intervertebral disk and the outer fibrous ring is called the annulus fibrosus. *(5:786)*

76. **(B)** The supraclavicular nerves innervate the top of the shoulder and originates from the cervical plexus. The axillary nerve also innervates the skin of the shoulder, but more distally. *(5:836)*

77. **(E)** The organization of the brachial plexus begins with the roots of C5-T1, which then organize into three trunks, followed by the

anterior and posterior divisions. Below the level of the clavicle the divisions organize into three cords and then finally transition into the branches of the brachial plexus. *(5:828-9)*

78. **(C)** The sural, saphenous, and superficial peroneal nerves provide exclusively cutaneous innervation to the foot. The tibial nerve, in addition to providing cutaneous innervation, also provides innervation to the deeper structures of the foot. *(5:845-7)*

79. **(A)** The saphenous nerve is a branch of the femoral nerve and travels down the medial aspect of the lower leg to innervate the ankle. *(5:841)*

80. **(A)** The sciatic nerve is composed of the ventral rami of L4-S3 from the sacral plexus. The ventral rami of T12-L4 comprise the lumbar plexus. *(5:843)*

81. **(E)** The first rib is easily imaged when performing ultrasound-guided supraclavicular blocks. It may provide some level of protection from a possible pneumothorax when advancing a needle. *(5:832)*

82. **(D)** Branches of the sciatic nerve and femoral nerve need to be blocked for a transmetatarsal amputation. An ankle block will anesthetize the tibial, deep peroneal, superficial peroneal, and sural nerves that are all branches of the sciatic nerve. In addition the saphenous nerve, which is a branch of the femoral nerve, is part of a complete ankle block. *(5:840-7)*

83. **(E)** Ultrasound has been shown to facilitate needle placement in neuraxial techniques, especially in patients with difficult epidural localization. *(5:851)*

84. **(C)** This is an ultrasound image of the femoral nerve after injection of local anesthetic. The femoral nerve innervates the quadriceps muscles that are responsible for extending the lower leg at the knee joint. The sciatic nerve is responsible for plantar flexion, dorsiflexion, eversion, and inversion of the foot. The sciatic nerve innervates the hamstring muscles

allowing for flexion at the knee joint. The femoral nerve does not innervate the hip flexors. *(4:69-72)*

85. **(B)** The cutaneous innervation of the medial aspect of the lower leg is from the saphenous nerve that is a branch of the femoral nerve. The cutaneous innervation of the lateral aspect of the thigh is from the lateral femoral cutaneous nerve and the posterior thigh from the posterior femoral cutaneous nerve. The sciatic nerve innervates the lateral aspect of the lower leg and dorsum of the foot. *(5:842)*

86. **(B)** The ventral rami of the spinal nerves from C5-T1 comprise the brachial plexus. There is variable contribution from C4 and T2. The cervical plexus is comprised of the ventral rami of C2, C3, and C4. *(5:828)*

87. **(B)** Typically the interscalene approach results in a nearly 100% incidence of blockade of the phrenic nerve. The incidence of phrenic nerve blockade from a supraclavicular approach has ranged from 3050%. *(5:831)*

88. **(A)** The ulnar nerve provides dorsal and ventral innervation to the cutaneous as well as intrinsic components of the 5th metacarpal and digit. Ulnar nerve blockade at the level of the forearm will provide complete postoperative analgesia. *(5:837)*

89. **(B)** The saphenous nerve provides cutaneous innervation to the medial aspect of the lower leg and ankle with a variable extension on the medial aspect of the foot. The innervation distal to the knee joint is predominately from the sciatic nerve with the saphenous nerve being the only contribution from the femoral nerve. *(5:841)*

90. **(A)** The predominate innervation to the ankle joint comes from the sciatic nerve and therefore a sciatic nerve block would be appropriate. Although the saphenous nerve provides some innervation to the ankle joint, it has a minor role. For postoperative analgesia, the sciatic block should be the first block performed and in many instances a saphenous

nerve block may not be necessary. However for complete surgical anesthesia, in addition to a sciatic nerve block, a saphenous nerve block is required. *(5:843-5)*

91. **(C)** Available evidence suggests that a supraclavicular block can take the place of an interscalene block for anesthetizing the shoulder joint. The suprascapular nerve and axillary nerve innervate the shoulder joint. The suprascapular nerve typically branches from the upper trunk of the brachial plexus while the axillary nerve is a branch nerve of the brachial plexus. Since the supraclavicular block is a block at the trunk level of the plexus, both of these nerves would be anesthetized. *(5:831-3)*

92. **(B)** The ventral and lateral aspect of the forearm is innervated by the lateral antebrachial cutaneous nerve (LACN). The LACN is an extension of the musculocutaneous nerve. Therefore a musculocutaneous nerve block would need to be performed. *(4:849)*

93. **(A)** The medial aspect of the forearm is innervated by the medial antebrachial cutaneous nerve (MACN). The nerve fibers of this nerve are derived from the C8-T1 spinal nerves or the inferior trunk of the brachial plexus. If sensation were intact on the medial aspect of the forearm, this would suggest that these fibers were missed when performing the supraclavicular block. The ulnar nerve, radial nerve, and median nerve innervate the hand. The ulnar nerve fibers are also derived from the C8-T1 spinal nerves or inferior trunk. Therefore if sensation were intact on the medial aspect of the forearm, this would also suggest that the ulnar nerve would also be intact. *(5:837)*

CHAPTER 13

Anesthesia for Cardiothoracic and Vascular Surgery
Questions

DIRECTIONS (Questions 94-174): Each of the numbered items or incomplete statements in this section is followed by answers or by completions of the statement. Select the ONE lettered answer or completion that is BEST in each case.

94. A 72-year-old patient who underwent successful CABG is extubated 2 hours after arrival in the ICU. The next morning, the patient experiences the acute onset of sinus bradycardia with associated hypotension. The next best step in management is to

    (A) initiate artificial cardiac pacing
    (B) start isoproterenol
    (C) start epinephrine
    (D) perform a stat TTE
    (E) administer adenosine

95. Afterload is reduced while diastolic perfusion pressure is increased by

    (A) dopamine
    (B) epinephrine
    (C) nitroglycerin
    (D) nitroprusside
    (E) intraaortic balloon counterpulsation

96. Ischemia from a right coronary artery lesion would most likely be evident on electrocardiographic lead

    (A) I
    (B) II
    (C) VR
    (D) AVL
    (E) V5

97. Increased amplitude of **v** waves in a central venous pressure recording indicates

    (A) junctional rhythm
    (B) atrial fibrillation
    (C) tricuspid regurgitation
    (D) hypovolemia
    (E) heart block

98. At 17°C

    (A) EEG activity is unchanged
    (B) cellular integrity is lost
    (C) cerebral blood flow increases
    (D) cerebral metabolic rate of oxygen consumption ($CMRO_2$) is less than 10% of normothermic value
    (E) the brain switches to anaerobic metabolism

99. Which one of the following modalities for artificial pacing will result in ventricular, as opposed to atrial, pacing only?

    (A) Transvenous endocardial leads
    (B) Epicardial leads
    (C) External noninvasive electrodes
    (D) Esophageal electrodes

100. A 62-year-old male with a past medical history of alcohol abuse, smoking, and COPD is admitted to the hospital with severe substernal chest pain after an episode of binge drinking during which he reportedly threw up violently. He is brought to the operating room for emergent exploration of the chest for suspected esophageal rupture. His physical examination is notable for signs and symptoms consistent with severe sepsis, tachypnea, and SpO_2 of 89% while breathing O_2 through a nonrebreather facemask. Airway exam is notable for a Mallampati III score and a full beard. The surgeon informs you that one-lung ventilation will be required to facilitate esophageal repair. The anesthetic plan most likely to result in safe induction of anesthesia and adequate lung separation in addition to rapid-sequence induction includes

(A) placement of right-sided double-lumen tube

(B) placement of left-sided double-lumen tube

(C) placement of single-lumen tube followed by right mainstem intubation

(D) placement of Univent tube followed by selective bronchial blockade

(E) placement of single-lumen tube followed by left mainstem intubation

101. The best drying effect before fiberoptic endoscopy is performed is achieved by the administration of

(A) neostigmine

(B) pyridostigmine

(C) edrophonium

(D) atropine

(E) glycopyrrolate

102. A patient undergoing right upper lobectomy for lung cancer in the left lateral decubitus position is experiencing hypoxemia while receiving an FIO_2 of 1.0 during one-lung anesthesia with a double-lumen tube. Which one of the following options is the most appropriate next step in the treatment of hypoxemia?

(A) Application of continuous positive airway pressure (CPAP) to the non-dependent lung

(B) Application of PEEP to the dependent lung

(C) Intermittent reinflation of the non-dependent lung

(D) Reinstitute two-lung ventilation

(E) Administration of oxygen via suction catheter to the collapsed lung

103. During cardiopulmonary bypass, patients

(A) need large doses of muscle relaxants at 25°C

(B) require neuromuscular blockade during cooling and warming

(C) should have $PaCO_2$ maintained at about 30 mm Hg

(D) should have their lungs hyperinflated

(E) should have continued pulmonary ventilation

104. Nitroglycerin causes vasodilation that is markedly potentiated by

(A) metoprolol

(B) remifentanil

(C) labetalol

(D) magnesium sulfate

(E) sildenafil

105. An 82-year-old patient with a cardiac rhythm-management device (ICD/pacemaker) in place requires surgery that entails the use of electrocautery. Which one of the following statements is true?

(A) The cutaneous electrode (skin pad) of a unipolar electrocautery unit should be as close to the pulse generator as possible.

(B) Electrocardiographic monitoring is necessary only if the patient is being paced.

(C) Placing a magnet over the device can deactivate the pacing function of an ICD.

(D) The risk for interference is negligible if the pacer is a demand unit.

(E) Electrocautery can electrically reset the pacemaker.

DIRECTIONS: Use the following scenario to answer Questions 106-107: A 42-year-old woman is referred by a thoracic surgeon from the clinic for mediastinoscopy. On evaluation, the patient is sitting up on the stretcher, and the respiratory pattern is notable for tachypnea that according to the patient has been present for the past two weeks. The patient's voice sounds hoarse, and she tells you that she sleeps with two pillows at night.

106. Based on the description of symptoms, which one of the following findings is likely to be present on physical exam?

   (A) Pain of the shoulder and medial aspect of forearm
   (B) Rubor of face, and arm veins fail to empty on elevation
   (C) Lower extremity edema, and rales on auscultation
   (D) Pursed lips, prolonged expirium, and bilateral wheezing on auscultation
   (E) Paraesthesias, tetany, and dizziness

107. Based on the patients' presentation, which one of the following is the safest approach to induction of anesthesia?

   (A) Upper extremity IV access and rapid-sequence induction with placement of a single-lumen tube
   (B) Upper extremity IV access and rapid-sequence induction with placement of double-lumen tube
   (C) Lower extremity IV access, standard IV induction, mask ventilation, placement of single-lumen tube
   (D) Lower extremity IV access, placement of arterial blood pressure monitor, maintenance of spontaneous breathing, placement of single-lumen tube
   (E) Upper extremity IV access, placement of arterial blood pressure monitor, maintenance of spontaneous breathing, placement of single-lumen tube

108. The patient with a pacemaker in place may develop competing rhythms when a normal sinus rhythm is present and the unit has been converted to the asynchronous mode. If the pacing stimuli fall on the T wave of the previously conducted beats,

   (A) ventricular fibrillation will follow
   (B) there is little danger, since the energy output is low with current pulse generators
   (C) ventricular fibrillation is less likely if hypoxemia is present
   (D) ventricular fibrillation is less likely with catecholamine release
   (E) ventricular fibrillation is less likely with myocardial infarction

109. Intraaortic balloon counterpulsation is a circulatory assist method that

   (A) is used for patients with aortic aneurysms
   (B) is used for patients with aortic insufficiency
   (C) causes an intraaortic balloon to be inflated during systole
   (D) increases coronary blood flow
   (E) increases impedance to the opening of the left ventricle

110. The clamping of the thoracic aorta in aneurysm repair is followed by

   (A) immediate hypotension
   (B) immediate hypertension
   (C) cardiac standstill
   (D) no change
   (E) loss of blood pressure in the right arm

111. A 72-year-old patient is undergoing thoracic aortic surgery. When the patient is extubated on the first postoperative day, he is noted to have paraplegia on neurological exam. This complication of aortic surgery is most commonly due to

   (A) pressure on the spinal cord during surgery
   (B) long periods of hypotension
   (C) hypothermia associated with the surgery
   (D) spinal cord ischemia
   (E) loss of cerebrospinal fluid

112. Hypovolemia may occur during abdominal aneurysm procedures as a result of all of the following EXCEPT

(A) blood loss

(B) inadequate fluid replacement

(C) use of vasodilators

(D) loss of fluid into the bowel

(E) expansion of the vascular bed during occlusion

113. The blood flow rate for an adult on total cardiopulmonary bypass is generally

(A) 15 mL/kg/min

(B) 35 mL/kg/min

(C) 55 mL/kg/min

(D) 85 mL/kg/min

(E) 115 mL/kg/min

114. When an adult patient is on total cardiopulmonary bypass,

(A) arterial pressure is generally maintained above 50 mm Hg

(B) blood is pumped from the venae cava and drains by gravity into the aorta for circulation

(C) the level of blood in the venous reservoir of the pump reflects the central venous pressure of the patient

(D) venous pressure elevation is of no consequence

(E) venous return to the pump is always started before arterial infusion

115. A 48-year-old female with a history of 40 pack-years of smoking, hypertension, and hypercholesterolemia is to undergo right carotid endarterectomy for symptomatic, high-grade stenosis. Which one of the following statements regarding the anesthetic care for carotid artery surgery in this patient is true?

(A) Blood pressure during carotid occlusion should be maintained at, or above the patient's baseline.

(B) The use of a BIS monitor will reliably detect intraoperative cerebral ischemia.

(C) The use of volatile anesthetics would result in superior brain protection as compared to propofol.

(D) The surgical procedure should be preceded by tests to show if carotid clamping can be tolerated.

(E) The use of regional anesthesia would minimize the risk of perioperative stroke.

116. The most reliable monitor for detection of intraoperative myocardial ischemia is

(A) creatine phosphokinase levels

(B) changes in the ST-T segment on ECG

(C) transesophageal echocardiography

(D) troponin concentrations

(E) exhaled nitric oxide

117. A 72-year-old male is presenting for endovascular stent graft repair of a 6.8 cm descending thoracic aortic aneurysm. The patient's past medical history is significant for insulin dependent diabetes, hypertension, hypercholesterolemia, coronary artery disease, and myocardial infarction. The patient's past surgical history is significant for infrarenal aortic aneurysm repair. In order to decrease the risk of spinal cord ischemia, part of the anesthetic management should be

(A) the preoperative placement of a lumbar drain

(B) intraoperative EEG monitoring

(C) deep hypothermic circulatory arrest (DHCA)

(D) deliberate hypotension

(E) a "high-dose narcotic" technique

118. An 84-year-old female with known severe mitral stenosis is to undergo urgent left hip hemiarthroplasty after suffering a femur fracture after a fall. The patient had a failed spinal anesthetic in the past and is refusing neuraxial anesthesia. The hemodynamic goal after induction of anesthesia should include

(A) increased heart rate

(B) increased contractility

(C) increased preload

(D) decreased contractility

(E) increased afterload

119. In comparing patients undergoing esophagectomy against those undergoing pulmonary resection, it is generally TRUE that esophagectomy patients

(A) have better nutritional status

(B) have less risk of aspiration

(C) have better pulmonary function

(D) are less likely to be hypoxic during single lung ventilation

(E) are less likely to need postoperative ventilation

120. The human larynx

(A) lies at the level of the 1st through 4th cervical vertebrae

(B) in the adult is narrowest at the level of the cricoid cartilage

(C) is innervated solely by the recurrent laryngeal nerve

(D) is protected anteriorly by the wide expanse of the cricoid cartilage

(E) lies within the thyroid cartilage

121. A patient is undergoing a mediastinoscopy when there is a sudden loss of pulse and pressure wave being monitored at the right wrist. The mediastinoscope is withdrawn, with resumption of normal vital signs. The most likely cause of the problem is

(A) cardiac arrest

(B) superior vena cava obstruction

(C) air in the mediastinum

(D) compression of the innominate artery

(E) anesthetic overdose

122. A 71-year-old man is admitted with a complaint of hoarseness and sore throat. On indirect laryngoscopy, a supraglottic mass is noted with edema of the cords. He is scheduled for a direct laryngoscopy under general anesthesia. The approach to this procedure should be

(A) kept simple, since it is a short procedure

(B) induction, paralysis, and laryngoscopy

(C) induction, paralysis, intubation, and laryngoscopy

(D) paralysis, intubation, induction, and laryngoscopy

(E) to establish an airway before paralysis or instrumentation

123. A patient with esophageal obstruction is to have a general anesthetic for esophagoscopy. He has had a barium swallow on the previous day. One of the greatest dangers of the planned procedure is

(A) bleeding

(B) hypotension

(C) difficult intubation

(D) aspiration

(E) arrhythmia

DIRECTIONS: Use the following figure to answer Questions 124-127:

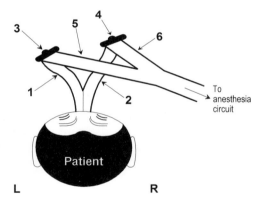

124. The figure shows a view of a patient with a double-lumen tube viewed from the head of the bed. To ventilate the right lung and deflate the left lung, one should

(A) clamp at 1 and uncap at 3

(B) clamp at 6 and uncap at 3

(C) clamp at 5 and uncap at 3

(D) clamp at 5 and uncap at 4

(E) clamp at 1 and 6 and uncap at 3

125. After the tube has been correctly positioned, a bronchoscope is used. By opening at 4 and looking down the lumen of 2, one should see

    (A) the left upper lobe with a right-sided tube
    (B) the carina with a right-sided tube
    (C) the trachea with a right-sided tube
    (D) the carina with a left-sided tube
    (E) the left upper lobe with a left-sided tube

126. To lavage the right lung while ventilating the left lung, one would perform all the following EXCEPT

    (A) clamp at 6
    (B) clamp at 2
    (C) pour fluid into 4

    (D) inflate the bronchial cuff
    (E) inflate the tracheal cuff

127. All of the following are true about the double-lumen tube in the figure EXCEPT

    (A) lumen 1 is the bronchial lumen in a left-sided tube
    (B) the pressures are equal at 1 and 2 when no clamps are applied
    (C) CPAP to the right lung is applied at 4
    (D) clamping at 6 isolates the left lung from the anesthesia circuit
    (E) clamping at 5 and uncapping at 3 will allow the left lung to collapse

DIRECTIONS: Use the following figure to answer Questions 128-129:

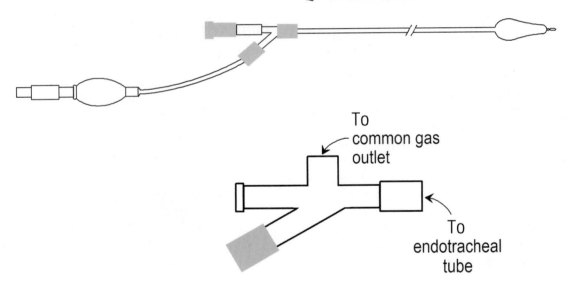

128. The device depicted in the figure is

    (A) a Univent bronchial blocker tube
    (B) a Fogarty catheter
    (C) a Sengstaken-Blakemore tube
    (D) an independent (Arndt) endobronchial blocker
    (E) an airway exchange catheter

129. Which one of the following statements about the device depicted is true?

    (A) It is useful to obtain one-lung ventilation in patients who are already intubated or have a difficult airway.
    (B) Positive pressure ventilation has to be interrupted for proper placement.
    (C) There is no need for fiberoptic bronchoscopy to verify correct positioning of the device.
    (D) It can only be used in patients undergoing right sided surgery.
    (E) With this device, the endotracheal tube has to be exchanged at the end of surgery if the patient is to remain intubated.

130. During apneic oxygenation

    (A) the time elapsed before desaturation occurs is independent of the patient's pulmonary status
    (B) all arrhythmias are due to hypoxemia
    (C) the carbon dioxide tension is not important
    (D) the carbon dioxide level rises about 3-6 mm Hg/min
    (E) pulse oximetry is not helpful

131. The bronchial venous systems drains into all of the following vascular beds EXCEPT

    (A) Thebesian veins
    (B) hemiazygos veins
    (C) azygos veins
    (D) pulmonary veins
    (E) mediastinal veins

132. A 58-year-old male with past medical history significant for moderate to severe aortic regurgitation is undergoing laparoscopic ventral hernia repair under general anesthesia. Assuming that the patient's blood pressure is normal and at baseline, administration of which one of the following drugs is likely to result in improved forward flow?

    (A) Norepinephrine
    (B) Glycopyrrolate
    (C) Esmolol
    (D) Phenylephrine
    (E) Vasopressin

133. The administration of fentanyl in large doses (0.1 mg/kg) generally results in

    (A) increased pulmonary vascular resistance
    (B) decreased heart rate
    (C) histamine release
    (D) more profound hypotension than is seen with morphine (1 mg/kg)

134. Which one of the following interventions is most likely to result in preservation of renal function during aortic aneurysm surgery?

    (A) Administration of furosemide
    (B) Keeping aortic cross clamp time less than 120 min
    (C) Administration of dopamine
    (D) Endovascular approach to aortic aneurysm repair
    (E) Administration of mannitol

DIRECTIONS: Use the following scenario to answer Questions 135-136: A 75-kg patient is undergoing elective repair of an aortic aneurysm. Twenty minutes after incision the patient develops tachycardia, hypotension, and subsequent ST elevations in lead V, as well as a rise in the pulmonary artery (PA) pressures. An infusion of vasopressor is started to correct hypotension.

135. In addition to correcting the hypotension, the most effective intervention for the treatment of elevated PA pressures in this scenario is

    (A) infusion of milrinone
    (B) addition of inhaled nitric oxide
    (C) infusion of nitroglycerin
    (D) start hyperventilation
    (E) increase in F_{IO_2} to 1.0

136. With respect to the patient's tachycardia, the next best step in management is

    (A) observation only
    (B) administration of metoprolol
    (C) administration of nicardipine
    (D) administration of neostigmine
    (E) administration of glycopyrrolate

137. A 72-year-old patient underwent an uncomplicated CABG for severe three-vessel coronary artery disease four hours ago and is now requiring increasing levels of hemodynamic support. The patient was started on an epinephrine infusion, currently at 2 mcg/kg/min. Vital signs are blood pressure (BP) 80/50, heart rate 130, pulmonary artery pressure 50/25, central venous pressure 24, cardiac index 1.6, and the ECG shows variations in amplitude. A bedside transthoracic echocardiogram shows right atrial collapse and abnormal ventricular septal motion. Based on the patient's presentation, the next best step in management is to

    (A) add norepinephrine
    (B) stop epinephrine and start milrinone
    (C) return immediately to the operating room for reexploration of the chest
    (D) add nitroglycerin
    (E) stat CT of the chest with pulmonary embolism protocol

138. An anesthetic consideration for Marfan syndrome is

    (A) atlanto-axial instability
    (B) aortic stenosis
    (C) possible difficult intubation
    (D) mitral regurgitation
    (E) ventricular septal defect (VSD)

139. A 29-year-old male suffered a motorcycle crash and is undergoing intramedullary nailing of the left femur. The accident occurred 24 h ago. Shortly after intramedullary reaming, the patient develops tachycardia, hypotension and hypoxemia. There are no ST-segment changes on the five-lead EKG. What is the most likely finding on the patient's transesophageal echocardiogram?

    (A) Fluid collection around the heart without any diastolic collapse
    (B) Regional wall motion abnormalities in the anterolateral wall of the left ventricle
    (C) Large color flow via the intra-atrial septum

    (D) Distended right atrium and ventricle, collapsed left atrium and ventricle
    (E) Large color flow via the intraventricular septum

140. When $Paco_2$ and pH are managed by the alpha-stat method during hypothermic cardiopulmonary bypass,

    (A) the corrected pH is 7.4
    (B) ABG results will be corrected to current patient temperature
    (C) the uncorrected $Paco_2$ is 40 mm Hg
    (D) the corrected $Paco_2$ is 40 mm Hg

141. A 77-year-old woman with coronary artery disease and significant aortic stenosis develops myocardial ischemia shortly after induction of anesthesia. She is being treated with beta blockers and nitroglycerin, and her blood pressure is being supported with an infusion of norepinephrine. Throughout this event the patient's oxygen saturation is 100%. The patient continues to be ischemic. What statement about the use of an intraaortic balloon pump (IABP) in this patient is true?

    (A) An IABP is not indicated and the patient should be put on cardiopulmonary bypass.
    (B) An IABP is contraindicated because the patient has aortic stenosis.
    (C) An IABP should be placed immediately.
    (D) The tip of the IABP balloon has to be placed just distal to the coronary arteries.
    (E) An IABP is contraindicated due to the risk of leg ischemia.

142. A 65-year-old female with a history of severe aortic stenosis requires urgent laparoscopic cholecystectomy. An important hemodynamic goal during anesthetic care is

    (A) decreased afterload
    (B) slow heart rate
    (C) decreased preload
    (D) high heart rate
    (E) decreased contractility

143. Cannon waves in the central venous pressure tracing

    (A) are caused by atrial fibrillation

    (B) can be seen with atrioventricular nodal rhythms

    (C) result from left atrial contraction against the closed mitral valve

    (D) will resolve with ventricular pacing

    (E) represent an artifact caused by air in the pressure transducer system

144. The right lung, in the upright position

    (A) is the smaller of the two

    (B) has a single fissure

    (C) has three lobes

    (D) receives 45% of total lung blood flow

    (E) is less frequently involved in aspiration compared to the left

145. A 74-year-old patient is to undergo for right-sided thoracotomy for resection of lung cancer. The patient's past medical history is significant for myocardial infarction four months ago at which time the patient underwent the placement of two drug-eluting stents and was started on antiplatelet therapy with clopidogrel. According to the patient's cardiologist, the patient is to continue clopidogrel throughout the perioperative period. The surgeon is requesting an analgesic strategy that would provide the patient with about 36 h of postoperative pain control to facilitate extubation and early mobilization. Which one of the following is the most effective and safest method of analgesia for this patient?

    (A) postoperative right intercostal block

    (B) lumbar epidural catheter

    (C) patient controlled analgesia with IV opioid

    (D) thoracic epidural catheter

    (E) right paravertebral block via continuous catheter

146. A patient with severe COPD and severe pulmonary hypertension is to undergo bilateral lung transplant. The en-bloc double-lung transplant, as compared to bilateral sequential single-lung transplantation

    (A) has a decreased need for blood transfusions

    (B) has a lower incidence of ischemia at the site of tracheal anastomosis

    (C) results in a higher need for cardiopulmonary bypass

    (D) is technically easier

    (E) does not require cardiac arrest

147. A 68-year-old patient is to undergo a Whipple procedure for resection of a tumor of the head of the pancreas. The patient's past medical history is significant for myocardial infarction and the placement of a bare metal stent, hypertension, hypercholesterolemia, and COPD secondary to tobacco abuse. The preoperative ECG is significant for a right bundle branch block, and the preoperative TTE is significant for diastolic dysfunction with an ejection fraction of 45% as well as moderate to severe aortic regurgitation. In addition to arterial blood pressure, a decision is made for intraoperative monitoring with a pulmonary artery catheter for estimation of left ventricular preload. Based on this patient's presentation, left ventricular preload as assessed by pulmonary artery catheter measurements will likely be

    (A) underestimated because of aortic regurgitation

    (B) overestimated due to the right bundle branch block

    (C) underestimated due to decreased left ventricular compliance

    (D) underestimated because the patient will be on positive pressure ventilation

    (E) accurately reflected by LAP, LVEDP, and PAOP

DIRECTIONS: Use the following figure to answer Questions 148-149:

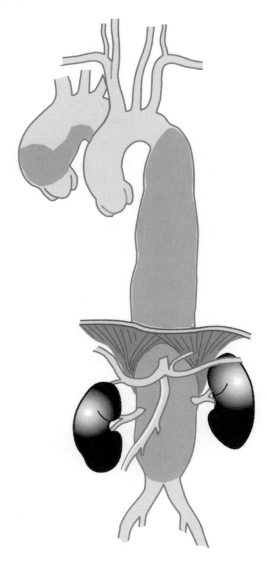

148. A 58-year-old male comes to the emergency department with diffuse chest pain that is radiating into his back. His past medical history is significant for tobacco and alcohol abuse, hypertension, and hypercholesterolemia, as well as peripheral vascular disease. A workup for acute coronary syndrome is negative, and the patient undergoes CT imaging of chest and abdomen with IV contrast that reveals a thoracoabdominal aneurysm that is deemed symptomatic and the patient is scheduled to undergo urgent surgical repair. Based on the drawing, which one of the following classifications of this patient's aneurysm is accurate?

(A) Stanford A
(B) DeBakey II
(C) Stanford B
(D) Crawford I
(E) Crawford II

149. The risk of spinal cord ischemia with surgical repair of this type of lesion is approximately

(A) 2%
(B) 10%
(C) 20%
(D) 30%
(E) 40%

150. An 82-year-old patient with anterior two-vessel coronary artery disease and unstable angina is referred by the cardiologist for CABG. Her past medical history is otherwise significant for type I diabetes, chronic renal insufficiency, peripheral vascular disease, COPD, and atherosclerotic ascending aortic disease. The cardiac surgeon decides to perform off-pump CABG to the LAD and the RCA. Considering this patient's comorbidities and the proposed procedure, it is true that

(A) minimally invasive coronary artery bypass grafting would be a suitable alternative
(B) the surgeon will require a stabilization device for the distal anastomoses
(C) cooling of the patient is required as part of the procedure
(D) hemodynamic goals are easier to achieve as compared to CABG with cardiopulmonary bypass
(E) the use of propofol for maintenance of anesthesia will result in equivalent myocardial protection as compared to volatile anesthetics

151. The patient population most likely to benefit from transcatheter aortic valve implantation is

(A) children and young adults with congenital, noncalcific aortic stenosis
(B) adult patients with severe aortic regurgitation

(C) asymptomatic adult patients with calcific aortic stenosis and severe obstruction

(D) adult patients with symptomatic severe aortic stenosis deemed too high risk for surgery

(E) adult patients with symptomatic severe aortic stenosis without other associated comorbidities

152. A 60-year-old female was admitted with a large goiter and a history of hoarseness. An incidental finding on the chest x-ray was tracheal deviation with questionable narrowing of the tracheal lumen. After induction was complicated by a difficult intubation requiring multiple attempts, the thyroid was removed with some difficulty and at the end of the procedure the patient was breathing spontaneously. Immediately after extubation, breathing was labored and retraction was noted. Causes of this may include all of the following EXCEPT

(A) bilateral recurrent laryngeal nerve injury

(B) laryngospasm

(C) tracheal collapse

(D) bronchospasm

(E) thyrotoxicosis

153. Hypoxic pulmonary vasoconstriction

(A) occurs when regional atelectasis mechanically obstructs blood flow

(B) is primarily triggered by alveolar carbon dioxide tension

(C) leads to diversion of blood away from poorly ventilated areas of the lung

(D) is potentiated by administration of nitrous oxide

(E) is augmented by an increase in pulmonary artery pressure

154. At the conclusion of an aortic aneurysm repair associated with significant blood loss, diffuse bleeding and the absence of clot formation is noted in the surgical field. A thromboelastogram shows decreased maximum amplitude. The appropriate treatment includes administration of which one of the following?

(A) Protamine

(B) Cryoprecipitate

(C) Fresh frozen plasma

(D) Aminocaproic acid

(E) Platelets

155. Structures that pass anteriorly to the trachea include all of the following EXCEPT

(A) pulmonary artery

(B) thyroid isthmus

(C) innominate artery

(D) aortic arch

(E) left brachiocephalic vein

156. Indications for one-lung ventilation include all of the following EXCEPT

(A) infection with purulent secretions

(B) massive pulmonary hemorrhage

(C) bronchopleural fistula

(D) unilateral bronchopulmonary lavage for alveolar proteinosis

(E) Ivor-Lewis esophagectomy

157. During awake, closed chest ventilation in the lateral decubitus position,

(A) the lung relationships are the same as in the semirecumbent position, i.e., the apex is in zone 1 and the bases are in zone 3

(B) ventilation is highest at the apex

(C) perfusion is greater in the nondependent lung

(D) compliance is unequal in the two lungs

(E) the nondependent lung receives most of the tidal ventilation

158. A 35-year-old man is admitted to the emergency department following an automobile accident. It is noted that there is a contusion over the anterior thorax, he is tachypneic, and he has a scaphoid abdomen. Auscultation reveals poor breath sounds on the left side. Chest x-ray shows a large air cavity in the left side of the thorax. Blood pressure is 80/60, and heart rate is 120 per minute. Diagnoses that must be considered include all of the following EXCEPT

(A) ruptured spleen
(B) pneumothorax
(C) diaphragmatic hernia
(D) cardiac contusion
(E) fat embolism syndrome

159. A 69-year-old woman is scheduled for routine CABG. Since her preoperative cardiac catheterization, her platelet count has dropped from 312 to 252 × 10^3/mm^3. A heparin-induced thrombocytopenia (HIT) immunoassay has been ordered and it resulted in a positive HIT antibody. She has a large bruise at the site of her catheterization. There are no signs of deep venous thrombus or any other thrombotic events. You should

(A) delay surgery for 2 months
(B) proceed with surgery and use a direct thrombin inhibitor instead of heparin
(C) proceed with surgery and use heparin
(D) use only 50% of the regular heparin dose and proceed with surgery
(E) use a combination of warfarin and low-dose heparin to achieve adequate anticoagulation

160. A 73-year-old patient is undergoing emergent three-vessel CABG for symptomatic left main coronary artery disease. Upon completion of the surgical procedure, the patient develops the need for high dose inotropic support, and the decision is made to implant a left ventricular assist device (LVAD) to facilitate weaning from cardiopulmonary bypass (CPB). After discontinuation of CPB, the patient is noted to be hypotensive with low pump flow rates apparent on the LVAD device. Immediate TEE examination does not show any evidence of inflow cannula obstruction, but is significant for systolic collapse of the right atrium and diastolic collapse of the right ventricle. The ECG shows low QRS voltage. The most likely cause for this patient's hypotension is

(A) graft failure
(B) acute hypovolemia
(C) right ventricular failure
(D) pulmonary embolus
(E) pericardial tamponade

161. The advantages of ultrasound-guided central venous catheter placement, as compared to the landmark technique, include all of the following EXCEPT

(A) prevention of arterial injury
(B) direct visualization of the target vessel
(C) decreased time required for internal jugular vein catheterization
(D) decreased number of attempts required
(E) decreased overall complication rate

DIRECTIONS (Questions 162-164): Each group of items below consists of lettered headings followed by a list of numbered phrases or statements. For each numbered phrase or statement, select the ONE lettered heading or component that is most closely associated with it and fill in the circle containing the corresponding letter on the answer sheet. Each lettered heading or component may be selected once, more than once, or not at all.

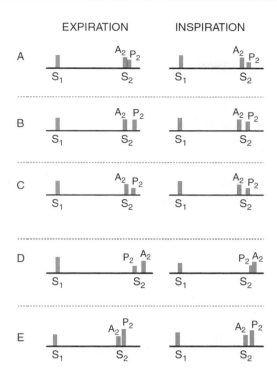

EXPIRATION   INSPIRATION

A

B

C

D

E

For each patient, select the appropriate diagram of the heart sounds.

162. A 64-year-old patient with a history of rheumatic fever presenting for elective aortic valve replacement.

163. A 21-year-old female with Down syndrome and echocardiographic evidence of right ventricular overload.

164. A 70-year-old male with a 60 pack-year history of smoking and a history of pneumonectomy for lung cancer with mild respiratory insufficiency and evidence of right ventricular strain on echocardiography.

DIRECTIONS (Questions 165-174): Each group of items below consists of lettered headings followed by a list of numbered phrases or statements. For each numbered phrase or statement, select the ONE lettered heading or component that is most closely associated with it. Each lettered heading or component may be selected once, more than once, or not at all.

(A) Mid-esophageal four chamber
(B) Mid-esophageal two chamber
(C) Mid-esophageal long axis
(D) Transgastric two chamber
(E) Transgastric mid-papillary short axis
(F) Mid-esophageal aortic valve short axis
(G) Mid-esophageal aortic valve long axis
(H) Mid-esophageal bicaval
(I) Mid-esophageal right ventricular inflow-outflow
(J) Deep transgastric long axis
(K) Upper esophageal aortic valve short axis
(L) Upper esophageal aortic valve long axis
(M) Transgastric long axis
(N) Mid-esophageal ascending aortic short axis
(O) Mid-esophageal ascending aortic long axis

For each photograph of a transesophageal echocardiogram, select the standard, two-dimensional tomographic view.

165.

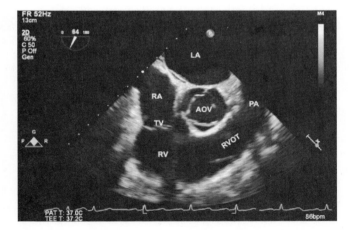

166.

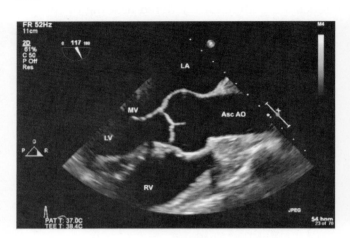

167.

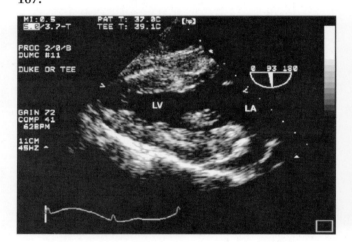

168.

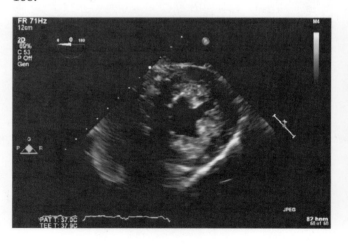

169.

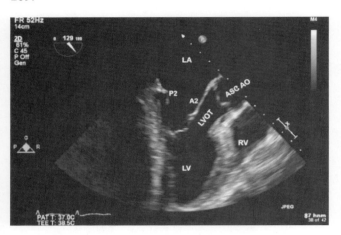

170.

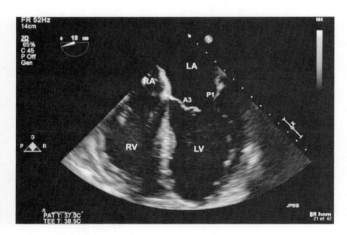

171.

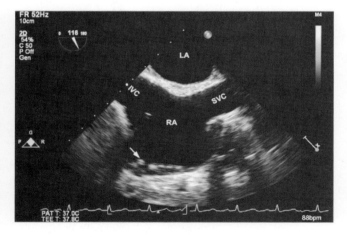

172.

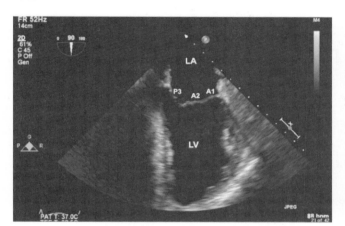

174.

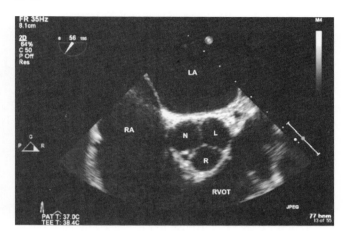

173.

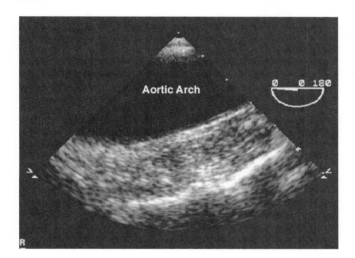

Answers and Explanations

94. **(A)** The best next step in management is to initiate artificial cardiac pacing, either via pacer cables still in situ, or via transcutaneous pads. Indications for artificial pacing include, but are not limited to: SA node dysfunction with symptomatic bradycardia as described in this case, junctional rhythm that can sometimes be corrected by means of overdrive pacing, symptomatic chronotropic incompetence, and atrial fibrillation with bradycardia and pauses greater than 5 sec. In settings outside the cardiac ICU, administration of chronotropic agents such as epinephrine might be indicated on a temporary basis as a bridge to pacer therapy. *(6:1876)*

95. **(E)** No pharmacological alternative meets both goals. *(6:2235)*

96. **(B)** The inferior wall of the left ventricle is supplied by the right coronary artery and is most apparent in leads II, III, and AVF. *(6:1836)*

97. **(C)** An incompetent tricuspid valve permits right ventricular pressure to be transmitted to the right atrium, causing increased amplitude of the **v** wave. Increased **a** waves occur in heart block and junctional rhythm, while **a** waves are absent in atrial fibrillation. *(5:409; 6:1905)*

98. **(D)** At 17°C, cerebral oxygen consumption is reduced to about 8% of the normothermic value and, while metabolic activity is decreased, cellular integrity is maintained. This accounts for the brain's tolerance to modest periods of cardiac arrest during hypothermia. Both cerebral blood flow and electrical activity decrease during hypothermia. *(6:166)*

99. **(C)** The external noninvasive units are ventricular pacing devices. *(1:896; 4:817; 5:1084; 6:72)*

100. **(D)** The patient described in this vignette likely has mediastinitis from esophageal rupture, acute lung injury, and very little, if any, tolerance for apnea during airway instrumentation. The safest choice among the options listed to secure the airway and be able to provide single lung ventilation is rapid-sequence induction, followed by placement of a Univent tube. The Univent is a single lumen tube with built in bronchial blocker that passes through a small channel within the wall of the endotracheal tube. Other choices would include the Arndt, or Cohen, endobronchial blockers, that are guided with fiberoptic bronchoscopy, or a wire-guided mechanism respectively. If a double-lumen tube is chosen, a left-sided double-lumen tube is the tube of choice, however unlikely to be tolerated by this patient due to baseline hypoxemia. Placement of a standard single-lumen tube is unlikely to result in adequate lung separation, thus making surgical exposure far more difficult. *(5:967, 985)*

101. **(E)** Of the anticholinergic agents, glycopyrrolate and scopolamine are better antisialagogues than atropine. The other medications listed are cholinesterase inhibitors that have increased salivation as a major side effect. *(5:973)*

102. **(A)** CPAP with oxygen to the collapsed lung will decrease shunt and improve the hypoxemia. The remaining choices B, C, and D are listed in the order the clinician should proceed if application of CPAP to the non-dependent

lung does not resolve the hypoxemia. Option E would likely be less effective, and might lead to overdistention of the operative lung. *(5:972)*

103. **(B)** Shivering is blocked with muscle relaxants during warming and cooling but does not occur in very cold muscle. *(5:908)*

104. **(E)** Nitroglycerin is metabolized to nitric oxide, an activator of guanylate cyclase in vascular smooth muscle. The enzyme produces intracellular cyclic-GMP. The cyclic-GMP is degraded by a specific phosphodiesterase (PDE-5) that is inhibited by sildenafil. Profound hypotension can occur when a sublingual dose of nitroglycerin is given within several hours of an oral dose of sildenafil. Intravenous nitroglycerin must be slowly titrated in that setting. *(1:752; 6:2025)*

105. **(E)** Magnets cause most pacemakers to pace asynchronously at a preset rate, however some devices may be deactivated permanently and have to be reprogrammed. Magnets do not affect the pacing rate of ICD's. Since newer devices are very complex, the use of magnets should be reserved for emergency situations, and the devices have to be interrogated after completion of surgery. The indifferent plate should be placed away from the pacemaker or ICD. If the pacer is in demand mode, it may sense the cautery current as depolarization and shut off. *(5:63, 1281)*

106. **(B)** This patient has symptoms consistent with superior vena cava (SVC) syndrome. In addition to the symptoms described in (B), these patients may have multiorgan involvement including neurologic, respiratory, cardiac, gastrointestinal, and renal symptoms. The other findings described here might be found in a patient with thoracic outlet syndrome in (A), congestive heart failure in (C), acute asthma or a COPD exacerbation in (D), and hyperventilation syndrome in (E). *(5:993-4; 6:2185)*

107. **(D)** Patients with SVC syndrome should be kept upright to facilitate venous drainage of the upper vessels, and if a general anesthetic is required be induced while maintaining

spontaneous respirations due to the high risk of airway compression and cardiovascular collapse resulting from the loss of muscle tone associated with administration of muscle relaxants and the supine position. In many cases these patients require fiberoptic intubation. Due to the impaired venous drainage from the SVC to the heart, intravenous lines should be placed in the lower extremities. *(5:993-4)*

108. **(B)** With modern pacemaker units, the energy output is so low that there is little danger of fibrillation. However, ventricular fibrillation is more common in the patient with a high catecholamine concentration, myocardial infarction, or hypoxemia. *(6:1899)*

109. **(D)** The intraaortic balloon pump is deflated during systole. It is rapidly inflated during diastole, thereby increasing coronary blood flow. It decreases impedance to left ventricle ejection. It is contraindicated in the patient with aortic insufficiency. *(6:2235-6)*

110. **(B)** Clamping of the thoracic aorta leads to an immediate increase in blood pressure. Assuming the heart can withstand the markedly increased afterload, there should not be standstill or hypotension. Blood pressure readings may be lost in the left arm, but the pulse in the right arm should be present, depending on the placement of the clamp relative to the take-off of the vessels to the arms. *(5:1025-7)*

111. **(D)** A complication of aortic surgery is spinal cord ischemia due to compromise of the radicular arteries. These arteries are not constant, and the large artery to the spine, the artery of Adamkiewitz, may be compromised leading to ischemia. Pressure on the cord can also lead to ischemia. Hypothermia may be protective. Loss of cerebrospinal fluid is not a factor. Long periods of hypotension may lead to ischemia. *(5:1025-8)*

112. **(E)** The expansion of the vascular bed that occurs follows the release of the clamps. It is due to a reactive vasodilatation. Other factors, such as blood loss, inadequate fluid replacement,

vasoactive drugs, and extravasation of fluid, are all important. *(5:1028-9)*

113. **(C)** The flow rate on total bypass can be varied to achieve the perfusion pressure that is desired. This must be varied with the state of resistance. *(5:899)*

114. **(A)** When the patient is on bypass, the pressure is usually kept above 50 mm Hg. Lower pressures can be tolerated, but there is no agreement on any specific perfusion pressure. *(5:899)*

115. **(A)** The overriding goals of anesthetic care for carotid endarterectomy (CEA) surgery are hemodynamic stability and prompt emergence from anesthesia at the conclusion of the procedure to facilitate neurologic examination. There is universal agreement that the patient's blood pressure should be maintained at, or 20% higher, than the highest recorded awake blood pressure to maintain adequate collateral cerebral perfusion during carotid clamping. Experience with processed EEG monitors such as the BIS is still lacking, and the raw EEG provides higher sensitivity for the detection of intraoperative cerebral ischemia. There is no conclusive evidence in the literature suggesting an advantage of volatile anesthetics over propofol with regard to brain protection during CEA. Preoperative clamp tests are not indicated, and general anesthesia compared to regional anesthesia appears to result in identical outcomes, with the possible exception of patients with contralateral carotid occlusion who might benefit from regional anesthesia. *(5:1018-21)*

116. **(C)** Wall motion abnormalities detected by TEE generally precede ischemic ST-changes detected on ECG. None of the other options is suitable for the detection of intraoperative ischemia. *(5:1867)*

117. **(A)** Strategies to mitigate the risk of spinal cord ischemia in this high-risk patient include placement of a lumbar drain, as well as neurophysiologic monitoring such as SSEP's or MEP's. Intraoperative EEG monitoring will not

provide information about spinal cord ischemia, and is considered the gold standard for monitoring the brain during CEA. Hypotension is to be avoided since it would increase the risk of ischemia. DHCA is a technique employed during open repair or replacement of the thoracic aorta. Patients undergoing successful stent graft repair of the thoracic aorta are routinely extubated at the end of the procedure, and a high-dose opioid technique does not provide spinal cord protection. *(5:915, 940, 1019)*

118. **(C)** The hemodynamic goals for this patient should include a slow heart rate and augmentation of preload to ensure preservation of forward flow through the stenosed valve. Tachycardia and increase in afterload and contractility could decrease cardiac output and increase myocardial oxygen demand respectively. *(5:910)*

119. **(C)** Esophagectomy patients are generally malnourished. They are at risk for aspiration, since esophageal function is frequently compromised. Their pulmonary function is equal between their lungs, and thus they are more likely to have a significant shunt during one-lung ventilation. The surgery is more extensive than most thoracotomies, and the patients more frail, so postoperative ventilation is common. *(5:983)*

120. **(E)** The larynx lies at the level of the 3rd--6th cervical vertebrae, and in the adult, the narrowest portion is at the level of the vocal cords. The larynx is innervated by the recurrent laryngeal nerve and the superior laryngeal nerve. It lies within the thyroid cartilage. The wide margin of the cricoid cartilage is posterior. *(5:548)*

121. **(D)** The innominate artery passes anterior to the trachea and can be compressed by the mediastinoscope. The right subclavian artery is a branch of the innominate artery, while the left subclavian artery comes off the aorta directly and does not cross in front of the trachea. Compression of flow in the innominate will also obstruct flow to the right carotid

artery, and may compromise cerebral perfusion in patients with cerebrovascular disease or an incomplete circle of Willis. Air in the mediastinum should have little hemodynamic effect. Cardiac arrest, superior vena cava obstruction, and anesthetic overdose can all cause pulselessness, but rarely as suddenly or reversibly. Having a monitor of perfusion on the other arm, such as an oximeter probe, can help differentiate innominate compression from other causes of circulatory compromise. *(5:988)*

122. **(E)** In any patient with hoarseness and a documented supraglottic mass, it is mandatory to establish the airway before proceeding with the anesthesia. Awake fiberoptic intubation, awake tracheostomy (all with topical anesthesia), or spontaneous ventilation with an inhaled anesthetic are the only safe methods. *(5:1234-5)*

123. **(D)** Aspiration is possible, since the esophagus may contain barium from the examination as well as other oral intake. The esophagus should be suctioned before induction, although the thick barium suspension may not be completely removed. *(5:983)*

124. **(C)** By clamping at 5, gas cannot flow into the left lumen, and thus to the left lung. Uncapping at 3 allows the gas in the left lung to escape. Clamping at 1 would prevent flow to the left side, but uncapping would cause a leak in the anesthetic circuit. Assuming good tube position and isolation, the handedness of the tube doesn't matter. *(5:963-5)*

125. **(D)** Through position 4, one is looking down the right lumen. From the right lumen, no left lung segmental bronchi can be seen with any type of properly positioned double-lumen tube. The right lumen will be the tracheal lumen on a left-sided tube, in which case the carina can be seen. *(5:965)*

126. **(B)** All the steps are correct for ventilating via the left lumen while pouring fluid into the right lumen except that clamping at 2 will

block the fluid flow. The cuffs should be up to ensure lung isolation. *(5:978)*

127. **(D)** Clamping at 6 isolates the right lung. *(5:963-5)*

128. **(D)** The Arndt bronchial blocker can be used in patients who are already intubated, so there is no need to change the endotracheal to a double-lumen tube should one-lung ventilation be required. It can also be used for patients with a difficult airway and patients with trauma who require one-lung ventilation. The Univent tube is a single lumen endotracheal tube with an integrated, movable bronchial blocker. The Sengstaken-Blakemore tube is an esophageal device used for temporary control of intractable variceal bleeding. *(5:967)*

129. **(A)** Positive pressure ventilation does not have to be interrupted during placement of the bronchial blocker because of the multiport adapter that will accommodate the breathing circuit, a fiberoptic bronchoscope and the endobronchial blocker. The device has to be placed under fiberoptic bronchoscopic guidance and its use is not limited to only the left or right lung. If the patient continues on mechanical ventilation upon conclusion of surgery, the endobronchial balloon is deflated and the device removed while the endotracheal tube remains in place. *(5:967)*

130. **(D)** The carbon dioxide tension rises about 6 mm Hg during the first minute of apneic oxygenation and about 3-6 mm Hg per minute thereafter. It will rise more quickly in individuals with a low FRC. All arrhythmias are not due to hypoxemia but may be due to increased catecholamines. These in turn may be increased due to increased carbon dioxide. Pulse oximetry has been of definite benefit in these procedures. *(5:551)*

131. **(A)** The Thebesian veins are the smallest veins in the heart and drain directly into the ventricles, whereas the remainder of the coronary arterial blood is drained via the venous system into the coronary sinus and eventually into the

right atrium. All other options are correct. *(5:902, 951)*

132. **(B)** The hemodynamic goal of anesthetic care is the reduction of the regurgitant fraction that can be achieved by augmentation of preload, mildly increased heart rate (i.e., administration of low-dose glycopyrrolate), and avoidance of increased afterload. *(5:910)*

133. **(B)** Administration of high-dose fentanyl will result in bradycardia, but blood pressure will remain relatively stable. Fentanyl, as opposed to morphine, does not release histamine. The cardiac output will decrease to a mild degree. Morphine-induced changes are more pronounced. *(5:711-2)*

134. **(D)** While some of the pharmacological strategies mentioned have been shown to preserve renal function in animal models, this has not been conclusively shown in humans. Among the strongest predictors of postoperative renal dysfunction is aortic cross clamp time, particularly if the aorta is clamped for more than 50 min. Of note, even the infrarenal location of the aortic cross clamp can cause changes in renal blood flow that in turn can contribute to postoperative renal dysfunction. The most significant progress in prevention of acute kidney injury during aortic surgery has come from the widespread adoption of endovascular techniques. *(5:1027-8)*

135. **(C)** The rise in PA pressure is due to left ventricular dysfunction resulting in a rise in left ventricular end diastolic pressure (LVEDP). The goal in this situation is to decrease LVEDP, which will translate into lower PA pressures, in order to improve myocardial perfusion. Nitroglycerin induces venodilation, thus decreasing ventricular filling, transmural pressure, and myocardial work. A side effect of nitroglycerin is hypotension that is counterproductive and often treated simultaneously with phenylephrine. While milrinone decreases PA pressure it leads to an increase in myocardial oxygen consumption. Nitric oxide decreases the PA pressure as well, but it might not have a significant effect on LVEDP. Since the

patient in this vignette is neither hypoxic nor hypercarbic, increased ventilation and oxygenation are unlikely to decrease PA pressure. *(1:747-55)*

136. **(B)** Tachycardia in patients with coronary artery disease is controlled with beta blockers. They decrease heart rate and myocardial contractility, resulting in better coronary perfusion and less oxygen demand. Observation only is not indicated. Nicardipine may lower the heart rate, but does not reduce contractility. *(1:326)*

137. **(C)** This patient has the symptoms of immediate postoperative cardiac tamponade: hypotension, tachycardia, equalization and elevation of PA diastolic pressure and CVP, and low cardiac index. While norepinephrine might help to support the blood pressure, it delays definitive care. Milrinone would add to the hypotension, and so would nitroglycerin. Chest CT is not indicated based on the hemodynamic abnormalities and would delay definitive therapy. *(5:458, 913; 6:1975)*

138. **(C)** Marfan syndrome is associated with aortic changes making dissection more common. Hypertension should be avoided. The high-arched palate may make intubation more difficult. Aortic stenosis is not seen, but aortic insufficiency is common. Atlanto-axial instability and/or ventricular septal defect are seen with congenital syndromes such as Down and achondroplasia. *(5:271-2)*

139. **(D)** The most likely diagnosis is fat embolism syndrome. The typical TEE picture for any large (pulmonary) embolus is an overfilled right side of the heart, and significantly underfilled left side. Fluid around the heart is indicating a pericardial effusion or tamponade; this patient is already 24 h post-trauma and there is no collapse of the patient's heart chambers that renders the diagnosis of tamponade unlikely. Regional wall motion abnormalities indicate a possible ischemic event that is unlikely due to this patient's age and the lack of ST-changes on a 5 lead EKG. Large color flows across the septa on echocardiography

indicate an ASD or a VSD that are unlikely to appear acutely in this situation. *(5:1203)*

140. (C) The other responses pertain to the pH-stat method. *(5:532)*

141. (C) Because pharmacologic attempts at reversing ischemia have failed, insertion of an intraaortic balloon is indicated. The treatment of myocardial ischemia includes correcting the hemodynamics (slow-normal heart rate, high-normal blood pressure, and lowering of the PA pressure) and treatment of severe anemia and hypoxemia. Since the event occurred shortly after induction, large blood loss and severe anemia are unlikely. Immediate initiation of cardiopulmonary bypass in this situation is an option, but is impractical since the surgery is just beginning. Absolute contraindications for placement of an IABP are aortic regurgitation and aortic dissection. The pump can be placed with the help of TEE, x-ray or even by approximation, if TEE and x-ray are not available. The tip of the balloon has to be placed in the proximal thoracic aorta just distal to the left subclavian artery. IABP therapy may cause leg ischemia, however in this situation the benefits of IABP (increased coronary blood flow) outweigh the potential for leg ischemia, for which the patient needs careful postoperative observation. *(6:2234-5; Kar B, et al., Circulation 2012; 125:1809-17).*

142. (B) Slow heart rate and maintenance of afterload are the hemodynamic goals for the patient with severe aortic stenosis, while decreased afterload and higher heart rate are preferred in patients with aortic and mitral regurgitation. Decreased contractility is desired in hypertrophic obstructive cardiomyopathy (HOCM) to avoid left ventricular outflow obstruction. *(5:910)*

143. (B) Cannon waves appear when the right atrium contracts after closure of the tricuspid valve, and is not due to artifact. The **a**-wave is not present with atrial fibrillation and can be caused by ventricular pacing and resulting AV-dissociation. Effective restoration of AV-synchrony with atrial or AV-pacing will

restore the normal CVP trace. Loss of the atrial component of ventricular filling during junctional rhythm may be poorly tolerated. *(5:409; 6:1823)*

144. (C) The right lung is the larger of the two. It has three lobes (upper, middle, and lower) and two fissures (horizontal and oblique). Since it is the larger of the two, it receives 55% of total blood flow. Since the axis of the right mainstem bronchus is more in line with the trachea, the right lung is more frequently involved in cases of aspiration as compared to the left. *(5:951, 959, 1002)*

145. (E) Because the patient is on antiplatelet therapy with clopidogrel, neuraxial techniques are contraindicated. An intercostal block will only last from 4–8 h; an intrapleural catheter would be more suitable but is not listed as an option in the question. IV PCA is unlikely to provide the same level of analgesia and is associated with greater side effects as compared to a paravertebral catheter that is considered safe in patients on antiplatelet therapy. *(5:1007-8)*

146. (C) With the exception of option C, all of the options listed are advantages of bilateral sequential single-lung transplantation that has the additional advantage of not requiring full anticoagulation. *(5:1091)*

147. (A) Left ventricular preload in this patient will likely be underestimated due to aortic regurgitation, which leads to a discrepancy between LAP and LVEDP, due to continued ventricular filling after mitral valve closure. A right bundle branch block and decreased pulmonary vascular bed such as in COPD will also make underestimation of left ventricular preload more likely, while positive pressure ventilation and decreased left ventricular compliance will lead to overestimation of left ventricular preload. *(5:414-5)*

148. (E) The figure shows a thoracoabdominal aneurysm classified as Crawford type II that involves the entire descending thoracic aorta with extension across the diaphragm through the abdominal aorta to the aortic bifurcation.

Stanford A and B as well as BeBakey I through III are classifications of aortic dissections. *(5:918; 6:2063)*

149. **(C)** The risk of spinal cord ischemia with either open or endovascular repair is approximately 20% for this type of lesion. *(5:917)*

150. **(B)** While off-pump CABG is a suitable approach for anterior, inferior, and lateral vessels, minimally-invasive CABG, utilizing the internal thoracic (mammary) artery, is suitable for one- or two-vessel disease on the left side of the heart. While the hemodynamic goals for patients undergoing CABG with cardiopulmonary bypass, and those undergoing off-pump CABG are the same, they are harder to attain with the latter approach due to the mobilization of the heart that may cause arrhythmia and hemodynamic instability, particularly when the distal anastomoses are performed. Myocardial protection appears to be better with the use of volatile anesthetics as compared to propofol, reflected in less myocardial injury in the first 24 h postoperatively. Patients undergoing off-pump CABG procedures are kept normothermic. *(5:907-8)*

151. **(D)** Current indications for transcatheter aortic valve implantation include adult patients with severe aortic stenosis deemed too high risk for surgery. The procedure is currently being evaluated as an alternative to reoperation in patients with prosthetic valve failure not due to paravalvular regurgitation. The patient population described in option A is usually referred for percutaneous balloon aortic valvuloplasty, while asymptomatic patients with severe obstruction are usually followed carefully with serial echocardiograms until they meet operative criteria. *(6:1941)*

152. **(E)** Nerve injury is common with difficult dissections. Laryngospasm may be present due to secretions or injury to the vocal cords during difficult intubation. Tracheal collapse may be present due to tracheomalacia. Bronchospasm may be a reason for the dyspnea due to airway sensitivity. While thyrotoxicosis can cause respiratory failure secondary to increased

production of carbon dioxide and increased work of breathing, its onset would be more gradual. *(5:151, 575-6)*

153. **(C)** Hypoxic pulmonary vasoconstriction (HPV) is a constriction of pulmonary arteries in response to alveolar hypoxia. Atelectatic lungs have identical degrees of HPV to those ventilated with nitrogen, excluding mechanical factors. HPV can occur in denervated lungs (e.g., after transplantation). Hypocapnia decreases HPV, but hypercapnia has no effect. Hypoxia is the primary trigger of HPV. Alkalosis and acidosis both decrease HPV, as does administration of nitrous oxide. The pulmonary vasoconstrictor response to hypoxia is decreased with increases in pulmonary artery pressure, cardiac output, left atrial pressure, or central blood volume. *(5:612-3, 967-70)*

154. **(E)** A thromboelastogram (TEG) measures the clot strength over time. The amplitude of the graph refers to the clot strength at a given time during the clot formation. The maximum strength (or amplitude) correlates with platelet function. Protamine would be given to reverse the effects of heparin. To differentiate between the effects of heparin administered intraoperatively and other causes of coagulopathy, two TEG samples need to be analyzed: one with, and one without, heparinase. Plasma and cryoprecipitate would be indicated for slow onset and slow formation of clotting on the TEG, respectively (prolonged R-value and diminished angle A). Aminocaproic acid is administered for states of hyperfibrinolysis. *(5:194)*

155. **(A)** The pulmonary artery is caudal to the carina. *(5:988)*

156. **(E)** The other options are indications for one-lung ventilation. In the setting of infection with purulent secretions, the goal is to avoid spillage and contamination of the contralateral lung. During surgery for bronchopleural fistula, the goal is to control the distribution of ventilation to the unaffected lung. Other procedures with high priority for one-lung ventilation include thoracic aortic aneurysm repair, pneumonectomy, upper lobectomy and video-assisted thoracoscopic surgery (VATS), however the indication is not absolute. *(5:963, 1038)*

157. **(D)** In the lateral position, lung relationships change. While there are three distinct zones as in the upright patient, these are distributed along a vertical gradient in the lateral position. Perfusion is therefore greater in the dependent lung that also receives most of the tidal ventilation. Compliance differs between the lungs because the dependent lung is at a lower FRC due to the weight of the abdominal contents and mediastinum. The dependent alveoli therefore are on the steep portion of the transpulmonary pressure-alveolar volume curve that explains their greater share of the tidal ventilation *(5:961-2)*

158. **(E)** In the patient with blunt anterior chest injury, respiratory distress, and hypotension, all of the diagnoses listed with the exception of option E must be considered. Fat embolism syndrome is more likely to affect patients with major lower extremity or pelvic fractures. *(5:1351, 1362)*

159. **(C)** Surgery should proceed with using heparin. It remains the first-line anticoagulant for patients undergoing cardiac surgery and can be readily reversed with protamine at the conclusion of surgery. The patient described in this vignette does not fit the diagnosis for HIT. The large hematoma described might explain the drop in platelets that is less than 50% from baseline. Antibody seroconversion in the absence of clinical signs does not confirm the diagnosis of HIT. The patient's surgery should not be delayed nor should alternative methods of anticoagulation be pursued. Direct thrombin inhibitors such as argatroban and bivalirudin cannot be reversed. Lower doses of heparin are not indicated, and would increase the risk of clotting within the cardiopulmonary bypass machine. *(5:900)*

160. **(E)** The most common causes for hypotension in the setting of low LVAD pump flow rates in addition to inflow cannula obstruction are options B through E. The latter is most likely in this scenario given the TEE findings as well as the low voltage ECG. Additional findings on TEE evaluation may include pericardial effusion as well as equalization of chamber pressures on pulmonary artery catheter monitoring. Graft failure is less likely based on the scenario given. *(5:925)*

161. **(A)** The use of ultrasound technology, while providing several advantages, does not completely prevent arterial injury. A thorough understanding of anatomy as well as formal training in ultrasound technique is paramount in avoiding these types of complications. *(5:411)*

162. **(D)** Depicted here is reversed or paradoxical splitting of the second heart sound that can be found in aortic stenosis, as well as LBBB. Examination findings consistent with severe AS would include parvust et tardus carotid upstrokes, a late-peaking grade 3 or greater midsystolic murmur, as soft A_2, a sustained LV apical impulse, and an S_4. *(6:1827-8)*

163. **(B)** The patient has a congenital atrial septal defect that is common in Down syndrome, often first encountered in the adult life, and more common in female patients. The associated murmur is mid-systolic in nature. *(6:1827-8, 1921)*

164. **(E)** The patient has pulmonary hypertension after pneumonectomy that will manifest as narrow splitting of S_2. Pre-existing impairment of pulmonary vascular compliance associated with CHF, and cor pulmonale may be exacerbated after extensive lung resection, leading to serious pulmonary hypertension and right-sided heart failure. *(5:954; 6:1827-8)*

165. **(I)** *(Lauer R, Mathew JP. Transesophageal tomographic views. In: Mathew JP, et al., eds., Clinical Manual and Review of Transesophageal Echocardiography, 2nd ed., New York: McGraw-Hill, 2010, Figure 5-27)*

166. **(G)** *(Lauer R, Mathew JP. Transesophageal tomographic views. In: Mathew JP, et al., eds., Clinical Manual and Review of Transesophageal*

Echocardiography, 2ⁿᵈ ed., New York: McGraw-Hill, 2010, Figure 5-20)

167. **(D)** *(Lauer R, Mathew JP. Transesophageal tomographic views. In: Mathew JP, et al., eds., Clinical Manual and Review of Transesophageal Echocardiography, 2ⁿᵈ ed., New York: McGraw-Hill, 2010, Figure 5-14)*

168. **(E)** *(Lauer R, Mathew JP. Transesophageal tomographic views. In: Mathew JP, et al., eds., Clinical Manual and Review of Transesophageal Echocardiography, 2ⁿᵈ ed., New York: McGraw-Hill, 2010, Figure 5-11)*

169. **(C)** *(Lauer R, Mathew JP. Transesophageal tomographic views. In: Mathew JP, et al., eds., Clinical Manual and Review of Transesophageal Echocardiography, 2ⁿᵈ ed., New York: McGraw-Hill, 2010, Figure 5-9)*

170. **(A)** *(Lauer R, Mathew JP. Transesophageal tomographic views. In: Mathew JP, et al., eds., Clinical Manual and Review of Transesophageal Echocardiography, 2ⁿᵈ ed., New York: McGraw-Hill, 2010, Figure 5-7)*

171. **(H)** *(Lauer R, Mathew JP. Transesophageal tomographic views. In: Mathew JP, et al., eds., Clinical Manual and Review of Transesophageal Echocardiography, 2ⁿᵈ ed., New York: McGraw-Hill, 2010, Figure 5-25)*

172. **(B)** *(Lauer R, Mathew JP. Transesophageal tomographic views. In: Mathew JP, et al., eds., Clinical Manual and Review of Transesophageal Echocardiography, 2ⁿᵈ ed., New York: McGraw-Hill, 2010, Figure 5-8)*

173. **(L)** *(Lauer R, Mathew JP. Transesophageal tomographic views. In: Mathew JP, et al., eds., Clinical Manual and Review of Transesophageal Echocardiography, 2ⁿᵈ ed., New York: McGraw-Hill, 2010, Figure 5-34)*

174. **(F)** *(Lauer R, Mathew JP. Transesophageal tomographic views. In: Mathew JP, et al., eds., Clinical Manual and Review of Transesophageal Echocardiography, 2ⁿᵈ ed., New York: McGraw-Hill, 2010, Figure 5-19)*

CHAPTER 14

Anesthesia for Neurosurgery
Questions

DIRECTIONS (Questions 175-227): Each of the numbered items or incomplete statements in this section is followed by answers or by completions of the statement. Select the ONE lettered answer or completion that is BEST in each case.

175. As the temperature of the brain decreases

    (A) MAC increases
    (B) autoregulation of blood flow is lost
    (C) cerebral metabolic rate decreases 6% to 7% per degree Celsius
    (D) cerebral Q_{10} decreases
    (E) brain oxygen extraction increases

176. Of the many factors affecting intracerebral blood flow, which one of the following is a correct description?

    (A) Vasomotor paralysis: vasoconstriction of vessels in or near ischemic areas
    (B) Autoregulation: ability of vessels to respond in a manner consistent with maintaining homeostasis
    (C) Luxury perfusion: metabolic requirements in excess of blood flow
    (D) Intracerebral steal: decrease of blood flow in normal areas with increased flow to ischemic areas
    (E) Inverse steal: diversion of flow to normal areas from ischemic areas

177. Which one of these is the best agent to decrease cerebral oxygen requirement?

    (A) A muscle relaxant
    (B) A glucose solution
    (C) An anticonvulsant

    (D) A barbiturate
    (E) Oxygen by mask

178. Use of succinylcholine to facilitate endotracheal intubation in patients with increased intracranial pressure is associated with

    (A) increased intracranial pressure
    (B) no change in intracranial pressure
    (C) incomplete muscle relaxation
    (D) conditions more satisfactory than those with the use of pancuronium
    (E) hyperkalemia

DIRECTIONS: Use the following scenario to answer Questions 179-180: A 45-year-old woman is undergoing a coil embolization procedure to obliterate a basilar tip aneurysm. She suffers from mild hypertension for which she takes hydrochlorothiazide. She is anesthetized with 2% sevoflurane in oxygen and vecuronium for muscle relaxation. The catheter approaches the aneurysm through the vertebral artery. On deploying the coil, there is a sudden increase in arterial blood pressure and global depression of ST segments detected by ECG.

179. The most likely diagnosis is

    (A) hypertensive crisis
    (B) dissection of the vertebral artery and brain stem ischemia
    (C) arterial air embolism to the posterior circulation and hind brain ischemia
    (D) pain from manipulation of the intra-arterial catheter
    (E) rupture of the aneurysm with subarachnoid hemorrhage

180. Treatment should include all of the following EXCEPT

(A) hyperventilation

(B) emergent placement of an external ventricular drainage catheter

(C) propofol bolus followed by continuous infusion

(D) immediate increase in sevoflurane concentration to reduce arterial blood pressure

(E) immediate angiography and continued placement of coils

181. In the artificially ventilated neurosurgical patient, PEEP

(A) should be used routinely

(B) should be used only on selected patients with the head of the patient never elevated

(C) has no effect on intracranial pressure

(D) should be withheld in all cases

(E) should be titrated against requirements for oxygenation and neurologic status

182. Treatment of the neurosurgical patient with mannitol may be followed by all of the following EXCEPT

(A) initial hypervolemia

(B) decreased urine volume

(C) hypovolemia

(D) decreased central venous pressure

(E) a decrease in arterial pressure

183. Nitrous oxide should be avoided in patients with

(A) brain tumor

(B) subarachnoid hemorrhage

(C) closed head injury

(D) pneumocephalus

(E) subdural hematoma

184. To obtain maximum benefit from hyperventilation during a neurosurgical procedure, the Pa_{CO_2} should be maintained at

(A) 15 to 20 mm Hg

(B) 20 to 25 mm Hg

(C) 25 to 30 mm Hg

(D) 35 to 40 mm Hg

(E) 40 to 45 mm Hg

185. Following closed head injury, systemic sequelae may include all of the following EXCEPT

(A) disseminated intravascular coagulation

(B) diabetes insipidus

(C) syndrome of inappropriate secretion of antidiuretic hormone

(D) hyperglycemia

(E) hypocarbia

186. An intraoperative "wake up" test performed during surgery on the spine

(A) assesses integrity of the dorsal spinal cord

(B) is not necessary if somatosensory evoked potentials are monitored

(C) assesses sensory function of the upper extremity

(D) is intended to assess recall

(E) can be associated with venous air embolism

187. Electroconvulsive therapy (ECT)

(A) is relatively contraindicated in patients with known cerebral or aortic aneurysms

(B) never produces a seizure

(C) is not contraindicated in patients with intracranial mass lesions

(D) does not require hemodynamic monitoring

(E) cannot be performed with muscle relaxants

188. Attention must be given to the value of intracranial pressure on induction because increased intracranial pressure may lead to

(A) herniation of brain tissue

(B) increased cerebral blood flow

(C) elevation in cerebral perfusion pressure

(D) brain retraction

(E) increased CSF volume

DIRECTIONS: Use the following scenario to answer Questions 189-192: A patient undergoing a craniotomy in the sitting position has both a radial artery and a right atrial pressure catheter in place. The external auditory canal is 26 cm above the level of the right atrium (5 cm below the manubrium). The cranium is open and the brain exposed.

189. With the arterial pressure transducers located at the level of the right atrium, the mean arterial blood pressure is 90 mm Hg and the central venous pressure is 5 mm Hg. What is the cerebral perfusion pressure?

(A) 95

(B) 85

(C) 70

(D) 59

(E) Cannot be determined directly

190. If the arterial catheter transducer were repositioned to the level of the external auditory canal, then

(A) the MAP would not require correction to measure perfusion pressure at the base of the brain

(B) the measured MAP would remain the same if the arm were not elevated

(C) the same effect could be accomplished by elevating the arm to the level of the external auditory canal

(D) CPP would equal measured MAP–CVP

(E) blood pressure determined with a cuff on the upper arm would be less than the measured pressure

191. When electronically "zeroing" the transducer system, the stopcock immediately above the transducer diaphragm is opened to air and

(A) the transducer should be positioned at the point where pressure is measured

(B) the position relative to the patient is irrelevant

(C) the transducer should be positioned at the level the catheter enters the radial artery

(D) the arm must be positioned at the level of the right atrium

(E) the transducer should be re-zeroed whenever the position is changed

192. During the procedure the arterial catheter fails; cuff pressures are monitored. Cerebral perfusion pressure

(A) cannot be determined unless the head is lowered to the level of the heart

(B) can be determined only from a cuff pressure determined at the radial artery

(C) cannot be determined unless limb with the cuff is elevated to the level head

(D) equals the systolic blood pressure determined at the brachial artery irrespective of location

(E) is determined from the mean blood pressure corrected for the difference in height where measured from the position of the external auditory canal

193. During a craniotomy, after the dura mater is opened, the intracranial pressure

(A) increases

(B) equals zero

(C) changes directly proportional to blood flow

(D) decreases only if the head is elevated

(E) is unchanged

194. Jugular venous oxygen saturation monitoring

(A) assesses global oxygen extraction from brain

(B) requires bilateral placement to fully assess the brain

(C) is unchanged during hyperventilation

(D) is highly sensitive to all cerebral ischemia

(E) is directly affected by cardiac output

DIRECTIONS: Use the following scenario to answer Questions 195-197: A 15-year-old girl had a spinal fusion with Harrington rod instrumentation. Motor and somatosensory evoked potentials were obtained throughout. On emergence, the patient was unable to move her left lower extremity.

195. The causes of this may include all of the following EXCEPT

(A) overcorrection of the scoliotic curve
(B) cord compression due to hematoma
(C) direct surgical damage to the cord
(D) hypothermia
(E) traction of the anterior spinal artery

196. The best course of action on discovery of this loss of function is

(A) extubate the trachea, begin blood transfusion
(B) observe for 24 h
(C) establish baseline neurologic function and observe for changes
(D) immediate imaging of spine by CT or MRI
(E) initiate somatosensory evoked potentials

197. Motor evoked potentials for the left lower extremity were reduced during surgery but improved with induced hypertension. The appropriate initial maneuver on discovery of the deficit would be

(A) avoid pressors that could increase vascular constriction
(B) increase mean arterial blood pressure with pressors
(C) induce hypercarbia
(D) administer mannitol
(E) administer hypertonic saline infusion

198. All of the following are complications associated with the sitting position for cervical surgery EXCEPT

(A) sciatic and cranial nerve trauma
(B) pneumocephalus
(C) quadriplegia
(D) airway edema
(E) blindness

199. The advantage of the sitting position for craniotomy is

(A) reduced intraoperative blood loss
(B) easier positioning
(C) preservation of cranial anatomy
(D) easy access to the airway
(E) hypertension

200. Hypertonic saline administered to a patient with elevated ICP

(A) may lead to hyperosmolar coma
(B) removes water from the normal brain tissue while increasing filling pressure
(C) may lead to cerebral edema if the blood–brain barrier is impaired
(D) is effective in doses of 0.25 g/kg
(E) is contraindicated in patients with renal failure

201. When administered to the neurosurgical patient, dexamethasone

(A) will reduce cerebral edema surrounding a brain tumor
(B) is effective because of its osmolar property
(C) is more effective in control of edema caused by traumatic injury
(D) is contraindicated in patients with Addison disease
(E) produces hypoglycemia

202. Administration of nitrous oxide 66% in oxygen

(A) reduces intracranial pressure
(B) depresses responsiveness of cerebral blood flow to carbon dioxide
(C) produces cerebrovascular dilatation
(D) slows EEG
(E) increases metabolic suppression produced by propofol

203. Air embolism may be a fatal complication depending upon

    (A) the site of entry
    (B) the amount of air and rate of entry
    (C) volume status
    (D) presence of a properly positioned pulmonary artery catheter
    (E) patient position

204. Concerning magnetic resonance imaging

    (A) motion artifacts are rare
    (B) objects containing ferromagnetic material are propelled within the magnetic field
    (C) routine monitoring is impossible
    (D) large prosthetic metal implants are completely contraindicated
    (E) automatic implanted cardiac defibrillators should be switched off before imaging

205. Sensitive methods to detect venous air embolism include all of the following EXCEPT

    (A) precordial Doppler
    (B) mass spectrometry
    (C) capnograph
    (D) electrocardiograph
    (E) transesophageal echocardiography

206. Concerning induced hypothermia all of the following are true EXCEPT

    (A) cerebral metabolism is decreased
    (B) cerebral vascular resistance increases
    (C) cerebral vasculature remains responsive to carbon dioxide
    (D) cerebral blood flow remains coupled to metabolism
    (E) more glucose is required by the brain for metabolism

207. If surgery is to be performed on a patient in the sitting position

    (A) the legs should be wrapped with elastic bandages
    (B) the legs should be positioned below the level of the heart
    (C) the patient can only be positioned awake
    (D) the neck should be hyperextended
    (E) the patient should be positioned as quickly as possible to avoid loss of monitors

208. Morphine as a premedication is indicated to facilitate induction in

    (A) infants
    (B) patients with increased intracranial pressure
    (C) comatose patients
    (D) very anxious patients
    (E) pulmonary hypertension

209. During a cerebral aneurysm clip obliteration, sodium nitroprusside is infused. The expected results include

    (A) short duration of action when infusion is terminated
    (B) bradycardia
    (C) alkalosis
    (D) elevated sodium thiosulfate levels
    (E) methemoglobinemia

210. When a precordial Doppler ultrasonic transducer is used to detect air embolus, it

    (A) can detect 0.5 mL of air
    (B) functions at 15 Hz
    (C) requires central venous access
    (D) is positioned over the point of maximum intensity
    (E) is less sensitive than capnography

DIRECTIONS: Use the following scenario to answer Questions 211-213: A patient with a convexity meningioma and several month history of severe headaches has a ventriculostomy for intracranial pressure monitoring in place preoperatively. Induction of general anesthesia with oxygen and nitrous oxide administered to the patient lead to an increased intracranial pressure.

211. The increase in intracranial pressure may be mitigated by administration of

(A) isoflurane
(B) vecuronium
(C) fentanyl
(D) ketamine
(E) propofol

212. The effect of agents or drugs to modify a response of increased intracranial pressure

(A) remains independent of individual and brain state
(B) is consistent across situations
(C) depends on the summation of influences on cerebrovascular tone
(D) can be determined with imaging
(E) is independent of ventilation state

213. Which one of the following will reduce the increase in intracranial pressure?

(A) Open the ventriculostomy to drain
(B) Positive pressure hypoventilation
(C) Reducing blood pressure with nitroglycerin
(D) Facilitate venous drainage
(E) Lowering the transducer from the level of the external auditory canal to the mid axillary line

214. During surgery for excision of an intradural tumor in the lower thoracic level, integrity of the spinal cord may be confirmed by

(A) performing an intraoperative "wake-up" to test motor function in lower extremities
(B) monitoring brainstem-evoked potentials

(C) monitoring somatosensory and motor evoked potentials
(D) monitoring the train-of-four on all four limbs
(E) intraoperative MRI of the spine

215. Therapy for neurogenic pulmonary edema includes all of the following EXCEPT

(A) reduce intracranial hypertension
(B) α-adrenergic antagonists
(C) supportive respiratory care
(D) central nervous system depressants
(E) naloxone 4 mg IV

216. Cervical spine instability should be considered in any patients with

(A) ankylosing spondylitis
(B) Down syndrome
(C) Marfan syndrome
(D) spinal stenosis
(E) neurofibromatosis

DIRECTIONS: Use the following scenario to answer Questions 217-219: A previously healthy 42-year-old woman is admitted to the neurological intensive care unit after suddenly losing consciousness while sitting at her desk at work. A CT scan showed a subarachnoid hemorrhage, and a cerebral angiogram revealed that the hemorrhage was due to rupture of an aneurysm of the right middle cerebral artery. Her caregivers are concerned that she may develop vasospasm.

217. Detection of cerebral vasospasm includes all of the following EXCEPT

(A) transcranial Doppler
(B) assessment of mental status
(C) jugular bulb venous oxygen saturation
(D) angiography
(E) assessment of motor function

218. Cerebral vasospasm is most likely to occur after subarachnoid hemorrhage on days

(A) 0-6
(B) 4-14
(C) 7-21

(D) 12-20

(E) up to one month

219. Endovascular treatment for cerebral vaso-spasm after subarachnoid hemorrhage includes all of the following EXCEPT

(A) intraarterial injection of mannitol

(B) angioplasty

(C) intravenous infusion of nicardipine

(D) induced hypertension

(E) intracerebral stenting

220. A patient returns to surgery to treat a CSF leak after transsphenoidal resection of the pituitary. Induction of general anesthesia should include

(A) inhalational induction with nitrous oxide and sevoflurane

(B) head down positioning to prevent CSF drainage

(C) rapid sequence endotracheal intubation

(D) placement of a ventriculostomy to prevent CSF drainage

(E) placement of an nasogastric tube to empty the stomach of blood and CSF

221. During carotid endarterectomy with EEG monitoring, both hemispheres demonstrate profound slowing of frequency and burst suppression. The anesthetic technique consists of continuous infusions of propofol and remifentanil. The most likely diagnosis is

(A) propofol overdose

(B) hypothermia

(C) hypotension

(D) inadequate perfusion to both hemispheres

(E) elevated ICP

222. Signs of venous air embolism include all of the following EXCEPT

(A) arrhythmia

(B) hypertension

(C) heart murmur

(D) bubbles at the operative site

(E) decreased end-expired carbon dioxide

DIRECTIONS (Questions 223-225): Each group of items below consists of lettered headings followed by a list of numbered phrases or statements. For each numbered phrase or statement, select the ONE lettered heading or component that is most closely associated with it. Each lettered heading or component may be selected once, more than once, or not at all.

(A) Amyotrophic lateral sclerosis

(B) Multiple sclerosis

(C) Cauda equina syndrome

(D) Guillain-Barre syndrome

(E) Myasthenia gravis

(F) Muscular dystrophy

(G) Familial periodic paralysis

(I) Myasthenic syndrome (Eaton-Lambert syndrome)

For each patient with muscle weakness, select the most likely disease process.

223. A 64-year-old woman has undergone thoracotomy for lobectomy to resect small cell carcinoma of the lung. On emergence she appears weak. She cannot maintain a sustained head lift and cannot generate sufficient tidal volumes to be extubated. Muscle relaxation had been maintained with vecuronium; there were three small twitches with fade elicited with a blockade monitor set to train-of-four before administration of neostigmine and glycopyrrolate. She reported a history of easy fatigue with exertion particularly when climbing stairs. There was no history of diplopia or dysphagia. There was no improvement with additional neostigmine.

224. A 47-year-old man has a six-month history of progressive dysarthria and dysphagia, and is presenting for a gastrostomy tube for weight loss from inadequate nutrition. He has difficulty managing oral secretions and has to sleep with the height of the bed at 45 degrees because of obstructive sleep apnea. He demonstrates no symptoms of weakness either with walking or movement of hands or arms.

225. A 27-year-old woman presents with sudden onset of loss of bowel and bladder function and weakness in both legs. She cannot stand or walk but can sit. She has an elevated white blood cell count with an abnormal smear; white blood cell differential is predominantly lymphocytes with the presence of multiple immature lymphocytes and blast cell. She is afebrile and free of pain.

DIRECTIONS (Questions 226-227): Each group of items below consists of lettered headings followed by a list of numbered phrases or statements. For each numbered phrase or statement, select the ONE lettered heading or component that is most closely associated with it. Each lettered heading or component may be selected once, more than once, or not at all.

(A) Atelectasis

(B) Pulmonary embolism

(C) Pneumothorax

(D) Patent foramen ovale

(E) Aspiration

(F) Neurogenic pulmonary edema

(G) Spinal shock

For each patient with intraoperative coughing, select the appropriate diagnosis.

226. A 65-year-old man presents for spinal decompression and bilateral foraminotomies at multiple levels for spinal stenosis extending from T8 to L4. He has been incapacitated by pain and leg weakness, and has been largely bedridden for several weeks before surgery. He has undergone uneventful awake fiberoptic intubation after topical anesthesia of the airway with lidocaine while sitting upright. He has positioned himself prone on the operating room table and moved his legs on command before induction of general anesthesia. Anesthesia is maintained with remifentanil and nitrous oxide; no muscle relaxants have been administered. During laminectomy in the thoracic region he begins to cough. He becomes hypotensive and the SaO_2 falls from 98% to 89%. Positive pressure ventilation with 100% oxygen and high inflation pressure do not improve oxygen saturation.

227. A 16-year-old otherwise healthy male is undergoing Harrington rod placement to correct scoliosis. Anesthesia consists of continuous infusions of propofol and remifentanil; no muscle relaxants have been administered since induction. Standard monitoring with noninvasive blood pressure, ECG, SaO_2, and esophageal temperature probe are applied to the patient. He is prone and both somatosensory and motor evoked potentials have been unchanged since induction. Immediately after rod placement and distraction of the spine, a motor evoked potential is performed and the patient coughs several times. During closure the surgeon notices air bubbles in the arterial circulation in the epidural space.

Answers and Explanations

175. (C) Cerebral metabolic rate decreases with a fall in temperature. This decrease is quantitated as the Q_{10}, or changes in metabolic rate for a 10°C change in temperature. While the first Q_{10} is 2.2, the second Q_{10} is about 5; the difference between the first and second Q_{10} values is thought to be due to cessation of brain electrical activity. Temperature has no effect either on autoregulation or on oxygen extraction from blood. MAC decreases with a fall in temperature. *(5:916, 1469-71; 6:166)*

176. (B) The definition of autoregulation is correct. Vasomotor paralysis involves vasodilatation. Luxury perfusion is perfusion in excess of requirements. Intracerebral steal involves blood flow away from ischemic areas. Inverse steal involves diversion of flow from normal areas to ischemic areas. *(5:871-4; 6:2255)*

177. (D) The best agent for decreasing cerebral oxygen requirement is a barbiturate. A muscle relaxant may be useful by preventing the patient from coughing and moving. Phenytoin reduces cerebral oxygen consumption caused by seizures; in the absence of seizures it has little effect on cerebral metabolic rate. *(1: 535-6; 5:876,886; 6: 2257)*

178. (A) Intracranial pressure may increase after succinylcholine. The increase is attenuated with prior administration of a small dose of a nondepolarizing muscle relaxant to prevent fasciculations. Both ventilation to reduce $PaCO_2$ and administration of thiopental reduce the rise in ICP. Increased ICP does not predispose to hyperkalemia; serum potassium will not rise above the usual 0.5 to 1.0 mEq/L. *(5:878)*

179. (E) Systemic hypertension and ECG changes often accompany cerebral aneurysm rupture and resulting intracranial hypertension. This is a dreaded complication of endovascular procedures. Dissection or occlusion of the vertebral artery can occur but is more likely during catheter placement. Arterial air embolism that occludes cerebral blood flow can occur but will not cause hypertension. Vessels are insensate but pain on manipulation is more common with dural vessels. *(5:889-93)*

180. (D) Treatment of intraprocedural rupture focuses on immediate diagnosis with angiography and obliteration of the aneurysm to stop the hemorrhage. Placement of an external ventricular drainage catheter facilitates reduction in ICP by drainage of CSF. Maneuvers to reduce ICP are appropriate including hyperventilation and propofol. Hypertension is reflexive and supports cerebral circulation during high ICP; increasing sevoflurane decreases perfusion pressure both by elevating ICP through vasodilation and reducing blood pressure. *(5:889-93)*

181. (E) Although PEEP may be necessary in the ventilation of the neurosurgical patient, its use should not be routine. The level of PEEP should be titrated to the need and effect. It is helpful to monitor intracranial pressure to ascertain possible deleterious effects. The head should be elevated. *(5:873)*

182. (B) Urinary volume will increase with mannitol administration. At first the patient may become hypervolemic both from administration of the volume of mannitol and the increase in intravascular volume from shifting of free water from the intracellular and extravascular spaces. Hypovolemia may develop after diuresis with a fall in both venous and arterial pressure. *(1: 681-2; 5:880)*

183. (D) While not an absolute contraindication to use, nitrous oxide has been reported to increase cerebral blood flow; this may be a consideration in patients with increased ICP from head injury, intracranial hemorrhage, and tumor. Since nitrous oxide diffuses into air-containing spaces, the presence of pneumocephalus is a contraindication to use because of the potential to increase ICP. *(5:878, 882)*

184. (C) The cerebral vasoconstrictive effect is diminished by reducing $PaCO_2$ below 25 mm Hg. In addition, at a $PaCO_2$ below 20 mm Hg, the effect is self-defeating with potential development of cerebral ischemia. *(5:87, 1468-9; 6:2255-7)*

185. (E) There are many systemic sequelae of closed head injury. Coagulopathy and disseminated intravascular coagulation may result from cerebral trauma, possibly from the release of brain thromboplastin into the systemic circulation. Posterior pituitary dysfunction is common and manifests as disturbances in antidiuretic hormone secretion. Hyperglycemia with nonketotic hyperosmolar coma can also occur. These patients often suffer from respiratory compromise and are hypoxemic and hypercarbic. *(5:1462-78; 6:2255-7)*

186. (E) Awakening the patient intraoperatively is a means to assess motor function in the lower and occasionally upper extremities after distraction of the vertebral column in spine surgery. Compromise of blood supply may occur from surgical manipulation or straightening of the cord. The use of somatosensory-evoked potentials assesses only sensory function, primarily a dorsal spinal cord function, and does not rule out a motor deficit, primarily a ventral cord function. Negative inspiratory force generated during spontaneous ventilation can cause the common problem of venous air embolism. *(5:489)*

187. (A) In order to be effective in treating depression, electroconvulsive therapy must induce a seizure. Because of the rapid and unpredictable changes in blood pressure accompanying the seizure, patients with aneurysms may not be candidates for this therapeutic modality. In addition, the increases in cerebral metabolic activity and concomitant rise in blood flow can increase ICP and, therefore, may cause cerebral herniation in patients with decreased intracranial compliance from mass-occupying lesions. Therefore, these conditions represent relative contraindications to ECT. *(1:266; 5:1267-8)*

188. (A) If intracranial pressure increases on induction, global or areas of focal ischemia may occur from herniation and/or decreased perfusion pressure. Brain retraction may cause ischemia during surgery. Hydrocephalus is a cause of increased ICP, not a consequence. *(5:871-3; 6:2255-7)*

189. (C) The cerebral perfusion pressure is mean arterial blood pressure less the intracranial pressure (MAP – ICP). In this case the ICP is 0 since the cranium is open. Since the MAP is measured at the level of the right atrium, the pressure would be less at the circle of Willis (located at the level of the external auditory canal) because the head is elevated. Thus the MAP at the base of the brain would be 70 mm Hg; 90 mm Hg − (26 cm ÷ 1.3 mm Hg/cm) in order to correct for the height. *(5:406-9, 882-3)*

190. (A) With the transducers positioned at the level of the circle of Willis, the measured pressure is the arterial pressure at the base of the brain. Position of the arm containing the arterial catheter with respect to the transducer will not alter the value of the measured pressure. Arterial pressure of any structure below the level of the transducer will be higher than the measured value. *(5:406-9, 882-3)*

191. **(B)** Electronic zeroing merely sets a pressure of 0 mm Hg to the electrical output of the transducer when the zeroing maneuver is performed. Opening the stopcock to ambient pressure (air pressure) exerts a pressure on the transducer diaphragm equal to the height of the column of fluid between the opened stopcock and the diaphragm. By convention, the stopcock opened is the one directly above the diaphragm and the column height is 1–2 cm. The position of the transducer relative to the patient will not affect the electronic zero and is irrelevant to the procedure (opening the stopcock disconnects the patient from the system). Once the electronic zero is established, there is no need to re-zero the instrument unless to correct for electronic drift that can occur with time. *(5:406-9, 882-3)*

192. **(E)** Arterial blood pressure can be determined by cuff from any location. Cerebral perfusion pressure is calculated from the mean pressure corrected for the difference in height from where measured to the external auditory canal by the equation given in the explanation to Question 189 *(5:406)*

193. **(B)** Once the skull is open and the dura mater incised, the brain is no longer confined within the cranium, and intracranial pressure is zero. *(5:871-3)*

194. **(A)** Jugular bulb venous oximetry detects changes in brain oxygen extraction from blood. The catheter is positioned retrograde in a single jugular bulb and reflects venous drainage from predominantly a single hemisphere; if positioned extracranially, contamination with noncerebral venous blood dilutes effectiveness as a monitor. Changes in oxygen delivery, either from content or blood flow, are reflected in the percent saturation of the draining venous blood. Focal ischemia may not be detected. Cardiac output, unless in extreme shock, has no effect. *(5:875)*

195. **(D)** Hypothermia is a systemic effect and would not present as a focal deficit. The deficit described may be the result of any of the other

situations. Peripheral nerve damage is an unusual complication. *(5:484-9, 1200-1)*

196. **(D)** If the patient awakens with a deficit that cannot be explained either immediate imaging or exploration of the surgical site is indicated for potential cord compression from a hematoma. The patient should be left intubated pending a decision to facilitate speed of reoperation. Somatosensory evoked potentials do not provide motor information. *(5:484-9, 1200-1)*

197. **(B)** Traction on the anterior spinal artery produced by straightening of the spine can cause ischemia in selected regions of the spinal cord. Induced hypertension may improve perfusion. Systemically administered pressors do not cause vasoconstriction in the central nervous system. Edema treated with mannitol or hypertonic saline is an unlikely cause of inadequate perfusion in this setting. *(5:484-9, 1200-1)*

198. **(E)** Blindness is a rare complication of the prone position; the etiology is obscure but may involve increased intraocular pressure. With the sitting position, the sciatic nerve is at risk for compression from inadequate padding or traction injury from improper positioning. Traction of cranial nerves, especially the abducens (VI), can result from caudal displacement of the brain. Air trapped over the superior surface of the brain produces pneumocephalus. Quadriplegia has been reported due to cord compression from extreme flexion of the neck. Similarly, airway edema can occur from obstruction of venous drainage. *(5:896)*

199. **(A)** Intraoperative blood loss is reduced in the sitting position due to increased venous drainage. The positioning is more difficult than with a supine position and access to the patient and airway is limited. Hypotension is frequently a complication. Anatomy is not preserved and cranial nerve traction is a problem. *(5:365-6)*

200. **(B)** Hypertonic saline effectively reduces ICP by removing water from normal tissues. It may be administered in the setting of renal failure. Unlike mannitol there is no potential

for hyperosmolar coma if given in large doses and does not cause cerebral edema by diffusing intracellularly if the blood–brain barrier is impaired. Mannitol is effective in doses as low as 0.25 g/kg. *(5:174, 511, 537; 6:2256-8, 2271)*

201.   **(A)** Dexamethasone is effective in the treatment of cerebral edema in patients with brain tumors. It has been shown to be less effective in the patient with brain injury from acute closed head trauma. The mechanism is probably from a decrease in inflammatory processes caused by the tumor. There is no contraindication in Addison disease. Hyperglycemia is a commons side effect. *(1:1232; 5:881; 1126-7; 6:2256-8, 2271)*

202.   **(C)** Induction of anesthesia with nitrous oxide as the sole agent has been shown to increase cerebral blood flow and intracranial pressure. Although nitrous oxide produces cerebrovascular dilatation, the cerebral blood flow response to carbon dioxide is preserved. These effects on cerebral hemodynamics are altered by the addition of other anesthetic agents; barbiturates and benzodiazepines blunt the increase in intracranial pressure. *(1:546-7; 5:873-4)*

203.   **(B)** Both the amount and rate of entry of air are important factors in determining consequences of venous air embolism. The site of entry is unimportant. Although a pulmonary artery catheter may be useful for monitoring, the port is too small to be helpful in the withdrawal of air. Volume status has no effect on severity of response. While some positions increase likelihood of embolism, patient position during entrainment does not impact outcome. *(5:881-2)*

204.   **(B)** All ferromagnetic material can create artifacts in the image and can be drawn into the magnetic field. While some metal implants may shift position in the field and heat during scanning, some implants are safe for imaging. The patient must remain motionless for several minutes during scanning; movement artifacts from breathing and arterial pulsation are common. Pacemakers and AICD's remain contraindicated for imaging. *(5:896-7)*

205.   **(D)** Arrhythmias and cardiovascular collapse are late signs of venous air embolism. The precordial Doppler in conjunction with a capnograph or pulmonary artery catheter will usually detect air before physiologic consequences occur. *(5:881-2)*

206.   **(E)** During hypothermia, the brain requires less glucose and oxygen because of reduced metabolic demand. Cerebral blood flow remains coupled to metabolism and decreases; cerebral vascular resistance increases. Responsiveness to changes in $PaCO_2$ is unchanged. *(5:1469-71; 6:2258-9)*

207.   **(B)** Positioning the patient in the sitting position requires planning and is performed after induction of anesthesia. In order to minimize venous pooling in the lower extremities, a potential cause of hypotension, the legs should be wrapped and positioned level with the heart. The head should never be hyperextended. Positioning should be done slowly to avoid hypotension. *(5:365-6, 881-3)*

208.   **(D)** Morphine as a sedating premedication is useful in anxious patients but can depress ventilation. It is contraindicated in the very young, patients with increased intracranial pressure, and comatose patients. *(1: 501-2; 5:703-5, 709-10, 713)*

209.   **(A)** Sodium nitroprusside has a short duration of action. It may cause an acidemia and is usually associated with tachycardia. Cyanide toxicity may also occur; intravenous sodium thiosulfate is the antidote. *(1:782-3; 6:1913; 5:746-7)*

210.   **(A)** Precordial Doppler is one of the most sensitive monitors of venous air embolism clinically available and can detect air in quantities as small as 0.5 mL. The ultrasonic probe, which functions at 2.0 MHz, is placed over the right side of the heart. Central venous access can be used to withdraw entrained air from the right atrium; it is not required for monitoring. *(5:874-5)*

211. **(E)** Propofol may block increases in intracranial pressure produced by nitrous oxide. Isoflurane and ketamine are potent cerebral vasodilators and increase intracranial pressure. Vecuronium will have no effect on ICP. Opioids increase ICP by depressing ventilation. *(1: 536-7; 5:875-8)*

212. **(C)** Drug effects on intracranial pressure are not constant but vary among individuals, with ventilation, and the state of the brain at the time applied. The total effect on cerebrovascular tone will determine the effect on cerebral blood volume and intracranial pressure. Imaging does not predict ICP. *(5:871-3, 875-8; 6:2255-7)*

213. **(A)** ICP can be lowered by opening the ventriculostomy to remove some CSF. While hyperventilation may reduce ICP, simple mechanical ventilation without a change in Pa_{CO_2} will have no effect. Nitroglycerin is a vasodilator and increases ICP. Moving the transducer will only change the value but the ICP remains the same. ICP is measured with the transducer at the level of the external auditory canal. Obstructing venous drainage increases ICP but simple facilitating drainage will not overcome the increase produced by nitrous oxide. *(5:871-3; 6:2255-7)*

214. **(C)** An intraoperative wake-up test demonstrates upper and lower limb movement on command and assures integrity of the ventral spinal cord containing the corticospinal tracts. Monitoring of somatosensory-evoked potentials tests the integrity of the dorsal portion of the spinal cord, whereas motor evoked potential monitoring detects integrity of corticospinal tracts. Brain stem-evoked potentials are useful on intracranial procedures involving the posterior fossa but have no values for monitoring spinal cord function. The train-of-four monitor only evaluates the function of a peripheral nerve and the neuromuscular junction. Intraoperative MRI is time consuming and images may not detect ischemic damage. *(5:490)*

215. **(E)** Neurogenic pulmonary edema is thought to involve massive sympathetic discharge from injured brain in response to intracranial hypertension. It is treated by both reduction of intracranial pressure and supportive care to maximize oxygenation. Naloxone in high doses can produce pulmonary edema. *(5: 886; 6: 3359)*

216. **(B)** Patients with Down syndrome and rheumatoid arthritis are at high risk for atlantoaxial instability. Patients with ankylosing spondylitis may have their cervical vertebrae fused in flexion. Such patients may develop cervical spine instability after attempts to extend the neck during intubation. Neurofibromatosis may present as schwannoma within the spinal canal but does not produce cervical instability. *(5: 137-47, 895, 1201; 6: 135)*

217. **(C)** Cerebral vasospasm is segmental narrowing of the cerebral vessels most commonly the large conduit vessels at the base of the brain. Extreme spasm may impair blood flow and cause ischemia. The presence of spasm can be monitored by transcranial Doppler to detect increased blood flow velocity and neurological exam for mental status and motor function. Cerebral angiography detects loss of vessel caliber. Jugular bulb venous oxygen saturation is too insensitive to detect small regions of ischemia. *(5:889-90)*

218. **(B)** Cerebral vasospasm occurs most commonly on days 4 through 14 after subarachnoid hemorrhage with a peak on day 7. *(5:885-7; 6:2204, 2263)*

219. **(E)** Endovascular treatment of cerebral vasospasm after subarachnoid hemorrhage typically involves angioplasty of the stenotic segments or intraarterial injection of vasodilators including papaverine or calcium channel antagonists verapamil or nicardipine. Intraarterial mannitol is used to treat larger vessel spasm during angiography. Intracerebral vessel stenting is unnecessary to restore flow. *(1:757-60; 5:889-90)*

220. **(C)** Active drainage of CSF indicates an open conduit from the nose to the sella turcica. Positive pressure ventilation carries the risk of

passage of gas into the cranium and should be avoided. Nitrous oxide is avoided because of the risk of expanding a pneumocephalus often accompanying a CSF leak. Drainage of the CSF with a ventriculostomy does not correct these issues. A nasogastric tube will obscure the surgical field and carries the potential for passage into the cranial cavity. *(5:884-5)*

221. **(A)** Burst suppression on EEG is produced most commonly by excessive doses of hypnotic medications including propofol, barbiturates, isoflurane, or etomidate. Hypothermia or hypotension resulting in inadequate brain perfusion produce slowing of the EEG or electrical silence. Similarly, elevated ICP could compromise cerebral perfusion and slow the EEG. *(1:333-46; 5:479, 611, 694, 696-8, 710)*

222. **(B)** Air embolism is associated with arrhythmia, heart murmur (when there is a large amount of air), bubbles at the operative site, and decreased end-tidal CO_2. Hypotension occurs after a large volume of air is entrained. *(5:881-2)*

223. **(I)** Myasthenic syndrome is associated with neoplasms including small cell carcinoma of the lung. Administration of neostigmine rarely results in improvement of symptoms. The proximal muscle groups are more commonly affected, while bulbar symptoms from cranial nerve involvement are rare. *(1:234; 5:958; 6:3482-3)*

224. **(A)** Amyotrophic lateral sclerosis can present with predominantly bulbar symptoms of dysarthria and dysphagia while muscle strength in the extremities may be preserved. Collapse of the pharyngeal muscular during sleep is common, as well as difficulty handling secretions. *(5:139-40; 6:3345-7)*

225. **(C)** Cauda equina syndrome is caused by compression of the spinal nerves below the termination of the cord. It can be produced by many different etiologies including lymphoma. Bowel and bladder symptoms are common. *(5:1156; 6:2269)*

226. **(B)** Coughing, even during general anesthesia, may be associated with pulmonary embolism. Inactivity associated with lower extremity weakness and back pain predisposes to deep vein thrombosis. *(5:1257, 1288-9; 6: 104-5, 2170-7)*

227. **(D)** During surgery in the prone position the wound is above the heart and negative intrathoracic pressure predisposes to venous air embolism. Exposure of the trabecular bone during instrumentation of the spine generates a route for the entrainment of air. Coughing or strong inspiration during light anesthesia may produce negative intrathoracic pressure. The presence of air within the arterial system indicated a paradoxical embolism via a patent foramen ovale. *(5:881-2; 6: 3275)*

CHAPTER 15

Obstetric Anesthesia
Questions

DIRECTIONS (Questions 228-309): Each of the numbered items or incomplete statements in this section is followed by answers or by completions of the statement. Select the ONE lettered answer or completion that is BEST in each case.

228. A parturient presents to labor and delivery complaining of decreased fetal movement at 34 weeks gestational age. The most likely next step to evaluate the well-being of the fetus is to perform a(n)

   (A) oxytocin contraction test (OCT)
   (B) biophysical profile (BPP)
   (C) non-stress test (NST)
   (D) umbilical artery Doppler flow study
   (E) fetal scalp pH analysis

229. You receive a page for an emergent cesarean section in a 27-year-old parturient in labor with a functioning epidural for fetal distress. You rush to the bedside, and after aspirating the epidural catheter, inject which one of the following agents or combination of agents while accompanying the patient to the operating room?

   (A) 2% lidocaine with 1:200,000 epinephrine
   (B) 3% 2-chloroprocaine
   (C) 2% lidocaine with 1:200,000 epinephrine and bicarbonate

   (D) 0.5% bupivacaine with bicarbonate
   (E) 3% 2-chloroprocaine with sodium bicarbonate

230. Absolute contraindications to major conduction anesthesia in parturients include all of the following conditions EXCEPT

   (A) preexisting neurologic disease of the spinal cord
   (B) patient refusal
   (C) infection at the site of needle insertion
   (D) hypovolemic shock
   (E) severe coagulopathy

231. As compared with regional anesthesia for cesarean section, general anesthesia results in a/an/the

   (A) approximately 17-fold increased risk of maternal death
   (B) higher incidence of maternal hypotension
   (C) approximately twofold increased risk of maternal death
   (D) majority of recent maternal deaths related to failed intubation rather than in the postoperative period
   (E) lower incidence of uterine atony

232. A 30-year-old G1P1 patient underwent an emergent cesarean section under epidural anesthesia. She received 4 mg epidural morphine for pain control prior to removal of the catheter. Four hours postpartum she begins to complain of incisional pain. The most likely explanation for this is

(A) the dose of morphine is insufficient for epidural administration

(B) morphine has a high lipid solubility resulting in an expected analgesic period of 1-4 h

(C) 2-chloroprocaine was used for the urgent cesarean section

(D) 2% lidocaine with bicarbonate was used for the urgent cesarean section

(E) she received nalbuphine for relief of pruritus

233. You receive a phone call from an obstetrician who has just seen a patient with von Willebrand disease (vWD) for her first prenatal visit. He inquires as to the anesthetic-related implications of the patient's disease during pregnancy and the use of neuraxial anesthesia in this patient. All of the following responses are true of vWD EXCEPT

(A) vWD is the most common inherited coagulopathy and affects 1-2% of the general population

(B) evidence-based recommendations for neuraxial anesthesia in the setting of vWD can be made

(C) specific treatment strategies may be determined in consultation with a hematologist

(D) the treatment of vWD depends on its severity and subtype

(E) vWD is not necessarily a contraindication to neuraxial anesthesia

DIRECTIONS: Use the following scenario to answer Questions 234–236: A 26-year-old G1P0 patient presents to the labor and delivery department at 35 weeks gestational age complaining of a headache and scotomata. Her blood pressure is 150/100, pulse is 84, and her oxygen saturation is 100% breathing room air. Physical examination reveals marked facial edema and a Mallampati 4 airway. Her cervix is 2 cm dilated. Laboratory values include a platelet count of $90,000/mm^3$, a 24-hour urine specimen containing more than 5 g of protein, and normal liver function tests. Physical examination reveals epigastric pain.

234. All of the following are consistent with a diagnosis of severe preeclampsia EXCEPT

(A) platelet count of $90,000/mm^3$

(B) headache

(C) scotomata

(D) diastolic blood pressure of 100 mm Hg

(E) epigastric pain

235. The obstetrician begins an infusion of magnesium sulfate and decides to induce labor in the patient given her diagnosis of severe preeclampsia. She then calls you to request an epidural. You inform the obstetrician that

(A) severe preeclampsia is a contraindication to epidural placement

(B) the platelet count is an absolute contraindication to the placement of an epidural

(C) the epidural should be placed later in active labor after a repeat platelet count is obtained

(D) you will obtain informed consent and place an epidural

(E) the patient should receive a spinal to reduce the risk of hematoma

236. The most common cause of mortality in a patient like this one is

(A) cardiac arrest

(B) renal failure

(C) hepatic rupture

(D) respiratory arrest after inability to intubate

(E) cerebrovascular accident

237. A 26-year-old G2P0 patient requests an epidural. The epidural placement is uneventful. Twenty minutes later you are called to the labor room because the patient is complaining of

shortness of breath and is still in pain. A quick sensory exam reveals a much higher level on the right side of the patient with a patchy sensory block. There is no fetal distress and the patient is oxygenating well. Your next step in the management of this patient should be to

(A) pull the catheter back 1 cm and administer another bolus of local anesthetic solution

(B) stop the epidural infusion, observe the patient, and administer another bolus of local anesthetic solution when the sensory level recedes

(C) stop the epidural infusion, observe the patient, replace the epidural catheter, and administer another bolus of local anesthetic solution once the level has receded.

(D) intubate the patient and provide supportive measures

(E) administer a bolus of fentanyl through the epidural catheter to enhance the block

238. You are called by an obstetrician to see an HIV-positive patient on her first postpartum day. She underwent an uneventful vaginal delivery under epidural anesthesia. She is now complaining of a positional headache and neck stiffness. You have a discussion about an epidural blood patch (EBP). You tell her

(A) given her HIV status an EBP is contraindicated and you recommend conservative treatment

(B) an EBP has a success rate of approximately 70% after the first attempt

(C) if she were to have a wet tap in the future, evidence-based medicine supports the placement of a prophylactic EBP

(D) severe complications of EBP are rare and may include transient bradycardia, facial palsy, and arachnoiditis.

(E) the absence of a documented wet tap makes the diagnosis of postdural puncture headache (PDPH) unlikely in this patient

239. Regarding placental physiology, which one of the following drugs crosses the placenta in appreciable amounts?

(A) Atropine

(B) Glycopyrrolate

(C) Succinylcholine

(D) Vecuronium

(E) Heparin

DIRECTIONS: Use the following scenario to answer Questions 240-241: An 18-year-old G2P1 patient presents for repeat cesarean section. She is 59 inches tall and underwent a previously uneventful primary cesarean section. Shortly after the administration of spinal anesthesia, the patient begins to complain of shortness of breath. Her blood pressure is 80/40 and her heart rate is 48 bpm. The patient tells you she is nauseated, short of breath, and her hands are tingling.

240. Initial management of this patient should include all of the following EXCEPT

(A) administration of ephedrine

(B) asking the patient to squeeze your hands with hers

(C) IV fluid bolus administration

(D) supplemental administration of oxygen

(E) placing the patient in the Trendelenburg position

241. Within a few minutes the patient becomes unresponsive, profoundly hypotensive, and apneic. Appropriate management would include all of the following EXCEPT

(A) positive pressure ventilation via endotracheal intubation

(B) left uterine displacement

(C) support of maternal circulation with IV fluids and ephedrine

(D) administration of 100% oxygen

(E) prompt administration of epinephrine to support maternal circulation

242. A 32-year-old G1P0 patient presents to the labor and delivery department in early labor. Her prenatal course is unremarkable except for a history of multiple sclerosis (MS). True statements regarding her care include all of the following EXCEPT

(A) an increase in body temperature of as little as 0.5°C can result in an exacerbation or relapse

(B) exaggerated responses to inhaled anesthetics can occur due to autonomic dysfunction

(C) pregnancy is associated with an improvement in symptoms, but relapse can occur postpartum

(D) epidural anesthesia is associated with greater risk of relapse than spinal anesthesia

(E) a hyperkalemic response to succinylcholine can be seen in patients with significant muscle atrophy

243. A 30-year-old G2P1 female presents for a repeat cesarean section at 40 weeks gestational age. Her prenatal course is complicated by recurrent pregnancy loss and she is positive for the lupus anticoagulant. She has been on unfractionated heparin 10,000 units subcutaneously twice a day throughout her third trimester. Her last dose was last evening (twelve hours ago). True statements regarding her care include

(A) regional anesthesia is safe and no further testing is necessary

(B) regional anesthesia is contraindicated in this patient

(C) a general anesthetic is indicated

(D) a partial thromboplastin time and platelet count should be obtained prior to performing a regional anesthetic

(E) the peak effect of subcutaneous heparin is 4 h after subcutaneous injection

DIRECTIONS: Use the following scenario to answer Questions 244-245: A 27-year-old G2P1 female presents with a history of profound depression at 34 weeks gestational age. She had a recent suicide attempt and her psychiatrist now recommends

electroconvulsive therapy (ECT). You are asked to counsel the patient regarding the use of ECT in pregnancy.

244. Which one of the following statements is true about ECT during pregnancy?

(A) The American Psychiatric Association recommends that ECT be deferred until the third trimester of pregnancy.

(B) Most of the psychotropic medicines have a long history of safe use in pregnancy.

(C) The overall incidence of miscarriage is higher with the use of ECT than in the general population.

(D) Your recommendation to the patient can be based on prospective, randomized controlled trials.

(E) The anesthetic agents used for ECT have a long history of safe use in pregnancy.

245. Appropriate measures for parturients undergoing ECT would include all of the following EXCEPT

(A) preoperative obstetric consultation

(B) monitoring of the fetal heart rate before and after ECT

(C) endotracheal intubation

(D) monitoring of uterine contractions after ECT

(E) left uterine displacement after 14 weeks gestational age

246. All of the following drugs may cause worsening of myasthenic symptoms EXCEPT

(A) oxytocin

(B) aminoglycoside antibiotics

(C) magnesium sulfate

(D) terbutaline

(E) carboprost tromethamine

247. A 27-year-old G2P1 female presents to you for consultation regarding a vaginal birth after cesarean section (VBAC). Her first cesarean was a low transverse incision for breech presentation. You tell her that

(A) VBAC is successful in less than half of patients in whom a low-transverse cesarean section was made during previous cesarean delivery

(B) epidural analgesia does not delay the diagnosis of uterine rupture

(C) epidural analgesia decreases the likelihood of successful VBAC

(D) the risk of uterine rupture is approximately 2%

(E) according to the American College of Obstetricians and Gynecologists (ACOG), anesthesia providers must be available within 30 min to provide emergency care for patients attempting VBAC

248. Which one of the following is the most common cause of severe postpartum hemorrhage?

(A) Lacerations

(B) Retained placental tissue

(C) Coagulopathy

(D) Uterine atony

(E) Uterine inversion

249. A 38-year-old G0 patient opts for in vitro fertilization (IVF). She has undergone hormonal stimulation and is about to receive human chorionic gonadotropin (hCG) to induce oocyte maturation. She will present for transvaginal egg retrieval 36 h after administration of human chorionic gonadotropin (hCG). Which one of these anesthetic considerations is true?

(A) She will not need to fast if she is given conscious sedation.

(B) Paracervical block may be used as the sole anesthetic.

(C) Conscious sedation is the most commonly utilized anesthetic technique.

(D) Adding 10 mcg of fentanyl to intrathecal lidocaine solution improves postoperative analgesia but increases time to ambulation and discharge.

(E) General anesthesia decreases the successful fertilization rate of the retrieved oocytes.

DIRECTIONS: Use the following scenario to answer Questions 250-251: A 38-year-old G1P0 female at 39 weeks gestational age is being induced for pre-eclampsia. She is given a 4-g bolus of magnesium sulfate followed by an intravenous infusion at 2 g/h.

250. Which one of the following statements regarding the use of magnesium sulfate in this patient is true?

(A) Magnesium sulfate is eliminated primarily through the liver.

(B) Patellar reflexes are lost at serum magnesium levels of approximately 2 mg/dL.

(C) Magnesium sulfate may antagonize the effects of neuromuscular blocking agents.

(D) Therapeutic blood concentrations are 4-8 mg/dL.

(E) Magnesium sulfate does not cross the placenta.

251. The patient undergoes an uneventful delivery and is sent to the postpartum floor on an infusion of magnesium sulfate for twenty-four hours. A nurse discovers the patient is having breathing difficulty and you are paged stat to the room. Upon arrival, you note that the patient is lethargic. Her blood pressure is 110/60, heart rate is 70, and she is in severe respiratory distress. Management of this patient would include all of the following EXCEPT

(A) administration of epinephrine 1 mg intravenously

(B) support of respiration with bag-mask and possible endotracheal intubation

(C) discontinuing the infusion of magnesium sulfate

(D) administration of calcium gluconate 1 g intravenously

(E) obtaining a serum magnesium level

252. A 30-year-old G1P0 patient presents for antenatal counseling regarding her history of a malignant hyperthermia (MH) episode. Which one of the following recommendations is true?

(A) MH is inherited in an autosomal recessive fashion.

(B) There is a 25% chance that the fetus will be MH-susceptible.

(C) Ester, but not amide, local anesthetic agents are safe in MH-susceptible patients.

(D) Her child will need to be treated with non-triggering anesthetics in the future unless the child undergoes caffeine-halothane contracture testing and the testing is negative.

(E) Once labor begins, she will be given prophylactic dantrolene that does not cross the placenta.

253. An infant with a heart rate of 70, a weak cry, minimal muscle flexion, a grimace to oropharyngeal suctioning and acrocyanosis at five minutes would receive an Apgar score of

(A) 2

(B) 4

(C) 5

(D) 6

(E) 7

DIRECTIONS: Use the following scenario to answer Questions 254-255: You are called to the trauma room where you encounter a 31-year-old G2P1 patient at 34 weeks estimated gestational age. She was involved in a motor vehicle accident and has suffered multiple injuries. She is actively being resuscitated. Fetal heart tones are present. Shortly after your arrival, the patient goes into cardiac arrest during the resuscitation. The obstetrical team is present in the trauma room.

254. All of the following statements regarding the resuscitation of this patient are true EXCEPT

(A) left uterine displacement should be maintained during the resuscitation

(B) chest compressions should be performed slightly above the center of the sternum

(C) cardioversion has been used in all stages of pregnancy without significant complications

(D) vasopressor agents may decrease blood flow to the uterus

(E) standard ACLS drug dosages should be adjusted upward for pregnant patients

255. It has been four minutes since resuscitative measures were instituted. The patient remains asystolic. You should now consider

(A) administering a biphasic shock of 200 J

(B) administering a monophasic shock of 360 J

(C) asking the obstetrician to perform a perimortem cesarean section

(D) administering a second dose of vasopressin

(E) calling the code

256. Well known gastrointestinal changes that occur during pregnancy include all of the following EXCEPT

(A) the combination of esophageal displacement into the thorax and progestin result in a lowering of the lower esophageal sphincter tone

(B) gastric emptying of liquid and solid materials is not altered during pregnancy

(C) a higher risk of gallbladder disease secondary to biliary stasis and an increased secretion of bile

(D) gastric emptying is slowed during labor

(E) epidural anesthesia using local anesthetics only delays gastric emptying

257. The most reliable means of detecting uterine rupture in this patient is

(A) maternal tachycardia

(B) uterine tenderness

(C) severe hemorrhage

(D) a non-reassuring fetal heart rate pattern

(E) maternal complaint of pain during labor

258. Regarding placental transfer of drugs, which one of the following favors increased maternal to fetal drug transfer?

(A) Molecular weight less than 1,000 Daltons
(B) Hydrophilic substance
(C) Charged substance
(D) High bound drug fraction
(E) Lower portion of unionized drug in maternal plasma

259. In order for an epidural to relieve the second stage of labor, the epidural must cover which one of these dermatomes?

(A) T10-L1
(B) T11-T12
(C) L2-L4
(D) L3-L5
(E) S2-S4

260. Well known endocrine changes that occur during pregnancy include all of the following EXCEPT

(A) the thyroid gland enlarges during pregnancy
(B) estrogen induces an increase in thyroid-binding globulin which results in a relative hyperthyroid state during pregnancy
(C) free T3 and free T4 concentrations remain unchanged
(D) pregnant patients are insulin resistant primarily due to placental production of lactogen
(E) cortisol levels are increased during pregnancy

DIRECTIONS: Use the following figure to answer Question 261:

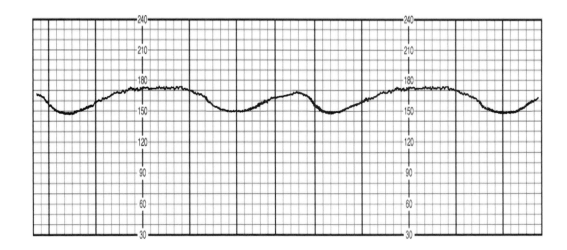

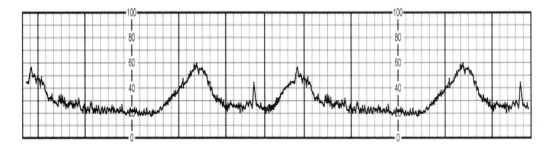

261. You are finishing a routine preoperative evaluation on a patient for an elective repeat cesarean section in the antepartum assessment area when you view the following fetal heart tracing on a patient in the next room who is being assessed for decreased fetal movement at 36 weeks. She is contracting spontaneously. This is an example of

    (A) early decelerations
    (B) a reactive non-stress test
    (C) variable decelerations
    (D) fetal bradycardia
    (E) a positive oxytocin contraction test (OCT)

262. A variety of physiologic changes in uteroplacental blood flow occur during pregnancy and include which one of the following characteristics?

    (A) The uterus accounts for roughly 12% of the cardiac output at term.
    (B) Uteroplacental blood flow is widely autoregulated during pregnancy.
    (C) Uterine blood flow increases dramatically to approximately 200 to 300 mL/min at term.
    (D) The main supply of blood to the uterus is from the uterine arteries that arise from the aorta.
    (E) General anesthetic doses typically used decrease uterine blood flow.

263. A 27-year-old G2P1 female presents for anesthetic consultation at 16 weeks gestational age. Her prenatal course is significant for a history of mild mitral stenosis (MS). She is currently asymptomatic (NYHA Class 1 disease). You tell her that all of the following statements about her condition are true EXCEPT

    (A) approximately 25% of patients with mitral stenosis first experience symptoms during pregnancy
    (B) mitral stenosis is the most commonly encountered valvular lesion in pregnancy

    (C) epidural anesthesia is preferred for vaginal or cesarean delivery
    (D) ephedrine is the pressor of choice to treat hypotension
    (E) maternal expulsive efforts during the second stage of labor are discouraged

264. Which one of the following statements concerning the management of a parturient with an unanticipated difficult airway is consistent with the ASA difficult airway algorithm?

    (A) In an elective cesarean section, proceed under mask ventilation if the patient has had nothing by mouth.
    (B) Never attempt blind nasal intubation because of the risk of bleeding from engorged airways.
    (C) If able to ventilate with mask and the fetus is in serious distress, no additional steps should be taken to obtain a secure airway and delivery should proceed immediately.
    (D) Never attempt cricothyrotomy in a pre-eclamptic patient because of potential coagulopathy.
    (E) If unable to ventilate or intubate, attempt to place an LMA with cricoid pressure and if successful consider proceeding to cesarean section in the presence of fetal distress.

265. Which one of the following changes in lab values is expected during pregnancy?

    (A) Decreased hematocrit
    (B) Increased P_{CO_2}
    (C) Increased pH
    (D) Increased creatinine
    (E) Decreased factors VII, VIII, X, and fibrinogen

266. Nonobstetric surgery during pregnancy occurs with an estimated frequency of 0.3% to 2.2%. Anesthetic concerns regarding nonobstetric surgery during pregnancy include all of the following EXCEPT

(A) rapid sequence induction should be performed after 16 weeks gestational age when general anesthesia is required

(B) regional anesthesia, when appropriate, is a reasonable alternative

(C) aspiration prophylaxis should be accomplished with either a nonparticulate antacid and/or a histamine H_2 antagonist combined with a gastric prokinetic agent

(D) benzodiazepines are contraindicated due to the increased incidence of cleft palate

(E) left uterine displacement for the prevention of aortocaval compression is not necessary in the first trimester

DIRECTIONS: Use the following photograph to answer Questions 267-268:

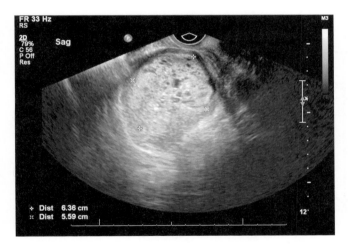

A 27-year-old patient presents at ten weeks gestation with abnormal uterine bleeding, hyperemesis, and bilaterally enlarged ovarian cysts. On exam her uterus is greater than expected size and her beta-hCG is markedly elevated (100,000 mIU/mL). An ultrasound is obtained and is shown above.

267. The most likely diagnosis in this patient is

(A) ectopic pregnancy

(B) incomplete spontaneous abortion

(C) twin gestation

(D) molar pregnancy

(E) septic abortion

268. Proper anesthetic management of this patient would include all of the following EXCEPT

(A) blood products should be immediately available

(B) two large bore intravenous catheters should be placed

(C) an intravenous infusion of oxytocin should be started after evacuation of the uterus has been completed

(D) close observation of the patient post procedure for evidence of hemorrhage or cardiopulmonary distress

(E) general anesthesia is preferred

269. A parturient is diagnosed with retained placenta after delivery and requires manual exploration of the uterus. All of the following are acceptable management strategies EXCEPT

(A) intravenous analgesia

(B) epidural analgesia

(C) saddle block

(D) intravenous nitroglycerine, 400 mcg

(E) induction of general anesthesia with 1 mg/kg ketamine

DIRECTIONS: Use the following figure to answer Questions 270-271:

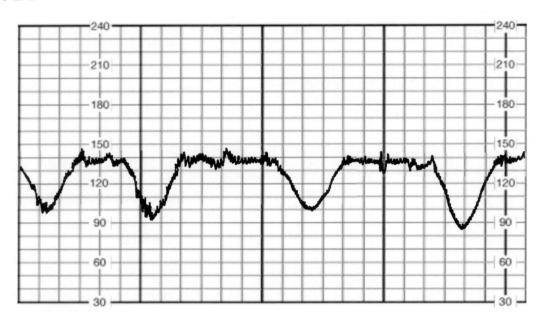

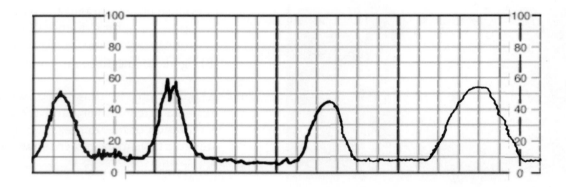

270. The tracing in the graph shows a pattern referred to as

(A) late deceleration
(B) variable deceleration
(C) early deceleration
(D) maximal deceleration
(E) late acceleration

271. The type of heart rate tracing shown in the graph is usually associated with

(A) cord compression
(B) placental insufficiency
(C) head compressions

(D) acute fetal asphyxia
(E) tetanic contraction

272. You are asked to place an epidural in a patient who is laboring with a singleton in breech presentation. All of the following are true regarding breech presentation EXCEPT

(A) a higher incidence of congenital abnormality
(B) a lower frequency of prolapsed umbilical cord
(C) fetal head entrapment may necessitate the need for rapid induction of general anesthesia

(D) causes of breech presentation include preterm delivery, multiple gestation, and uterine abnormalities

(E) it accounts for approximately 3-4% of all pregnancies

273. The usual blood loss associated with an uncomplicated vaginal delivery of twins is approximately

(A) 400 mL

(B) 600 mL

(C) 800 mL

(D) 1000 mL

(E) 1200 mL

274. A 27-year-old G1P0 patient is being treated for preterm labor with terbutaline. An adverse effect of terbutaline used for preterm labor is

(A) cardiac arrhythmia

(B) hyperkalemia

(C) bradycardia

(D) hypertension

(E) hypoglycemia

275. Nerve injury during labor and delivery can result from all of the following EXCEPT

(A) compression of lumbosacral trunk by the head of fetus

(B) peroneal nerve injury by lithotomy stirrup

(C) epidural hematoma secondary to block

(D) femoral nerve compression by the lithotomy stirrup

(E) chemical contamination of the subarachnoid space

276. A 35-year-old heroin-addicted parturient in labor is requesting pain relief. Which one of the following options is LEAST desirable?

(A) Meperidine

(B) Continuous epidural analgesia

(C) Nitrous oxide

(D) Butorphanol

(E) Lumbar sympathetic block

277. Uterine rupture is an obstetrical emergency often necessitating general anesthesia. It is

associated with significant maternal morbidity and increases neonatal mortality by 60-fold. Conditions associated with uterine rupture include all of the following EXCEPT

(A) previous uterine surgery

(B) trauma

(C) grand multiparity

(D) intrauterine manipulation

(E) twin gestation

278. Well-known changes that occur in the central nervous system of the parturient include all of the following conditions EXCEPT

(A) nerve fibers have increased sensitivity to local anesthetics

(B) MAC for inhalational agents is decreased by approximately 40%

(C) activation of the endorphin system

(D) no change in dose requirement for local anesthetic in the first trimester

(E) spinal CSF volume is reduced

DIRECTIONS: Use the following scenario to answer Questions 279-280: You are called emergently to a delivery room where a patient has just undergone a natural childbirth. The nurse informs you that the patient is bleeding and asks for your assistance. The obstetrician states there is a uterine inversion. The patient is pale with a blood pressure of 60/40. Her pulse is 125. She is actively bleeding. She has a single 18-gauge IV that is infusing lactated Ringer solution containing 20 U/L of oxytocin. The IV is running wide-open.

279. Initial steps in the management of this patient include all of the following EXCEPT

(A) obtain large-bore IV access

(B) place the patient in the Trendelenburg position and administer vasopressors as needed

(C) obtain a blood sample for CBC, type and cross match, and DIC screen

(D) continue infusing the IV solution containing oxytocin

(E) immediate attempt at replacement of the uterus

280. The obstetrician's initial attempts to replace the uterus are unsuccessful. He asks for your assistance. While preparing to move to the operating room, which one of the following maneuvers may be of most benefit?

(A) IV bolus of 2 g of magnesium sulfate
(B) IM injection of 5 mg of ritodrine
(C) IV injection of 0.2 mg of terbutaline
(D) IV bolus of 50–100 mcg of nitroglycerine
(E) placement of a saddle block

281. Prophylactic measures taken to prevent maternal hypotension during and following spinal anesthesia include all of the following EXCEPT

(A) administration of 500-1000 mL of crystalloid solution
(B) left lateral displacement of the uterus
(C) Trendelenburg position after spinal injection
(D) placement of the spinal anesthetic with the patient in the lateral position
(E) infusion of a vasopressor

282. An obstetrician asks you to stand by in case he needs to perform an urgent cesarean section. His patient is 8 cm dilated. The fetal heart rate pattern is nonreassuring and there is no fetal response to fetal scalp stimulation. The patient is comfortable with a working epidural in place. He states he is going to perform fetal blood capillary pH testing. All of the following statements are true regarding fetal blood capillary pH testing EXCEPT

(A) it is a method that cannot be used to assess fetal well-being during labor of a breech presentation
(B) a fetal scalp pH of 7.25 or higher is considered normal
(C) a fetal scalp pH less than 7.20 is indicative of significant asphyxia and the need for immediate delivery
(D) a fetal scalp pH of 7.20-7.24 is intermediate and requires close monitoring and repeat sampling
(E) it requires adequate dilation of the cervix

283. The one finding present in eclamptic patients and not in preeclamptics is

(A) hyperreflexia
(B) decreased uteroplacental perfusion
(C) presence of seizure activity
(D) treatment with magnesium sulfate
(E) general vasoconstriction

284. A change in the anatomy or physiology of the stomach that is associated with pregnancy is

(A) decreased acid secretion
(B) decreased gastric emptying time
(C) downward displacement of the pylorus
(D) incompetence of the lower esophageal sphincter beginning in the first trimester
(E) epidural analgesia using only local anesthetics slows gastric emptying

285. You are called to the postpartum floor to perform an epidural blood patch (EBP) on a patient who had a wet tap two days prior during the placement of her labor epidural. You explain to her that all of the following are true of an epidural blood patch EXCEPT

(A) the success rate for a first EBP approaches 85%
(B) prophylactic epidural saline bolus is effective in decreasing the incidence of postdural puncture headache (PDPH)
(C) if the site of dural rent is unknown, the lowermost interspace should be used
(D) 15–20 mL of aseptically obtained autologous blood is typically used for the EBP
(E) 95% of postdural puncture headaches last less than one week

286. You are called to the delivery room and are asked to assist in the resuscitation of a newborn term infant. The infant is not breathing and the heart rate is less than 100. Steps to take include all of the following EXCEPT

(A) provide warmth, clear the airway and dry, stimulate, and reposition the infant
(B) if the infant remains apneic or the heart rate is less than 100, provide positive pressure ventilation

(C) 100% oxygen should be used during assisted ventilation

(D) during the first assisted, breath positive pressure at 20 cm H$_2$O should be maintained for 4-5 sec at the end of inspiration to overcome the surface tension of the lungs and open up the alveoli

(E) if mask ventilation lasts more than 2-3 min, the stomach should be emptied with an orogastric tube

287. A 27-year-old paraplegic patient with a T6 lesion presents to the labor and delivery suite in early labor. She is 4 cm dilated and requests an epidural. Which one of the following statements regarding her anesthetic management is true?

(A) Spinal anesthesia is contraindicated in this patient.

(B) Neuraxial anesthesia is unnecessary in this patient since the patient has no sensation below the T6 level.

(C) The test dose used after placement of an epidural will identify unintentional subarachnoid injection.

(D) Patients with a spinal cord injury are more prone to orthostatic hypotension that can contribute to a decrease in uteroplacental perfusion.

(E) If general anesthesia is necessary, a depolarizing agent may be used without reservation.

288. The local anesthetic that attains the lowest fetal concentration relative to maternal concentration is

(A) lidocaine

(B) ropivacaine

(C) 2-chloroprocaine

(D) mepivacaine

(E) bupivacaine

DIRECTIONS: Use the following scenario to answer Questions 289-290. You are asked to evaluate a 30-year-old G4P3 female who presents at 37 weeks gestation for her third cesarean section as well as tubal ligation. Her prenatal course is complicated by known placenta previa. She has had no antepartum bleeding. She currently weighs 250 pounds and is 62 inches tall. Her airway exam reveals a Mallampati class 4 with normal range of motion.

289. During the anesthesia interview you advise the patient that

(A) her risk of placenta accreta is 25%

(B) her risk of placenta accreta is 11%

(C) her risk of placenta accreta is over 50%

(D) spinal anesthesia is contraindicated

(E) she must undergo general anesthesia for her repeat cesarean section

290. During your preoperative interview, you advise her of all of the following EXCEPT

(A) two large-bore intravenous catheters will be placed

(B) she will be typed and crossmatched for blood

(C) combined spinal-epidural (CSE) will be performed

(D) an obstetrical hysterectomy may be required

(E) the procedure will be performed under spinal anesthesia to avoid a potentially difficult airway

291. A neuropathy manifested as numbness, tingling, burning, or other paresthesia that is probably the most commonly encountered neuropathy related to childbirth is

(A) compression of the lumbosacral trunk

(B) obturator nerve palsy

(C) femoral nerve palsy

(D) sciatic nervy palsy

(E) lateral femoral cutaneous nerve palsy

292. You are called by a colleague who has tried multiple times to place an epidural in a laboring patient who had corrective surgery for scoliosis. She asks about the placement of a caudal anesthetic. You reply that all of the following statements are true about her condition EXCEPT

(A) caudal anesthesia is an acceptable alternative in this patient

(B) identification of the sacral hiatus is necessary

(C) a test dose similar to that used during lumbar epidural placement is not necessary prior to administration of local anesthetic

(D) accurate placement of the caudal needle is confirmed by the "feel" of the needle passing through the sacrococcygeal ligament that overlies the sacral hiatus between the sacral cornua

(E) the needle should only be advanced 1 to 2 cm into the caudal canal

293. Patient-controlled analgesia (PCA) is a viable alternative for pain management during labor in patients with a contraindication to or unsuccessful attempt at neuraxial analgesia. Remifentanil PCA has more recently been used. True statements regarding remifentanil PCA include all of the following EXCEPT

(A) plasma concentrations of remifentanil in pregnant patients are about half those found in nonpregnant patients

(B) remifentanil rapidly crossed the placenta

(C) there is more nausea and vomiting compared to meperidine PCA

(D) the context-sensitive half-time of 3.5 min is not affected by the duration of infusion

(E) remifentanil is rapidly metabolized by plasma and tissue esterases to an inactive metabolite

294. In a pregnant woman at term, you would expect an increase in all of the following values EXCEPT

(A) functional residual capacity

(B) dead space

(C) tidal volume

(D) lung compliance

(E) inspiratory reserve volume

295. A 30-year-old G3P2 female presents for an anesthesia consultation. Her prenatal course is significant for a history of HSV-2 infection. All of the following statements regarding her care are true EXCEPT

(A) primary herpes infection is associated with viremia

(B) asymptomatic shedding of the virus may occur in the genital tract

(C) the presence of either active lesions or prodrome are an indication for cesarean section

(D) neuraxial anesthesia is contraindicated in a patient with active recurrent HSV-2 infection in labor

(E) epidural or intrathecal administration of morphine increases the risk of recurrence of HSV-1, but not HSV-2, infection in obstetrical patients

296. A 30-year-old G1P0 female at 18 weeks estimated gestational age has just been diagnosed with a pheochromocytoma and presents for an anesthetic consultation. You tell her that all of the following statements are true EXCEPT

(A) early laparoscopic resection of the tumor is possible prior to the third trimester

(B) pheochromocytoma is associated with an increased incidence of both fetal death and intrauterine growth restriction (IUGR)

(C) if surgical resection is not accomplished prior to delivery, spontaneous vaginal delivery is the preferred method of delivery

(D) phenoxybenzamine is the most commonly prescribed α-adrenoceptor antagonist used

(E) nicardipine may be used intraoperatively to prevent hypertension during resection of the tumor

297. True statements regarding fetal electronic monitoring during nonobstetric surgery include all of the following EXCEPT

(A) the American College of Obstetricians and Gynecologists (ACOG) acknowledge there are no data to allow specific recommendations for fetal heart rate (FHR) monitoring for obstetric patients undergoing nonobstetric surgery

(B) monitoring should be performed before and after surgery

(C) intraoperative monitoring is recommended when possible, especially after 24 weeks gestational age

(D) a decrease in FHR variability during general anesthesia is an indication of fetal compromise and an indication for cesarean delivery

(E) an experienced obstetric provider should be present to monitor and interpret the FHR tracing and uterine activity

298. Plasma cholinesterase concentrations during pregnancy are

(A) highest at term

(B) unchanged from normal levels

(C) increased

(D) decreased resulting in a clinically significant prolongation of amide type local anesthetics

(E) decreased to a degree not resulting in a clinically significant prolongation of succinylcholine

299. You are confronted with a 28-year-old G1P0 female with achondroplasia. She presents for an elective cesarean section at 39 weeks gestational age. True statements regarding her

achondroplasia and obstetrical anesthetic management include all of the following EXCEPT

(A) marked lumbar lordosis and scoliosis may cause technical difficulties during attempts at neuraxial anesthesia

(B) it may be difficult to estimate the appropriate dose of local anesthetic for single-shot spinal anesthesia

(C) spinal may be preferred to epidural injection of local anesthetic

(D) achondroplasia is inherited as an autosomal dominant mode, although most cases occur as a result of spontaneous mutation

(E) although a higher incidence of difficult intubation has been reported in achondroplastic patients, most reports note no difficulty in airway management.

300. A 27-year-old G1P0 woman is admitted at term for an ex utero intrapartum therapy (EXIT) procedure. The surgeons plan to excise a large embryonic cervical tumor. All of the following are characteristics of the maternal and fetal anesthetic care EXCEPT

(A) placement of an epidural catheter for postoperative maternal pain control

(B) pulmonary denitrogenation, rapid sequence induction, and endotracheal intubation of the mother

(C) fetal anesthesia provided by intramuscular injection of opioid and a paralytic agent either by ultrasound guidance prior to uterine incision or directly after hysterotomy and delivery of the fetus

(D) 1 to 1.5 MAC of volatile inhalational agent is required for the procedure

(E) fetal tracheal intubation after hysterotomy with maintenance of fetoplacental circulation until the procedure is completed.

DIRECTIONS: Use the following figure to answer Question 301:

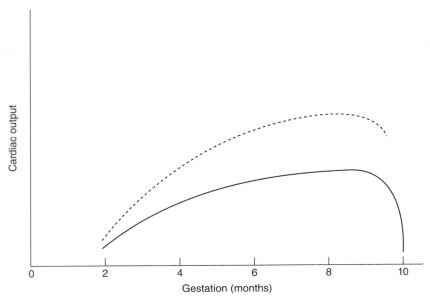

301. The figure above shows the change in cardiac output with pregnancy. The discrepancy in the two lines is due primarily to the effect

   (A) on respiration
   (B) on uterine blood flow
   (C) on venous return
   (D) of pressure on the aorta
   (E) on the central nervous system

302. Adjuvants such as epinephrine or bicarbonate are often used during obstetrical epidural anesthesia. True statements regarding the use of these adjuvants include all of the following EXCEPT

   (A) epinephrine is more effective at prolonging the action of short-acting local anesthetics than longer-acting agents
   (B) the addition of sodium bicarbonate hastens the onset of the block by increasing the pH closer to the pKa of the local anesthetic
   (C) hypotension occurs less frequently with epidural administration of an alkalinized local anesthetic
   (D) epinephrine has intrinsic analgesic effects via stimulation of pre-synaptic α_2-adrenoceptors that contribute to

greater reliability and intensity of the block
   (E) alkalization of bupivacaine must be performed carefully because the margin between satisfactory alkalization and precipitation is narrow

303. Which one of the following is the correct statement regarding drug action and placental transfer in a parturient?

   (A) Placental transfer is minimal with muscle relaxants.
   (B) Opioids do not cross the placenta.
   (C) Inhalational anesthetics increase uterine muscle tone.
   (D) Nitrous oxide is contraindicated for cesarean section secondary to interference with vitamin B_{12} synthesis.
   (E) Thiopental does not cross the placenta.

304. True statements regarding total spinal anesthesia include all of the following EXCEPT

   (A) it is a rare complication that can result from both intrathecal or epidural administration of local anesthetic
   (B) it cannot result from subdural administration of local anesthetic

(C) supportive measures to provide oxygenation and prevent aspiration, including endotracheal intubation, may be necessary

(D) preventative measures may include waiting for a partial spinal to wear off and then administering a second spinal in the case of elective cesarean section

(E) conversion to general anesthesia may be necessary

305. Well-known cardiovascular changes that occur at term in pregnancy include which one of the following parameters?

(A) A 25% decrease in heart rate

(B) A 20% increase in systemic vascular resistance

(C) An increase in myocardial contractility

(D) A decrease in left ventricular end-diastolic volume

(E) A decrease in left ventricular end-systolic volume

DIRECTIONS (Questions 306-307): Each group of items below consists of lettered headings followed by a list of numbered phrases or statements. For each numbered phrase or statement, select the ONE lettered heading or component that is most closely associated with it. Each lettered heading or component may be selected once, more than once, or not at all.

(A) Placenta previa
(B) Placenta accreta
(C) Uterine inversion
(D) Ruptured uterus
(E) Placental abruption
(F) Amniotic fluid embolus
(G) Severe preeclampsia

For each patient, select the most likely etiology.

306. A 27-year-old primipara at term in labor at 8 cm ruptures her membranes spontaneously, sits up, and states, "My heart." She then becomes hypotensive and unresponsive. She begins to have significant vaginal bleeding shortly afterwards.

307. A 30-year-old parturient at 32 weeks gestational age presents to the labor and delivery suite complaining of decreased fetal movement and abdominal pain. She admits to chronic cocaine use throughout her pregnancy. Her blood pressure is 120/60. Her abdomen is firm. A non-stress test is non-reassuring. An ultrasound is performed which reveals no abnormal placental findings.

DIRECTIONS (Questions 308-309): Each group of items below consists of lettered headings followed by a list of numbered phrases or statements. For each numbered phrase or statement, select the ONE lettered heading or component that is most closely associated with it. Each lettered heading or component may be selected once, more than once, or not at all.

(A) Oxytocin
(B) Mifepristone
(C) Carboprost tromethamine
(D) Vasopressin
(E) Methysergide
(F) Misoprostol
(G) Methylergonovine
(H) Methylprednisolone

For each patient, select the most appropriate medication.

308. You are called to a room where a 27-year-old G6P6 female has just delivered via natural childbirth and is bleeding. The patient has a history of severe reactive airway disease and upon entering the room she is actively wheezing. The obstetrician states the uterus remains boggy and the patient continues to bleed despite the administration of oxytocin and methylergonovine.

309. In a patient with excessive postpartum bleeding, this medication is intended to be administered solely as an intramuscular or intramyometrial injection because it may cause severe hypertension when injected as an IV bolus.

Answers and Explanations

228. (C) A non-stress test is the easiest test to perform with few contraindications. The mother is placed on an electronic fetal monitor. A reassuring non-stress test would demonstrate two fetal heart rate accelerations within a 20-min period of at least 15 bpm for at least a 15-sec duration. A reassuring NST has a high negative predictive value meaning a low risk of fetal death within one week of testing. A non-reassuring NST would require additional testing with either an OCT or BPP. *(5:292-3)*

229. (E) 2-Chloroprocaine has the fastest onset, especially when combined with sodium bicarbonate. It is also rapidly metabolized by both mother and fetus resulting in little fetal accumulation. Systemic toxicity is low making it one of the safest local anesthetics used in pregnancy. *(1:579, 5:1157)*

230. (A) All of the options are absolute contraindications except preexisting neurologic disease that may be a relative contraindication. *(5: 1151)*

231. (C) General anesthesia is associated with an increased risk of maternal death. This is partly due to the physiologic changes associated with pregnancy. The introduction of alternative airway devices in the recent past as well as the development of the difficult airway algorithm has contributed to the decreased risk of maternal death with general anesthesia as compared to regional anesthesia from a 16.7- to a 1.7-fold increased risk. *(5:1148, 1159)*

232. (C) 2-chloroprocaine is known to have an impact on the efficacy of neuraxial opioids.

In this case, the most likely agent used for the emergent cesarean section would be 2-chloroprocaine with or without bicarbonate due to its rapid onset and low systemic toxicity. *(5: 1159)*

233. (B) There are varying types of vWD, type 1 being the most mild and common form seen in pregnancy. Most recommendations for neuraxial anesthesia are based on expert opinions (level of evidence 5). Neuraxial anesthesia has been used safely in the past in patients with vWD, however, minimal "safe" factor levels remain undefined in the obstetrical population and evidence-based recommendations cannot be made. *(5:209-10; Choi S, et al. Anesth Analg 2009; 109:648-60)*

234. (D) Blood pressure criteria for severe preeclampsia include a systolic blood pressure of greater than or equal to 160 mm Hg or a diastolic blood pressure of greater than or equal to 110 mm Hg. The rest would be consistent with severe preeclampsia. *(5:294)*

235. (D) The patient's airway exam is concerning. This is a patient who might very well not tolerate labor and require an emergent cesarean section. While it is controversial regarding an absolute platelet count below which neuraxial anesthesia should be avoided, epidural analgesia has been successfully placed in patients with platelet counts below 100,000/mm^3 if there is no other existing coagulopathy. The placement of an epidural in this patient with a potentially difficult airway is reasonable after informed consent has been obtained. In addition, it may help to avoid a difficult airway scenario. Waiting until the patient is in active labor will only give more time for the platelet count to drop. While a spinal may decrease the incidence of hematoma formation, the patient is in labor and may require repeat spinal anesthetics. This is not only impractical, but also does not help to avoid a difficult airway scenario should emergent cesarean section be required. *(5:296)*

236. (E) Magnesium sulfate is used in preeclampsia to prevent seizures. Acute treatment of elevated blood pressure, most commonly with hydralazine or labetalol, is used to prevent cerebrovascular complications cited as the most common cause of mortality in patients with severe preeclampsia. *(2:987; 5:295)*

237. (C) This most likely represents a subdural placement of an epidural catheter. The block does not follow the typical pattern and may be characterized as patchy or extensive and is often higher than expected. It can be confused with subarachnoid injection of local anesthetic. Treatment consists of recognizing the subdural placement, supportive measures, and replacement of the catheter. *(5:860-1)*

238. (D) Postdural puncture headache (PDPH) typically consists of a postural headache in the frontal or occipital areas. Nausea, vomiting, neck stiffness, photophobia, and auditory changes have all been reported. EBP is the definitive treatment for PDPH. EBP has been used successfully in HIV-positive patients and is unlikely to introduce HIV into the CNS as this occurs early in the clinical course of the disease. Success rates are quoted at approximately 85% after a single blood patch. The most frequent complication is back pain, but rare complications including facial palsy, bradycardia, and arachnoiditis have been reported. Prophylactic EBP is controversial. *(5:862-3)*

239. (A) The anticholinergic agents atropine and scopolamine do readily cross the placenta. In contrast, glycopyrrolate does not. Muscle relaxants do not readily cross the placenta. *(2:62-3)*

240. (E) The patient is experiencing a high spinal block. Initial evaluation and treatment would include assessing the level of the spinal by having the patient squeeze her hands and by demonstrating her ability to speak in full sentences. Vasopressors, fluid administration, and supplemental oxygen are all indicated. Ephedrine is a better choice than phenylephrine given the bradycardia. Placing the patient in the Trendelenburg position to treat the hypotension may increase the height of the block and result in a total spinal. *(5:860)*

241. (C) The patient has progressed to a total spinal anesthetic. Immediate airway and circulatory support are vital. Securing the airway via endotracheal tube with 100% oxygen, left uterine displacement, and prompt administration of epinephrine are all critical to the care of this patient. Ephedrine would not be as efficacious as epinephrine at this point. *(5:860)*

242. (D) Both spinal and epidural anesthesia has been used safely in parturients with MS. Some evidence suggests there may be a higher incidence of relapse with spinal anesthesia. Avoidance of stress and hyperthermia are essential. *(5:139-41)*

243. (D) The guidelines from the American Society of Regional Anesthesia (ASRA) state that 5000 units of unfractionated heparin subcutaneously twice a day does not increase the risk of epidural/spinal hematoma. If the patient is on three times a day dosing or greater than 10,000 units/day subcutaneously, ASRA states the safety of neuraxial blockade in these patients has not been established. ASRA recommends a platelet count be obtained in patients on heparin for more than four days to rule out heparin-induced thrombocytopenia (HIT). A normal aPTT would also be prudent prior to needle placement. The peak effect of a subcutaneous dose of heparin is two hours. *(4:954-5; 5:1023; Horlocker T, et al. Reg Anesth Pain Med 2012; 35: 64-101)*

244. (E) Data from case studies show the incidence of miscarriage to be 1.6%. This is lower than the incidence of miscarriage in the general population. Many psychotropic medications are believed to increase the risk of birth defects. ECT can be safely administered during all trimesters of pregnancy. *(2:351-2)*

245. (E) The uterus does not contribute to aortocaval compression until approximately 18-20 weeks gestation. Endotracheal intubation should be considered after the first trimester. Monitoring of the fetal heart rate and uterine contractions should be considered. Consultation with the patient's obstetrician should also be considered. *(2:351-2)*

246. (E) Many drugs can exacerbate the symptoms of myasthenia gravis. Of the drugs listed above, carboprost tromethamine has not been shown to worsen the symptoms. *(2:1060; 5:996)*

247. (B) VBAC is successful in 60-80% of women in whom a low-transverse incision was made during previous cesarean delivery. The major risk of VBAC is uterine rupture that is estimated to occur in less than 1% of patients undergoing a trial of labor. ACOG states that physicians, anesthesia providers, and other personnel must be immediately available to provide emergency care for patients attempting VBAC. *(2:375-85)*

248. (D) Uterine atony is the most common cause of severe postpartum hemorrhage accounting for approximately 80% or more of cases of primary (within the first 24 h of delivery) postpartum hemorrhage. Despite preventative measures, postpartum hemorrhage occurs in 4%-6% of pregnancies. *(2:818-821)*

249. (C) Paracervical block may be used during transvaginal oocyte retrieval, however, since this technique incompletely blocks sensation from the vaginal and ovarian pain fibers, additional analgesia will be required. Conscious sedation, neuraxial anesthesia, and general anesthesia have all been used successfully. Standard fasting guidelines should be used, however, careful consideration should be undertaken prior to canceling the procedure. Failure to retrieve the oocytes can increase the risk of ovarian hyperstimulation syndrome. In addition, if the window for maximal oocyte retrieval is missed (34-36 h after administration of hCG), spontaneous ovulation will occur with resultant loss of oocytes, invalidating the significant effort and expense incurred during hormonal stimulation. *(2:306-13)*

250. (D) Magnesium sulfate is primarily eliminated by the kidneys. Preeclamptic patients with significant renal impairment may develop magnesium toxicity more easily and should be monitored more closely (with serial patellar reflex exams and serum measurements). Patellar reflexes are lost at serum magnesium levels of approximately 12 mg/dL. Magnesium potentiates the effects of both depolarizing and nondepolarizing neuromuscular blocking agents. Magnesium does cross the placenta and may cause fetal respiratory compromise. *(2:769-71, 986)*

251. (A) The patient is experiencing magnesium toxicity. This may be due to a mechanical malfunction of the infusion pump or an error in the preparation of the infusion. Initial management should be directed toward treating the respiratory compromise with either bag-mask ventilation or obtaining a definitive airway when available. Calcium gluconate should be administered as soon as possible in this patient with presumed magnesium overdose. The magnesium infusion should be shut off immediately and a magnesium serum level should be obtained to confirm the diagnosis. The patient's cardiovascular status is not compromised and therefore epinephrine is not indicated at this time. *(2:986; 5:521-2)*

252. (D) MH is an autosomal dominant disease with incomplete penetrance. There are very few reports of the development of MH during pregnancy. Dantrolene does cross the placenta and may be associated with fetal hypotonia. There is also one report of uterine atony after administration of dantrolene, although this was thought to be secondary to the effects of mannitol. Neuraxial anesthesia should be encouraged in all parturients with MH, however, standard preparations should be made in case general anesthesia is required. All local anesthetics are safe in MH patients. *(2:1023-31)*

253. **(C)** The Apgar score is based on five parameters that are assessed at one and five minutes after birth. Further assessments may be made at five-minute intervals if the initial scores are low. Although the usefulness of the Apgar score is still being debated, it is used throughout the world to assess fetal wellbeing at birth. *(2:159-61)*

254. **(E)** The drug protocols used for ACLS in nonpregnant patients should also be used in pregnant patients. A slightly higher placement of the hands for compressions, left uterine displacement, and early endotracheal intubation are all indicated in pregnant patients. While vasopressor agents may decrease blood flow to the uterus, optimal care of the mother is the best therapy for the fetus. The amount of current that reaches the fetus in cardioversion is negligible. *(2:900-4)*

255. **(C)** If resuscitative efforts are unsuccessful, there is some evidence to support the performance of a perimortem cesarean section (hysterotomy). Evacuation of the uterus allows for relief of aortocaval compression and restoration of venous return to the heart and may aide in maternal resuscitative efforts. It may also allow for delivery of a viable fetus depending on the gestational age and time from onset of cardiac arrest. Asystole is not a shockable rhythm. A second dose of vasopressin is not part of the ACLS protocol. *(2:900-4)*

256. **(E)** Gastric emptying is not altered during pregnancy, but is slowed during labor. In addition, the use of opioids (intravenously or neuraxially) can also delay gastric emptying. Epidural administration of only local anesthetic has been shown not to delay gastric emptying. *(2:23-5)*

257. **(D)** Continuous fetal heart rate monitoring represents the best way of detecting uterine rupture. Pain, uterine tenderness, and maternal tachycardia have both low specificity and sensitivity as diagnostic symptoms or signs of lower uterine segment rupture. Most cases of lower uterine segment rupture do not lead to severe hemorrhage as the lower uterine scar is relatively avascular. *(2:380-3)*

258. **(A)** Factors affecting drug transfer across the placenta include drug size, lipid solubility, protein binding, pKa, pH, and blood flow. It is the free unbound drug fraction that more easily crosses the placenta. *(2:62-4)*

259. **(E)** The second stage of labor involves the distention of the vaginal vault and perineum. These impulses arise from the pudendal nerves that are composed of lower sacral fibers (S2-S4). *(2:223)*

260. **(B)** Estrogen does induce an increase in the production of thyroid-binding globulin resulting in an increase in the total T3 and T4 concentrations. However, it is the unbound free T3 and free T4 that are the active hormones and these remain unchanged during pregnancy. The patient thus remains euthyroid. *(2:25-6)*

261. **(E)** An OCT can be performed with either spontaneous contractions, administration of intravenous oxytocin, or by direct nipple stimulation. The definition of a positive oxytocin contraction test is three adequate contractions in a ten-minute period with repetitive late decelerations. A negative OCT is associated with a 99% fetal survival within one week. A positive OCT has been associated with an adverse fetal outcome in approximately 40% of cases. This combination of positive OCT and lack of fetal heart rate variability is especially ominous. *(2:97-9)*

262. **(A)** The nonpregnant uterine circulation demonstrates autoregulation. In contrast, the pregnant uterus has both placental and nonplacental circulations. The uteroplacental circulation is a widely dilated, low resistance system where perfusion is largely pressure-dependent with little or no ability for autoregulation. Clinically, uteroplacental flow is dependent upon maternal blood pressure. In contrast, a smaller portion of uterine blood flow supplies the myometrium and nonplacental endometrium that may maintain autoregulatory responses in both the pregnant and nonpregnant state. The doses of general anesthetics used clinically have minimal effects on uterine blood flow unless there is significant maternal hypotension. The uterine arteries arise from the internal iliac (hypogastric) arteries. *(2:37-40; 5:292)*

263. **(D)** The goals of anesthetic management for this patient should include: (1) maintenance of a slow heart rate and sinus rhythm; (2) aggressive treatment of acute atrial fibrillation; (3) avoidance of aortocaval compression; (4) maintenance of adequate venous return; (5) maintenance of adequate systemic vascular resistance; and (6) prevention of pain, hypoxia, hypercarbia, and acidosis, all of which can exacerbate pulmonary hypertension. Epidural use allows for careful titration of local anesthetic and may help reduce the incidence of hypotension. The epidural also decreases maternal tachycardia that may be poorly tolerated. Phenylephrine is preferred over ephedrine to treat hypotension given the direct chronotropic effect of ephedrine. Vacuum or low outlet forceps delivery is preferred to maternal expulsive efforts during the second stage of labor thus avoiding the deleterious effects of the Valsalva maneuver. The postpartum period is of particular concern for these patients as the sudden increase in preload may flood the central circulation and result in the development of pulmonary edema. Intensive monitoring should be continued for at least twenty-four hours after delivery of any woman with mitral stenosis. *(2:891-4)*

264. **(E)** The unanticipated difficult airway in obstetric anesthesia has the potential for very serious consequences with two patients at risk. The mother's life has priority, but every effort must be made to deliver a viable infant. Airway assessment should be reevaluated prior to cesarean section because significant changes can occur during labor. In the presence of fetal distress and the inability to intubate and ventilate the patient, placement of an LMA with cricoid pressure and proceeding to emergency

cesarean section is an acceptable alternative. *(2:655-69)*

265. **(A)** Pregnancy is associated with many laboratory deviations from "normal." Hemoglobin and hematocrit decrease, platelets remain unchanged or decrease, and most coagulation factors increase, BUN and creatinine decrease, and both bicarbonate and P_{CO_2} decrease resulting in little change in pH. *(2:120-3)*

266. **(D)** Benzodiazepines are no longer felt to cause facial cleft defects and therefore may be used safely in pregnancy. Incompetence of the lower esophageal sphincter and anatomic changes associated with pregnancy both increase the risk of aspiration pneumonia. Although it is unclear at what stage of pregnancy this becomes significant, aspiration prophylaxis is prudent in the pregnant patient. Regional anesthesia is a reasonable alternative to general anesthesia and potentially limits drug exposure during surgery. The uterus does not become an intraabdominal organ until 12-13 weeks gestation and therefore left uterine displacement is not necessary in the first trimester. *(2:342-6; 5:1150)*

267. **(D)** Molar pregnancy occurs in 1 of 1500 pregnancies in the United States. Clinically the patient presents with vaginal bleeding after delayed menses. The absence of fetal cardiac activity, a uterus large for gestational age, and a marked elevation of beta-hCG are all highly suggestive of hydatidiform mole. The ultrasound demonstrates the presence of hydropic villi that is pathognomonic for molar pregnancy. *(2:329-32)*

268. **(C)** Molar pregnancies tend to bleed profusely. Oxytocin infusion is advocated either before or during the evacuation of the uterus to help reduce the amount of blood loss. Acute cardiopulmonary distress has been observed in as many as 27% of patients after evacuation. While there are multiple causes, trophoblastic embolization is responsible in more than half the cases. General anesthesia is preferred over neuraxial anesthesia given the potential for massive hemorrhage. *(2:329-32)*

269. **(D)** Small doses of nitroglycerine (50-100 mcg) have been shown to relax the uterus to allow for manual extraction of the placenta. Caution should be used with the use of regional anesthesia in the presence of significant postpartum bleeding to avoid hypotension. Ketamine is a good induction drug in the presence of maternal bleeding, but has been shown to produce a dose-related increase in uterine tone. *(2:822-23)*

270. **(C)** The pattern represented is that of early decelerations, in which the heart rate decreases with the onset of contraction, reaches the low point with the peak of contraction, and then returns to baseline as the uterus relaxes. In contrast, late decelerations start after the contraction is underway, and the low point occurs after the contraction is over. Variable decelerations are variable in shape and onset. *(2:143-6; 5:292-3)*

271. **(C)** The early deceleration pattern is seen with fetal head compression, which leads to increased vagal tone. Cord compression leads to variable decelerations, whereas placental insufficiency leads to late decelerations. *(2:144-5; 5:293)*

272. **(B)** There is a higher frequency of prolapsed cord, especially with a footling or complete breech presentation, because the fetal head no longer occupies the lower uterine segment. A higher incidence of congenital abnormalities has been found. The fetal head is the largest presenting part and it is last to present, therefore, fetal head entrapment can occur and is a life threatening complication of vaginal breech delivery that may require rapid induction of general anesthesia or the use of either sublingual or intravenous nitroglycerine. *(2:779-786)*

273. **(D)** The usual blood loss in an uncomplicated vaginal delivery of twins is approximately 1000 mL. *(2:23; 4:789)*

274. **(A)** Tocolytic agents, such as ritodrine and terbutaline, relax uterine smooth muscle by direct stimulation of β-adrenoceptors. These patients are at increased risk for fluid overload, tachycardia, dysrhythmia, hyperglycemia,

hypokalemia, hypotension, and pulmonary edema. The etiology of pulmonary edema is controversial and has been reported to be both cardiac and noncardiac in origin. *(2:765-769; 5:293-94)*

275. **(D)** Compression of the lumbosacral trunks by the fetal head is probably the most common cause of postpartum foot drop. Incorrect patient positioning can cause peroneal nerve injury secondary to the lithotomy stirrups. Femoral nerve compression can occur secondary to excessive flexion of the hip in the lithotomy position. Epidural hematoma or chemical contamination of the subarachnoid space fortunately are rare complications. *(2:701-21)*

276. **(D)** Opioid agonist–antagonists may trigger withdrawal symptoms when administered to opioid-tolerant patients. *(2:1142)*

277. **(E)** Predisposing conditions for uterine rupture include previous uterine surgery, especially vertical incisions and prolonged intrauterine manipulation. Trauma and grand multiparity have also been associated with uterine rupture. According to the American College of Obstetricians and Gynecologists (ACOG), a patient with a twin gestation who is a candidate to undergo a vaginal birth after cesarean section (VBAC) is at no greater risk of uterine rupture than a singleton pregnancy. There has been concern about regional anesthesia masking signs of rupture, especially in patients attempting vaginal birth after cesarean. The experience seems to support the safety of epidural anesthesia if continuous electronic monitoring of uterine activity and the fetal heart rate is performed. *(2:817)*

278. **(D)** Anesthetic requirements are decreased in pregnancy, with 25% less local anesthetic needed for regional anesthesia. Anatomic changes, such as distended epidural veins or decreased volume of CSF, increase spread of local anesthetics. However, these changes are also seen in the first trimester, well before significant mechanical changes have occurred. It is postulated that pregnancy-induced hormonal changes in nerve tissue sensitivity are

also responsible for the altered sensitivity to local anesthetics. Increased progesterone concentrations may be responsible for the 25% to 40% reduction in MAC to general anesthetics. Endorphin concentrations rise during pregnancy thus contributing to an elevated pain threshold. *(2:27-31)*

279. **(D)** All uterotonics should be discontinued until after the uterus is replaced. Uterine relaxation is necessary to replace the uterus. Additional help should be summoned as blood loss can be massive resulting in hypovolemic shock and maternal death. *(Dayan S, et al., Anesth Analg 1996; 82:1091-3)*

280. **(D)** IV administration of nitroglycerine has both a rapid onset (30-40 sec) and a short-lived effect (approximately 1 min) on uterine relaxation. Hypotension is minimal at this dose. Ritodrine, terbutaline, and magnesium sulfate have all been used, but none are as rapid in onset and their effects may need to be reversed. A saddle block would be impractical and contraindicated given the profound hypotension. *(Dayan S, et al., Anesth Analg 1996; 82:1091-3)*

281. **(C)** Methods to prevent maternal hypotension include fluid administration, lateral displacement of the uterus, placing the patient on her side as opposed to the sitting position during placement of the spinal anesthetic, and infusion of a vasopressor. A head-down tilt may result in more cephalad spread of a hyperbaric local anesthetic solution. This will potentially increase the level of the block and cause more hypotension. *(2:531; 5:1155)*

282. **(A)** Fetal blood capillary testing may be used to assess fetal well-being during labor. It requires adequate cervical dilation to allow for sampling of the presenting part. It may be used in both vertex and breech presentations. If the resulting pH is intermediate, continued close monitoring and repeat sampling within thirty minutes is required if delivery has not been accomplished. *(2:148)*

283. **(C)** All the findings are present in preeclampsia and eclampsia, except the presence of seizure

activity. Eclampsia is defined as the new onset of seizures or unexplained coma during pregnancy or the postpartum period in a woman with signs and symptoms of preeclampsia and without a preexisting neurologic disorder *(2:998)*

284. **(D)** The stomach is displaced upward and toward the left side of the diaphragm and its axis is rotated 45 degrees to the right. This displaces the intraabdominal portion of the esophagus into the thorax, thus reducing lower esophageal sphincter tone. In addition, progestins also contribute to a relaxation of the lower esophageal sphincter tone. *(2:23-5)*

285. **(B)** Prophylactic epidural saline bolus has not been shown to be effective in decreasing the incidence of PDPH. MRI studies obtained after EBP have confirmed a predominantly cephalad spread of injected blood, therefore the lowermost interspace should be used. Most anesthesia providers inject 10-20 mL of blood. Success rates of up to 85% have been cited after performance of a single EBP with a 98% success rate after a second EBP. Ninety-five percent of postdural puncture headaches last less than one week, although rarely symptoms may last months or even years. *(2:682-95; 5:862-63)*

286. **(D)** During the first assisted breath, positive pressure at 30-40 cm H_2O should be maintained for 4-5 sec at the end of inspiration to overcome the surface tension of the lungs and open the alveoli. Subsequently, the maximal pressure generated should be between 20-30 cm H_2O. *(2:164-70)*

287. **(D)** Loss of sympathetic tone below the level of the lesion does render the patient more susceptible to orthostatic hypotension. These patients often have low baseline blood pressure and this can be worsened by administration of neuraxial or general anesthesia. Women with spinal cord lesions at or above T6 are at increased risk of autonomic hyperreflexia and therefore neuraxial anesthesia is appropriate and indicated in this patient. Noxious stimuli, bladder distention or uterine contractions can all cause malignant hypertension in a patient with autonomic hyperreflexia. A standard test dose of 3 mL

1.5% lidocaine will not identify an accidental subarachnoid injection as the patient is already paraplegic. The administration of succinylcholine to a paraplegic patient may result in a hyperkalemic response. *(2:1056-9)*

288. **(C)** 2-chloroprocaine is metabolized rapidly by plasma and tissue esterases, therefore it does not attain a high concentration in the fetus. The other agents also cross the placenta but are broken down more slowly resulting in higher maternal:fetal ratios. *(2:248-9; 5:1157)*

289. **(C)** The risk of placenta accreta is 1:2500 in the general population. This risk increases in the presence of placenta previa and further increases with each subsequent history of previous cesarean section. In this case, the risk of placenta accreta is approximately 60%. *(5:296)*

290. **(E)** This patient is at significant risk for postpartum hemorrhage. She is also potentially at risk for a difficult airway. A CSE would allow for excellent anesthesia with the ability to extend the anesthetic should it be warranted. Large-bore IV access and the immediate availability of blood is mandatory. If placenta accreta is encountered, obstetrical hysterectomy may be required. Although the procedure could be done under spinal anesthesia, this method would not allow for extension of the neuraxial block and could necessitate general anesthesia in a patient with a suspected difficult airway. *(5:296)*

291. **(E)** Meralgia paresthetica is a neuropathy of the lateral femoral cutaneous nerve and is probably the most commonly encountered neuropathy related to childbirth. It may arise during pregnancy or intrapartum. The most likely cause is entrapment of the nerve as it passes around the anterior superior iliac spine beneath or through the inguinal ligament. *(2:705-7)*

292. **(C)** In this patient with surgically corrected scoliosis, epidural analgesia may not be possible. Caudal anesthesia may be more technically feasible and is an acceptable alternative. Unintentional dural puncture and intravascular cannulation are possible with caudal

anesthesia, especially when the needle is advanced further into the caudal canal. A test dose is therefore recommended. If a continuous caudal is placed, there is possibly a higher risk of infection and larger volumes of drugs are required. *(2:236-9, 432-3)*

293. **(C)** PCA with meperidine, morphine, or fentanyl have all been used for labor. More recently, remifentanil has been used because of its potential advantages resulting from its pharmacokinetic properties that include rapid onset and rapid metabolism via plasma and tissue esterases. Remifentanil has been shown to cause less nausea and vomiting compared to other opioids such as meperidine. Although remifentanil readily crosses the placenta, it is rapidly redistributed and metabolized by the fetus. The context-sensitive half-time is unaltered by the duration of administration. *(2:420-3; 5:713)*

294. **(A)** FRC decreases at term. There is an increase in dead space, tidal volume, lung compliance, and inspiratory reserve volume at term. *(2:19-21; 5:290-1)*

295. **(D)** Recurrent genital herpes infection does not contraindicate the administration of neuraxial anesthesia. Unlike primary herpes infection, maternal antibodies are present with secondary infection and therefore viremia is unlikely. There are insufficient data to allow a definitive recommendation regarding neuraxial anesthesia in patients with primary infection. Patients with a history of HSV-2 are often placed on prophylactic antiviral medication in hopes of preventing a recurrent outbreak as this necessitates the performance of a cesarean section in order to decrease the incidence of neonatal herpes infection. *(2:806-7; 5:713)*

296. **(C)** Pheochromocytoma is rare during pregnancy with an estimated incidence of less than 0.2 per 10,000 pregnancies. Patients present with a variety of paroxysmal symptoms including headache, sweating, and palpitations. Hypertension and orthostatic hypotension are common. Definitive therapy is surgical resection of the tumor. Patients are placed on α- and β-adrenoceptor antagonists prior to

resection. The second trimester is the ideal time for laparoscopic or open resection. Alternatives include cesarean section at term with concurrent tumor resection, cesarean at term with open or laparoscopic resection 2–8 weeks later, or vaginal delivery with laparoscopic resection 6 weeks later. To prevent increased abdominal pressure on the tumor during labor, cesarean section is the preferred method of delivery in patients with unresected pheochromocytoma. *(2:929-34; 5:1124-6)*

297. **(D)** General anesthetic agents readily cross the placenta and affect the fetus. In addition, FHR variability does not become consistently reactive until approximately 27 to 28 weeks gestational age. Therefore, a decrease in FHR variability alone is not necessarily a cause for concern. However, sustained fetal tachycardia, bradycardia, or recurrent FHR decelerations do suggest fetal compromise. *(2:1161)*

298. **(E)** Plasma cholinesterase levels are typically decreased by 25% during pregnancy. The decreased concentrations do not result in clinically significant effects on ester-type local anesthetics or succinylcholine in the doses generally used. *(2:338-9)*

299. **(C)** Achondroplasia occurs with a prevalence of 1 in 26,000 live births. Most cases do occur from a spontaneous mutation. Neuraxial anesthesia may be difficult because of the associated changes involving the spinal column. These patients may have decreased cervical range of motion and a higher incidence of difficult intubation has been reported in achondroplastic patients. Although steps should be taken to deal with a potentially difficult airway, most reports show no difficulty with airway management. It can be very difficult to predict the correct dose of local anesthetic to be used during neuraxial anesthesia and these patients are at increased risk for either inadequate or high/total spinal. It has been suggested that epidural anesthesia be used as this allows the anesthesiologist to titrate the dose of local anesthetic to the desired level of anesthesia. *(2:1048-49)*

300. **(D)** EXIT procedures are used for a variety of situations including thoracotomy for cystic adenomatoid malformation, transition from placental gas exchange to ECMO for expected pulmonary insufficiency, excision of giant cervical teratoma, and laryngeal atresia. Anesthetic technique includes the placement of an epidural catheter for postoperative analgesia. The same principles apply to induction of general anesthesia for an EXIT procedure as those for cesarean delivery. However, sufficient time must be allowed after induction of anesthesia to achieve high-end tidal concentrations of volatile agent (2–3 MAC) prior to surgery to ensure uterine relaxation and fetal anesthesia. Fetal anesthesia can be supplemented with opioid and/or paralytic agent administered via ultrasound guidance prior to hysterotomy or directly after delivery of the fetus. Intubation is performed after delivery of the fetal head and shoulders, but the fetus is not ventilated and fetoplacental circulation is maintained. After the surgical procedure is completed, the fetus is given surfactant if indicated through the endotracheal tube and ventilated. Once the fetus' oxygenation is adequate, the umbilical cord is cut and the infant is given to the neonatology team. Once the infant is delivered, uterine relaxation is rapidly reversed, the uterus is closed, and the patient is extubated at the end of the procedure. The epidural is then used for postoperative pain management. *(2:123-31)*

301. **(C)** There is an increase in cardiac output as pregnancy progresses until about the eighth month, at which time the increase is attenuated. When studying cardiac output in the pregnant patient, one must know whether the study was made with the patient in the supine or lateral position. In the supine position, cardiac output will be decreased because of the weight of the uterus primarily on the inferior vena cava although compression of the aorta also occurs. Up to 15% of term parturients will experience bradycardia and a substantial drop in blood pressure when supine resulting in supine hypotension syndrome. A 10-15 degree left lateral tilt is recommended in parturients beyond 17 to 20 weeks gestational age. *(2:18, 531)*

302. **(C)** Hypotension occurs more frequently with epidural administration of an alkalinized local anesthetic likely due to the more rapid onset of sympathetic blockade. *(2:271-4)*

303. **(A)** Many drugs administered to the parturient cross the placenta and have neonatal effects ranging from fetal heart rate changes to neonatal depression. Opioids are the most commonly used agents during labor and may produce neonatal depression depending upon the total dose and time interval from administration to delivery of the fetus. Inhalational agents rapidly cross the placenta and cause uterine relaxation. Muscle relaxants have minimal transfer. *(2:62-6)*

304. **(B)** Total spinal anesthesia is a very serious and rare complication of intrathecal, epidural, or subdural administration of local anesthetic. Several mechanisms have been proposed after failed epidural including expansion of the epidural space resulting in compression of the spinal canal and further cephalad spread of intrathecal anesthetic, rapid transfer of anesthetic from the epidural space through the dural hole, and sufficient coverage of the neural roots that decreases the dose requirements of subsequent spinal anesthesia. Supportive measures including vasopressors and fluids should be instituted. Endotracheal intubation and general anesthesia may be required. *(2:462-3)*

305. **(C)** There is an increase in left ventricular end-diastolic volume and no change in left ventricular end-systolic volume resulting in an increased ejection fraction. Cardiac contractility is increased, SVR decreases, and heart rate increases. *(2:16-9; 5:290)*

306. **(F)** Amniotic fluid embolism occurs when fetal tissue gets into the maternal circulation. It is reported to occur during tumultuous labor.

It is now thought to be secondary to a massive autoimmune response to the fetal tissue rather that a true embolus to the pulmonary artery. Patients experience cardiovascular collapse and become coagulopathic. Immediate delivery of the fetus along with aggressive resuscitation and extracorporeal membrane oxygenation may be indicated. Despite these efforts, the mortality rate remains high and intact survival remains low. *(Gist R, et al., Anesth Analg 2009; 108:1599-1602)*

307. **(E)** Placental abruption occurs with premature separation of the placenta from the uterine wall. Multiple risk factors exist including smoking, cocaine use, trauma, hypertension, preeclampsia, diabetes, multiple pregnancies, and advanced maternal age. Classic findings include abdominal pain, bleeding (sometimes concealed), uterine irritability, and tenderness. Concealed bleeding may not be seen by ultrasound in up to 50% of cases. *(5:296)*

308. **(F)** Although carboprost tromethamine is the preferred prostaglandin treatment for refractory uterine atony, it is relatively contraindicated in patients with reactive airway disease. Misoprostol is a prostaglandin E_1 analogue that may be used in place of carboprost tromethamine in patients with reactive airway disease or pulmonary hypertension. The recommended dose is 800-1000 mcg per rectum for cases unresponsive to other uterotonic agents. *(2:818-22; 5:1155-7)*

309. **(G)** Ergot alkaloids are a class of drugs used to treat uterine atony. Ergonovine and methylergonovine are the two most commonly used ergot alkaloids used to treat uterine atony. In cases of life-threatening hemorrhage, a slow intravenous injection may be considered in an attempt to treat both postpartum hemorrhage and hypotension. *(2:821)*

CHAPTER 16

Pediatric Anesthesia
Questions

DIRECTIONS (Questions 310-396): Each of the numbered items or incomplete statements in this section is followed by answers or by completions of the statement. Select the ONE lettered answer or completion that is BEST in each case.

310. Preoperative evaluation of a 4-year-old boy for myringotomy and placement of tympanostomy tubes is concerning for possible difficulty with airway management. Physical exam reveals micrognathia, glossoptosis, and cleft palate. What is the most likely diagnosis?

    (A) Beckwith Syndrome
    (B) Goldenhar Syndrome
    (C) Pierre-Robin Syndrome
    (D) Treacher Collins Syndrome
    (E) Trisomy 21

311. A 2-year-old child is rushed to the trauma room for a laparotomy after sustaining multiple injuries in a motor vehicle accident. The child arrives intubated and pharmacologically paralyzed. The child is tachycardic, mildly hypotensive, and hypothermic. All of the following may be consequences of unintended, intraoperative hypothermia EXCEPT

    (A) decreased oxygen consumption
    (B) increased metabolic rate
    (C) systemic hypotension
    (D) pulmonary hypertension
    (E) hypoglycemia

312. A newborn infant born at 33 weeks gestational age presents for gastroschisis repair. In preparing medications for this patient, all of the following are considerations that will affect your medication selection EXCEPT

    (A) increased ventilatory depression from maternally administered opioids
    (B) immature blood brain barrier
    (C) lower protein availability for drug binding
    (D) increased sensitivity to CNS toxicity of lidocaine
    (E) immature enzyme systems for drug metabolism

313. A 3-week-old infant, born at 38 weeks gestational age, weighing 4 kg, presents for a Ladd's procedure. In order to request the appropriate amount of blood, you would like to know the allowable blood loss for this patient. What is the blood volume of this patient?

    (A) 160 mL
    (B) 200 mL
    (C) 400 mL
    (D) 280 mL
    (E) 320 mL

314. A 6-year-old boy presents to the holding area for elective repair of an inguinal hernia. He is a mild asthmatic and has not taken any daily asthma medications for 5 weeks. He is currently wheezing throughout on physical exam. You inform the mother that you will

    (A) proceed with surgery without treatment
    (B) postpone until tomorrow after 2 doses of montelukast
    (C) refer the patient to his pediatrician for evaluation and treatment
    (D) proceed with surgery after albuterol
    (E) perform surgery with sedation and analgesia with local infiltration

315. A 2-year-old child has suffered extensive burns to his head, neck, and torso. What percentage of his body has been affected?

   (A) 30% of total surface area
   (B) 35% of total surface area
   (C) 40% of total surface area
   (D) 45% of total surface area
   (E) 50% of total surface area

316. A neonate presents with respiratory distress, a scaphoid abdomen, and absent breath sounds on the left side of the chest. The incidence of this congenital lesion is 1 in 2000-5000 live births. Which one of the following statements is true?

   (A) Mortality in infants with this lesion is 50-70%.
   (B) 70% of all lesions involve the foramen of Bochdalek.
   (C) 30% of infants with this lesion have an accompanying congenital urologic abnormality.
   (D) 30% of infants with this lesion have an accompanying congenital cardiac lesion.
   (E) Approximately 5% of infants with this lesion present with symptoms of bowel obstruction.

317. A 3-month-old African-American baby is scheduled for elective repair of an inguinal hernia. He has an older brother with sickle cell anemia, but he has not had any diagnostic tests for sickle cell anemia. His hematocrit is 30%. This baby

   (A) almost certainly has sickle cell anemia
   (B) should receive a preoperative transfusion
   (C) should undergo a screening test for HbS prior to anesthesia
   (D) may undergo anesthesia safely without further testing
   (E) has a 50% chance of having sickle cell anemia

318. A 10-day-old infant, born at 27 weeks gestational age, weighing 1,100 g at birth, is noted to have clinical signs and symptoms of peritonitis and intestinal obstruction. The patient has had increasing oxygen requirements over the past 48 h, and has been becoming progressively more tachypneic. The patient is also thrombocytopenic, and has developed metabolic and respiratory acidosis. Which one of the following statements is true of this patient's likely diagnosis?

   (A) It is an anomaly found predominantly in premature infants.
   (B) Umbilical artery catheterization should be performed in order to monitor hematologic and metabolic abnormalities.
   (C) The mortality is about 50%.
   (D) Cardiovascular collapse usually occurs early in the course of the illness.
   (E) Metabolic abnormalities include hypoglycemia resulting from intestinal malabsorption.

319. A 4-year-old child requires postoperative intubation and sedation in the PICU. It is expected that the child will remain intubated for more than 1-2 d. Which one of the following is the least desirable medication to use for sedation for this period of time?

   (A) Midazolam
   (B) Morphine
   (C) Ketamine
   (D) Propofol
   (E) Dexmedetomidine

320. A 4-day-old, full term neonate presents for repair of imperforate anus. The baby has no other abnormalities. All of the following are true regarding transitional circulation in this patient EXCEPT

   (A) the patient's pulmonary vascular resistance has decreased relative to the pressures in utero
   (B) the patient's pressures on the left side of the heart have increased relative to the pressures in utero
   (C) completion of closure of the ductus arteriosus requires adequate arterial muscle tissue

(D) mechanical closure of the ductus arteriosus has occurred in this patient

(E) events during anesthesia may cause a return to fetal circulation

321. A 1-month-old infant, born at 35 weeks gestational age, presents for inguinal hernia repair. The patient no longer requires oxygen and no longer demonstrates episodes of apnea and bradycardia. A spinal anesthetic is performed with tetracaine and then the patient is positioned for surgery. During positioning the patient's legs are inadvertently raised up above the patient's torso. What is the most likely clinical sign that will be seen in the patient?

(A) A decrease in oxygen saturation
(B) Agitation or irritability
(C) Hypotension
(D) An increase in heart rate
(E) Loss of consciousness

322. A 2-year-old child (weight 13 kg) is scheduled for circumcision. The most suitable dose of local anesthetic for a dorsal penile block is

(A) bupivacaine 0.25% 8 mL
(B) lidocaine 1% 8 mL
(C) lidocaine 1.5% with epinephrine 1:200,000 8 mL
(D) bupivacaine 0.25% 15 mL
(E) bupivacaine 0.125% 15 mL

323. Preoperative assessment of a healthy pediatric patient shows the patient to be normotensive with a blood pressure of 82/54. What is the likely age of this patient?

(A) full term neonate
(B) 4 months
(C) 8 months
(D) 12 months
(E) 18 months

324. A 3-year-old healthy child presents preoperatively for elective repair of an umbilical hernia. The mother informs you that the child had 4 ounces of apple juice 2 h ago. You recommend

(A) to cancel surgery
(B) to delay surgery by 2 h
(C) to delay surgery by 4 h
(D) to delay surgery by 6 h
(E) to proceed with surgery now

325. In the delivery room, after birth, an infant is noted at 1 min to be blue, motionless and unresponsive, with minimal respiratory effort, and heart rate of 70 bpm. At 5 min after birth, the infant is centrally pink with blue extremities, demonstrates some flexion at the hips and slight grimacing to stimulation, still has minimal respiratory effort, and a heart rate of 80 bpm. Initial resuscitation should include all of the following EXCEPT

(A) oxygen
(B) radiant heat
(C) intubation
(D) glucose
(E) bicarbonate

326. A newborn has Apgar scores of 4 and 5 at 1 and 5 min, respectively, and requires resuscitation, including intubation, after birth. Which one of the following is the most significant factor associated with lack of closure of the ductus arteriosus in this patient?

(A) Increased Pa_{CO_2}
(B) Decreased Pa_{CO_2}
(C) Increased Pa_{O_2}
(D) Decreased Pa_{O_2}
(E) Increased pulmonary artery pressure

327. A 5-month-old infant is anesthetized for correction of an eye condition. Immediately after intubation, bilateral breath sounds and chest excursion are noted and there is 100% oxygen saturation with an F_{IO_2} of 0.5. After positioning for surgery, the oxygen saturation is noted to have dropped to 94%, no other changes having been made. The most likely cause for this fall in oxygen saturation is

(A) a kinked endotracheal tube
(B) bronchospasm
(C) migration of the endotracheal tube into the right mainstem bronchus
(D) inspissated secretions plugging the tube
(E) anesthesia machine failure

328. A 20-month-old child presents for removal of a swallowed foreign body. The child is crying intermittently, and is reluctant to separate from his father for any length of time. The child is drooling significantly and appears unable to swallow his secretions, but is not in respiratory distress. He complains of a sore throat. Which one of the following is the most appropriate premedication and route for this patient?

(A) Oral midazolam
(B) Nasal midazolam
(C) Rectal midazolam
(D) Oral fentanyl
(E) Oral ketamine

329. A neonate is noted to have a murmur. The patient is not cyanotic, but is noted to have dyspnea, tachypnea, and diaphoresis with eating. What is the most likely congenital cardiac defect?

(A) Atrial septal defect
(B) Ventricular septal defect
(C) Tetralogy of fallot
(D) Coarctation of the aorta
(E) Transposition of the great arteries

330. An infant is undergoing general anesthesia for pyloromyotomy. A rapid sequence induction was performed with propofol and succinylcholine. Anesthesia was maintained with sevoflurane in oxygen and air. After induction the patient was noted to be tachycardic. During the surgery, the patient is noted to become more tachycardic with a rise in end tidal CO_2, and an increase in temperature as measured with nasopharyngeal temperature probe. You are concerned that this could be malignant hyperthermia. Of the following signs and symptoms, which one is the most common first sign of malignant hyperthermia?

(A) Cyanosis
(B) Dark-colored urine
(C) Hypercarbia
(D) Arrhythmia
(E) Hot circle absorber

331. An 11-month-old, 10-kg infant presents for hypospadias repair. The child is otherwise healthy. An LMA is placed after induction and the patient is then ventilated with tidal volumes of 80 mL. What percentage of that volume is respiratory dead space in this patient?

(A) 5%
(B) 10%
(C) 20%
(D) 30%
(E) 40%

332. Your institution is evaluating various pediatric warming devices in order to choose the most effective for use in your operating room. Which one of the following statements is true of the available pediatric warming devices?

(A) When using radiant warmers, core temperature should be measured to prevent skin burns.
(B) Circulating water blankets are not very useful in children smaller than 10 kg due to the decreasing ratio of body surface area to body mass.
(C) A warm air mattress is the most useful device to keep a child warm.
(D) Use of heat moisture exchangers is an efficient way to increase a child's body temperature.
(E) Circulating water blankets work by convection and therefore, they should not be directly in contact with the skin.

333. A healthy 5-month-old presents for repair of an umbilical hernia. Induction of anesthesia is uneventful and surgical preparation and draping are completed. At incision it is noted that the patient's temperature is 34.9°C. The patient had a normal temperature in the preoperative area. The most important factor in the operating room contributing to the patient's current temperature is which one of the following?

(A) Body temperature on arrival to the operating room
(B) Room temperature
(C) Lack of a warming blanket
(D) Use of cold fluids
(E) Temperature of prep solutions

334. A neonate presents for repair of an inguinal hernia. The plan is for a spinal anesthetic. The parents are agreeable to a spinal but are concerned about injury to the infant's spinal cord. You explain to the parents the technique for spinal in a neonate and how to minimize the chance of injury to the spinal cord, emphasizing that the conus medullaris is located at which one of the following levels in the neonate?

(A) First lumbar vertebra
(B) Second lumbar vertebra
(C) Third lumbar vertebra
(D) Fourth lumbar vertebra
(E) Fifth lumbar vertebra

335. A 4-year-old previously healthy child presents for repair of a femur fracture. The plan is for an inhalational induction followed by placement of a peripheral IV and then intubation. Which one of the following is the most appropriate size uncuffed endotracheal tube for this child?

(A) 3.5 mm
(B) 4.0 mm
(C) 4.5 mm
(D) 5.0 mm
(E) 5.5 mm

336. An 18-month-old child presents for repair of tetralogy of Fallot. During the procedure, prior to cardiopulmonary bypass, the child's blood

pressure is noted to decrease over several minutes from 88/57 to 76/41. All of the following are true EXCEPT

(A) the patient's SpO$_2$ will likely decrease with this decrease in blood pressure
(B) phenylephrine is a useful medication to increase blood pressure in this patient
(C) epinephrine is a useful medication to increase blood pressure in this patient
(D) if the blood pressure continues to fall, the surgeon should be asked to apply pressure to the aorta.
(E) ephedrine is not a useful medication to increase blood pressure in this patient

337. A child is admitted with an incarcerated inguinal hernia. The child has nasal congestion and discharge, with a productive cough. The child is afebrile and lung sounds are clear to auscultation bilaterally. Which one of the following is the most appropriate way to proceed?

(A) The surgery should be cancelled.
(B) The surgery should be allowed to proceed, but the child should not be intubated.
(C) The child should be started on antibiotics, and the surgery should proceed.
(D) The surgery should proceed with careful monitoring.
(E) The patient should be operated on only under spinal anesthesia.

338. A neonate presents for repair of myelomeningocele. The neonate was born full term. All of the following are true regarding anesthetic technique and surgery for this patient EXCEPT

(A) supine position should be avoided and therefore the patient should be intubated in the lateral position
(B) succinylcholine may be used safely in this patient
(C) extubation at the conclusion of the surgery is desirable
(D) spinal anesthesia is a possible technique for this patient
(E) this patient will likely need a ventriculoperitoneal shunt

339. A 6-year-old, 24-kg child presents for a cyst removal. The child has been NPO since midnight and it is now 0800. What is this child's approximate fluid requirement for the fasting deficit?

(A) 190 mL

(B) 240 mL

(C) 380 mL

(D) 510 mL

(E) 580 mL

340. A 12-year-old patient with sickle cell disease presents for an exploratory laparoscopy and possible laparotomy. The patient is otherwise healthy and has not had a vaso-occlusive crisis in several months. Preparation of this patient for surgery should include all of the following EXCEPT

(A) transfuse to a hemoglobin level of 15 g/dL

(B) treat infection

(C) maintain good hydration

(D) provide good pulmonary care

(E) avoid stasis of blood flow

341. A 6-week-old baby born at 34 weeks gestation presents in the holding area for elective repair of an inguinal hernia. The parents believe that they will be taking their child home today after surgery. You inform them

(A) they may take their child home today

(B) the child may have to stay for several hours

(C) the surgery will be postponed until the child reaches 60 weeks postconceptual age

(D) the child will be admitted for 23 h of apnea monitoring

(E) the child will need apnea monitoring at home tonight

342. A 7-year-old, 35-kg girl is scheduled for excision of a large intraabdominal mass. Her starting hematocrit is 36% and the minimally acceptable hematocrit is 24%. How much blood could the patient lose before transfusion is necessary?

(A) 250 mL

(B) 450 mL

(C) 650 mL

(D) 950 mL

(E) 1100 mL

343. A 3-year-old child presents emergently for repair of an incarcerated inguinal hernia. The patient was recently diagnosed with hypothyroidism and started treatment less than one week ago. All of the following may be encountered in this patient while undergoing anesthesia EXCEPT

(A) hypothermia

(B) hypoventilation

(C) sensitivity to opioids

(D) small mouth and large tongue

(E) hyperkinetic myocardium

344. A 7-year-old patient with Down syndrome is admitted for dental extractions. Additional medical history includes well-controlled asthma. The patient had myringotomy and ear tubes in the past without problems. In providing anesthesia for this patient, which one of the following is true?

(A) Atropine should be avoided.

(B) Opioids should be avoided.

(C) Preoperative neck mobility should be documented.

(D) Intubation should be avoided.

(E) Neuromuscular blockers should be avoided.

345. A 5-year-old boy is admitted with an open eye secondary to severe globe laceration. He had eaten 1 h before his accident. General anesthesia is required for the repair. The intubation should be accomplished

(A) by an awake intubation

(B) after injection of 100 mg of succinylcholine

(C) after administration of rocuronium followed by succinylcholine

(D) after vecuronium administration

(E) after inhalation induction with sevoflurane

346. A 1-day-old child presents with coughing and choking at his first feed. Following investigation, a diagnosis of tracheoesophageal fistula (TEF) is made. Which one of the following statements is true?

(A) Esophageal atresia is associated with tracheoesophageal fistula in 10% of cases.

(B) Air leak through the fistula is minimized with paralysis.

(C) Postoperative intubation is necessary to protect the airway from aspiration.

(D) Sump suction is maintained in the esophageal pouch to lessen the risk of aspiration.

(E) 10% of infants with TEF have the associated anomalies of VATER syndrome.

347. Nonanesthetized newborns and infants rely on nonshivering thermogenesis to help maintain body temperature. All of the following are true of nonshivering thermogenesis EXCEPT

(A) it refers to the increased metabolism of brown fat

(B) brown fat is highly vascularized and contains an abundance of mitochondria

(C) brown fat metabolism results in up to 25% of the cardiac output being diverted through the brown fat

(D) brown fat comprises 25% of the infant's total body weight

348. A neonate develops respiratory distress soon after birth. A chest radiograph demonstrates hyperinflation of the left lung, with herniation across the midline and mediastinal shift, and atelectasis of the right lung. Which one of the following statements is true?

(A) The right lower lobe is most commonly affected in patients with this congenital malformation.

(B) Neonates with this congenital malformation usually present with cardiovascular collapse due to mediastinal shift.

(C) This congenital malformation coexists with congenital heart disease in about 50% of cases.

(D) Neonates with this congenital malformation should be treated with assisted ventilation as soon as possible in order to improve gas exchange.

(E) Differential diagnosis of this congenital malformation includes congenital cystic lesions and congenital diaphragmatic hernia.

349. A full term neonate is scheduled for inguinal hernia repair. The anesthetic plan is for spinal anesthesia. Which one of the following statements is true of spinal anesthesia in the neonate?

(A) It is suitable as the sole technique of anesthesia for procedures lasting 2 h or more.

(B) The apex of the conus medullaris is usually at L2-L3.

(C) Epinephrine should never be added to local anesthetics.

(D) Tetracaine 0.4 mg/kg is a suitable dose for subarachnoid block.

350. A newborn, born at 31 weeks gestational age, develops nasal flaring, chest retractions, and grunting soon after birth. Chest radiograph demonstrates diffuse atelectasis. The most likely diagnosis is

(A) bronchopulmonary dysplasia
(B) patent ductus arteriosus
(C) congenital lobar emphysema
(D) hyaline membrane disease
(E) tracheoesophageal fistula

351. A 32-year-old woman with recently diagnosed preeclampsia delivers a baby at 39 weeks gestational age. During labor and delivery, it was noted that the amniotic fluid was heavily stained with meconium. Apgar scores for this neonate are 7 and 8 at 1 and 5 min, respectively. Which one of the following statements is true?

(A) This neonate will most likely develop respiratory difficulties in the first few days of life.

(B) This neonate has a very high risk for developing radiographic evidence of pneumothorax.

(C) Meconium is best removed by suction via an endotracheal tube.

(D) Absence of meconium in the mouth and pharynx precludes the presence of meconium in the trachea.

(E) Meconium is an indication of fetal distress.

352. A neonate, who was born at 36 weeks gestational age with gastroschisis and has undergone staged reduction of the defect, presents for final closure in the operating room. When planning for fluid management for this patient, all of the following are important considerations for this patient EXCEPT

(A) maturation of renal function is more rapid in full term compared to preterm infants

(B) the glomerular filtration rate of this patient is less than 20% of the adult value

(C) the glomerular filtration rate does not affect the neonate's ability to handle free water

(D) the glomerular filtration rate reaches the adult value by about 1-2 years of age

(E) potassium excretion is much less efficient in neonates compared to adults

353. A 4-year-old child is brought to the emergency department at 1 a.m. She was put to bed in apparently good health, but awoke four hours later crying and having difficulty breathing. Physical examination reveals that the child is flushed, drooling, sitting upright, and has severe inspiratory stridor. Which one of the following statements is true?

(A) The most likely diagnosis is acute laryngotracheobronchitis.

(B) A possible diagnosis is croup.

(C) Rectal temperature should be checked.

(D) The child should be taken straight to the operating room for intubation/emergency tracheostomy.

(E) It is important to place an IV prior to induction in this patient.

354. A neonate undergoes inhalation induction with 7% sevoflurane. A peripheral IV is placed and the patient is then intubated. Soon after induction and intubation the patient is noted to be mildly hypotensive. The hypotension may be explained by the fact that the cardiac output

(A) may decrease significantly because of decreases in stroke volume

(B) is not very sensitive to changes in afterload

(C) is relatively insensitive to volume loading

(D) is reflected by a rightward shift of the cardiac function curve as compared to the adult

(E) may decrease significantly due to decreases in heart rate

355. A full term neonate presents for bilateral inguinal hernia repair. General anesthesia with an endotracheal tube is planned. All of the following are true of this patient's airway EXCEPT

(A) a 3.0-mm endotracheal tube is a suitable first choice for this patient

(B) pressures of 30 cm H_2O are usually required for adequate IPPV

(C) this patient's glottis is located at the level of C2

(D) positive pressure ventilation should be conducted at a rate of about 30-60 breaths per minute

(E) the narrowest part of this patient's airway is at the cricoid ring

356. A newborn presents for repair of omphalocele. All of the following are true of this defect EXCEPT

(A) it is a central midline defect
(B) it is a congenital defect originating in the first trimester of pregnancy
(C) it is usually associated with infection and loss of extracellular fluid
(D) it is associated with a high incidence of congenital abnormalities
(E) the herniated bowel is covered by the amnion

357. A newborn presents for repair of myelomeningocele. During maintenance of anesthesia, end tidal isoflurane is 0.9%. A colleague offering you a break comments on the end tidal isoflurane and expresses concern that the patient is not receiving adequate anesthesia. You explain that the concentration is adequate for the patient for all of the following reasons EXCEPT

(A) neonates have an immature nervous system
(B) neonates have an immature blood–brain barrier
(C) neonates have elevated progesterone levels
(D) neonates have elevated blood levels of β-endorphin
(E) neonates have immature liver function

358. A 10-month-old with septic arthritis presents for placement of a central venous catheter for a course of antibiotics. The patient has a peripheral IV in place. The patient is preoxygenated, undergoes IV induction followed by intubation. During intubation it is noted that the SpO_2 decreases from 100% to 86%. The reason for this rapid desaturation compared with adults is due to which one of the following?

(A) High respiratory rate
(B) High oxygen consumption

(C) Small endotracheal tube
(D) Small expiratory reserve volume
(E) Small tidal volume (TV)

DIRECTIONS: Use the following scenario to answer Questions 359-360: A 2-year-old child presents for repair of a ventricular septal defect. Preoperative evaluation reveals congestive heart failure, failure to thrive, and a pulmonary:systemic flow ratio greater than 2:1.

359. Which one of the following is the most appropriate induction technique?

(A) Halothane dialed to 6% on the vaporizer in 100% oxygen.
(B) Sevoflurane dialed to 6% on the vaporizer in 100% oxygen
(C) Propofol 5 mg/kg with fentanyl 2 mcg/kg
(D) Ketamine 2 mg/kg with fentanyl 2 mcg/kg

360. If shunt reversal occurs intraoperatively, which one of the following is an appropriate treatment?

(A) Ketamine
(B) α-adrenoceptor agonists
(C) 50% oxygen and 50% nitrous oxide
(D) High inhaled concentrations of volatile anesthetics

361. In a full term, 4-kg neonate, which one of the following is true regarding body fluid?

(A) Total body water (TBW) constitutes approximately 3 kg of this patient's weight.
(B) Extracellular fluid (ECF) accounts for approximately 2.5 kg of this patient's weight.
(C) Adipose tissue accounts for less than 1 kg of this patient's weight.
(D) Intracellular fluid accounts for approximately 2.5 kg of this patient's weight.

362. Fetal circulation is characterized by right to left shunting across the ductus arteriosus and the foramen ovale. Fetal circulation progresses to transitional circulation with birth that is characterized by which one of the following?

(A) Complete closure of the ductus arteriosus

(B) Complete closure of the foramen ovale

(C) Decreased pulmonary vascular resistance

(D) Decreased systemic vascular resistance

363. A 3-week-old neonate, born at 32 weeks gestational age presents for exploratory laparotomy for likely bowel obstruction. During the procedure vecuronium is used for muscle relaxation. After the initial dose of vecuronium given at induction, the patient was noted to be breathing spontaneously during preparation and draping for surgery. An additional dose of vecuronium was given prior to the start of surgery, and it was noted that the patient did not recover from this dose as rapidly as from the initial dose. Which one of the following explains the reason for the prolonged recovery from the second dose of muscle relaxant?

(A) Blood brain barrier

(B) Volume of distribution

(C) Albumin concentrations

(D) Metabolism

(E) α_1-acid glycoprotein concentrations

364. A 5-week-old, 4-kg infant presents for open pyloromyotomy. Electrolyte abnormalities were corrected preoperatively. The patient was born full term and is otherwise healthy. General anesthesia is induced with propofol 15 mg and rocuronium 6 mg. No opioid is administered and the surgeon injects local anesthesia at the incision site. At the conclusion of the case, neostigmine 0.1 mg and glycopyrrolate 0.02 mg are administered. The patient is awake, but appears weak and with spontaneous breathing has tidal volumes of 6-8 mL. All of the following could explain this patient's persistent weakness EXCEPT

(A) musculature is poorly developed

(B) muscle mass is less

(C) the myoneural junction is not well developed

(D) total body water is greater

(E) inadequate dose of neostigmine

365. At the conclusion of a gastroschisis repair, arrangements are made to transport the patient, intubated, to the ICU. The surgeon requests that the patient remains paralyzed and that you continue with controlled ventilation. Which one of the following is the best circuit to use for transport of this patient to the ICU?

(A) Mapleson A

(B) Mapleson B

(C) Mapleson C

(D) Mapleson D

(E) Mapleson E

366. During resuscitation of a newborn with an Apgar score of 2 at 2 min, sodium bicarbonate is administered. All of the following are potential side effects of sodium bicarbonate EXCEPT

(A) metabolic alkalosis

(B) hypernatremia

(C) hepatic necrosis if given through a venous catheter whose tip is in the liver

(D) hyperglycemia

(E) hyperosmolality

367. You are called to help evaluate a neonate who has presented to the emergency department with respiratory distress. The child is breathing >50 breaths per min and has sternal and subcostal retractions. All of the following contribute to increased work of breathing in this neonate EXCEPT

(A) overcoming elastic forces

(B) overcoming resistive forces

(C) laminar air flow

(D) increased respiratory rate

(E) radius of the infant's airway

368. During anesthesia for a previously healthy infant having a spica cast placed, you note that the patient periodically has mild desaturations that respond well to recruitment maneuvers. Which one of the following best explains why infants are prone to airway collapse and atelectasis?

(A) Closing capacity is greater than functional residual capacity.

(B) Closing capacity is greater than residual volume.

(C) Closing capacity increases with increased age.

(D) Closing capacity is greater than expiratory reserve volume.

(E) Closing capacity is greater than vital capacity.

369. An infant presents for emergent repair of coarctation of the aorta. The infant was born full term, had no problems after delivery and went home on day 2 of life. All of the following are associated with coarctation of the aorta EXCEPT

(A) ventricular septal defect

(B) bicuspid aortic valve

(C) Turner syndrome

(D) mitral valve abnormalities

(E) pulmonic stenosis

370. A 4-year-old child with a history of upper airway obstruction undergoes tonsillectomy and adenoidectomy. The child is otherwise healthy. The surgery and anesthesia are uneventful and the patient is extubated easily and without complication in the operating room at the conclusion of surgery. In recovery, the patient is noted to have symptoms consistent with postintubation laryngeal edema. The treatment for this should include all of the following EXCEPT

(A) inhalation of mist

(B) parenteral glucocorticoids

(C) nebulized racemic epinephrine

(D) sedation

(E) head up position

371. A 4-week-old, 4-kg child presents with several days of nonbilious, projectile vomiting and inability to tolerate feeds. The child was born full term, had no problems after birth and went home on day 2 of life. The patient has had decreased urine output and a metabolic panel demonstrates multiple metabolic derangements. The next step in management is

(A) proceed to the operating room for emergent repair of the lesion

(B) start an IV and give 20 mL/kg of lactated Ringer solution, then proceed to the operating room for repair of the lesion

(C) administer an IV solution containing bicarbonate ion

(D) admit the patient to the floor, start IV hydration, and check a metabolic panel several hours later

(E) administer an antiemetic such as ondansetron

DIRECTIONS: Use the following scenario to answer Questions 372-373: A 4-year-old child presents to the emergency department with acute onset of a high fever, sore throat, stridor, dysphagia, and drooling. The patient is sitting up and appears anxious.

372. The most likely diagnosis is

(A) laryngotracheobronchitis

(B) epiglottitis

(C) aspirated foreign body

(D) laryngeal papillomatosis

373. Treatment includes all of the following EXCEPT

(A) humidified oxygen

(B) glucocorticoids

(C) antibiotics

(D) intubation

(E) hydration

374. A 14-year-old girl presents to the emergency department with wheezing and hemoptysis. A history reveals solvent abuse. All of the following are possible physiological derangements in this patient due to solvent abuse EXCEPT

(A) hepatic dysfunction
(B) peripheral neuropathy
(C) renal dysfunction
(D) neutropenia
(E) methemoglobinemia

375. A 20-month-old child with a ventricular septal defect presents with dyspnea, tachypnea, and decreased activity tolerance. The patient is tachycardic with SpO_2 of 90-93%. All of the following are mechanisms that may explain this patient's presentation EXCEPT

(A) decreased pulmonary vascular resistance
(B) obstruction of the left main stem bronchus by the left atrium
(C) compression of bronchi by distended pulmonary vessels
(D) increased interstitial and alveolar lung water
(E) elevated left atrial pressure

376. A neonate with a diagnosis of Pierre Robin syndrome presents for anesthesia. Which one of the following preoperative evaluations is indicated in this patient in the setting of this syndrome?

(A) Cardiac echo
(B) Chest x-ray
(C) Renal ultrasound
(D) MRI of the spine
(E) Lumbar puncture

377. An infant born at 29 weeks is brought to the operating room for laser treatment for retinopathy of prematurity. The infant was intubated for the first two weeks of life. Which one of the following statements about retinopathy of prematurity (ROP) is true?

(A) ROP is related to incomplete vascularization of the retina at birth.
(B) ROP is directly related to the FIO_2.
(C) ROP occurs in 90% of extremely low birth weight infants.
(D) ROP occurs only after exposure to hyperoxemia for at least 24 h.
(E) ROP does not occur in full term infants.

378. A 5-year-old patient exhibits symptoms of subglottic edema in the recovery area. The patient has a history of mild asthma, abdominal pain, chronic constipation, and is obese. The patient underwent an upper endoscopy and colonoscopy under general anesthesia. The patient was intubated after three attempts and the remainder of the procedure and anesthesia was uneventful. All of the following statements about subglottic edema are true EXCEPT

(A) it is more common in pediatric than adult patients
(B) it may be prevented with use of steroid cream on the endotracheal tube
(C) it may be prevented by ensuring a leak around the endotracheal tube at <30 cm H_2O pressure
(D) it is associated with changes in position during the procedure
(E) it is associated with multiple attempts at intubation

379. A 2-week-old neonate presents for repair of tracheoesophageal fistula (TEF). The patient has proximal esophageal atresia and blind pouch and a distal TEF. All of the following statements are true EXCEPT that

(A) this patient has the most common type of TEF
(B) the incidence of TEF in premature babies is higher than in term infants
(C) it is contraindicated to pass an naso/orogastric tube in this type of TEF
(D) the congenital anomalies associated with TEF occur in 30% to 50% of patients
(E) the most common congenital defect associated with TEF is cardiac

380. A 2-year-old child presents for urgent rigid bronchoscopy for likely foreign body aspiration. The child was eating popcorn and was noted to have an episode of choking followed by intermittent coughing. The patient is currently not in any distress. On physical exam, there is diffuse wheezing over the right lung field and it is suspected that the food particle is located in the right mainstem bronchus. Which one of the following is true regarding the management of this child?

(A) After retrieval of the food particle from the right main stem bronchus, investigation of the left mainstem bronchus is still indicated in this case even if no particulate matter is found in the trachea.

(B) As the patient is not in any distress, the procedure should be postponed until the patient is appropriately fasted.

(C) Positive pressure ventilation should not be used as it may cause the foreign body to move more distally in the airway.

(D) The patient should be paralyzed during the removal of the foreign body in order to prevent coughing at that time.

(E) A propofol based total intravenous anesthetic technique should not be used as the patient may become apneic with this.

381. A 5-year-old boy with hypotonic cerebral palsy presents for gastrostomy tube revision. All of the following are complications associated with this disease EXCEPT

(A) joint contractures
(B) scoliosis
(C) cardiomyopathy
(D) epilepsy
(E) recurrent respiratory dysfunction

382. A neonate is found to have a congenital cardiac lesion. The child is cyanotic, has intracardiac shunting, but is not exhibiting signs or symptoms of congestive heart failure. Which one of the following is the most likely diagnosis for this child?

(A) Patent ductus arteriosus
(B) Total anomalous pulmonary venous drainage
(C) Atrioventricular canal
(D) Ventricular septal defect
(E) Transposition of the great arteries

383. A 3-year-old child presents with acutely raised intracranial pressure from a blocked ventriculoperitoneal shunt. Surgical alleviation of the problem is planned. Which one of the following is true regarding anesthesia for this patient?

(A) Premedication with intramuscular opioids is beneficial, minimizing further increases in intracranial pressure due to agitation and induction of anesthesia.

(B) Induction of anesthesia with intravenous ketamine 0.5-1 mg/kg is a suitable technique.

(C) Rapid sequence induction should be avoided.

(D) Concentrations of isoflurane of up to 1% result in minimal increases in cerebral blood flow.

DIRECTIONS: Use the following scenario to answer Questions 384-385: A 2-year-old child presents to the emergency department with low grade fever, cough, stridor, and dyspnea. The patient had been well until 3 d ago when she developed symptoms of an upper respiratory tract infection.

384. The most likely diagnosis is

(A) laryngotracheobronchitis
(B) epiglottitis
(C) aspirated foreign body
(D) laryngeal papillomatosis

385. Treatment typically includes which one of the following?

(A) Humidified oxygen
(B) Glucocorticoids
(C) Antibiotics
(D) Intubation

386. A 4-year-old child with Down syndrome presents for tonsillectomy and adenoidectomy for upper airway obstruction. The child had a ventricular septal defect repaired in the past that was well tolerated. The patient does not have any other congenital abnormalities and neck radiographs are negative for atlantoaxial subluxation. On arrival to the operating room, the child is very agitated and crying. You induce general anesthesia with sevoflurane dialed to 8% and then establish IV access. You note that the patient's heart rate has decreased from 140 bpm prior to induction to 102 bpm now. You administer propofol 4 mg/kg, fentanyl 1 mcg/kg, and rocuronium 0.5 mg/kg. Just after the patient has been intubated, you note that the heart rate is now 55 bpm with sinus rhythm. What is the most likely cause of this bradycardia?

   (A) Propofol
   (B) Fentanyl
   (C) Vagal response from direct laryngoscopy
   (D) Sevoflurane
   (E) Rocuronium

387. A 4-year-old child with a genetic syndrome presents for tonsillectomy for upper airway obstruction. The child has elfin facies, hypothyroidism treated with levothyroxine, neuro-developmental delay, repaired aortic stenosis and coarctation of the aorta, and generalized muscle weakness. This child most likely has which one of the following syndromes?

   (A) DiGeorge syndrome
   (B) Down syndrome
   (C) Trisomy 18
   (D) Trisomy 13
   (E) Williams syndrome

388. A 2-year-old boy is undergoing an inguinal hernia repair. As part of the anesthetic, you have discussed a single-shot caudal injection with the parents. After an uneventful inhalation induction of general anesthesia, the patient is positioned for the caudal injection. You palpate the patient's lower back to identify the site for injection. All of the following are landmarks that may be palpated to aid in performing a caudal injection EXCEPT

   (A) posterior superior iliac spine
   (B) sacrococcygeal ligament
   (C) sacral hiatus
   (D) sacral cornu
   (E) L4-L5 intervertebral space

389. A 5-year-old boy with cerebral palsy, a seizure disorder controlled with medication, mild asthma, and controlled gastroesophageal reflux presents for ventriculoperitoneal shunt revision. The patient is asymptomatic at this time, but increased head circumference was noted on routine exam. Regarding the anesthetic plan and medications to be used, all of the following are true for this patient EXCEPT

   (A) an inhalational induction is contraindicated for this patient
   (B) it is acceptable to use succinylcholine for this patient
   (C) this patient will require less propofol than a child without cerebral palsy
   (D) this patient will require less volatile agent than a child without cerebral palsy

390. You are planning to use normovolemic hemodilution in a 14-year-old patient who will be undergoing correction of idiopathic scoliosis. The child has a history of mild asthma, alpha-thalassemia, and has had surgery and anesthesia before without any problems. In determining weather of not it would be safe to use normovolemic hemodilution in this patient, you consider that all of the following are either relative or absolute contraindications to use of normovolemic hemodilution EXCEPT

   (A) sickle cell disease
   (B) sepsis
   (C) large amount of expected blood loss
   (D) moderate anemia
   (E) renal insufficiency

391. You are seeing a 12-year-old girl, accompanied by her mother, preoperatively prior to her having an arthroscopy of her knee. When asking about family history of problems with anesthesia, the patient's mother state that she has severe postoperative nausea and vomiting (PONV) after general anesthesia and she would like to know what the likelihood is that her daughter will have problems with this after her surgery today. You have a discussion with the patient and her mother about PONV. Which one of the following is true of PONV in pediatric patients?

(A) The incidence of PONV is inversely related to age.
(B) PONV is common in young children.
(C) The incidence of PONV in adolescents is less than that in adults.
(D) The type of surgery does not affect the incidence of PONV in children.
(E) The type of anesthesia used does not affect the incidence of PONV in children.

392. An 11-year-old girl presents for laparoscopic cholecystectomy. She is otherwise healthy. Carbon dioxide will be used for insufflation of the abdomen to facilitate surgery. All of the following are side effects of insufflation with carbon dioxide EXCEPT

(A) 25% increase in $PaCO_2$
(B) increased ventilation/perfusion mismatch
(C) increased pulmonary vascular resistance
(D) increased venous return
(E) increased systemic vascular resistance

DIRECTIONS (Questions 393-396): Each group of items below consists of lettered headings followed by a list of numbered phrases or statements. For each numbered phrase or statement, select the ONE lettered heading or component that is most closely associated with it. Each lettered heading or component may be selected once, more than once, or not at all.

(A) Apert syndrome
(B) Beckwith-Wiedemann syndrome
(C) Budd-Chiari syndrome
(D) Ehlers-Danlos syndrome
(E) Gilbert syndrome
(F) Kawasaki disease
(G) Peutz-Jeghers syndrome
(H) Reiter syndrome
(I) Sjögren syndrome
(J) Stevens-Johnson syndrome
(K) Sturge-Weber syndrome
(L) Turner syndrome
(M) von Hippel-Lindau syndrome

For each pathological state, select the associated disease or syndrome.

393. Pheochromocytoma

394. Coarctation of the aorta

395. Hypoglycemia

396. Seizures

Answers and Explanations

310. (C) Pierre-Robin syndrome is characterized by mandibular hypoplasia and pseudomacroglossia (the tongue protrudes from the mouth but is not actually enlarged). It is associated with high arched and cleft palate. Macroglossia is a feature of Beckwith Syndrome and Trisomy 21. Trisomy 21 is also associated with congenital cardiac defects. Goldenhar Syndrome is characterized by hemifacial microsomia, congenital cardiac defects, and vertebral instability. Treacher Collins syndrome is associated with micrognathia, choanal atresia, vertebral abnormalities, and cardiac defects. *(5:271-2)*

311. (B) Cold stress may cause hypoxia, acidosis, depletion of glycogen stores, hypoglycemia, pulmonary vasoconstriction and hypertension, shock, disseminated intravascular coagulation, altered drug metabolism, and delayed emergence. *(5:260)*

312. (D) The preterm infant is particularly susceptible to maternally-administered drugs. They have immature enzyme systems, an incomplete bundle branch block, and decreased protein for binding. The preterm infant metabolizes both ester and amide local anesthetics and is actually less sensitive to the CNS toxicity of lidocaine than full-term infants. *(5:1170, 1173)*

313. (E) The normal blood volume in a full term infant is 80 mL/kg (4 kg × 80 mL/kg = 320 mL). A premature infant has a higher volume per unit of weight, 90-100 mL/kg. *(5:258)*

314. (C) The patient's caregivers have been non-compliant with asthma medications. He clearly is not at baseline nor optimized for elective surgery. The patient should be referred to his pediatrician. He should be placed back on a maintenance dose of montelukast for a minimum of 2 weeks. Sedation and analgesia with local anesthesia is usually not a reasonable choice in this age group. *(5:131)*

315. (E) The head constitutes 10% of total body surface area in the adult, 13% in a 10- to 14-year-old child, 15% in a 5- to 9-year-old child, and about 19% in a 1- to 4-year-old child. The torso constitutes 26% of total body surface area in adults and children of all ages. *(5:1339)*

316. (E) The infant presents with symptoms consistent with congenital diaphragmatic hernia (CDH). Mortality in these patients is 20-50%. Approximately 90% of these herniations occur through the foramen of Bochdalek, although they may occur through the substernal sinus (foramen of Morgani). Less than 1% of cases have bilateral herniations. Affected infants present with respiratory distress related to lung hypoplasia. There is no known association with congenital urologic abnormalities. Cardiovascular abnormalities accompany CDH in about 23% of cases. Apart from congenital heart lesions, the increase in intrathoracic components may also cause obstruction of the inferior vena cava and decreased preload resulting in decreased cardiac output. Bowel obstruction may occur and cause the presenting symptoms in 5% of cases. *(5:1177)*

317. (D) This baby has a 25% chance of having sickle cell anemia. He is not anemic for his age and does not require a transfusion. Screening tests for HbS cannot differentiate between homozygous HbS patients and heterozygous HbS/HbA patients. Furthermore, even if this baby were homozygous for HbS, at three months of age he would have an amount of HbF (fetal hemoglobin) that would make a sickle crisis very unlikely. *(5:206-7, 274-5; 6:855-7)*

318.   **(D)** Necrotizing enterocolitis is a disease, not an anomaly. It occurs predominantly in premature infants under 1,500 g birth weight and the mortality is 10% to 30%. Associations include birth asphyxia, hypotension, systemic infections, early feeding, and umbilical vessel catheterization. Umbilical artery catheters are usually replaced with peripheral arterial catheters so that mesenteric blood flow is not compromised. Metabolic and hematologic abnormalities include hyperglycemia, thrombocytopenia, coagulopathy, and anemia. Infants usually lose vast quantities of fluid into the extracellular space leading to clinical shock and the need for cardiovascular support. *(5:1178-9)*

319.   **(D)** This patient will require prolonged intubation and sedation. Of all these medications, propofol is least desirable for this purpose due to the risk of developing propofol infusion syndrome (PRIS) that is characterized by lipemia, metabolic acidosis, hyperkalemia, and rhabdomyolysis that may progress to myocardial instability and refractory cardiovascular collapse. The risk of developing PRIS is more likely if the duration of use is greater than 48 h, and if the dose is greater than 5 mg/kg/h. *(3:122)*

320.   **(D)** At birth, the pulmonary vascular resistance decreases dramatically in response to lung expansion, increased pH, and a rise in alveolar oxygen tension. This reduces the pulmonary artery pressure and increases pulmonary blood flow. The increased amount of blood returning to the left atrium raises the pressures in the left atrium closing the foramen ovale. The ductus arteriosus closes primarily in response to increased oxygen tension. This is functional closure, but complete mechanical closure requires adequate arterial muscle and occurs after 10 d or more. Arterial hypoxemia, hypercarbia, or acidosis can all cause return to fetal circulation. *(5:250-1)*

321.   **(A)** Total spinal anesthesia, produced either with a primary spinal technique or secondary to an attempted epidural anesthetic, presents as respiratory insufficiency rather than as hypotension. The reason for this is the lack of sympathetic tone in neonates. The first indication of trouble is a decreasing oxygen saturation value rather than a decreasing blood pressure. *(3:879)*

322.   **(A)** Bupivacaine 0.25% is the most suitable choice of agent because it has the longest duration of action and may therefore give some postoperative pain relief. It may be used in doses up to 1 mL/kg, but a volume of 8 mL is quite sufficient. Epinephrine-containing solutions should not be used for this type of block because of the risk of ischemia to the penis. *(5:1188-9)*

323.   **(B)** *(5:257)*

324.   **(E)** Proceed with surgery. Most institutions allow a 2-h fast for clear liquids, 4-h fast for breast milk, 6-h fast for formula or a light meal, and an 8-h fast for solids. *(5:275-6)*

325.   **(D)** In the newborn infant, the glucose level is normally lower than in an older child, the value normally being 30 mg/dL. Resuscitation will require intubation, oxygen, heat, and bicarbonate. *(3:737-3)*

326.   **(D)** The major factor that causes closure of the ductus arteriosus is the Pao_2. Hypoxia in the early newborn period may delay closure. *(3:364)*

327.   **(C)** When a small but persistent change in oxygen saturation is noted, the position of the endotracheal tube must be reassessed. The other causes noted above are also possibilities in this situation but are less likely. *(5:1186-87)*

328. **(C)** An oral medication is not ideal in this situation because the child is having difficulty swallowing his secretions and will not likely be able to swallow an oral premedication. Furthermore, ketamine will increase salivation that is not desirable in this situation, and fentanyl may cause nausea and vomiting. Nasal midazolam burns on administration and is not as effective if the patient has been crying and has a significant amount of nasal secretions. *(5:1184)*

329. **(B)** This child has a noncyanotic lesion, but is exhibiting signs of congestive heart failure. Atrial septal defect and coarctation of the aorta are both noncyanotic lesions, but they are not typically associated with congestive heart failure. Tetralogy of Fallot and transposition of the great arteries are cyanotic lesions and are not typically associated with congestive heart failure. *(5:928-33)*

330. **(C)** Hypercarbia is often the first sign of malignant hyperthermia. Other early signs and symptoms include tachycardia, masseter muscle rigidity, and increased body temperature. *(5:1497)*

331. **(D)** The ratio of dead space to tidal volume, V_D/V_T, is approximately 30% and is the same in neonates and adults. This has always been one of the problems inherent in the equipment used for pediatrics. If the dead space of the equipment exceeds the infant's dead space, providing effective ventilation is more difficult. *(5:256, 1171)*

332. **(C)** When using radiant warmers, skin temperature should be measured and should not exceed 37°C to avoid skin burns. Circulating water blankets are most useful in children smaller than 10 kg due to the greater ratio of body surface area to body mass. Use of heat moisture exchangers is a way to add humidity to the circuit, but is not a useful way to raise body temperature. Circulating water blankets

work by conduction and for that reason they should not have direct contact with the patient's skin. *(3:1100)*

333. **(B)** Most operating rooms are kept at a low temperature for the comfort of the staff. The infant loses heat by conduction to the cold table, by convection from the cold air, by evaporation, and by radiation. Total heat loss by these mechanisms is as follows: radiation 39%, convection 34%, evaporation 24%, and conduction 3% of heat loss. Once the child is covered, some of the heat loss decreases, but if a body cavity is opened, more surface area is available for heat loss, particularly evaporative. *(5:259; 3:560-2)*

334. **(C)** The spinal cord extends to the L3 level in the newborn. When performing spinal anesthesia, this must be kept in mind. In the adult, the spinal cord ends at the level of the upper edge of L2. *(3:874-5)*

335. **(D)** The typical 4-year-old child should be intubated with an endotracheal tube of 5.0 mm internal diameter. This is determined by the formula 4 + age/4 for the internal diameter of the endotracheal tube. In this case, 4 + 4/4 = 5. *(3:1104-5; 5:1186)*

336. **(C)** This patient is experiencing an intraoperative hypercyanotic episode or "tet spell." With a decrease in blood pressure, right to left intracardiac shunting increases leading to a decrease in SpO_2. Methods to increase blood pressure involve increasing systemic vascular resistance such as administration of phenylephrine. Or, if blood pressure continues to decrease despite administration of phenylephrine, surgical pressure on the aorta to temporarily increase systemic vascular resistance and improve oxygenation is indicated. *(3:483-4)*

337. **(D)** The child who has an incarcerated hernia is going to need surgery to reduce the hernia lest strangulation occur. An upper respiratory

infection is not an ideal situation, but since the procedure must be done, it should be done with careful attention to detail, including monitoring. Since the infection is most likely viral, antibiotics should not be given. *(3:60-2; 5:1250)*

338. **(A)** The patient should be transported to the OR in the prone position but may be carefully positioned supine for intubation. Succinylcholine does not cause hyperkalemia in this patient population. Spinal anesthesia alone or in conjunction with general anesthesia may be performed. This involves placing local anesthetic into the open sac or injecting it into the sac. 90-95% of these patients have Arnold-Chiari malformation and will require a ventriculoperitoneal shunt. *(5:1180-1)*

339. **(D)** Maintenance fluids are calculated as follows: for the first 10 kg of body weight, the hourly fluid is 4 mL/kg. The second 10 kg of body weight has an hourly fluid need of 2 mL/kg. For each kg of body weight above 20 kg, the maintenance fluid need is 1 mL/kg. Thus for the 24-kg child in this question, the deficit fluid requirement is 510 mL (40 mL + 20 mL + 4 mL) × (8 h). *(3:164; 5:1187)*

340. **(A)** Studies have demonstrated that patients transfused to hemoglobin values of 10 g/dL have a lower incidence of sickle cell-related complications. Many centers are now transfusing, (direct, partial exchange, or exchange), to lower the percentage of sickle cells present. The preparation should strive for good hydration, good pulmonary care, and during the procedure, avoidance of hypothermia and stasis. *(3:182-6; 5:206-7)*

341. **(D)** Former premature infants are at risk for postanesthesia apnea if they are younger than 55-60 weeks postconceptual age (PCA). The incidence of apnea is inversely proportional to both gestational age and PCA. In addition, the risk of postanesthesia apnea increases if the infant has a history of apnea or if anemia is present. The incidence of apnea is quite low in ages greater than 45-50 weeks PCA, however, most institutions use 55 or 60 weeks PCA as a cutoff for day surgery in this population. *(3:64-6; 5:250)*

342. **(D)** To calculate the allowable blood loss (ABL), one must determine the patient's blood volume using 70 mL/kg body weight. The most common formula is listed below:

$$ABL = \text{Blood Volume} \times (Hct_I - Hct_T)/Hct_{mean}$$

where Hct_I = initial hematocrit, Hct_T = target hematocrit, Hct_{mean} = mean of Hct_I and Hct_T.

Thus,
$$ABL = (35 \text{ kg} \times 70 \text{ mL/kg}) \times 12/30$$
$$ABL = 2450 \text{ mL} \times 12/30 = 980 \text{ mL}$$

(5:258)

343. **(E)** Hypoventilation, hypothermia, and difficult intubation are potential problems for the anesthesiologist in treating the baby with myxedema. The children are sensitive to opioids. The mouth is of normal size, and the tongue may appear large. The heart is not hyperkinetic as in hyperthyroidism. *(3:549-50)*

344. **(C)** About 13% to 18% of patients with Down syndrome have atlantoaxial subluxation. These patients should have neck mobility evaluated prior to anesthesia to determine if any manifestations of cord compression develop with particular neck movement. Sensitivity to atropine was thought to be present in these children, but that was later disproved. The children can receive neuromuscular blockers and opioids if needed. Children with Down syndrome may be intubated if needed. However, care should be taken in all patients with Down syndrome to avoid excessive flexion, rotation or extension of the neck. *(3:996-7)*

345. (C) This is a difficult management problem. Both succinylcholine alone and an awake intubation will cause an increase in intraocular pressure, possibly causing expulsion of the contents of the globe. The use of succinylcholine preceded by a defasciculating dose of rocuronium will rapidly provide good intubating conditions and has not been reported to cause expulsion of the globe contents. The practitioner should be aware of the side effects and implications associated with the use of succinylcholine in children, especially young boys in whom hyperkalemic cardiac arrests have been reported. The use of this drug in pediatric patients has largely been restricted to emergencies. An inhalational induction may be required in the extremely uncooperative child, however, the risk of aspiration may be increased as compared to a rapid-sequence induction. *(3:694; 5:1223)*

346. (D) In 90% of cases, esophageal atresia is associated with TEF, but esophageal atresia may be an isolated occurrence. Careful positioning of the endotracheal tube with the tip just above the carina but below the fistula may help to minimize gastric insufflation, as will a gastrostomy. Positive pressure ventilation with or without paralysis is likely to increase the air leak through the fistula but is often necessary. Early extubation after surgery is desirable because it prevents prolonged pressure of the endotracheal tube on the suture line. Constant sump suction from the upper esophageal pouch decreases the accumulation of saliva and reduces the potential for aspiration. 30-50% of these infants have the associated anomalies of VATER syndrome. *(3:755-7; 5:1179-80)*

347. (D) Nonshivering thermogenesis is an increase in metabolic heat production that is not associated with muscle activity. It primarily involves the metabolism of brown fat that is highly vascularized and gets its brown color from the abundance of mitochondria present. Brown fat comprises 2-6% of the infant's total body weight. Up to 25% of the cardiac output is diverted through the brown fat to allow for direct warming of the blood. *(3:562-3)*

348. (E) Congenital lobar emphysema most commonly affects the left upper lobe but may involve the whole lung. It usually presents with progressive respiratory failure but mediastinal shift and cardiovascular collapse may occur. Anesthetic care is aimed at minimizing expansion of the emphysema; spontaneous respiration should be maintained if possible until the thorax is open, low peak inspiratory pressures should be used if assisted ventilation is required, and nitrous oxide should be avoided. Cardiac defects coexist in about 15% of patients. *(3:287, 760)*

349. (D) The duration of any spinal anesthetic drug is shorter in the neonate than the adult, and for this reason epinephrine is usually added. However, even with tetracaine 0.4-0.5 mg/kg with epinephrine the block usually lasts only about 90 min, therefore spinal anesthesia is unsuitable as the sole technique for longer procedures. The spinal cord often ends as low as L3-L4 in neonates so blocks should be performed at L4-L5 or L5-S1 in patients of this age. *(3:877-80; 5:1189)*

350. (D) This presentation is most consistent with hyaline membrane disease. Bronchopulmonary dysplasia occurs later and is a result of exposure to high levels of oxygen and ventilation therapy. Patent ductus arteriosus presents with symptoms of congestive heart failure. Congenital lobar emphysema presents with progressive respiratory failure, unilateral thoracic hyperexpansion, atelectasis of the contralateral lung, and possible mediastinal shift. Tracheoesophageal fistula presents with excessive oral secretions, regurgitation of feedings, and occasionally respiratory distress. *(3:748-9, 755, 760)*

351. (C) Respiratory difficulties occur in about 15% of cases. If the airway is not suctioned adequately before or shortly after the onset of breathing, meconium in the airways will move distally into the small airways and alveoli, causing respiratory difficulties and intrathoracic gas leaks. Fortunately, these gas leaks are usually small, but large pneumothoraces can occur in about 10% of cases. Meconium is best removed by endotracheal intubation and suction using a specially designed device. It is also useful to suction the stomach to remove meconium that might be regurgitated and aspirated later. Meconium is not an indication or cause of fetal distress. Rather it reflects a fetus with a mature intestinal tract. *(5:247-8; 3:21)*

352. **(C)** Renal function is markedly diminished in the neonate because of low perfusion pressure and immature glomerular filtration and tubular function. The ability to handle antibiotics (largely excreted by glomerular filtration) is therefore reduced. Glomerular filtration rate is about 20 mL/min/1.73 m² at birth (adult value ≈ 120) but develops rapidly thereafter reaching near complete maturation at 5 months of age and complete maturation at 1 to 2 years. However, maturation may be delayed in premature infants. Neonates are much less able to conserve or excrete free water, and they are much less efficient at excreting potassium loads than adults. Therefore, the normal range of serum potassium is greater in neonates compared to adults. *(3:569-70; 5:252)*

353. **(D)** The most likely diagnosis is acute epiglottitis that characteristically has a swift onset without a preceding upper respiratory tract infection. The differential diagnosis includes acute laryngotracheobronchitis (slower onset over days, not hours) and inhaled foreign body. Croup appears typically in younger children, age 3 months to 3 years, 2-3 d after a respiratory tract infection. The clinical presentation is a patient with stridor, dyspnea, and a "barking cough." This is a true pediatric emergency, and securing the airway is the first priority. The child is quite toxic, unable to swallow her own saliva, and has severe stridor. The child should not undergo any procedure that might provoke crying and complete obstruction of the airway (such as inserting a thermometer into the rectum or insertion of an IV line). Once facilities are ready for emergency intubation in an OR setting, and tracheostomy should this fail, the child should undergo general anesthesia and intubation. *(5:1230-1)*

354. **(E)** The myocardial structure of the heart, particularly the volume of cellular mass devoted to contractility, is significantly less in the neonate than in the adult. These differences and others produce a leftward displacement of the cardiac function curve and less compliant ventricles. This accounts for the tendency toward biventricular failure, sensitivity to volume loading, poor tolerance to increased afterload, and rate-dependent cardiac output. *(5:251, 1171.)*

355. **(B)** Positive pressure ventilation should normally be commenced at a rate of 30 to 60 breaths per minute and a PEEP of 1-3 mm Hg maintained. Most asphyxiated neonates do not have lung disease and rarely require inflation pressures greater than 25 cm H₂O. The glottis is at C2 in infants and C4-5 in adults. The narrowest part of the infant's airway is the cricoid cartilage and remains this way until puberty at which time the narrowest part of the airway is the glottis. *(5:250, 254-5)*

356. **(C)** Omphalocele and gastroschisis should not be confused. Omphalocele is a midline defect, whereas in gastroschisis the herniated bowel is to the side of the umbilical cord. Between the 5th and 10th week of fetal life, abdominal contents are extruded into the extraembryonic coelom. Failure of part of these contents to return to the abdomen at about week 10 results in an omphalocele that is covered by a membrane, the amnion. This protects the abdominal contents from infection and loss of extracellular fluid. In contrast, gastroschisis develops later in fetal life. It results from interruption of the omphalomesenteric artery at the base of the umbilical cord. The gut herniates out through this tissue defect and the degree of herniation may be slight, or almost all of the abdominal contents may be outside the peritoneal cavity. The intestines and viscera are not covered by any membrane and so are highly susceptible to infection and fluid loss. There is a high incidence of other congenital abnormalities with omphalocele but not with gastroschisis. *(5:1178)*

357. **(E)** The neonate has an immature central nervous system with attenuated responses to nociceptive cutaneous stimuli. These responses mature in the first few months of an infant's life, along with an increase in MAC. Progesterone has been shown to reduce the MAC of the pregnant mother. The newborn infant has elevated progesterone levels, and animal studies have suggested that these are related to reduced MAC values. High concentrations of β-endorphin are present in the first few days of postnatal life and may cross the immature blood–brain barrier of the neonate, thus increasing the pain threshold and reducing MAC values. Liver function does not affect MAC in neonates. *(5:1171)*

358. **(B)** The oxygen consumption in neonates and infants, at 7 mL/kg, is nearly double that of adults. In combination with a small dynamic FRC, desaturation during apnea occurs much faster as compared to adults. *(5:355-6)*

359. **(D)** The preoperative evaluation suggests that this child's VSD is large and that there may be problems encountered on induction of anesthesia. Only low concentrations of potent inhalational anesthetic agents can be tolerated by these patients without significant systemic hypotension. Therefore, high inspired concentrations of halothane or sevoflurane or high dose propofol for induction are probably less safe than an induction with intravenous agents such as ketamine and fentanyl that maintain systemic arterial pressure. It may also be important to use an F_{IO_2} of less than 1.0 in order to avoid a rapid decrease in pulmonary vascular resistance and subsequently increased left-to-right shunting. *(3:479-80)*

360. **(B)** If right ventricular pressures are close to systemic pressures, relatively mild systemic hypotension (such as during induction of anesthesia) may cause the shunt to reverse (now becoming right-to-left) with systemic desaturation and further myocardial dysfunction. If shunt reversal does occur, 100% oxygen and use of an α-adrenergic agonist such as phenylephrine to increase systemic vascular resistance usually results in resumption of left-to-right shunting. *(5:934)*

361. **(A)** TBW accounts for ≈ 70-75% of weight at birth, and falls to ≈ 65% of weight by the age of 1 year. TBW is divided into two compartments: ICF and ECF. In the full term neonate ECF and ICF each constitutes ≈ 40% of weight. Adipose tissue affects water content. It accounts for roughly 16% of a newborn's weight and ≈ 23% of weight in a one-year-old. *(5:1170)*

362. **(C)** Pulmonary vascular resistance decreases with breathing room air, lung expansion, improved oxygenation, and clamping of the umbilical cord. Functional closure of the foramen ovale and ductus arteriosus occurs with birth, but anatomical closure takes up to 72 h for the foramen ovale and weeks for the ductus arteriosus. With birth, systemic vascular resistance increases. *(3:364; 5:250-1)*

363. **(B)** Blood brain barrier is immature in neonates slowing some medications greater access to the brain. Total body water is greater in the infant, making the apparent volume of distribution larger. The increased apparent volume of distribution results in diluted concentrations of parenterally administered medications, and explains why some medications must be given in larger doses to achieve therapeutic effect. Neonates have an immature neuromuscular system. Therefore, the first dose of neuromuscular blocker may have the same effect and duration in a child as in an adult. However, due to the larger apparent volume of distribution, subsequent doses may have a prolonged duration of action. The albumin and α_1-acid glycoprotein concentrations are lower, leading to more unbound drug available to bind to receptors. The immaturity of the liver leads to decreased drug metabolism of some drugs. *(5:1171-2)*

364. **(E)** Lower doses of muscle relaxant are needed for the neonate because of poorly developed musculature, smaller muscle mass, and an immature myoneural junction. The greater total body water causes a dilutional effect that leads to a requirement for larger doses. This patient may have up to 0.28 mg of neostigmine. *(3:125, 131)*

365. **(D)** The Mapleson D system is the most efficient circuit for controlled ventilation. It may also be used for spontaneous ventilation, though it is not as efficient as the Mapleson A system is for spontaneous ventilation. *(5:638-40)*

366. **(D)** Administration of sodium bicarbonate to a newborn may increase the PaO$_2$ through a decrease in pulmonary vascular resistance if the pH is increased above 7.10-7.20. Sodium bicarbonate is very hypertonic; care must be taken to avoid liver damage from injection into the liver. Hypernatremia, hyperosmolality, hypercapnia, and metabolic alkalosis are all potential side effects. *(3:840-1)*

367. **(C)** The work of breathing involves overcoming both elastic and resistive forces. The neonate's chest wall is largely cartilaginous and therefore, highly compliant. This promotes chest wall collapse when work of breathing requires more negative intrathoracic pressure as evidenced by retractions. As the child breathes very fast, the work is increased, since turbulent, not laminar, flow is more prevalent. Resistance to flow is governed by Poiseuille's Law:

$$\text{Resistance} = \frac{8vl}{\pi r^4}$$

where r is the radius of the tube, in this case, the airway, l is the length of the tube, and v is the viscosity of the gas. *(5:255)*

368. **(A)** Closing capacity (CC) is greater than functional residual capacity (FRC) at birth and gradually decreases from infancy to adulthood at which time CC is less than FRC. As CC is greater than FRC in infants, airway closure may occur even during normal tidal volumes resulting in atelectasis. *(5:255)*

369. **(E)** Coarctation may occur in isolation or may be associated with all of the lesions listed except pulmonic stenosis, and it is associated with Turner syndrome. *(3:303, 483)*

370. **(D)** Posttraumatic or postintubation croup is treated with head up position, mist inhalation, parenteral glucocorticoids, and nebulized racemic epinephrine. Glucocorticoids are not immediately effective, and some question their use at all, but they are usually given. Sedation of the child is based on the decision of whether or not the child's anxiety may be contributing to the problem. Sedation should not be a routine order. *(5:576, 1286)*

371. **(D)** Pyloric stenosis is not a surgical emergency. Infants may be significantly hypovolemic, hypokalemic, hypocalcemic, and alkalotic. It is necessary to rehydrate the patient and correct the metabolic abnormalities prior to proceeding with surgery. Administering an antiemetic is not indicated in this situation, as the cause of vomiting is mechanical obstruction to gastric emptying. *(3:761-2)*

372. **(B)** This is the classic presentation of epiglottitis. The child is typically sitting up to allow better handling of the secretions. Since the child has pain on swallowing, drooling is common. The onset is sudden, and the child is febrile. *(5:1230-1)*

373. **(B)** The treatment of epiglottitis is primarily securing the airway in a controlled environment, usually the operating room, with a surgeon available to provide a surgical airway. As the cause of this is bacterial, antibiotics are indicated. Hydration and humidified oxygen are desirable, but glucocorticoids are not indicated. *(3:676; 5:1230-1)*

374. **(D)** Patients who have a history of solvent abuse may have a peripheral neuropathy (common after prolonged exposure to hexane or methyl ethyl ketone). Halogenated hydrocarbons may cause acute or chronic hepatic and renal disease, depending on the amount inhaled and the duration of the abuse. Neutropenia is unlikely. Methemoglobinemia may be caused by abuse of amyl nitrate. *(5:326)*

375. (A) Excessive pulmonary blood flow is common in patients with congenital heart disease. Increased pulmonary artery pressure and blood flow can limit gas exchange by several mechanisms leading to the symptoms described in this patient. Distended pulmonary vessels may compress bronchi and increase work of breathing. Increased venous return distends the left atrium that may compress the left main stem bronchus. Increased pulmonary blood flow and pressure along with elevated left atrial pressure cause pulmonary venous congestion. Lung compliance decreases and airway resistance increases. Areas of the lung with atelectasis and shunting then lead to desaturation even in this child with an noncyanotic congenital lesion. *(5:932)*

376. (A) The Pierre Robin syndrome is usually not associated with renal, lung, or vertebral problems. Children with this syndrome may have congenital cardiac disease and a preoperative cardiac echo for nonemergent surgery is indicated. *(5:249)*

377. (A) There is controversy concerning the role of oxygen in retinopathy of prematurity. The retina is at risk until the vascularization is complete at about 44 weeks. It is not related to FIO_2 but is related to oxygen tension and also to other factors as well. It occurs in 50% of extremely low birth weight infants. Retinopathy has been reported in full-term infants and in premature infants never given oxygen therapy. *(3:738)*

378. (B) Subglottic edema is more common in pediatric patients, especially between the ages of 1 and 4 years old. It may be prevented by the use of an appropriate-sized endotracheal tube and ensuring an adequate leak around the tube and by minimizing intubation attempts. The use of creams on the tube has not been shown to be effective. It is associated with changes in position during the procedure and there is increased risk with positions other than supine. *(3:253)*

379. (C) This type of TEF accounts for 80-90% of cases. Esophageal atresia and TEF are often associated with other congenital abnormalities,

in particular the VATER association (vertebral abnormalities, imperforate anus, tracheoesophageal fistula, radial aplasia, and renal abnormalities), cardiac defects, and duodenal atresia. Of these, cardiac is the most common. Infants with TEF should be maintained prone or in the lateral position with a 30° head-up tilt to decrease the risk of pulmonary aspiration and a large bore naso/orogastric tube should be placed to help prevent aspiration. *(5:1179-80)*

380. (A) The left mainstem bronchus should also be investigated as aspirated food can crumble and can potentially be located in both bronchi even in the absence of wheezing on the left. Although the patient is in no distress, organic matter, such as popcorn or peanuts, tends to swell and fragment or crumble over time, making retrieval even more difficult. Spontaneous ventilation is usually preferred when possible, but if ventilation and oxygenation are inadequate, assisted and even controlled ventilation may be necessary. With the actual removal of the foreign body, it is important that the patient does not cough or respond in any other way that may cause the surgeon to drop the foreign body. However, this can be accomplished without muscle relaxation if the child is deeply anesthetized. There are many possible techniques that may be used for a case like this including total intravenous anesthesia with propofol. The patient may become apneic, but this is possible with any of the other techniques as well. *(3:679-80, 774-5)*

381. (C) Cardiomyopathy is not a complication associated with hypotonic cerebral palsy. *(3:492-3)*

382. (E) Newborn infants with significant congenital heart disease commonly present with either cyanosis or congestive cardiac failure. Cyanosis occurs when there is a significant degree of intracardiac shunting. Transposition of the great arteries always results in cyanosis and sometimes presents with congestive heart failure. The remainder of the lesions rarely results in cyanosis. Patent ductus arteriosus sometimes results in congestive heart failure. Total anomalous pulmonary venous drainage, atrioventricular canal, and ventricular septal defect frequently present with congestive heart failure. *(3:928-33)*

383. **(D)** In the presence of increased intracranial pressure (ICP), these patients may be vomiting and are at risk for pulmonary aspiration. Therefore, preoperative sedation with opioid analgesics may be unsafe and a rapid sequence induction (despite the risks of further raising ICP) may be the procedure of choice. Ketamine would be a poor choice in this situation because it can lead to intracranial hypertension and it also increases $CMRO_2$. If intravenous access is a problem, inhalational induction with halothane or sevoflurane and cricoid pressure may be performed but is less desirable. Once induction is complete, the trachea intubated, and intravenous access secured, anesthesia may be maintained with intravenous agents or low concentrations of isoflurane. Of the commonly used potent volatile anesthetic agents, isoflurane appears to produce the smallest increase in cerebral blood flow for the depth of anesthesia produced and is usually used freely in neurosurgical procedures up to a minimum alveolar concentration of about 1. *(5:873-4)*

384. **(A)** This is the classic presentation of laryngotracheobronchitis (croup). These patients have a gradual onset of symptoms including a barking cough, a low-grade (if any) fever, and a subglottic obstruction. *(5:1230-31)*

385. **(A)** Treatment of laryngotracheobronchitis is primarily medical and supportive and includes humidified oxygen, hydration, and nebulized racemic epinephrine. The use of glucocorticoids is controversial, and antibiotics are not indicated as the etiology is viral and not bacterial. Intubation is usually not necessary and is only indicated for respiratory fatigue and/or cyanosis. *(3:676; 5:1230-1)*

386. **(D)** High inspired concentrations of sevoflurane may cause bradycardia, particularly in susceptible patients. This patient is at risk for this effect due to the diagnosis of Down syndrome and due to having had a ventricular

septal defect repair in the past. Propofol and rocuronium are more likely to cause tachycardia. Fentanyl may cause bradycardia but is unlikely to cause this degree of bradycardia at the dose used. A vagal response could cause bradycardia, but the heart rate was already decreasing making sevoflurane the most likely cause. *(3:303, 476; 5:1187)*

387. **(E)** Williams syndrome is a congenital gene deletion syndrome typically involving the long arm of chromosome 7. Features of this syndrome include elfin facies, outgoing personality, endocrine abnormalities such as hypercalcemia and hypothyroidism, neurodevelopmental delay, growth deficiency, muscular weakness, valvular and supravalvular aortic stenosis, coarctation of the aorta, abnormalities of the origin of the coronary arteries, diffuse narrowing of the abdominal aorta, and renal artery stenosis. *(3:303-4)*

388. **(B)** The needle pierces the sacrococcygeal ligament to enter the epidural space, but this is not a structure that is palpated in performing a caudal injection. *(3:880-1)*

389. **(A)** Although these patients often have decreased ability to swallow secretions, and have gastroesophageal reflux, there is no evidence that a rapid sequence induction is safer. Succinylcholine may be used safely in these patients because the muscles of these patients have never been denervated. These patients require less propofol and volatile agent than otherwise healthy children. *(3:652)*

390. **(C)** Normovolemic hemodilution is contraindicated in patients with sickle cell disease, sepsis, and compromised function of any major organ that may be affected by significant changes in perfusion and oxygenation. Patients with moderate anemia are not good candidates for this technique because not enough red cells can be removed from these patients to make the technique effective. This technique is specifically indicated in surgeries in which the amount of blood loss is expected to be greater than half the child's blood volume. *(3:218)*

391. **(A)** The incidence of PONV in children is inversely related to age. It is not common in very young children, then it increases throughout childhood, and in adolescents the incidence is greater than that in adults. Certain surgeries have a higher incidence of PONV, including tonsillectomy, strabismus repair, hernia repair, orchiopexy, microtia repair, and middle ear procedures. The type of anesthetic does influence the incidence of PONV. For example, propofol-based anesthesia when used in procedures with a high incidence of PONV has been shown to result in a much lower incidence of PONV than isoflurane-based anesthesia. *(3:1017-8)*

392. **(D)** Venous return decreases with pneumoperitoneum contributing to decreased cardiac output. *(3:587-9)*

393. **(M)** In addition to pheochromocytoma, the syndrome is associated with angiomas of the retina and hemangioblastomas of the cerebellum and/or spinal cord, and cysts in various organs including the kidney and pancreas. *(6:793)*

394. **(L)** In addition to gonadal dysgenesis, Turner syndrome is associated with coarctation of the aorta. *(5:271; 6:1925)*

395. **(B)** The syndrome is associated with overproduction of insulin-like growth factor II that leads to chronic and severe hypoglycemia. *(5:293, 1261)*

396. **(K)** The syndrome is associated with vascular tumors of the face (port-wine stain) and severe seizures. *(5:1223)*

CHAPTER 17

Anesthesia for Miscellaneous Procedures
Questions

DIRECTIONS (Questions 397-456): Each of the numbered items or incomplete statements in this section is followed by answers or by completions of the statement. Select the ONE lettered answer or completion that is BEST in each case.

397. A 58-year-old, 5'8", 138-kg male is brought emergently to the operating room for exploration of an open tibial fracture with vascular compromise under general anesthesia. Vital signs are BP 112/64, HR 94, RR 22, SpO_2 96%. A rapid sequence induction with propofol, fentanyl, and succinylcholine is performed. Upon loss of consciousness, the patient desaturates precipitously, requiring positive pressure ventilation to maintain oxygenation. The LEAST effective means of preventing this desaturation would be preoxygenation with

(A) the application of positive pressure ventilation

(B) four vital capacity breaths with 100% O_2 within 30 sec

(C) 100% O_2 for 3 min

(D) placement of the patient's head, neck, and upper body in the "ramped" position

(E) placement of the patient in the reverse Trendelenburg position

398. A 53-year-old, 5'10" 142-kg patient underwent an 8-h excision of a pancreatic cyst under combined general/epidural anesthesia. The epidural, placed at the T8 level, was dosed preoperatively with good effect. In the PACU, the patient has no incisional pain, but complains of severe bilateral buttock, upper back, and shoulder pain. On physical examination, there is tenderness to palpation of the affected areas. The most appropriate initial step in management should be to

(A) begin broad spectrum antibiotics

(B) add an anti-inflammatory to patient's analgesic regimen

(C) remove the epidural catheter and culture the tip

(D) seek a consult from the neurology service

(E) assure adequate volume repletion

399. You are asked to evaluate a 47-year-old male with advanced alcoholic cirrhosis, now placed on the liver transplant waiting list. In reviewing his chart, you note that he has a MELD score of 13 and is listed as a Child-Pugh class B. The criterion that is common to both classification models is

(A) serum creatinine

(B) degree of ascites

(C) serum bilirubin

(D) serum albumin

(E) severity of encephalopathy

DIRECTIONS: Use the following scenario to answer Questions 400-401: A 28-year-old, 5'3", 124-kg woman, who underwent Roux-en-Y gastric bypass surgery four months ago, presents to your preoperative testing unit for evaluation prior to a scheduled laparoscopic cholecystectomy. You notice her gait seems unsteady as she walks into your office, and that her handshake seems weak. On questioning, she describes a several week history of vomiting and muscle weakness that she attributes to a recent flu-like illness. On exam she exhibits both a slight foot and wrist drop bilaterally. Medical history is otherwise unremarkable.

400. All of the following conditions should be part of your differential diagnosis EXCEPT

(A) Wernicke's encephalopathy
(B) vitamin A deficiency
(C) Guillain-Barre syndrome
(D) APGARS neuropathy
(E) vitamin B_{12} deficiency

401. The single best predictor of problematic intubation in this patient is

(A) Mallampati class 4 airway
(B) body mass index
(C) neck circumference
(D) history of obstructive sleep apnea
(E) thyromental distance

DIRECTIONS: Use the following scenario to answer Questions 402-403: A 64-year-old, 5'11", 156-kg male is brought to the operating room for an emergent laparoscopic appendectomy under general endotracheal anesthesia. Induction is performed with midazolam, sufentanil, propofol, and succinylcholine.

402. The anesthetic agent that should be dosed according to lean body weight is

(A) propofol
(B) succinylcholine
(C) sufentanil
(D) midazolam

403. Anesthesia is maintained with O_2, N_2O, desflurane and sufentanil. Within 10 min of insufflation of the abdomen, the patient's oxygen

saturation has dropped slowly from 97% to 92%. The most appropriate initial step in management should be to

(A) increase tidal volume from 7 mL/kg to 10 mL/kg
(B) place the patient in reverse Trendelenburg position
(C) ask the surgeon to decrease the intraabdominal pressure by releasing carbon dioxide
(D) add 5 cm H_2O of PEEP
(E) change the ventilation mode from volume control to pressure control

404. A 52-year-old, 5'4", 118-kg male, previously healthy, is scheduled for excision of a pancreatic cyst. Prior to surgery, he undergoes pulmonary function testing. When comparing the results of this patient's study with those of a 5'8", 84-kg male with a similar medical history, one would expect the greatest difference in

(A) RV
(B) FRC
(C) TLC
(D) FVC
(E) FEV_1

405. You are called to the PACU to evaluate your patient, a previously healthy 51-year-old female who underwent an uneventful subtotal thyroidectomy for newly diagnosed papillary carcinoma that finished three hours ago, and who now appears to be in respiratory distress. On arrival, you immediately note her stridorous inspirations, her sternal retractions, and her agitation. The most likely cause of her symptoms is

(A) tracheomalacia
(B) unilateral recurrent laryngeal nerve injury
(C) hypocalcemia
(D) incisional hemorrhage
(E) bilateral recurrent laryngeal nerve injury

DIRECTIONS: Use the following scenario to answer Questions 406-407: A 67-year-old male with a diagnosis of acute cholangitis is brought to the operating room urgently for endoscopic sphincterotomy and drainage of the gallbladder. His past medical history is significant for a recent diagnosis of Graves disease for which he was started on antithyroid therapy 2 weeks before admission. He is now febrile (38.2°C) and tachycardic (104 bpm), with oxygen saturation of 96% and a stable blood pressure. He received antibiotics one hour prior to arriving in the operating room.

406. The laboratory value that will yield the most information about the patient's response to his antithyroid treatment is

(A) TSH

(B) free T3

(C) unbound T4

(D) radioiodine uptake

(E) total T3

407. After an uneventful general anesthetic with endotracheal intubation, the patient was transferred to the PACU. Initial vital signs included a HR 108, BP 94/48, SpO_2 98%, and T 38.4°C. You order a fluid bolus of 500 mL of crystalloid. One hour later, you are called to evaluate the patient who has just vomited and is now agitated, confused, and diaphoretic, with a temperature of 39.3°C, HR 152 bpm with ventricular ectopy, BP 86/42, SpO_2 97%. The least appropriate medication for initial management of this patient is

(A) methimazole

(B) aspirin

(C) dexamethasone

(D) cholestyramine

(E) propranolol

DIRECTIONS: Use the following scenario to answer Questions 408-409: A 46-year-old male is undergoing orthotopic liver transplant for end-stage liver disease secondary to alcoholic cirrhosis.

408. Risks during graft reperfusion include all of the following EXCEPT

(A) increased systemic vascular resistance

(B) paradoxical embolus

(C) right heart failure

(D) decreased coronary perfusion pressure

(E) pulmonary hypertension

409. Electrolyte disturbances commonly seen in patients undergoing liver transplantation include all of the following EXCEPT

(A) hyperkalemia

(B) hyperglycemia

(C) hypernatremia

(D) hypocalcemia

(E) hypoglycemia

410. 42-year-old male with end-stage renal disease secondary to a 25-year history of type I diabetes is scheduled for explant of a previously transplanted kidney followed by immediate renal transplant. The anesthetic maintenance technique that is most ideal in this situation is

(A) O_2, N_2O, desflurane, fentanyl, pancuronium

(B) O_2, N_2O, sevoflurane, fentanyl, cisatracurium

(C) O_2, air, isoflurane, fentanyl, vecuronium

(D) O_2, air, desflurane, fentanyl, cisatracurium

(E) O_2, air, desflurane, fentanyl, rocuronium

DIRECTIONS: Use the following scenario to answer Questions 411-412: A 71-year-old female is in your ICU following emergent repair of a rupture of her descending aorta following a motor vehicle accident. She is extubated 12 h after arrival to the unit. Shortly thereafter, she begins complaining of nausea, vomiting, and severe abdominal pain. Her abdominal exam is unimpressive. Laboratory results are pending.

411. The most likely etiology of her symptoms is

(A) acute cholecystitis

(B) small bowel obstruction

(C) ischemic colitis

(D) acute pancreatitis

(E) gastric perforation

412. Four hours later, the patient is becoming tachycardic, hypotensive, and unresponsive to fluid resuscitation. While awaiting a consult from the surgical service, pharmacologic support with which agent should be instituted?

(A) Dopamine
(B) Epinephrine
(C) Phenylephrine
(D) Dobutamine
(E) Norepinephrine

413. You are asked to evaluate a patient in the PACU who has undergone a TURP. On arrival, you find a 76-year-old agitated man yelling that he can't see anything. His past medical history is significant for smoking, hypertension, and coronary artery disease with recent stent placement. The most likely cause of the visual disturbance is

(A) sorbitol toxicity
(B) cortical blindness
(C) transient ischemic attack
(D) glycine toxicity
(E) hyperammonemia

414. A 74-year-old female is scheduled for ECT. Her past medical history is significant for chronic renal failure requiring dialysis three times per week. Her last dialysis was 3 d ago. You ask that a serum [K$^+$] be drawn prior to induction of anesthesia. After administration of succinylcholine, her serum [K$^+$] will rise approximately

(A) 0.5 mEq/L
(B) 1.5 mEq/L
(C) 3.0 mEq/L
(D) 0 mEq/L (no change)
(E) >3.0 mEq/L

DIRECTIONS: Use the following scenario to answer Questions 415-416: A 52-year-old male, involved in an MVA, is brought emergently to the operating room for exploratory laparotomy secondary to the presence of abdominal free air and fluid on CT scan. His past medical history is significant for alcoholic cirrhosis, Child's class B. Preoperative coagulation studies reveal a platelet count of 82,000/mm^3,

prothrombin time of 18 sec (control 13 sec), and partial thromboplastin time of 62 sec (control 27 sec).

415. His apparent coagulopathy from liver disease can be reversed with a combination of all of the following EXCEPT

(A) platelets
(B) fresh frozen plasma
(C) cryoprecipitate
(D) factor VIII
(E) vitamin K

416. During induction and maintenance of general anesthesia in this patient, it is important to remember that this patient may exhibit a(n)

(A) decreased response to catecholamines
(B) decreased volume of distribution
(C) decreased clearance of fentanyl
(D) increased hepatic blood flow during surgery
(E) increased protein binding

DIRECTIONS: Use the following scenario to answer Questions 417-418: A 64-year-old female with a history of hypertension and benign ventricular arrhythmias is scheduled for extracorporeal shock wave lithotripsy (ESWL) under general anesthesia. Your recommendation to the urologist is that he use synchronized ESWL.

417. The most accurate statement about synchronized ESWL is that

(A) it generates higher intensity waves than non-synchronized ESWL
(B) shock waves should be timed 20 msec before the R wave
(C) it requires deeper levels of analgesia
(D) it does not interfere with pacemakers
(E) it should be timed to correspond to the ventricular refractory period

418. You're told that the new lithotriptor recently purchased by the hospital has not yet been approved for use. Instead, the urologist will need to use the older model Dornier lithotriptor requiring a water bath. You are now concerned about which one of the following physiologic and hemodynamic changes that may occur once the patient is positioned and the procedure is underway?

(A) Transient hypertension followed by hypotension

(B) Decrease in venous return

(C) Rise in systemic vascular resistance

(D) Increased functional residual capacity

(E) Bradycardia

DIRECTIONS: Use the following scenario to answer Questions 419-420: An 82-year-old, 100-kg male with a history of hypertension and COPD is undergoing a transurethral resection of the prostate under spinal anesthesia at a T8 level. Thirty minutes into the procedure he complains that he is nauseated, and having trouble catching his breath. You note his blood pressure has increased from 100/68 mm Hg to 152/94 mm Hg, his heart rate has decreased from 74 to 56 bpm, and his ECG shows ST elevation in lead II. He is becoming restless and trying to sit up.

419. The management of this patient should include all of the following EXCEPT

(A) inform the surgeon

(B) check serum sodium, serum osmolality and hemoglobin

(C) start an infusion of a hypertonic saline solution

(D) administer intravenous furosemide

(E) stop the procedure

420. As you administer oxygen, draw blood for labs, and begin management of the patient, you note that he is becoming lethargic. His plasma [Na$^+$] is 119 mEq/L. The preferred maneuver to increase the plasma [Na$^+$] to 130 mEq/L is

(A) correcting his total body sodium deficit of 380 mEq

(B) infusing isotonic saline to increase [Na$^+$] 1-1.5 mEq/L/h

(C) infusing 0.5 liters of 3% saline over 2 h

(D) administering a potassium-sparing diuretic

DIRECTIONS: Use the following scenario to answer Questions 421-422: A 62-year-old woman with a history of severe gastroesophageal reflux is scheduled for a laparoscopic fundoplication. Past medical history is significant only for a 55 pack-year history of smoking. After an uneventful induction and intubation, she is anesthetized with isoflurane, oxygen, air, and fentanyl. After insertion of the trocar through the abdominal wall, she was placed in steep Trendelenburg position, carbon dioxide was insufflated, and the procedure begun. Three hours later, as the surgeon is preparing to remove the trocar, the patient becomes progressively more hypotensive, with a concomitant rise in peak inspiratory pressure and drop in oxygen saturation.

421. The most likely cause of the hypotension is

(A) compression of the inferior vena cava

(B) patient position

(C) carbon dioxide embolism

(D) pneumoperitoneum

(E) tension pneumothorax

422. After increasing inspired oxygen concentration, the priority should be to

(A) flatten the table

(B) place the patient into the left lateral position

(C) administer epinephrine

(D) auscultate the chest

(E) ask the surgeon to decompress the pneumoperitoneum

423. An otherwise healthy 36-year-old male is scheduled for an elective excision of vocal cord polyp utilizing CO$_2$ laser under general anesthesia. On exam patient is 5'11", 79 kg, with a normal airway exam. The most effective means to avoid an airway fire in this case is

(A) minimize inspired oxygen concentration

(B) wrap the endotracheal tube cuff with metal tape

(C) utilize an apneic oxygenation technique

(D) fill the cuff with a saline-blue dye mix

(E) add nitrous oxide

424. A 43-year-old previously healthy male presents for elective resection of a newly diagnosed pheochromocytoma. He began his phenoxybenzamine 10 d ago. All of the following statements are accurate about phenoxybenzamine EXCEPT

(A) dosing should be instituted before β-adrenoceptor blockade

(B) reversal depends on synthesis of α-adrenoceptors

(C) dosage should be adjusted according to the levels of urinary catecholamine metabolites

(D) it causes orthostatic hypotension and reflex tachycardia

(E) it is a non-competitive, non-selective alpha blocker that covalently binds to α-adrenoceptors

425. An 82-year-old patient is scheduled to undergo hip arthroplasty with a cemented prosthesis to repair a hip fracture secondary to a mechanical fall. The patient is anesthetized with a spinal anesthetic, in addition to a propofol infusion for sedation. Shortly after insertion of the prosthesis, the patient's blood pressure falls from 128/85 to 84/40, HR increases from 73 to 108 bpm, SpO_2 falls from 96% to 78%, and you notice a new right bundle branch block on ECG monitoring. The most likely cause of these changes is

(A) myocardial ischemia

(B) use of cement containing methylmethacrylate

(C) hypoventilation secondary to sedation

(D) increased intramedullary pressure

(E) hypovolemia

426. A 43-year-old otherwise healthy male, involved in a motorcycle accident on his way to work, presents to the operating room with a posteriorly displaced open tibial fracture. He is scheduled for emergent vascular exploration of the calf wound due to diminished distal pulses, with subsequent ORIF of the fracture. The most appropriate analgesic technique is

(A) sciatic nerve block with 1.5% mepivacaine

(B) patient controlled analgesia with morphine

(C) epidural analgesia with 0.5% bupivacaine and fentanyl infusion

(D) combined sciatic and femoral nerve block with 0.5% bupivacaine

(E) sciatic nerve block with 0.75% ropivacaine

427. A 24-year-old male was brought to the operating room intubated after suffering a closed head injury from a fall while hiking. He presented for an urgent ORIF of an open comminuted distal humerus fracture. An upper extremity tourniquet was inflated continuously at 100 mm Hg above the patient's systolic blood pressure, and remained inflated for 2.5 h during the case. The least likely effect from the use of the tourniquet is

(A) ulnar nerve palsy

(B) fibrinolysis with limb reperfusion

(C) microvascular thrombosis

(D) increased preload upon tourniquet inflation

(E) decrease in core temperature after tourniquet release

428. A 38-year-old male who had required a prolonged extrication after a motor vehicle accident is brought to the operating room for exploratory laparotomy for suspected ruptured spleen as well as fixation of multiple lower extremity fractures. After induction of general anesthesia and endotracheal intubation, an esophageal temperature probe is inserted showing an initial temperature reading of 32°C. All of the following may be encountered EXCEPT

(A) metabolic acidosis

(B) impairment of the intrinsic clotting cascade

(C) cardiac dysrhythmias

(D) platelet dysfunction

(E) profound peripheral vasodilation

DIRECTIONS: Use the following scenario to answer Questions 429-430: A 22-year-old 5'10", 110 kg otherwise healthy male was brought to the emergency department after being struck in the eye with a baseball. His exam revealed an open globe injury for which he is now brought emergently to the operating room. He states that he ate lunch just prior to the start of the ball game. On exam he has a large neck, 3-fingerbreadth thyromental distance, and a Mallampati Class 3 airway.

429. The safest anesthetic technique for this patient is

(A) retrobulbar block with intravenous sedation

(B) general anesthesia with laryngeal mask airway

(C) peribulbar block with intravenous sedation

(D) general anesthesia with awake fiberoptic intubation

(E) general anesthesia with rapid sequence induction

430. The best intubating conditions for this patient will be achieved using

(A) propofol, fentanyl, and succinylcholine 1.5 mg/kg

(B) propofol, lidocaine, and rocuronium 1.2 mg/kg

(C) propofol, fentanyl, and rocuronium 0.6 mg/kg

(D) propofol, fentanyl, rocuronium 0.5 mg, succinylcholine 1.5 mg/kg

431. You are asked to begin a case for your colleague. You introduce yourself to the patient, and note that he is a 63-year-old male scheduled for radical prostatectomy for prostate cancer. He is a very good historian, and tells you that his only medical problem is coronary artery disease, for which he underwent stent placement 2 years ago. His only medication is a beta blocker that he takes daily. When asked to sign the anesthesia consent, the patient informs you that he is a Jehovah's Witness, and that he refuses all blood therapy. He tells you that the surgeon is aware, and agrees. After extensive discussion with the patient in which you discuss the various options as well as possible complications from refusal of such therapy, he still refuses. You are uncomfortable caring for this patient. Your next step should be to

(A) proceed with the case, as you are ethically obligated to care for this patient

(B) speak with his health care proxy in an effort to obtain consent from him/her

(C) call a consult from the hospital ethics committee

(D) refuse to care for the patient, but obtain informed refusal

(E) call the hospital attorney to get a court order to give him blood if his life is at stake

432. A 55-year-old man has undergone an uneventful knee arthroscopy under general anesthesia. His only significant preoperative medical problem is osteoarthritis. The criterion LEAST important in determining appropriateness for discharge home from the Phase II postanesthesia care unit is

(A) pain score
(B) ability to void
(C) oxygenation
(D) blood pressure
(E) postoperative nausea and vomiting

433. A 78-year-old male is undergoing repair of a detached retina under general endotracheal anesthesia. The surgeon informs the anesthesiologist that he plans to inject a bubble of sulfur hexafluoride into the vitreal cavity to tamponade the retina. As the retina is re-attached, the anesthesiologist should

(A) discontinue nitrous oxide
(B) discontinue all fluorinated anesthetic gases
(C) ensure that all extraocular muscles are maximally paralyzed via the administration of a muscle relaxant
(D) elevate the head of the bed
(E) hyperventilate the patient

434. A 44-year-old patient underwent a 4-h operative procedure for emergency repair of a liver laceration and splenectomy following blunt abdominal trauma as a result of a motor vehicle accident. In the PACU the patient is noted to have worsening metabolic acidosis, poor urine output, and a tense and distended abdomen. The surgical team is questioning the possibility of abdominal compartment syndrome. Definitive diagnosis is made by

(A) measurement of cardiac output

(B) serial measurement of glomerular filtration rate

(C) measurement of pressure within the bladder

(D) measurement of simultaneous PCWP and CVP values

(E) serial measurements of abdominal girth

435. A 56-year-old, 84-kg patient is scheduled for outpatient knee arthroscopy for removal of loose intraarticular bodies. The patient has a 10 year history of severe obstructive sleep apnea for which he uses CPAP nightly. The single factor that would increase the safety of postoperative discharge of this patient is

(A) a surgical time of less than one hour

(B) placement of femoral nerve block to reduce postoperative pain

(C) use of CPAP by the patient at home

(D) adequate management of postoperative pain with ibuprofen

436. A 74-year-old patient is scheduled for an elective right hemicolectomy. During her preoperative evaluation, she tells your colleague that she was recently diagnosed with open angle glaucoma for which she was prescribed timolol eye drops that she uses faithfully. She will require a general anesthetic with a neuromuscular blocking agent. Your colleague's normal practice is to reverse neuromuscular blockade with atropine and neostigmine. Given this patient's history, your colleague should

(A) reverse with a combination of glycopyrrolate and neostigmine

(B) make no change in his practice

(C) avoid all nondepolarizing neuromuscular blocking agents

(D) use a short acting agent to allow spontaneous return of neuromuscular function

(E) reverse with a combination of atropine and edrophonium

437. A patient is brought to the operating room for repair of an open fracture sustained from a fall from a window during a house fire. The patient was intubated at the scene and ventilated with 100% oxygen via a bag-mask-valve device during transport to the hospital. The most reliable method for determining whether the patient has carbon monoxide poisoning while being ventilated with 100% O_2 is

(A) routine arterial blood gas analysis

(B) pulse oximetry

(C) capnometry

(D) arterial carboxyhemoglobin level

(E) capnography

438. You are asked to evaluate an 84-year-old patient scheduled for a right hemicolectomy. In comparison to a 44-year-old patient undergoing a similar procedure, you would expect to see a decrease in which one of the following physiologic parameters in the 84-year-old?

(A) Ventilation-perfusion mismatch

(B) Closing volume

(C) Vital capacity

(D) Alveolar dead space

(E) Residual lung volume

439. A 76-year-old female driver of a motor vehicle hit by a truck is brought to the operating room for emergent splenectomy and stabilization of a pelvic fracture. She arrives intubated, with a blood pressure of 80/40 and heart rate of 124. The patient's past medical history is unknown. Initial labs reveal a serum potassium concentration of 7.1 mEq/L. The serum potassium concentration will NOT be decreased by

(A) an intravenous bolus of calcium chloride

(B) hyperventilation

(C) infusion of glucose and insulin

(D) albuterol administered by nebulizer

(E) an intravenous bolus of sodium bicarbonate

440. A 62-year-old male with liver cirrhosis, currently on the liver transplant waiting list, is undergoing an emergency evacuation of subdural hematoma after a fall. The neurosurgeon is having difficulty controlling bleeding. The LEAST likely cause of the bleeding is

(A) disseminated intravascular coagulation

(B) splenic sequestration of platelets

(C) defective fibrin clot formation

(D) decreased synthesis of factor VIII

(E) reduced fibrinogen concentrations

441. A 68-year-old man who takes levodopa for management of Parkinson disease is scheduled to undergo an inguinal hernia repair. The patient has a history of type II diabetes as well as gastroesophageal reflux. The most appropriate perioperative anesthetic management includes

(A) droperidol as an antiemetic

(B) omission of levodopa on the morning of surgery

(C) metoclopramide for reduction of gastric volume

(D) spinal anesthesia with bupivacaine

(E) morphine for postoperative analgesia

442. A 16-year-old male, hit by a car while crossing the street, is brought emergently to the operating room for exploratory laparotomy for a presumed liver laceration, as well as extensive orthopedic injuries. You discuss with his parents the potential need to transfuse blood and blood products. When his mother asks what the greatest risk of transfusion is, you tell her

(A) mistransfusion due to human clerical error

(B) transfusion-related acute lung injury

(C) hepatitis C

(D) human immunodeficiency virus

(E) anaphylaxis

443. A 68-year-old woman with 40% second and third degree burns requires burn debridement twice daily. As she is being mechanically ventilated in the ICU, the surgical team has asked that the debridement be done at the bedside under general anesthesia. The LEAST appropriate agent for a brief general anesthetic in this patient is

(A) etomidate

(B) ketamine

(C) propofol

(D) midazolam

(E) methohexital

444. A 63-year-old man with cirrhosis is scheduled for a transjugular intrahepatic portosystemic shunt (TIPS) placement for management of severe portal hypertension with ascites. When lying flat he is short of breath that worsens when he sits up. He has a room air SpO_2 of 83%. The only physiologic derangement NOT seen in this patient would be

(A) impaired hypoxic pulmonary vasoconstriction

(B) elevated alveolar-arterial oxygen gradient

(C) intrapulmonary shunting

(D) decreased nitric oxide concentrations

445. An 88-year-old patient, who two weeks ago underwent aortic valve replacement, is noted during a postoperative clinic visit to have an unstable sternum and purulent drainage of his wound. Despite having had breakfast, he is scheduled for an emergent exploration of the wound. When planning this patient's anesthetic management, you recall that in the elderly

(A) MAC is increased for isoflurane

(B) metoclopramide is a useful adjunct to promote gastric emptying

(C) the effective dose for neuromuscular blockade is decreased

(D) thermoregulation is impaired

(E) glomerular filtration rate is increased

446. A 32-year-old woman sustains an injury to the left recurrent laryngeal nerve during a near total thyroidectomy. Which one of the following is the most likely postoperative finding?

(A) Adduction of the left vocal cord at rest

(B) Aphonia

(C) Laryngeal edema

(D) Stridor

(E) Paralysis of the left cricothyroid muscle

447. You are planning the anesthetic management of an 82-year-old man undergoing a carotid endarterectomy. He has a history of poorly controlled hypertension, as well as chronic renal failure requiring dialysis. The LEAST appropriate medication to manage intraoperative and postoperative hypertension would be

(A) esmolol

(B) hydralazine

(C) fenoldopam

(D) nitroglycerine

(E) nitroprusside

448. A 30-year-old patient presents for emergency appendectomy. He states that he was recently diagnosed with hypothyroidism but has been unable to afford the medication prescribed. The most likely manifestation of his disease in the perioperative period would be

(A) cardiac arrhythmias with ketamine administration

(B) decreased ventilatory response to hypoxia

(C) increased MAC of inhalational anesthetics

(D) decreased sensitivity to midazolam

(E) hypotension

449. A 46-year-old male is brought to the operating room for irrigation and debridement of an open tibial fracture. He had been trapped in his car after sliding off the road and hitting a tree during an ice storm. He remained alert and hemodynamically stable at the scene during a prolonged extrication. Evaluation in the emergency department reveals only an open tibial plateau fracture as well as a "seatbelt" bruise

on his anterior chest. He is hypothermic with a temperature of 34°C. All other vital signs, as well as EKG and laboratory values, were normal. MAC for isoflurane in this patient is approximately

(A) 0.8%

(B) 1%

(C) 1.25%

(D) 1.5%

(E) 1.75%

DIRECTIONS: Use the following scenario to answer Questions 450-451: A 22-year-old male is brought emergently to the operating room for exploration of multiple abdominal stab wounds. He was intubated at the scene due to loss of consciousness and respiratory compromise. BP on arrival to the operating room is 70/40, HR is 130 bpm, and oxygen saturation is 92%. Blood pressure responds minimally to volume resuscitation or vasopressors. Volatile anesthetic causes severe hypotension. Oxygen saturation drops each time the F_{IO_2} is decreased below 1.0.

450. The most appropriate medication to prevent intraoperative recall in this patient is

(A) remifentanil

(B) scopolamine

(C) midazolam

(D) droperidol

(E) rocuronium

451. You consider utilizing a BIS monitor to measure depth of anesthesia. The only factor that does not affect the accuracy of BIS monitoring is

(A) muscle activity

(B) hypoglycemia

(C) propofol

(D) electrical artifact

(E) ketamine

DIRECTIONS: Each group of items below consists of lettered headings followed by a list of numbered phrases or statements. For each numbered phrase or statement, select the ONE lettered heading or component that is most closely associated with it. Each lettered heading or component may be selected once, more than once, or not at all.

(A) Near miss
(B) Hazardous condition
(C) Sentinel event
(D) Latent error
(E) Preventable adverse event

For each situation, choose the appropriate patient safety concern.

452. An anesthesiologist new to the institution is asked to provide anesthesia for a 1-year-old requiring an urgent MRI. It has been several years since she has cared for a pediatric patient, and she has never before provided anesthesia in an MRI environment.

453. An 18-year-old patient was admitted to the emergency department after a bicycle accident. The Glasgow coma score at the scene was 12 that diminished to 7 in the emergency department. A CT scan of the head revealed an epidural hematoma compressing the left parietal lobe. The patient was brought emergently to the operating room for evacuation of the hematoma. Prior to induction of anesthesia, it was noted that his left pupil was now fixed and dilated. The patient was quickly prepped and draped, and a right craniotomy was performed.

DIRECTIONS: Each group of items below consists of lettered headings followed by a list of numbered phrases or statements. For each numbered phrase or statement, select the ONE lettered heading or component that is most closely associated with it. Each lettered heading or component may be selected once, more than once, or not at all.

(A) Plague
(B) Botulism
(C) Smallpox
(D) Brucellosis
(E) Anthrax
(F) Ebola
(G) Q fever
(H) Tularemia

For each patient suspected to be a victim of biologic terrorism, select the most likely biological agent.

454. A 46-year-old man presented with fever, fatigue, and shortness of breath 5 d after suspected exposure. Chest x-ray reveals mediastinal widening and bilateral pleural effusions. The patient was admitted to a regular ICU bed, and combination therapy begun with ciprofloxacin and clindamycin.

455. Twelve days after suspected exposure, a 28-year-old man presents with recent onset of fever, vomiting, backache, and a rash, which initially began on his face and extremities. Exam reveals vesicles and pustules on his face and extremities, and a maculopapular rash on his trunk, with lesions at the same stage at each location. He is immediately placed in a negative-pressure room on strict isolation precautions until resolution and scabbing of the lesions.

456. Twenty-four hours after suspected exposure, a 56-year-old woman develops symptoms of dry mouth, double vision, difficulty speaking, and swallowing. Because the diagnosis was made early, she was given a single dose of an equine antitoxin.

Answers and Explanations

397. **(D)** Application of positive pressure ventilation during preoxygenation decreases atelectasis formation and improves oxygenation. Four VC breaths with 100% oxygen within 30 sec have been suggested as superior to 3 min of 100% preoxygenation in obese patients. Preoxygenation in the head-up or sitting position is more effective and significantly extends the tolerance to apnea in obese patients when compared with the supine position. Placing the patient in the "ramped" position, with the head, neck, upper body, and shoulders elevated with folded towels or blankets, raises the chest to a point where an imaginary horizontal line can be drawn from the sternal notch to the external ear to better improve laryngoscopy and intubation, not to improve the effectiveness of preoxygenation. *(5:312)*

398. **(E)** Rhabdomyolysis has been documented in morbidly obese patients undergoing prolonged procedures; the main risk factor is prolonged duration of surgery. Elevations in serum creatinine and CPK levels unexplained by other reasons and complaints of buttock, hip, or shoulder pain in the postoperative period should raise the suspicion of rhabdomyolysis. Measurement of serum CPK pre- and postoperatively aids in early diagnosis and treatment. Early and aggressive volume replacement is mandatory in patients with rhabdomyolysis; alkaline fluids may be beneficial in preventing tubular necrosis and cast formation *(5:310, 2306)*

399. **(C)** The Child-Pugh classification has been used to assess prognosis in cirrhosis and to provide standard criteria for listing liver transplantation. Scoring is based upon the objective criteria of serum bilirubin, serum albumin, and prothrombin time as expressed by INR, as well as upon subjective criteria of degree of ascites and severity of encephalopathy. This system for assessing the need for liver transplantation has been replaced by the model for end-stage liver disease (MELD). The score is calculated using three objective variables only: serum bilirubin, prothrombin time expressed as INR, and serum creatinine. MELD scores of < 10, 10-14, and > 14 roughly correspond to Child-Pugh classes A, B, and C, respectively. *(5: 186-8, 2526)*

400. **(B)** Patients who have undergone previous gastric bypass surgery may exhibit signs and symptoms of metabolic and nutritional abnormalities related to malabsorption. Common deficiencies include vitamin B_{12}, iron, calcium, and folic acid. A collective form of postoperative polyneuropathy known as acute postgastric reduction surgery (APGARS) neuropathy could result. Patients with APGARS neuropathy present with protracted postoperative vomiting, hyporeflexia, and muscular weakness. Differential diagnoses of this disorder include thiamine deficiency (Wernicke encephalopathy, beriberi), vitamin B_{12} deficiency, and Guillain-Barre syndrome. Vitamin A is required for normal vision, as well as iron utilization and humoral and T-cell mediated immunity. Deficiency due to malabsorption may cause night blindness, as well as compromise immune defenses to infection. It does not, however, result in neuropathy. *(5:310, 600-1, 2260)*

401. **(C)** Neck circumference has been identified as the single biggest predictor of problematic intubation in morbidly obese patients. A larger neck circumference is associated with the male sex, higher Mallampati score, grade 3 views at laryngoscopy, and obstructive sleep apnea. Intubation difficulty correlates better with increased age, male sex, temporomandibular joint pathology, Mallampati classes 3 and 4, history of OSA, and abnormal upper teeth than with BMI. *(5:311)*

402. **(A)** Propofol's total clearance and volume of distribution at steady state correlate with total body weight; however, its negative cardiovascular effects combined with the negative physiologic effects of obesity on the cardiovascular system suggest induction dosing should be based on lean body weight. Succinylcholine should be dosed on total body weight due to the larger extracellular fluid compartment and linear increase in pseudocholinesterase activity seen in obese patients. Sufentanil and midazolam each have an increased volume of distribution and a prolonged terminal half-life in obese patients, but an unaffected plasma clearance, so that induction doses should be based upon total body weight. *(5:308-10)*

403. **(D)** Arterial oxygenation during laparoscopy in morbidly obese patients is affected mainly by body weight and not body position, pneumoperitoneum, or mode of ventilation, and oxygenation is not significantly improved by increasing either the respiratory rate or tidal volume. PEEP is the only ventilatory parameter that has consistently been shown to improve respiratory function in obese subjects, although it may decrease venous return, cardiac output, and subsequent oxygen delivery *(5:314)*

404. **(B)** Functional residual capacity will be decreased to approximately 65% of the value seen in a nonobese individual. Residual volume, total lung capacity, forced vital capacity, and the forced expiratory volume in 1 sec are minimally decreased in comparison with a nonobese individual. *(5:2093)*

405. **(D)** Postoperative hemorrhage can result in a rapidly expanding hematoma that can directly compress the trachea leading to signs of airway compression. Chronic compression by a large goiter can lead to tracheomalacia and subsequent tracheal collapse. Unilateral recurrent laryngeal nerve injury can cause unilateral vocal cord paralysis that manifests as hoarseness, breathlessness, glottic incompetence, poor cough, and aspiration. Bilateral recurrent laryngeal nerve injury produces bilateral vocal cord paralysis that will lead to airway obstruction and stridor; signs and symptoms, however, are noted almost immediately after extubation. Hypocalcemia may develop acutely secondary to inadvertent injury or removal of parathyroid glands during surgery. The hallmark of hypocalcemia is neuromuscular irritability (muscle weakness, numbness, tingling). If severe, it may lead to cause mental status changes, hypotension, and laryngospasm. *(5:156, 520, 1121-2, 1246)*

406. **(C)** Graves disease is marked by suppression of TSH and elevated concentrations of unbound T4. Thyroid function tests are reviewed 3-4 weeks after starting treatment with antithyroid drugs, and the dose is titrated based upon unbound T4 concentrations. Most patients do not achieve a euthyroid state until treated for 6-8 weeks. TSH concentrations remain suppressed for several months and therefore do not provide a sensitive index of treatment response. *(5: 2925-6)*

407. **(B)** Thyroid storm is an acute life-threatening form of hyperthyroidism. Symptoms include nausea, vomiting, diarrhea, agitation, confusion, diaphoresis, temperature greater than 38.5°C, tachycardia out of proportion to temperature, and arrhythmias. Multiple events may precipitate it, including acute illness (infection, CVA, trauma), surgery, and radioiodine treatment of patients with partially or untreated hyperthyroidism. Initial management includes large doses of methimazole that block hormone synthesis and partially inhibit peripheral conversion of T4 to T3; glucocorticoids that block conversion of T4 to T3 in the periphery and act as supportive therapy of possible adrenal insufficiency; β-adrenoceptor antagonists preferably propranolol (as it alone decreases conversion), to block cardiovascular effects; cholestyramine that binds thyroid hormone in the gut and enhances GI clearance; supportive measures (antipyretics, cooling, volume repletion); and management of precipitating illness. Salicylates are contraindicated as antipyretics as they decrease binding of thyroxine to thyroxine binding globulin, thereby aggravating the disease. *(1:1135, 1147-51; 5:115, 1118, 2927; Connery LE, Coursin DB, Anesthesiol Clin North Amer 2004; 22:526-8)*

408. **(A)** Reperfusion is the period of greatest hemodynamic instability during liver transplantation. Release of preservative solution, clot, air, debris, and acidemic blood (released from reperfused splanchnic circulation) into the pulmonary vasculature may cause severe pulmonary hypertension and resultant right heart failure. The resultant increase in central venous pressure (CVP) may open an occult patent foramen ovale, with risk of paradoxical embolus. Elevated CVP may also compromise graft reperfusion and contribute to early graft failure. Pulmonary hypertension and right heart failure will result in a decrease in systemic pressure and coronary perfusion pressure due to inadequate left ventricular preload. Although pulmonary vascular resistance will often increase, systemic vascular resistance

will decrease. *(5:1075-6; Steadman, RH, Anesthesiol Clin North Amer 2004; 22:687-711)*

409. **(C)** Serum sodium is often decreased in these patients secondary to the formation of ascites, renal failure, and the use of diuretics. Baseline potassium concentrations may vary, depending upon the use of potassium-sparing or potassium-wasting diuretics to control ascites, as well as patient's underlying renal function. Despite that, hyperkalemia is common intraoperatively due to the nature of the procedure itself. Splanchnic ischemia, the transfusion of large volumes of blood products, metabolic acidosis due to hypotension from depletion of circulating volume, and the preservative solution that is rich in potassium, all contribute to a significant rise in serum potassium. Serum ionized calcium tends to decrease due to vigorous administration of citrated blood products. Citrate is a chelating agent that binds to calcium. Hypoglycemia may be seen when the liver, the primary site of gluconeogenesis, is removed during the anhepatic phase, particularly when the phase is prolonged. Exogenous sources of glucose tend to mitigate this possibility, however. Dextrose containing IV fluids (drug-carrier infusions), as well as the use of methylprednisolone, often result in hyperglycemia. *(1:853, 5:1073-5)*

410. **(D)** Cisatracurium, rocuronium, and vecuronium do not depend on the kidney for elimination, have minimal hemodynamic effect, and have been used successfully in patients with marginal or no renal function. Because cisatracurium is metabolized in the plasma by Michael elimination, (often erroneously termed Hofmann elimination), its duration of action is not prolonged in renal failure. Although the liver is the primary metabolic site for rocuronium and vecuronium, the duration of blockade may be prolonged with these drugs if large doses are used, due to accumulation of metabolites that are excreted by the kidney. Pancuronium should not be used in kidney transplant recipients because it depends primarily on the kidney for elimination, causing a prolonged neuromuscular block. Neither desflurane nor isoflurane have nephrotoxic properties. N₂O may also be used, as it has minimal side effects, no renal toxicity, and rapid elimination. Sevoflurane is rarely used for renal transplantation due to concerns of fluoride and compound A toxicity. Although most human studies have not demonstrated deleterious effects of sevoflurane on the kidney, it has been deemed preferable to use one of the known safe alternatives. The pharmacokinetics and pharmacodynamics of fentanyl, sufentanil, alfentanil, and remifentanil are not significantly altered by kidney disease, and have been successfully used during renal transplantation *(1:543-7; 5:1098)*

411. **(C)** The most prevalent gastrointestinal disease complicating cardiovascular surgery is ischemic colitis; the incidence in patients requiring emergent aortic repair triples from that of elective aortic repair, about 5-9%. Mesenteric ischemia is typically seen in patients over 70 years old. It is categorized according to etiology: non-occlusive mesenteric ischemia, arterio-occlusive mesenteric ischemia, or mesenteric venous thrombosis. Non-occlusive ischemia is due to mesenteric arteriolar vasospasm in response to a severe physiologic stress such as dehydration or hypotension. The hallmark of mesenteric ischemia is severe acute, nonremitting abdominal pain completely out of proportion to physical findings, unlike other intrabdominal pathologies that often provides signs and symptoms including abdominal distention and/or peritoneal signs. *(5:288, 2510-1)*

412. **(D)** Management of patients with presumed mesenteric ischemia includes fluid resuscitation to counteract fluid sequestration within bowel wall, optimization of oxygen delivery, broad-spectrum antibiotics, and support of cardiac output with inotropic agents. Vasoconstrictors should be avoided; instead, dobutamine, a pure β-adrenoceptor agonist, is the preferred agent. *(5:2512)*

413. **(D)** Irrigation fluids with glycine are often used in TURP. The amino acid is an inhibitory neurotransmitter in the cortex and retina, and is most probably the causative agent of postoperative blindness and seizures in some TURP patients. Patients exhibit pupillary reflexes that are often sluggish or absent, unlike cortical blindness, in which reflexes are maintained. This suggests that the mechanism of blindness in these patients is direct inhibition of retinal potential transmission. Blindness resolves with decreasing blood concentrations of glycine. Blindness is bilateral, as opposed to TIA, in which visual disturbances are most commonly unilateral. Elevated concentrations of ammonia, a byproduct of glycine metabolism, cause symptoms of lethargy, muscle weakness, and encephalopathy. The absorption of sorbitol can result in the development of hyperglycemia and lactic acidosis related to the metabolism of sorbitol *(5:895, 1140, 2526)*

414. **(A)** Succinylcholine depolarizes muscle cells, causing an efflux of K⁺ through acetylcholine receptors. It will cause a transient rise in [K⁺] in normal individuals of 0.3-0.5 mEq/L. Succinylcholine may cause exaggerated hyperkalemic response in patients with conditions of muscle membrane degeneration (e.g., trauma, burns, primary muscle disorders) or neural denervation (e.g., stroke, multiple sclerosis, Guillain-Barre syndrome, spinal cord injuries). Patients with renal failure may have a higher baseline serum [K⁺] due to impaired potassium excretion, but the rise in [K⁺] is no different. *(5:273, 501, 517)*

415. **(D)** Causes of coagulopathy in patients with advanced liver disease include: (1) Vitamin K deficiency; (2) impaired synthesis of coagulation factors synthesized in liver (all factors except von Willebrand Factor VIII); and (3) splenic sequestration of platelets secondary to hypersplenism. These patients may also have decreased synthesis of coagulation inhibitors, and may not be able to clear activated coagulation factors or fibrin split products. Coagulopathy may therefore be treated with a combination of vitamin K, FFP, cryoprecipitate, and platelets. *(5:193-4, 215)*

416. (A) Patients with end-stage liver disease have multiple hemodynamic changes, including decreased SVR, increased cardiac output, and decreased β-adrenoceptor function with resultant decrease in response to catecholamines. Patients with severe liver disease have an increased volume of distribution secondary to an expanded extracellular volume space. As a result, clearances of morphine and alfentanil are reduced in cirrhosis, whereas fentanyl and sufentanil are not greatly affected. Because cirrhosis of the liver markedly decreases total hepatic blood flow as a result of fibrosis at the portal triad, patients with cirrhosis can be expected to have increased sensitivity to highly extracted drugs. Hepatic blood flow decreases during regional and general anesthesia secondary to direct and indirect effects of anesthetic agents, ventilatory mode, and type of procedure. Protein binding is decreased secondary to a decrease in albumin that increases the unbound fraction of ionized drugs. *(1:24; 5:186, 720, 1051)*

417. (E) Shock waves have the potential to trigger ventricular arrhythmias when they coincide with the repolarization period of the cardiac cycle. For this reason, ECG synchronization and shock delivery should be during the ventricular refractory period, 20 msec *after* the R wave. Shock waves from either gated (synchronized) or ungated (unsynchronized) ESWL may inhibit or reprogram cardiac pacemakers. Synchronization, or lack thereof, has no correlation with intensity of wave, or amount of analgesia required. *(5:1141-2)*

418. (C) The Dornier HM3 lithotriptor is an older electrohydraulic unit, requiring a water bath and generating high intensity waves requiring deeper analgesia. Immersion in a water bath initially results in transient vasodilation and hypotension, followed by rise in arterial blood pressure as venous blood redistributes centrally from the hydrostatic pressure of water on the lower extremities and abdomen. As SVR rises, cardiac output may decrease due to hydrostatic pressure on the lower extremities and the abdomen. The increase in venous return may shift blood to the intrathoracic vessels, precipitating congestive heart failure in susceptible individuals. FRC is decreased by 30-60%, predisposing some patients to hypoxemia. Water bath immersion has no direct effect on heart rate. *(5:1141-2)*

419. (C) During resection of the prostate, venous sinuses are opened, and large amounts of irrigation fluid can be absorbed into the systemic circulation, causing TURP syndrome. The syndrome has multiple manifestations characterized by fluid overload, hypoosmolality, hyponatremia, and neurologic disturbances, with onset as early as 15 min into the procedure. Symptoms may include nausea, confusion, hypertension, reflex bradycardia from volume overload, ECG changes from myocardial ischemia, desaturation, seizure, visual changes, and coma. When TURP syndrome is suspected, the procedure should be stopped; serum sodium, potassium, and osmolality should be measured, as should hemoglobin, as a measure of fluid absorption. Presumed pulmonary edema should be treated with diuresis. Hyponatremia does not need to be treated aggressively when it is not accompanied by hypoosmolality, or in the absence of neurologic symptoms. *(5:1139-41)*

420. (B) Rapid correction of hyponatremia may trigger demyelination of pontine or extrapontine neurons, leading to neurologic dysfunction that may include quadriplegia, pseudobulbar palsy, seizures, coma, and even death. For this reason, serum sodium is increased slowly, and hypertonic saline should be used only in the presence of life-threatening manifestations such as coma and seizures. Otherwise, sodium concentrations can be increased by administration of normal saline in combination with a loop diuretic or mannitol. Sodium correction should never exceed 1-1.5 mEq/L/h.

Na^+ deficit = TBW × (desired $[Na^+]$ − current $[Na^+]$). Total-body water of infants younger than 1 year of age is 75-80% of body weight, whereas that of adult males is 60% and that of females is 55%. Deficit = $100 \times 0.6 \times (130-119) = 60 \times 11 = 660$ mEq. It is common to correct only half the sodium deficit. *(1:31; 5:515, 1139-41)*

421. **(E)** Differential diagnosis of hypotension during a laparoscopic procedure includes carbon dioxide embolus, hemorrhage, compression of the vena cava from increased intraabdominal pressure, and pneumothorax. Relatively small CO_2 emboli are not uncommon and have been detected by TEE, while massive CO_2 embolus is a rare and catastrophic event. Hemorrhage would not increase PIP, while compression of the vena cava would be more likely during active insufflation of the abdomen with development of a significant pneumoperitoneum. Over time, however, a pneumothorax may develop, with associated hypoxemia, hypotension, and elevated airway pressures. The incidence of extraperitoneal insufflation of CO_2 has been reported to range from as little as 0.4%-2% to 20%-64%, and is more likely during lengthy procedures or procedures on the lower esophagus. *(5:1041-2)*

422. **(D)** When a pneumothorax is suspected, aggressive investigation (auscultation, chest radiograph) and management (e.g., chest tube for tension pneumothorax or conversion to an open procedure) should be undertaken. *(5:1041-2)*

423. **(C)** If the laser beam penetrates the endotracheal tube, the oxygen rich environment within the tube can cause an intense flame. Utilizing a tubeless technique (spontaneous ventilation, apneic oxygenation, or jet ventilation) will diminish the risk by decreasing the concentrated oxygen rich environment while removing a potentially flammable object from the airway. Combustion of PVC yields hydrogen chloride gas that is acidic, highly toxic, and irritating. Although an endotracheal tube may be wrapped with metallic tape to decrease the likelihood that it will catch fire, there is no way to wrap the tube cuff with metallic tape. Filling the cuff with tinted saline will alert one to a cuff rupture, but will not prevent fire. Nitrous oxide will support combustion. *(5:1236-9)*

424. **(C)** α-adrenoceptor blockade dose is increased every 3-4 d until either no symptoms of catecholamine excess are evident or the patient complains of side effects from postural hypotension and/or a stuffy nose, with a final dosage range of 40 to 100 mg/d. β-adrenoceptor agonists are administered for a persistent tachycardia and for control of other peripheral β-adrenergic effects of catecholamine excess. These drugs should never be given before α-adrenoceptor blockade because serious hypertensive sequelae may result. Adequate volume expansion after institution of the drug may take as long as 2 to 3 weeks. Thus patients presenting for surgery who have been on phenoxybenzamine for a shorter time period should have hypovolemia corrected preoperatively. *(5:158, 1124)*

425. **(D)** The main component of cement is methylmethacrylate (MMA) that has been linked to a clinical scenario consisting of hypotension, bronchoconstriction, hypoxia, cardiac arrest, and sudden death. It was at one time believed to be due to a hypersensitivity reaction to the MMA, resulting in acute vasodilatation and cardiac collapse. However, plasma concentrations in vivo during use of MMA have been found to be 10-20-fold below the concentrations required to cause clinically significant vasodilatation and hypotension. The actual cause is increased intramedullary canal pressure with resultant embolization of fat particles and debris into the medullary venous plexus during long bone manipulation, reaming, and cementing. Intramedullary pressure peaks are as high as 680 mm Hg in humans with cement use, compared to peaks below 100 mm Hg with the use of non-cemented implants. Clinical signs are similar to those found in PE or fat embolism: fever, tachycardia, hypotension, hypoxemia, and, in spontaneously breathing patients, dyspnea, and tachypnea. Other signs of fat emboli also may be seen on ECG, including right-axis deviation or right bundle branch block, reflecting increased pulmonary artery pressure and intrapulmonary shunt, potentially leading to right ventricular failure and cardiac arrest. *(5:1204)*

426. (B) In choosing the anesthetic technique for cases that may be associated with compartment syndrome, the anesthesiologist must avoid any postoperative technique, such as epidurals or peripheral nerve blocks that would delay diagnosis of the syndrome. If these techniques must be used in the setting of potential compartment syndrome, consideration should be given to continuously monitoring compartment pressures. The effect of techniques such as spinals and epidurals that cause sympathectomy (thus vasodilatation) is unclear. The increased blood flow to compartments may cause a further increase in compartment pressures. *(1:576-7, 579-80; 5:1205)*

427. (A) The complications of tourniquet use are many. Inflation of the tourniquet causes increases in preload and afterload; deflation causes decreases in preload and afterload; reperfusion causes a decrease in core temperature of up to 1°C, an increases in O_2 consumption, and increases in the partial pressure of CO_2 with resultant increase in cerebral blood flow, as well as metabolic and respiratory acidosis. Limb ischemia can cause ischemic capillaries leading to diffuse capillary leak upon reperfusion; tissue pressure leads to platelet aggregation and capillary obstruction, leading to release of inflammatory mediators that cause microvascular thrombosis. Tissue acidosis causes release of tissue plasminogen activator, causing a brief period of fibrinolysis. Pressure from the tourniquet can cause significant nerve injury, especially in the upper extremity. Radial nerve palsy is the most common nerve injury. *(5:1202-3)*

428. (E) Such patients have profound peripheral vasoconstriction induced by the thermoregulatory responses in an effort to conserve heat. The activation of arteriovenous shunts in the periphery decreases the effectiveness of applying heat to the extremities and the surface of the body in warming the patient. Cold-induced hypertension is accompanied by an increase in circulating catecholamines that augment cardiac irritability and lead to ventricular arrhythmias. Platelet function is impaired in even mild degrees of perioperative hypothermia, potentially related to a defect in the release of thromboxane A_2. Some impairment of clotting factor function is also noted. *(5:1505-7, 1510)*

429. (E) Repair of an open globe is a surgical procedure that is not considered amenable to regional anesthesia. The goals of general anesthesia for ophthalmic surgery include a smooth induction with a stable intraocular pressure, avoidance or treatment of the oculocardiac reflex, maintenance of a motionless field, a smooth emergence, and avoidance of postoperative nausea and vomiting. This can be accomplished in part by reducing the need for opioid analgesia through the use of a bulbar block in conjunction with general anesthesia. Efforts to quickly obtain good intubating conditions and prevention of coughing and straining are important for reducing the risk of extrusion of eye contents, thereby making awake fiberoptic intubation a suboptimal choice. Protection of the airway, especially in a patient with a full stomach, limits the use of an LMA. *(5:1222)*

430. (D) Although historic concerns exist about the safety of succinylcholine in the presence of an open globe, several retrospective studies show no link. Although succinylcholine does produce a temporary increase (7-10 min) in intraocular pressure (6-12 mm Hg), it is far less than that produced by coughing, straining (40 mm Hg), or direct pressure on the eye. Efforts to quickly obtain good intubating conditions and prevent coughing and straining are much more important for reducing the risk of extrusion of eye contents than the avoidance of succinylcholine. If the intubation is judged to be difficult but the eye is viable, succinylcholine (after pretreatment with a small dose of a nondepolarizing muscle relaxant,) is an appropriate option. If the patient is likely to be an easy intubation, a short- to intermediate-acting nondepolarizing agent, administered in greater-than-normal doses, such as 1 to 1.2 mg/kg of rocuronium, has proven effective. The use of propofol has been shown to improve intubating conditions if rocuronium is used. IV lidocaine and opioids may also reduce the risk of straining and coughing. *(5:122-3)*

431. (D) Anesthesiologists should obtain informed refusal when patients refuse recommendations or request a relevantly suboptimal technique. The concept underlying informed refusal is that these patients need to be more extensively informed about risks, benefits, and alternatives when they desire inadvisable techniques. Anesthesiologists are not ethically obligated to provide care for these patients in nonemergent situations, although they may wish to assist in finding a willing colleague. *(5:46)*

432. (B) Every PACU should have definite guidelines for discharge criteria that should account for the preoperative status of the patient and the expected postoperative morbidity. Generalized guidelines for PACU discharge include baseline mental status, stable vital signs within acceptable limits, and achievement of certain criteria, possibly through a clinical scoring system. Current practice, endorsed by the ASA, does not require delay of discharge until voiding; the patient's risk for failure to void must be assessed instead. Patients at high risk for urinary retention secondary to neuraxial blockade, colorectal or genitourinary surgery, or medical history, may be kept until voiding, or if bladder catheterization is necessary. *(5:1253-4, 1256)*

433. (A) Nitrous oxide is a very insoluble gas in blood, but is 117 times more soluble than sulfur hexafluoride. N_2O enters the intraocular gas bubble more rapidly that SF_6 can exit. If N_2O administration continues after injection of SF_6 gas into the vitreal cavity, the bubble can expand up to three times its volume, increasing intraocular pressure. If N_2O is then discontinued, the IOP can drop quickly, thereby causing re-detachment of the retina. Therefore N_2O should be discontinued at least 20 min before the injection of gas. *(5:1223)*

434. (C) Abdominal compartment syndrome often causes decreased cardiac output and increases in both PCWP and CVP. These changes are nonspecific and may be due to other causes. Intraabdominal pressure is monitored by instilling 50 mL of saline into the bladder, then measuring the pressure. Pressures >20 mm Hg in combination with organ failure are consistent with a diagnosis of abdominal compartment syndrome, although pressures as low as 12 mm Hg have been associated with systemic inflammatory response syndrome and multiorgan failure. Although increasing abdominal distension is also often present, serial measurements of abdominal girth do not provide an indication of intraabdominal pressure. *(5:1363)*

435. (D) The patient with obstructive sleep apnea is at increased risk for opioid-induced apnea. The ability to manage the patient's pain without opioids may permit the patient to have safe ambulatory surgery. A perioperative nerve block does not necessarily increase safety because the patient might require opioids when the block regresses. A short surgical time does not necessarily minimize postoperative pain. CPAP may prevent obstruction-related apneic episodes, but it does not necessarily affect the magnitude of opioid-induced ventilatory depression in these patients. *(5:710, 1257-8)*

436. (B) Topical administration of an anticholinergic like atropine into the eye can raise intraocular pressure (IOP) in a patient with glaucoma, particularly dangerous in those persons predisposed to the relatively rare narrow-angle glaucoma. Systemic administration of atropine to these patients may precipitate a first attack in unrecognized cases. It does not, however, result in intraocular concentrations of atropine adequate to cause mydriasis in a patient with open-angled glaucoma, particularly when treated appropriately. *(1:228-9)*

437. (D) The diagnosis of CO poisoning is made by measuring the carboxyhemoglobin concentration in arterial blood, expressed as a percentage saturation of hemoglobin. Pulse oximetry cannot distinguish between these two forms of hemoglobin as the absorbance spectrum of both are similar, leading to normal oximetry readings in the presence of very high amounts of carboxyhemoglobin in blood. The PaO_2 in an arterial blood gas sample measures the amount of oxygen dissolved in blood and does not indicate the quantity of oxygen bound to hemoglobin (saturation), leading to a normal PaO_2 even with high concentrations of carboxyhemoglobin. The oxygen saturation is a calculated value only. *(5:1336-7)*

438. (C) Vital capacity is significantly and progressively compromised by increases in thoracic rigidity and loss of ventilatory muscle power. Loss of lung elastic recoil is the primary anatomic mechanism by which aging degrades the efficiency of pulmonary gas exchange. Because the changes in elasticity are nonuniform, they disrupt the normal matching of ventilation and perfusion within the lungs, increasing both shunting and physiologic dead space. Small airway patency, normally maintained by elastic recoil, is compromised, and closing capacity increases. Residual lung volume increases because intrinsic lung elastic recoil is progressively reduced. *(5:277-82)*

439. (A) Emergency treatment is aimed at quickly stabilizing the myocardium by raising the action potential threshold and reducing excitability without changing the resting membrane potential. This can be accomplished by administering 0.5-1 g of calcium chloride. Although it protects the heart from the effects of elevated serum potassium, intravenous calcium has no effect on the serum potassium concentration. Hyperventilation, as well as the administration of sodium bicarbonate, nebulized albuterol, or insulin and glucose in combination, will all aid in decreasing the serum potassium concentration by driving potassium ion intracellularly. Increasing the availability of insulin enhances the activity of the Na,K-ATPase pump in skeletal muscle, as does the use of β_2-adrenoceptor agonists. Raising the systemic pH with sodium bicarbonate results in hydrogen ion release from cells that is accompanied by potassium ion movement into cells. The potassium-lowering action of sodium bicarbonate is most prominent in patients with metabolic acidosis. *(5:518, 6:357-9)*

440. (D) Coagulation disturbances are common in patients with chronic liver disease. The primary reasons include a decreased production of coagulation factors produced in the liver (all except factor VIII); and a congestive splenomegaly, or hypersplenism, resulting from portal hypertension. Thrombocytopenia is due to splenic sequestration of platelets that can result in platelet concentration of $70,000/mm^3$ or less. The development of DIC, a reduction in fibrinogen, and dysfibrinogenemia secondary to impaired fibrin polymerization, are all commonly seen in advanced liver disease. *(5:193; 6:980-1)*

441. (D) Regional anesthesia may offer significant advantages in patients with Parkinson disease by allowing an earlier return to oral intake, eliminating the use of neuromuscular blocking drugs and the risks of general anesthesia. Butyrophenones such as droperidol can lower the seizure threshold and cause extrapyramidal symptoms. Withdrawal of Parkinson disease medications in the perioperative period can cause significant worsening of their respiratory symptoms caused by upper airway dysfunction due to disease involvement of the intrinsic laryngeal muscles. Morphine has been reported to reduce dyskinesia at low doses but to induce akinesia at greater doses. *(5:701, 876; Nicholson G, et al., Br J Anaesth 2002; 89: 904-16)*

442. (B) Transfusion-related acute lung injury (TRALI) is the leading cause of transfusion-related mortality. Estimated TRALI incidence is once for every 3,000 to 70,000 plasma-rich components transfused and 1 per 50,000 units of low plasma volume components transfused. Human error accounts for the second highest incidence of adverse transfusion effects, whereas the transfusion-associated viral infectious risk is quite low, with the risk of hepatitis C being 1:1,935,000 and that of the human immunodeficiency virus being 1:2,135,000. Anaphylaxis and hemolytic transfusion reactions are both potentially fatal complications. *(5:149, 203-4)*

443. **(A)** Etomidate inhibits the enzyme responsible for performing the 11β-hydroxylation reaction in cortisol synthesis. A single induction dose of 0.3 mg/kg inhibits cortisol synthesis and the normal response to adrenocorticotropic hormone for up to 12 h. Because of the long duration of adrenal suppression associated with etomidate infusions, continuous administration has not been as extensively studied. There remains conflict about the issue of the reduction of cortisol after induction doses of etomidate, but it has been shown that infusions of several days' duration in ventilated intensive care unit patients were associated with increased mortality. Given that the duration of suppression of cortisol synthesis by etomidate is dependent on the cumulative dose, use of the agent in repeated procedural sedation in a critically ill patient is of concern. *(5:687, 696-7)*

444. **(D)** Hepatopulmonary syndrome is defined by the presence of hepatic dysfunction or portal hypertension, an elevated alveolar-arterial oxygen gradient, and intrapulmonary vasodilatation. Unlike portopulmonary hypertension, which is associated with pulmonary vascular vasoconstriction, hepatopulmonary syndrome results from vasodilatation and pulmonary vascular remodeling. Patients may present with digital clubbing, spider angiomata, arterial hypoxemia, and dyspnea that worsens upon moving from a recumbent to an upright position (orthodeoxia and platypnea). Intrapulmonary vasodilation may reflect true anatomical shunt, physiologic shunt, and precapillary or capillary dilation, leading to alterations in oxygen diffusion. Nitric oxide is elevated in the exhaled breath of patients with hepatopulmonary syndrome. *(5:194, 1051-5; 6:2601)*

445. **(D)** Decreasing lean tissue mass in the elderly reduces the capacity for body heat production, and impairment of thermoregulatory vasoconstriction places them at increased risk for inadvertent intraoperative hypothermia. Intraoperative core temperature decreases at a rate twice as great as that observed in young adults under comparable conditions, and the time needed for spontaneous postoperative rewarming increases in direct proportion to patient age. There exists an age-related increase in pharmacodynamic sensitivity to anesthetic agents, yet the cause remains unknown. With aging, relative minimum alveolar concentration values for the newer inhalational agents decline by approximately 30%. Decreases in the elderly brain neurotransmitter reserves are manifested by an increased sensitivity to drugs that might precipitate extrapyramidal symptoms or anticholinergic syndrome, including metoclopramide. Although the elderly have reduced skeletal muscle mass, disseminated neurogenic atrophy at the neuromuscular junction allows proliferation of extrajunctional cholinoreceptors. The median effective dose and steady-state plasma concentration required for half-maximal neuromuscular blocking effect (median effective concentration) remain virtually unchanged, or may actually increase slightly, in the elderly patient. Onset of blockade may be delayed, and duration prolonged, however. Renal plasma flow, glomerular filtration rate (GFR), and creatinine clearance all decline significantly. *(1:1326, 5:279-83)*

446. **(A)** Injury to the recurrent laryngeal nerve (RLN) prevents abduction of the ipsilateral vocal cord that becomes fixed in a paramedian position because of the unopposed action of the cricothyroid muscle. It commonly results in hoarseness. Bilateral nerve injury could result in apposition of the vocal cords and inspiratory obstruction with associated stridor and aphonia. Laryngeal edema would be seen with venous and lymphatic obstruction secondary to a hematoma, not injury to the RLN. *(5:1006, 1268, 1286)*

447. **(E)** Nitroprusside is rapidly metabolized to cyanide and thiocyanate, and accumulation of these metabolites can lead to cyanide or thiocyanate toxicity during prolonged administration, especially in patients with renal failure. *(5:1403)*

448. (B) Anesthetic implications of untreated hypothyroidism include an impaired ventilatory response to both hypoxia and hypercarbia. Atrial dysrhythmias, including atrial fibrillation, are seen in hyperthyroidism. Conventional anesthetic wisdom holds that thyroid status does not alter the minimum alveolar concentration. Data from animal studies using older volatile anesthetics supports that assumption, but there are no data relative to the newer potent inhalation agents. Similarly, conventional wisdom holds that hypothyroidism increases the sensitivity to sedative, analgesic, and anesthetic medications, but evidence is limited to older studies due to the lack of newer studies on current agents. Hypertension, particularly diastolic hypertension, is also commonly noted in hypothyroidism. *(5:1117)*

449. (B) A direct pharmacodynamic effect of hypothermia is its impact on minimum alveolar concentration (MAC). There is an approximately 5% reduction in MAC per degree drop in core body temperature. *(5:1510, 1653)*

450. (B) Scopolamine is a muscarinic receptor antagonist with greater permeation across the blood brain barrier. In therapeutic doses it causes CNS depression manifested as drowsiness and amnesia. The amnestic effects of midazolam (when given in the usual doses for premedication) are variable but usually short lived, and they should not be relied on to prevent recall of intraoperative events. Dexmedetomidine produces intense sedation, although it does not reliably produce amnesia, hypnosis, or general anesthesia. Neither droperidol nor muscle relaxants produce amnesia. *(1:227-30; 5:610, 698, 701, 1374)*

451. (C) The BIS is a proprietary algorithm (Aspect Medical Systems, Newton, MA) that generates a linear dimensionless number ranging from 0 to 100 that decreases in proportion to increased anesthetic depth. Evidence shows that it may be effective at reducing the incidence of intraoperative awareness when inhaled anesthetics are used to produce hypnosis. Confounding factors, which can alter BIS, include electrical artifact from electrocautery devices, physio-

logic alterations such as hypoglycemia, low-voltage EEG caused by genetic variation or drugs, neurologic abnormalities such as Alzheimer disease, and EMG (muscle). Finally, the value of BIS monitoring has been validated only for propofol and volatile anesthetics. When ketamine and N_2O are present, the relationship between BIS value and perceptive awareness can be significantly altered *(5:610)*

452. (D) James T. Reason is often cited for his conceptual thinking about system failure and human error. The process of accident evolution is widely referred to as the "Swiss cheese" model. The "Swiss cheese" model illustrates that accidents are typically the result of a series of events that include precursors that trigger or allow the chain of events that result in the final (active) adverse event. Reason termed these precursors latent errors. Latent errors have the potential for initiating or propagating an evolving accident. Examples are failure to maintain equipment or replace obsolete equipment, selection of low quality supply items, poor scheduling practices that promote haste or fatigue, and case scheduling and staffing models that allow assignment of relatively inexperienced clinicians to unfamiliar cases or high-risk patients. Latent errors rarely lead to an immediate accident, but are seen as a "lurking enemy," awaiting the circumstances that will combine to produce an unexpected catastrophic outcome, often in ways that are unusual and unpredictable. *(5:18)*

453. (C) As defined by the Joint Commission, a sentinel event is "an unexpected occurrence involving death or serious physical or psychological injury, or the risk thereof. Serious injury specifically includes loss of limb or function." JCAHO sentinel events that potentially involve anesthesia care include events that result in an unanticipated death or major permanent loss of function and are unrelated to the natural course of the patient's illness or underlying condition, surgery on the wrong patient or body part regardless of magnitude of procedure, unintended retention of a foreign body after surgery or other procedure, hemolytic transfusion reactions because of major blood group incompatibilities, and unanticipated death of a full-term infant. *(5:352-2)*

454. **(E)** Although there are three forms of anthrax (gastrointestinal, cutaneous, and inhalational), it is the inhalational form that is most likely to be the cause of death in a bioterrorist attack. The early symptoms include a viral prodrome with fever, fatigue, nausea and vomiting, and shortness of breath. CXR reveals characteristic findings of mediastinal widening and pleural effusions, as well as infiltrates. Symptoms tend to appear within 4-6 d of exposure. Patients are not contagious, and therefore do not need to be isolated. Therapy must be started quickly, with penicillin, doxycycline, and ciprofloxacin proven to be effective. Patients with active disease are often started on the above agents, in combination with either clindamycin or rifampin. *(6:1769-72)*

455. **(C)** Almost 50% of the U.S. population is susceptible to the smallpox virus, as immunization programs were stopped in the United States in 1972. Primary and secondary viremias occur within the first few days after exposure. Twelve to fourteen days after first exposure, patients develop high fever, vomiting, headache, and backache. A maculopapular rash forms, beginning on the face and extremities and extending to the trunk, with lesions in the same developmental stage within the same location. The lesions evolve into vesicles and pustules. Because it is highly infectious, patients must be kept in strict isolation until the pustules resolve and become scabs. *(6:1772, 1774-5)*

456. **(B)** Although botulinum toxin is not a live microorganism, it is one of the most potent toxins ever described, with estimates that 1 g of toxin would be enough to kill 1 million people if appropriately dispersed. Once absorbed into the bloodstream, it binds to the neuronal cell membrane, enters the cell, and cleaves one of the proteins required for intracellular binding of the synaptic vesicle to the cell membrane, thus preventing release of the neurotransmitter to the adjacent cell. Patients develop cranial nerve palsies followed by a descending flaccid paralysis. Most patients develop diplopia, dry mouth, dysphagia and dysarthria, and extremity weakness. Recovery requires regeneration of new motor neuron synapses that may take weeks to months. Treatment is mainly supportive, but if diagnosed early enough, administration of a heptavalent equine antitoxin may diminish symptoms and decrease severity of the disease. *(6:1776-8)*

CHAPTER 18

Critical Care Medicine
Questions

DIRECTIONS (Questions 457-530): Each of the numbered items or incomplete statements in this section is followed by answers or by completions of the statement. Select the ONE lettered answer or completion that is BEST in each case.

457. A previously healthy 18-year-old male presents to the emergency department with three days of dyspnea and facial swelling. He also reports a cough and hoarseness. His symptoms worsen with lying down. His chest x-ray reveals a widened mediastinum. Which one of the following is the most likely diagnosis?

    (A) Angioedema
    (B) Epiglottitis
    (C) Lymphoma
    (D) Pneumonia
    (E) Tracheomalacia

458. An 81-year-old male has been in the hospital for treatment of a urinary tract infection and delirium. During the night he got out of bed unassisted and sustained a fall. A subsequent evaluation revealed a C3 vertebral fracture. He went to the operating room for repair of his fracture. Postoperatively he was kept intubated for concerns about airway edema. The plan is to reassess his ability to be extubated in 24 h. In the interim, he requires sedation for safety. His vital signs are T 37.1°C, HR 58, BP 122/78, SpO$_2$ 100%. Which choice of sedative agent is most appropriate in this situation?

    (A) Dexmedetomidine
    (B) Etomidate
    (C) Midazolam
    (D) Propofol

459. A 66-year-old male is in the intensive care unit recovering from a ruptured abdominal aortic aneurysm repair. His postoperative course has been complicated by acute kidney injury and an NSTEMI. He remains intubated and mechanically ventilated. Four days into his course, his respiratory function worsens, and he is diagnosed with ventilator-associated pneumonia. Sputum culture grows *Haemophilus influenza*. Administration of which one of the following medications might have prevented this pneumonia?

    (A) Oral chlorhexidine
    (B) Systemic clindamycin
    (C) Systemic dexamethasone
    (D) Systemic omeprazole

460. Which one of the following statements about organ donation after cardiac death (DCD) is most accurate?

    (A) Requires declaration of brain death by a neurologist
    (B) Causes longer warm ischemic time than donation after brain death
    (C) Does not require patient/family consent
    (D) Does not involve extubation of the patient
    (E) Cannot involve ICU physician in end-of-life care of the patient

DIRECTIONS: Use the following figure to answer Question 461:

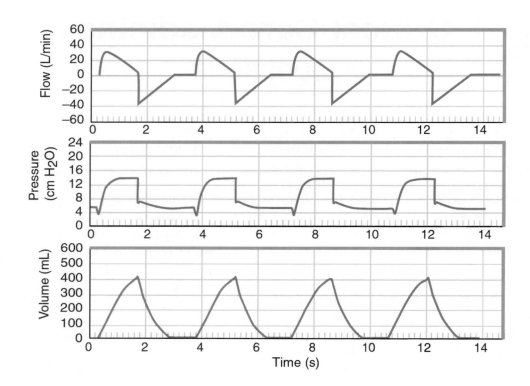

461. For the ventilatory mode depicted in the figure, which statement is correct?

   (A) The end of inspiration is determined by decrease to a set fraction of peak inspiratory flow.
   (B) Minute ventilation is independent of patient effort.
   (C) Pressure is the dependent variable.
   (D) A bronchopleural fistula will not affect inspiratory time.
   (E) Mandatory and spontaneous breaths are depicted.

DIRECTIONS: Use the following scenario to answer Questions 462-463: A 78-year-old man is admitted to the ICU following open repair of an abdominal aortic aneurysm. He has a history of coronary artery disease treated with a drug-eluting stent four years ago. His medications include aspirin, metoprolol, pravastatin, and lisinopril. A preoperative pharmacologic radionuclide myocardial stress test revealed no evidence of perfusion defects. His vital signs on arrival to the ICU are T 36.2°C, HR 68, BP 100/60, RR 12, oxygen saturation 99% on facemask oxygen. Pain score is 3/10. One hour later, his heart rate falls to 30 and blood pressure to 65/38; he is awake, alert, and has no complaints.

462. Which one of the following is the most appropriate first intervention?

   (A) Transvenous pacing
   (B) Endotracheal intubation
   (C) Cardiopulmonary resuscitation
   (D) Atropine

463. A few minutes later, the blood pressure is 180/110. An electrocardiogram is obtained and is shown in the figure below:

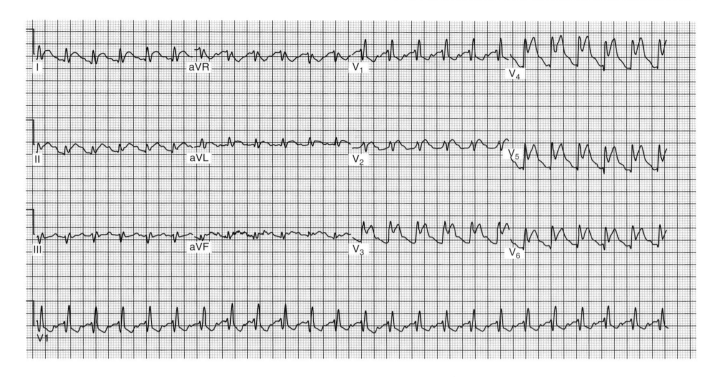

Appropriate interventions should include

(A) stat echocardiogram, dobutamine, blood transfusion

(B) thrombolysis, pulmonary artery catheter, dobutamine

(C) esmolol, nitroglycerin, transfer to cardiac catheterization suite

(D) stat CT angiogram, esmolol, cardiac surgery consult

(E) nitroprusside, intravenous heparin, transfer to cardiac catheterization suite

DIRECTIONS: Use the following scenario to answer Questions 464-469: A 77-year-old male is being treated for ascending cholangitis resulting in gram-negative bacteremia. He is intubated, sedated, and mechanically ventilated. A pulmonary artery catheter is placed five hours after presentation to assist with management of his hemodynamics and resuscitation. His vital signs are T 38.7°C, HR 91, BP 76/43 and SpO$_2$ 90%. CVP is 4 mm Hg. CO is 5 L/min.

His ABG is pH 7.29, PaCO$_2$ 37, PaO$_2$ 61. His hemoglobin is 9 g/dL.

464. Which one of the following would produce the greatest increase in oxygen delivery?

(A) An increase in arterial oxygen saturation to 100%

(B) An increase in heart rate to 110 beats/min

(C) An increase in hemoglobin to 10 g/dL

(D) An increase in stroke volume to 80 mL/beat

465. The cross sectional area of which one of the following is the primary determinant of systemic vascular resistance (SVR)?

(A) Arteries

(B) Arterioles

(C) Capillaries

(D) Venules

(E) Veins

466. Which one of the following correctly describes arteriolar and vascular smooth muscle receptors?

(A) α_1- and β_2-adrenoceptors mediate vasoconstriction

(B) α_1-adrenoceptors mediate vasoconstriction while β_2-adrenoceptors mediate vasodilation

(C) α_1-adrenoceptors mediate vasodilation while β_2-adrenoceptors mediate vasoconstriction

(D) α_1- and β_2-adrenoceptors mediate vasodilation

467. This patient would be expected to have which one of the following?

(A) Decreased angiotensin formation

(B) Decreased renin release

(C) Decreased vasopressin levels

(D) Increased aldosterone release

(E) Increased sodium excretion

468. Which one of the following provides an index of total body tissue perfusion?

(A) Cerebral oximetry

(B) Central venous oxygen saturation

(C) Mixed venous oxygen saturation

(D) Pulse oximetry

469. This patient would be expected to have which one of the following metabolic abnormalities?

(A) A decrease in hepatic lipogenesis

(B) A decrease in serum glucose concentrations

(C) A decrease in serum triglyceride concentrations

(D) An increase in pancreatic insulin release

(E) An increase in protein catabolism

470. A 47-year-old male is being treated for streptococcal pneumonia in the ICU. He is intubated and sedated for respiratory failure, and has had persistent fevers and an elevated white blood count. Diagnostic thoracentesis for a parapneumonic effusion revealed that the effusion was an empyema. As a result, he is scheduled to have a therapeutic thoracentesis in the interventional radiology suite. The patient has been on volume control ventilation with the following settings: TV 450, RR 20, PEEP 14, FIO_2 0.6. Prior to transport to the interventional radiology suite, you are called to the bedside. The patient has had worsening oxygenation with decreased oxygen saturation when he is turned or placed flat. He has required FIO_2 1.0 several times in the last several hours. Chest x-ray shows increasing size of the pleural effusion. Which one of the following is the most appropriate therapy?

(A) Arrange for open drainage of the effusion in the operating room

(B) Arrange for percutaneous drainage of the effusion at the bedside

(C) Continue with the scheduled procedure

(D) Delay thoracentesis until the patient is more stable

471. A 52-year-old male complains of nausea and a headache at work. He subsequently has an acute decline in wakefulness. His coworkers bring him to the emergency department. On evaluation, he opens his eyes to painful stimuli, makes incomprehensible sounds and localizes to pain. Select the patient's GCS from the list below.

(A) 6

(B) 7

(C) 8

(D) 9

(E) 10

472. A 47-year-old female was admitted to the ICU 18 h ago with pancreatitis and SIRS. She required intubation for increased work of breathing and large volume IV fluid resuscitation for hypovolemia. Her clinical picture has worsened over the last several hours. She has poor urine output, is hypotensive and has decreased minute ventilation due to high airway pressures. A chest x-ray shows mild bilateral pulmonary edema. Which one of the following is the most likely cause of the patient's symptoms?

(A) Abdominal compartment syndrome
(B) Cardiomyopathy
(C) Hypovolemia
(D) Infection
(E) Pulmonary embolism

473. A 23-year-old female presents to the labor triage unit with premature rupture of membranes at 34 weeks and 6 days gestational age. She reports that her pregnancy has been uncomplicated except for a DVT diagnosed in her first trimester. She is currently taking prenatal vitamins and enoxaparin (1 mg/kg BID). Her vital signs are T 37.1°C, HR 71, BP 112/68, RR 22, SpO_2 98%. A CBC, prothrombin time, partial thromboplastin time, and comprehensive metabolic panel done as part of her evaluation are unremarkable except for a platelet count of 57,000/mm^3. Fetal heart tones are reassuring. What is the most likely cause of her laboratory abnormality?

(A) Vitamin B_{12} deficiency
(B) Disseminated intravascular coagulation (DIC)
(C) Heparin induced thrombocytopenia (HIT)
(D) HELLP syndrome
(E) Placental abruption

DIRECTIONS: Use the following scenario to answer Questions 474-478: A 41-year-old male motorcyclist is struck by a car. He is unconscious at the scene and intubated en route. On arrival to the emergency department trauma bay, his systolic blood pressure is 60 mm Hg. Bilateral chest tubes are placed without an improvement in his hemodynamics. A chest x-ray, pelvic x-ray, long bone films and a FAST exam are rapidly obtained. The exams are positive for multiple left sided rib fractures, pulmonary contusions, an open-book pelvic fracture, a left femur fracture, and fluid in the hepatorenal fossa. Transfusion of two units O-negative packed red blood cells is initiated, and the patient is brought emergently to the operating room. A laparotomy is performed and the patient is found to have profuse bleeding from a ruptured liver as well as an expanding retroperitoneal hematoma. Over the course of the surgery, the patient receives 25 units of PRBCs, 15 units of FFP, and 4 single donor units of platelets. His current vital signs are T 35.7°C, BP 81/42, HR 127, SpO_2 95% on FIO_2 0.7. Laboratory values are remarkable for Hb 8.9 g/dL, platelets 103,000/mm^3, INR 1.7, fibrinogen 95 mg/dL, ABG pH 7.23, $PaCO_2$ 43 mm Hg, PaO_2 64 mm Hg, K 4.4 mEq/L, creatinine 1.6 mg/dL, and ionized calcium 0.81 mmol/L. A TEE-probe is inserted. There is no pericardial effusion. Both ventricles appear well filled with normal size, but the systolic function of both ventricles appears reduced.

474. Which one of the following is most likely to improve the patient's hemodynamic picture?

(A) Administration of bicarbonate
(B) Administration of calcium
(C) Increased PEEP
(D) Transfusion of packed red blood cells
(E) Warming the patient to > 36°C

475. The patient begins to bleed from his IV line sites and his nose. Which one of the following would be most likely to improve the patient's clotting ability?

(A) Administration of cryoprecipitate
(B) Administration of desmopressin
(C) Administration of fresh frozen plasma
(D) Administration of platelets
(E) Warming the patient to 37°C

476. The patient undergoes damage control laparotomy and embolization of bleeding pelvic vessels. He is brought to the ICU for further stabilization. Over the next 6 h, the patient's vasopressor requirement improves, and his transfusion requirement resolves. He is weaned from 32 to 7 mcg/min of norepinephrine. During that time frame, however, he develops oliguria. His laboratory data shows: Na 143 mEq/L, K 5.9 mEq/L, BUN 20 mg/dL, Cr 1.8 mg/dL, urine osmolality 332 mOsm/L H_2O, urine sodium 43 mEq/L, urine creatinine 18 mg/mL. Urinalysis is negative for leukocytes or red blood cells. What is the most likely cause of this patient's oliguria?

(A) Acute tubular necrosis
(B) Glomerulonephritis
(C) Interstitial nephritis
(D) Prerenal azotemia
(E) Urinary obstruction

477. There are peaked T waves on the ECG. Intravenous calcium is administered. What is the role of calcium in the treatment of hyperkalemia? Calcium

(A) antagonizes gastrointestinal absorption of potassium
(B) enhances renal excretion of potassium
(C) facilitates redistribution of potassium into cells
(D) increases cardiac myocyte excitability
(E) raises the cardiac action potential threshold

478. Two days later the patient returns to the operating room for fixation of a tibial fracture. During the procedure, he is found to have compartment syndrome of his lower leg, and a fasciotomy is performed. Postoperatively his CPK is 9,562 IU/L. Which of the following laboratory abnormalities are most likely?

(A) Elevated calcium, decreased potassium, decreased phosphorus
(B) Elevated calcium, increased potassium, decreased phosphorus
(C) Decreased calcium, decreased potassium, increased phosphorus
(D) Decreased calcium, increased potassium, increased phosphorus
(E) Decreased calcium, increased potassium, decreased phosphorus

479. A 26-year-old female presents to her oncologist's office with worsening dyspnea and chest pain. She is on warfarin for a history of DVT diagnosed six months ago, and she is being treated for breast cancer with chemotherapy. She is otherwise healthy. Physical exam reveals T 37.1°C, HR 122, BP 80/40, and peripheral edema. She is admitted urgently to the hospital. Her INR is 3.2. ECG shows sinus tachycardia with low QRS voltage and no ST changes. Which one of the following is most likely to lead to a diagnosis?

(A) Cardiac enzymes
(B) Chest x-ray
(C) D-dimer
(D) Echocardiography
(E) Urinalysis

480. A 35-year-old, previously healthy female is brought to the emergency department after a seizure. She has no memory of the event. She currently has no complaints. Her vital signs are T 37°C, HR 82, BP 126/75, RR 17, SpO_2 98%. Her neurologic examination is normal, including a GCS of 15. Her optic disks are sharp. Skin examination reveals a suspicious lesion on her right thigh. CBC and comprehensive metabolic panel (CMP) are unremarkable. Head CT shows a frontal mass consistent with metastasis. What is the most appropriate next step in management?

(A) CSF diversion
(B) Dexamethasone
(C) Intubation and hyperventilation
(D) Mannitol
(E) Decompressive craniectomy

481. Which one of the following measures is recommended during central venous catheter insertion, based on evidence supporting a reduction in the rate of central line-associated blood stream infection?

(A) Sterile head to toe draping of patient, chlorhexidine skin preparation, subclavian site

(B) Full barrier precautions, hand washing prior to line insertion, prophylactic antibiotic administration

(C) Sterile head to toe draping of patient, sterile rewire of catheter every 7 d, hand washing prior to line insertion

(D) Chlorhexidine skin preparation, removal of unnecessary catheters, avoidance of internal jugular site

(E) Hand washing prior to line insertion, head to abdomen draping of patient, removal of subclavian site catheters after 7 d

482. A 4-year-old boy with history of premature birth, asthma, and developmental delay is hospitalized in the PICU with respiratory failure due to respiratory syncytial virus (RSV). He has been intubated, sedated, and mechanically ventilated for 6 d. Vital signs are T 37.5°C, HR 92, BP 80/40. CVP is 6 mm Hg. He is ventilated in assist control pressure control mode at the following settings: FIO_2 0.7, PC 25 cm H_2O, PEEP 10, RR 30. On exam, he is unresponsive, has soft bilateral rales, and his urine is dark. ABG shows pH 7.18, $PaCO_2$ 56 mm Hg, PaO_2 65 mm Hg. Laboratory values are Na 146 mEq/L, K 5.4 mEq/L, Cl 110 mEq/L, BUN 28, Cr 1.9, CPK 6500 IU/L. Chest radiograph shows diffuse lobar infiltrates and low lung volumes. Which is the most appropriate next step in management?

(A) Transition from pressure control to pressure support ventilation

(B) Perform bedside echocardiogram

(C) Initiate neuromuscular blockade

(D) Discontinue propofol

(E) Begin continuous venovenous hemofiltration

DIRECTIONS: Use the following scenario to answer Questions 483-486: A 59-year-old man is admitted to the ICU following a hepatic resection complicated by hemorrhage. Surgery was aborted, the abdomen packed with laparotomy sponges, and he was transported intubated, sedated, and pharmacologically paralyzed to the ICU. Vital signs are T 34.5°C, HR 127, BP 80/45, RR 20, SpO_2 90% on FIO_2 0.8. He is oliguric with cool extremities; abdominal exam is significant for increasing distention. He is placed on mechanical ventilation in the mode depicted in the following figure:

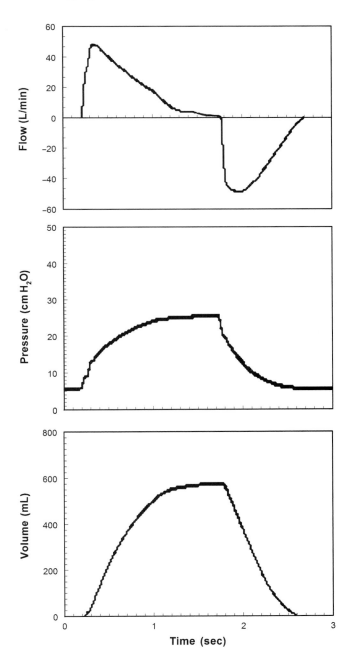

483. Following two hours of continuous resuscitation with blood products, which one of the following ventilatory alarms is most likely?

(A) Increased peak airway pressure over set limit
(B) Apnea > 30 sec
(C) Low minute ventilation
(D) High tidal volume
(E) Excessive inspiratory time

484. An arterial blood gas drawn on this patient shows pH 7.18, $Paco_2$ 55 mm Hg, Pao_2 60 mm Hg, base deficit 9. The patient's disorder is best described as

(A) respiratory acidosis
(B) mixed respiratory acidosis and metabolic alkalosis
(C) metabolic acidosis
(D) mixed respiratory acidosis and metabolic acidosis

485. The figure below depicts the patient's arterial waveform.

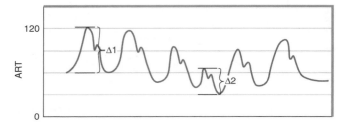

The following equation is derived from the measurements depicted in the figure:

$$\frac{\Delta 1 - \Delta 2}{\left(\dfrac{\Delta 1 + \Delta 2}{2}\right)} \times 100\%$$

The value determined by the equation is:

(A) stroke volume variation
(B) pulse pressure variation
(C) delta down
(D) respiratory variation
(E) systolic pressure variation

486. Based on the findings from the patient's arterial waveform, the next management should be

(A) inotrope administration
(B) vasopressor administration
(C) pericardiocentesis
(D) pulmonary artery catheterization
(E) fluid administration

487. A 44-year-old female presents to the emergency department with one hour of severe headache and mental status changes. Initial CT scan shows subarachnoid hemorrhage (SAH) that is likely due to aneurysmal rupture. Her initial Fisher Grade is 2. She is intubated in the emergency department due to concerns that she is unable to effectively manage her secretions. A subsequent repeat head CT shows that she has progressed to Fisher Grade 3. Which one of the following is the most likely mechanism for this change?

(A) Aneurysmal rebleeding
(B) Elevated intracranial pressure
(C) Seizures
(D) Vasospasm

488. Synchronized intermittent mandatory ventilation (SIMV) is associated with which beneficial effect as compared to controlled ventilation?

(A) Resting of the diaphragm
(B) Decreased work of breathing
(C) Improved V/Q matching
(D) Absence of patient-ventilator dyssynchrony
(E) Increased mean intrathoracic pressure

489. A 41-year-old woman underwent resection of an acoustic neuroma under total intravenous anesthesia (TIVA). The surgical procedure was notable for 12-h duration with 500 mL blood loss. She is admitted to the ICU postoperatively, is extubated, breathing comfortably, and is neurologically intact. Vital signs are normal. An ABG reveals pH 7.30, $Paco_2$ 42 mm Hg, Pao_2 150 mm Hg on supplemental oxygen, base deficit 4. A metabolic panel shows Na 143 mEq/L, K 3 mEq/L, Cl 115 mEq/L, HCO_3 20 mEq/L. Which one of the following is the most likely explanation for the patient's acid-base disturbance?

(A) Crystalloid resuscitation fluid administered during operation

(B) Loop diuretic administered to reduce brain swelling

(C) TIVA anesthetic agent

(D) Hypovolemia due to underresuscitation

(E) Nitroprusside treatment of intraoperative hypertension

490. Compared with norepinephrine in the treatment of septic shock, dopamine

(A) diminishes mortality

(B) diminishes incidence of renal failure

(C) has greater potency

(D) causes more tachydysrhythmias

DIRECTIONS: Use the following scenario to answer Question 491: A 19-year-old previously healthy man presents after crashing his moped into a stone wall. He was found without a helmet, ejected from the moped with GCS 4 (E1V1M2). Vital signs are T 35.8°C, HR 156, BP 79/45. He is being mask ventilated at rate 12 breaths per minute; SpO$_2$ 99% with bag mask ventilation at FIO$_2$ 1.0. A noncontrast brain CT is obtained with findings depicted below:

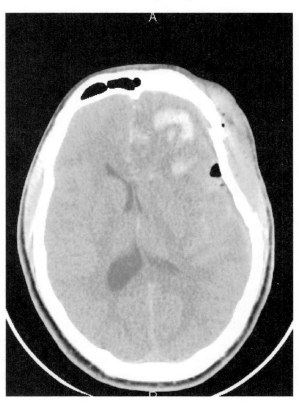

491. Following endotracheal intubation, which one of the following should be employed for immediate management of this patient?

(A) Mechanical ventilation to PaCO$_2$ 26 mm Hg, 23.4% saline bolus, furosemide bolus, head of bed elevation to 30 degrees

(B) Mechanical ventilation to PaCO$_2$ 35 mm Hg, ventriculostomy, 23.4% saline bolus, phenylephrine infusion to MAP > 80 mm Hg

(C) Mechanical ventilation to PaCO$_2$ 18 mm Hg, Trendelenberg position, emergent neurosurgical decompression, volume resuscitation with 0.9% saline

(D) Mechanical ventilation to PaCO$_2$ 35 mm Hg, methylprednisolone bolus, volume resuscitation with 0.9% saline, emergent neurosurgical decompression

(E) Mechanical ventilation to PaCO$_2$ 35 mm Hg, mannitol bolus, volume resuscitation with 5% albumin, emergent neurosurgical decompression

DIRECTIONS: Use the following scenario to answer Questions 492-494: A 74-year-old male presents to the emergency department from his nursing home with new onset confusion. His vital signs are T 38.5°C, HR 94, BP 92/61, RR 24, SpO$_2$ 96%. His white blood count is 14,000/mm^3. Blood, urine and CSF cultures are obtained. A urinary catheter is placed yielding scant dark urine. Gram stain of the urine specimen reveals many gram-negative rods. After volume resuscitation, the patient's heart rate and blood pressure are 87 and 104/65, respectively. A central venous line is placed, and the CVP is 12 mm Hg. Urine output remains low at 15 mL/h for 2 h.

492. This patient would most accurately be described as having:

(A) septicemia

(B) systemic inflammatory response syndrome (SIRS)

(C) sepsis

(D) severe sepsis

(E) septic shock

493. Which one of the following would be the most appropriate next step in management?

(A) Flush the urinary catheter

(B) Perform a head CT

(C) Give a bolus of IV fluids

(D) Perform a renal ultrasound

(E) Start antibiotics

494. Which one of the following resuscitation fluids has been associated with an increased incidence of acute renal failure in critically ill patients?

(A) Albumin

(B) Hydroxyethyl starch

(C) Normal saline

(D) Fresh frozen plasma

(E) Lactated Ringer solution

DIRECTIONS: Use the following scenario to answer Questions 495-498: A 44-year-old man with BMI = 40 kg/m^2 is now on postoperative day 1 following elective ventral hernia repair. The rapid response team is called to assess him for possible ICU transfer. His nurse reports that 3 h prior, he was sleepy, easily arousable, hemodynamically stable but complaining of 7/10 incisional pain that was treated with intravenous morphine delivered by PCA. One hour ago, he became disoriented and agitated, pulling out his intravenous access and urinary catheter. At that time, lorazepam 5 mg IM was administered and new intravenous access established. Now he is very somnolent. Vital signs show T 37.6°C, HR 92, BP 98/60, RR 7, SpO$_2$ 85% on supplemental oxygen via nonrebreather mask.

495. Which one of the following is the most likely finding on preoperative pulmonary function tests (PFTs) in this patient?

(A) Increased residual volume (RV)

(B) Decreased diffusing capacity (DLCO)

(C) Decreased forced expiratory volume in first second/forced vital capacity (FEV$_1$/FVC) ratio

(D) Increased total lung capacity (TLC)

(E) Decreased expiratory reserve volume (ERV)

496. The patient's wife volunteers a preoperative history of snoring at night, daytime sleepiness, and a referral for a sleep study that the patient has not yet undergone. Which one of the following combination of conditions is the most likely explanation for hypoxemia in the PACU in this patient?

(A) Atelectasis and anemia

(B) Intracardiac shunt and increased oxygen consumption

(C) Atelectasis and hypoventilation

(D) Hypoventilation and hypermetabolism

(E) Intrapulmonary shunt and decreased diffusing capacity

497. Which of the following are most appropriate in initial management of this patient?

(A) Administer flumazenil, provide noninvasive positive pressure ventilation (NIPPV), position head of bed at 45 degrees

(B) Position head of bed at 45 degrees, place nasogastric tube, draw ABG

(C) Administer naloxone, position head of bed at 45 degrees, discontinue supplemental oxygen

(D) Administer naloxone, provide noninvasive positive pressure ventilation (NIPPV), position head of bed at 45 degrees

(E) Change to hydromorphone analgesia, perform endotracheal intubation, and transfer to ICU

498. The patient fails to improve from the initial management strategy. He is transferred to the ICU. Following uneventful endotracheal intubation using etomidate, he becomes severely hypotensive, and unresponsive to fluid resuscitation. Vital signs are T 37°C, HR 110, BP 75/45, RR 18, SpO$_2$ 88% on FIO$_2$ 1.0. ABG reveals pH 7.40, PaCO$_2$ 60 mm Hg, PaO$_2$ 59 mm Hg, base excess 14. CXR shows no evidence of atelectasis or infiltrate. ECG reveals sinus rhythm, R axis deviation, and evidence of right ventricular strain. Which one of the following would be the most likely findings from bedside echocardiogram?

(A) Normal right ventricular size and function, dilated left atrium, small and hypercontractile left ventricle

(B) Normal right ventricle size and function, left ventricular apical ballooning

(C) Dilated and hypertrophied right ventricle, paradoxical intraventricular septal motion, small left ventricle

(D) Large pericardial effusion

(E) Normal right ventricular size and function, dilated, hypocontractile left ventricle with significant mitral regurgitation

DIRECTIONS: Use the following scenario to answer Questions 499-501: A 58-year-old man with COPD and diabetes mellitus is admitted to the ICU with the diagnosis of necrotizing fasciitis of the perineum. His vital signs are significant for T 39.1°C, HR 125, BP 79/52, RR 34, SpO$_2$ 88% on facemask oxygen.

499. Which one of the following is the explanation for a fall in mean arterial pressure following endotracheal intubation and mechanical ventilation?

(A) Catecholamine release associated with direct laryngoscopy

(B) Histamine release induced by ketamine administration

(C) Reduced venous return associated with positive pressure ventilation

(D) Decreased work of breathing causing a worsened lactic acidosis

(E) Increased left ventricular afterload associated with positive pressure ventilation

500. Mechanical ventilation of the patient is complicated by patient-ventilator dyssynchrony. What is the most likely cause?

(A) Rapid inspiratory flow rise time at the initiation of a breath

(B) Decelerating flow pattern with volume targeted ventilation

(C) Excessive sedation with propofol

(D) Auto positive end-expiratory pressure

(E) Ventilator inspiratory time matched to patient inspiratory time

501. During pressure assist/control mode ventilation, the endotracheal tube becomes partially obstructed by secretions. Which one of the following is most likely to result?

(A) Increased tidal volume

(B) Increased plateau pressure

(C) Apnea

(D) Decreased peak inspiratory pressure

(E) Decreased minute ventilation

DIRECTIONS: Use the following scenario to answer Questions 502-503: A 65-year-old man is admitted to the ICU following percutaneous nephrostomy tube placement to treat ureteral obstruction. Immediately following the procedure, he developed fever and hypotension. Vital signs upon arrival to the ICU are T 39.2°C, HR 130, BP 80/40, RR 38. Oxygen saturation is unobtainable. CVP is 3 mm Hg. He is awake and oriented and complains of 5/10 pain at the tube site. He has a Grade II/VI systolic ejection murmur at the left sternal border, cool extremities and poor peripheral pulses. Urine from the nephrostomy tube is cloudy yellow. Laboratory values show Na 138 mEq/L, K 4.6 mEq/L, Cl 108 mEq/L, BUN 32 mg/dL, Cr 2.2 mg/dL, WBC 22,000/mm^3, Hb 13 g/dL, platelet count 198,000/mm^3.

502. Which one of the following should be performed next?

(A) Fluid resuscitate to CVP 15 mm Hg

(B) Transfuse 1 unit packed red blood cells

(C) Place pulmonary artery catheter to measure SvO$_2$

(D) Fluid resuscitate to CVP 10 mm Hg

(E) Operative exploration for bleeding

503. Two hours later, the following vital signs are recorded: T 38°C, HR 118, BP 105/60, RR 32. CVP is 12 mm Hg, and ScvO$_2$ is 55%. Norepinephrine is infusing at 10 mcg/min to support the blood pressure. Which one of the following is the next most appropriate step?

     (A) Administer milrinone
     (B) Increase norepinephrine dose
     (C) Administer dobutamine
     (D) Administer vasopressin
     (E) Administer epinephrine

DIRECTIONS: Use the following scenario to answer Questions 504-505: A 34-year-old woman with systemic lupus erythematosus presents with dyspnea and chest pain. Vital signs are T 37.5°C, HR 128, BP 85/40, RR 36, SpO$_2$ 95% on nasal cannula oxygen. A bedside TTE is performed, with a subcostal image depicted below:

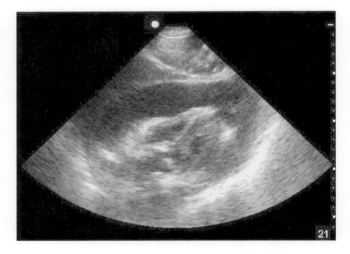

504. Which one of the following findings is most likely on physical examination?

     (A) Right ventricular heave along left sternal border
     (B) Diminished right sided breath sounds
     (C) Diastolic heart murmur
     (D) Palpable liver edge
     (E) Pulsus paradoxus > 12 mm Hg

505. Which one of the following treatments is most appropriate?

     (A) Thoracentesis
     (B) Thrombolysis
     (C) Pericardiocentesis
     (D) Diuresis
     (E) Inotropic support

DIRECTIONS: Use the following scenario to answer Questions 506-507: A 28-year-old woman with a history of Roux-en-Y gastric bypass presents with nausea, vomiting, and abdominal pain. Imaging suggests a small bowel obstruction. On induction of anesthesia for exploratory laparotomy, she has an observed aspiration of particulate contents. Following rapid intubation, her vital signs are T 37.2°C, HR 136, BP 80/40, SpO$_2$ 91% on mechanical ventilation with F$_{IO_2}$ 1.0. Physical exam reveals diffuse expiratory wheezing and rhonchi. A nasogastric tube drains copious feculent contents.

506. What is the next most appropriate intervention?

     (A) Bronchoalveolar lavage
     (B) Prone ventilation
     (C) Chest CT
     (D) Bronchoscopy with particulate removal
     (E) Hyperbaric oxygen

507. Which one of the following is the most appropriate pharmacologic intervention?

     (A) Sodium bicarbonate
     (B) Intravenous heparin
     (C) Antibiotics
     (D) Methylprednisolone
     (E) Inhaled nitric oxide

DIRECTIONS: Use the following scenario to answer Questions 508-513: You are responding to an overhead page reporting a code in the PACU. On arrival, you find a 47-year-old male who has just undergone a Whipple procedure. He had been doing well, but as the nurses were preparing his transfer to the ICU for further monitoring, he suddenly became unresponsive. They called a code, initiated CPR, and began reconnecting him to the monitors. You arrive as they are reconnecting the arterial line.

508. Critical myocardial blood flow is associated with an aortic diastolic blood pressure greater than which one of the following?

(A) 15 mm Hg
(B) 20 mm Hg
(C) 30 mm Hg
(D) 40 mm Hg
(E) 50 mm Hg

509. Which one of the following describes the attributes of effective chest compressions in adults?

(A) Rate 80, 2 cm depth, 25% compression time
(B) Rate 80, 5 cm depth, 50% compression time
(C) Rate 100, 2 cm depth, 25% compression time
(D) Rate 100, 5 cm depth, 50% compression time
(E) Rate 120, 2 cm depth, 25% compression time

510. The patient is placed back on telemetry. The rhythm is ventricular fibrillation (VF). What is the most appropriate next step in management?

(A) Administer amiodarone
(B) Administer epinephrine
(C) Biphasic cardioversion at 150 J
(D) Biphasic defibrillation at 200 J
(E) Endotracheal intubation

511. The respiratory therapist suggests end-tidal CO_2 monitoring. During CPR, end-tidal CO_2 correlates with which one of the following?

(A) Arterial CO_2
(B) Cardiac output
(C) Minute ventilation
(D) Arterial systolic blood pressure
(E) Venous CO_2

512. Patients who are intubated and receiving CPR should be ventilated at which one of the following rates?

(A) < 4 breaths/min
(B) 4-6 breaths/min
(C) 6-8 breaths/min
(D) 8-10 breaths/min
(E) 10-12 breaths/min

513. If a patient fails to regain consciousness after return of spontaneous circulation following VF arrest, which one of the following is the most appropriate next step in management?

(A) Administer mannitol
(B) Begin therapeutic hypothermia, if no contraindications
(C) Notify the family of the patient's poor prognosis
(D) Provide 100% FIO_2
(E) Schedule a cardiac catheterization to be performed after the patient regains consciousness

DIRECTIONS: Each group of items below consists of lettered headings followed by a list of numbered phrases or statements. For each numbered phrase or statement, select the ONE lettered heading or component that is most closely associated with it. Each lettered heading or component may be selected once, more than once, or not at all.

(A) Syndrome of inappropriate antidiuretic hormone (SIADH)
(B) Hepatorenal syndrome
(C) Congestive heart failure
(D) Cerebral salt wasting
(E) Hypovolemia
(F) Nephrogenic diabetes insipidus
(G) Central diabetes insipidus

For each of the following clinical scenarios, select the most likely diagnosis.

514. A 48-year-old woman presented 7 d ago with nausea, vomiting, and the worst headache of her life. She underwent a neurosurgical procedure, and is now obtunded with a Glasgow Coma Score (GCS) of 4 (E1VTM2). Her vital signs are T 37°C, HR 99, BP 120/80, RR 14. CVP is 2 mm Hg. Other relevant laboratory values include serum sodium 134 mEq/L, urine sodium 43 mEq/L, plasma osmolality 270 mOsm/kg, and urine osmolality 350 mOsm/kg.

515. A 67-year-old man is hospitalized in the ICU following colon resection for perforated sigmoid diverticulitis. He is intubated and mechanically ventilated. His vital signs are T 36.8°C, HR 88, BP 94/52, RR 16, SpO_2 92%, FIO_2 0.6. Systolic pressure variation from a radial arterial line is 4 mm Hg. He has pitting peripheral edema. He has serum sodium 133 mEq/L, urine sodium 10 mEq/L, plasma osmolality 270 mOsm/kg, and urine osmolality 600 mOsm/kg.

516. A 26-year-old man with a history of schizophrenia has suffered traumatic brain injury after jumping from a height of 50 feet. He has GCS 3(E1VTM1), no pupillary light reflexes, no corneal responses, and no gag or cough response. On apnea testing, arterial pH = 7.28 after 8 min with no observed respiratory effort. Several hours later, urine output is > 400 mL/h for 3 h, diminishing to 50 mL/h when intravenous vasopressin is administered. Laboratory values are serum sodium 158 mEq/L, urine sodium > 20 mEq/L, plasma osmolality 320 mOsm/kg, and urine osmolality 100 mOsm/kg.

517. A 56-year-old man with a history of non-alcoholic steatohepatitis (NASH) is hospitalized in the ICU following total colectomy to treat toxic megacolon. He is intubated and mechanically ventilated. His vital signs are T 37.5°C, HR 110, BP 90/52, RR 22, SpO_2 100%, FIO_2 0.4. Pulse pressure variation from a radial arterial line is 18%. He has a serum sodium 130 mEq/L, urine sodium 10 mEq/L, plasma osmolality 290 mOsm/kg, and urine osmolality 50 mOsm/kg.

518. A 66-year-old woman with a history of hepatitis C infection is transferred to the ICU on postoperative day 1 following laparoscopic cholecystectomy. Her vital signs are T 37.2°C, HR 125, BP 85/42, RR 18, SpO_2 94% on facemask oxygen. Urine output has been 5-20 mL/h for the past 12 h. She has received 1.5 L normal saline resuscitation over the past 4 h without increase in urine output or blood pressure. Her exam is notable for abdominal distention with shifting dullness. Laboratory values are notable for serum sodium 128 mEq/L, urine sodium 5 mEq/L, plasma osmolality 285 mOsm/kg, and urine osmolality 400 mOsm/kg.

DIRECTIONS: Each group of items below consists of lettered headings followed by a list of numbered phrases or statements. For each numbered phrase or statement, select the ONE lettered heading or component that is most closely associated with it. Each lettered heading or component may be selected once, more than once, or not at all.

(A) Anaphylactic shock
(B) Cardiogenic shock
(C) Hyperdynamic septic shock
(D) Hypovolemic shock
(E) Neurogenic shock
(F) Obstructive shock due to pulmonary embolism

For each patient with shock, select the most likely mechanism causing the symptoms.

519. A 46-year-old male is brought to the emergency department by paramedics. He was found down in his home after sustaining a 45% total body surface area burn. He was unresponsive at the scene and was intubated en route. His vital signs are T 36.1°C, HR 126, BP 81/42, RR 21, SpO_2 97%. A bedside hematocrit is 52%. A central line and an arterial line are placed to assist with care. His CVP is 6 mm Hg. Arterial waveform analysis suggests a decreased cardiac output. Central venous oxygen saturation is 47%.

520. A 26-year-old female is in the postpartum unit 12 h after delivering a healthy 39-week male via elective repeat cesarean section under spinal anesthesia. Her past medical history includes asthma, GERD and chronic low back pain. Her initial postoperative course was uneventful. She was ambulatory and had good oral intake. Over the past several hours, however, she has become increasingly fatigued and lethargic. Her vital signs are T 37.1°C, HR 118, BP 79/51, RR 22, SpO$_2$ 94% on room air. Her extremities are cool and edematous. Her hemoglobin is 9 g/dL. An intravenous fluid bolus did not improve her vital signs. Central venous and arterial lines are placed to assist with care. CVP is 15 mm Hg. Arterial waveform analysis suggests a decreased cardiac output. She begins to complain of dyspnea that worsens with lying flat.

521. A 62-year-old female is in a rehabilitation facility recovering from a right total hip replacement performed 3 weeks ago. Her past medical history is significant for obesity, hypertension, hypercholesterolemia, hypothyroidism and osteoarthritis. While working with the physical therapist, she develops dyspnea and chest pain. Emergency medical personnel arrive, finding her heart rate 105 bpm and blood pressure 89/59 mm Hg. She requires a nonrebreather oxygen mask to maintain her oxygen saturation > 90%. ECG done en route to the hospital shows sinus tachycardia without acute ST changes.

522. A 22-year-old male with a history of meningomyelocele is scheduled for correction of an Arnold-Chiari malformation. After an uneventful induction of anesthesia, arterial and central catheters are placed. The patient is then positioned, prepped and draped. One hour after incision, the patient develops hypotension, hypoxemia and increased airway pressures. The CVP is 1 mm Hg.

523. A 56-year-old male is brought to the emergency department by his brother due to progressive somnolence over the past 2 d. The patient is too lethargic to give a history but his brother reports that he avoids medical care. He is known to have a penicillin allergy since childhood. He had an ankle fracture repaired in the past. He smokes 2 packs/d and drinks a pint of whiskey daily. His vital signs are T 37.9°C, HR 113, BP 89/40, RR 26, SpO$_2$ 88% on 4 L/min by nasal cannula. There are rhonchi in the right lung. His feet are warm with bounding pulses.

524. A 16-year-old male is brought to the emergency department by paramedics. He was the unrestrained driver in a high speed motor vehicle accident. He was unresponsive at the scene and required intubation. On arrival, his vital signs are T 36.2°C, HR 61, BP 82/43, SpO$_2$ 100% while being ventilated with an Ambu bag. His GCS is 4 (E2VTM1). His initial chest x-ray and long bone films do not show any traumatic injuries. His FAST scan is negative. His feet are warm.

DIRECTIONS: Each group of items below consists of lettered headings followed by a list of numbered phrases or statements. For each numbered phrase or statement, select the ONE lettered heading or component that is most closely associated with it. Each lettered heading or component may be selected once, more than once, or not at all.

(A) Subarachnoid hemorrhage
(B) Hypercarbia
(C) Hypertensive encephalopathy
(D) Middle cerebral artery infarction
(E) Septic shock
(F) Meningitis
(G) Alcohol intoxication
(H) Epidural hematoma
(I) Concussion
(J) Postseizure state

For each patient with coma, select the most likely diagnosis.

525. A 79-year-old woman with COPD and abdominal pain underwent exploratory laparoscopy under spinal anesthesia. In the PACU, she is unresponsive with no focal or lateralizing signs. T 36.5°C, HR 110, BP 160/90, RR 6, SpO₂ 94% on supplemental oxygen.

526. A 22-year-old man presented to the emergency department following crashing his motorcycle into a utility pole. When emergency medical personnel responded, he reported that he struck his helmeted head into the pole without loss of consciousness. Vital signs at the scene were T 37.2°C, HR 130, BP 160/98, RR 22, SpO₂ 98% on room air, GCS 15 (E4V5M6). On arrival to the hospital, he is comatose with a left temporoparietal scalp laceration.

527. A-54-year old man with a history of glioblastoma is brought to the emergency room by family who found him unresponsive at home on the floor. Vital signs are T 37.8°C, HR 98, BP 150/80, RR 28, SpO₂ 98% on facemask oxygen. There are no visible traumatic injuries, but his clothing is saturated with urine. Head CT reveals no significant change from three weeks ago where a 2 cm lesion is seen in the right temporal lobe with minimal surrounding edema.

528. An 80-year-old woman with a history of prosthetic aortic valve and severe carotid stenosis who is prescribed warfarin anticoagulation presents after being found on her floor at home unresponsive. Her daughter reports that she had run out of her medications one week ago. T 35.2°C, HR 88 irregular, BP 170/90, RR 16, SpO₂ 95% on room air. Laboratory values are notable for sodium 145 mEq/L, glucose 130 mg/dL, BUN 40 mg/dL, creatinine 1.8 mg/dL, WBC 8,000/mm³, hemoglobin 12 g/dL, INR 0.9.

529. A 43-year-old woman presents with a history of subarachnoid hemorrhage 3 weeks prior due to ruptured cerebral aneurysm. She was treated with coil embolization of the aneurysm and subsequently developed obstructive hydrocephalus that has been treated since with an external ventricular drain. She was neurologically intact and recovering well until 8 h ago when her nurse noticed increasing drowsiness, progressing to obtundation and coma. Vital signs are T 39.2°C, HR 120, BP 110/70, RR 30, SpO₂ 100% on room air. She has no focal or lateralizing neurologic findings. Laboratory values show sodium 145 mEq/L, WBC 27,000/mm³, hemoglobin 9.2 g/dL, platelet count 110,000/mm³, INR 1.0.

530. A 21-year-old man has a history of bone marrow transplant 2 weeks ago presents with coma without focal or lateralizing neurologic findings. Vital signs show T 38.8°C, HR 100, BP 80/40, RR 32, SpO₂ 96% on room air. Exam is notable for alopecia, rigors, and cool extremities. Laboratory values reveal sodium 140 mEq/L, WBC 800/mm³ with differential count 50% neutrophils, 30% lymphocytes, 10% monocytes, 6% eosinophils, and 3% basophils.

Answers and Explanations

457. **(C)** This previously healthy young patient has developed symptoms referable to both the chest and the head/neck. Epiglottitis, pneumonia, or tracheomalacia could result in dyspnea, cough, and perhaps hoarseness, but they would be unlikely to cause facial swelling. Angioedema could account for this constellation of symptoms, but a three-day course would be unusual. This patient has symptoms of superior vena cava (SVC) syndrome, a clinical diagnosis based on symptomatology. Most cases of SVC syndrome are caused by malignancies such as lung cancer, lymphoma or metastases, but benign causes (strictures from intravascular devices, thyromegaly, and aortic aneurysm) also exist. SVC syndrome in a young man with a mediastinal mass is most commonly due to lymphoma or a mediastinal germ cell tumor. Patients with SVC syndrome commonly present with facial/neck swelling, dyspnea, and cough. Hoarseness, headache, congestion, hemoptysis, dysphagia, pain and syncope may also be seen. Symptoms worsen with a head down position. *(6:265-6, 2266-7, 2711-3)*

458. **(D)** Although nonpharmacologic interventions (such as a quiet environment, soothing music, or a familiar family member at the bedside) may reduce the need for sedatives, many mechanically ventilated patients require sedation for safety. The choice of sedative agent should be tailored to the patient, keeping in mind the patient's physiology and the side effect profiles of the sedative medications. Benzodiazepines can worsen confusion and delirium. As a result, their use should be limited to cases where side effects of other sedatives are unacceptable or where alcohol or benzodiazepine withdrawal may be contributing to confusion. Etomidate suppresses adrenocortical function. It is not appropriate for use as an infusion. Side effects of propofol include hypotension due to vasodilation, respiratory depression, and hyperlipidemia. Propofol infusion syndrome is a rare, but potentially fatal side effect of propofol administration. Dexmedetomidine is an α_2-adrenoceptor agonist. Administration causes sedation and analgesia with little respiratory depression. Side effects of dexmedetomidine include hypotension and bradycardia. Dexmedetomidine is rarely used for long-term sedation (> 1 day) due to cost. In this patient with bradycardia and an acceptable blood pressure, propofol would be the most appropriate sedative. Pain should also be treated, as untreated pain is associated with an increased incidence of delirium and worse outcomes. *(1:536-8, 548-9; 6:201)*

459. **(A)** Intensive care unit patients are at risk for multiple complications due to their critical illness. Prophylactic interventions have been developed to reduce morbidity from stress ulcers, ventilator associated pneumonia (VAP) and deep venous thrombosis. Oral decontamination with chlorhexidine is recommended to reduce the incidence of VAP. Other suggested interventions include head of bed elevation and daily assessment of readiness to wean. Clindamycin is an antibiotic that is active against gram positive and anaerobic bacteria. An infection with *Haemophilus* would not be treated by clindamycin. Dexamethasone is a glucocorticoid. It has no role in the treatment of VAP. Omeprazole (a proton pump inhibitor) is a reasonable choice for stress ulcer prophylaxis, but proton pump inhibitors are associated with increased rates of pneumonia. *(1:1434-5, 1755; 6:1114, 2448)*

460. **(B)** Donation after cardiac death (DCD) is an accepted method of organ donation that occurs after withdrawal of life support in a patient who is expected to die without such support. Recent renewed interest in DCD has been spurred by the mismatch between the number of patients awaiting organ transplantation and insufficient number of donors from the brain-dead procurement path. DCD donors are usually critically ill from irreversible neurologic illness, neuromuscular disease, or high spinal cord injury. Usually the patient and/or family, in collaboration with the treating ICU physicians, arrive at a decision to withdraw care in order to minimize suffering and allow the patient to die. Only in this context (after the decision to withdraw care has been made) should the patient or family be approached regarding the possibility of organ donation. If consent is rendered by the competent patient, or absent this by the family, DCD donation may proceed. In a controlled setting (either the ICU or the operating room), life support is withdrawn including removal of the endotracheal tube. The patient's symptoms of pain, anxiety, and dyspnea are treated appropriately to provide comfort during death. If asystole occurs within a set time interval (usually less than 2 h), the procurement team waits the prescribed time (usually 2-5 min) after cardiac death and then begins organ procurement. The dying process and wait period following asystole subject the organs to a longer warm ischemic time than brain dead donors, but thus far graft outcomes from DCD donors appear comparable to brain dead donors when appropriate selection criteria are satisfied. Even hearts have been reported to have been successfully transplanted following DCD donation. *(Fanelli V, et al. Curr Opin Anaesthesiol 2010; 23:406-10)*

461. **(A)** Pressure support ventilation (PSV) is depicted in the figure as evidenced by the negative pressure deflection before each inspira-

tion that triggers the delivered inspiratory flow. End of inspiration in PSV is determined by a decline to a certain percentage of peak inspiratory flow (usually 25%, although this may be adjusted). The figure shows only patient triggered inspirations without additional mandatory breaths. PSV may be problematic in the setting of a large bronchopleural fistula since flow through the defect may never drop, thereby resulting in continuous inspiration without termination. Minute ventilation in PSV is determined by patient effort; a higher respiratory rate will result in a higher MV if tidal volume remains approximately constant. *(5:1407-9; 6:2212)*

462. **(D)** In this setting, the bradycardia is causing asymptomatic hypotension. Atropine is an appropriate intervention to increase the heart rate rapidly. Transvenous pacing requires central venous access and subsequent placement of a wire. This cannot be performed quickly enough for this situation. Cardiopulmonary resuscitation (CPR) is not the appropriate first intervention in this patient who has a pulse, although CPR may be required if the patient's condition deteriorates or he is unresponsive to less invasive treatments. Similarly, endotracheal intubation is not necessary at this time. *(1:227-8, 5:1433; 6:2244)*

463. **(C)** The ECG demonstrates an acute ST elevation MI. Likely etiologies include coronary artery plaque rupture or in-stent thrombosis. The primary goal of therapy is rapid coronary reperfusion, preferably using catheter-based therapies directed at the involved coronary artery. Modern interventions may include thrombus extraction, balloon angioplasty, or coronary stenting using either bare metal or drug-eluting stents. Determination of the best intervention depends upon coronary anatomic findings and relative risk of potent anticoagulants inducing bleeding at the recent surgical site. Better outcomes from acute MI are achieved when the "door to balloon" time is less than 90 min. Thus, stat cardiology consultation and rapid mobilization of the patient to the catheterization suite are key. Pharmacologic measures to reduce myocardial oxygen consumption should be simultaneously employed. Thus, tachycardia should be treated with a beta-blocker, in this case a short-acting intravenous agent such as esmolol. Myocardial wall tension should be reduced by treating hypertension. Nitroglycerin is indicated for treatment in acute coronary syndrome (ACS) to diminish ischemic pain (if present), treat hypertension, reduce pulmonary congestion, and, when implicated, treat coronary vasospasm. Nitroglycerin has not been demonstrated, however, to diminish mortality due to ACS. Other pharmacologic therapies that should be rapidly administered include antiplatelet agents (aspirin ± a thieno-pyridine) depending upon the estimated risk of surgical bleeding from dual agents as well as the specific coronary artery intervention. A statin should be prescribed for patients not currently taking one, and an ACE-inhibitor considered for patients whose hemodynamics will tolerate the medication. Systemic thrombolytics for ACS are contraindicated for patients who have undergone recent surgery (<2 weeks). *(1:754; 5:750, 1385; 6:2025-8)*

464. (D) Oxygen delivery (DO_2) can be calculated using the following equations:

$$DO_2 = CO \times CaO_2 \times 10, \text{ and}$$

$$CaO_2 = (1.34 \times Hb \times HbO_2) + (0.003 \times PO_2)$$

where CO = cardiac output, and CaO_2 is the arterial oxygen content. The 10 is a factor that converts the final units to mL/min. HbO_2 is arterial oxygen saturation percentage, Hb is hemoglobin concentration, and PO_2 is the partial pressure of oxygen in arterial blood. His current DO_2 is:

$$DO_2 = 5 \text{ L/min} \times ((1.34 \text{ mL } O_2/\text{gm Hb} \\ \times 9 \text{ gm/dL} \times 0.9) + (0.003 \text{ mLO}_2/ \\ 100 \text{ mL/mm Hg} \times 61 \text{ mm Hg})) \times 10 \\ = 552 \text{ mL/min}$$

This can be approximated using just the first portion of the equation for CaO_2 as the contribution due to dissolved oxygen is generally small. Stroke volume is obtained using the formula:

$$CO = \text{heart rate} \times \text{stroke volume.}$$

The greatest increase in DO_2 occurs with an increase in the patient's stroke volume to 80 mL/beat (DO_2 = 803 mL/min). Be cautious with the units. *(5:415, 460)*

465. (B) Arteriolar luminal diameter is the primary determinant of SVR. *(6:2215)*

466. (B) α-adrenoceptors are found on arteriolar and venous smooth muscle cells. Stimulation of α_1-adrenoceptors results in vasoconstriction. β_2-adrenoceptors are found in smooth muscle and metabolic tissue. Stimulation of β_2-adrenoceptors causes skeletal and cardiac muscle vasodilation, bronchodilation, and decreased gastric motility. *(5:1401)*

467. (D) This patient is in septic shock. The kidneys respond to hypoperfusion by conserving salt and water. Renin is released from the juxtaglomerular apparatus and catalyzes the conversion of angiotensinogen to angiotensin I. Angiotensin I is subsequently converted to angiotensin II by angiotensin-converting enzyme. Angiotensin II causes vasoconstriction of the afferent arteriole, increasing glomerular hydrostatic pressure and filtration. Angiotensin II increases aldosterone release. Aldosterone is a mineralocorticoid that increases sodium reabsorption. Acute hypotension substantially increases vasopressin release. As shock continues, however, vasopressin levels decrease, resulting in a relative vasopressin deficiency. *(1:493, 703-12; 6:2044-5, 2217, 2281-2, 2930)*

468. (C) Mixed venous oxygen saturation (SvO_2) can be measured on blood taken from the distal tip of a pulmonary artery catheter. In states of hypoperfusion, extracted oxygen is a greater percentage of delivered oxygen. As a result, SvO_2 is typically reduced. Once a patient has been resuscitated, SvO_2 may be normal or elevated in inflammatory conditions. The normal value for SvO_2 is 70-75%. Mixed venous oxygen saturation is a function of oxygen delivery and extraction in the entire body, as the value is taken from blood in the pulmonary artery. Central venous oxygen saturation ($ScvO_2$), however, is taken from blood in the superior vena cava (via a central line), and thus reflects oxygenation of only the cephalad portions of the body. Under normal circumstances $ScvO_2$ is slightly less than SvO_2. In critically ill patients, oxygen extraction and consumption from the liver, kidneys, and GI tract is increased. As a result, SvO_2 may be less than $ScvO_2$. Cerebral oximetry and pulse oximetry would be expected to measure oxygen levels in local tissue beds. (5:1404, 426-8)

469.   **(E)** During shock states, there is disruption of normal metabolic cycles. Hepatic production of glucose is increased in the presence of decreased oxygen levels. Serum triglyceride levels are increased, due to decreased clearance of exogenous triglycerides and increased hepatic lipogenesis. Epinephrine is released from the adrenal medulla, causing increased glycogenolysis, increased gluconeogenesis, and reduced pancreatic insulin release. There is increased use of protein as an energy substrate. This results in a negative nitrogen balance. As a result, severe muscle wasting is a potential cause of morbidity in prolonged critical illness. (6:2216-7)

470.   **(B)** Critically ill patients are frequently subjected to intrahospital transport for diagnostic or therapeutic interventions. Such transport may be critical to patient management, but it also carries significant risk. Complications of transport are diverse including hemodynamic or respiratory deterioration, hypothermia, increased ICP, pain or anxiety, falls, and dislodgement of vascular access. The risks and benefits of patient transport must be considered on a patient- and situation-specific basis. This patient is likely to experience respiratory deterioration during transport and should not be subjected to transport for a procedure that can reasonably and safely be done at the bedside. The procedure should not be cancelled, however, as the patient's empyema is likely driving his critical illness. If transport is in the patient's best interest, then appropriate preparation and monitoring may reduce the risk of patient injury. (5:1375-87)

471.   **(D)** The Glasgow Coma Scale (GCS) is a scoring system used for communication and prognostication for patients with head injury. The patient score is the sum of the numbers given for the patient's best response in each of three categories:

Eye opening (E): spontaneous – 4, to loud voice – 3, to pain – 2, nil - 1

Verbal response (V): oriented – 5, confused/disoriented – 4, inappropriate words – 3, incomprehensible sounds – 2, nil – 1, intubated - T

Best motor response (M): obeys – 6, localizes to pain – 5, withdraws from pain – 4, abnormal flexion posturing – 3, extension posturing – 2, nil – 1

The highest potential score is E4V5M6 = 15. The lowest potential score is E1V1M1 = 3. This patient's score is E2V2M5 = 9. (6:3381)

472.   **(A)** Patients with acute pancreatitis often receive vigorous fluid resuscitation to maintain intravascular volume in the face of severe capillary leak. Ascites often develops, putting these patients at risk for the development of abdominal compartment syndrome. Elevated abdominal pressures worsen pulmonary compliance resulting in hypoventilation, atelectasis, hypoxemia, and elevated airway pressures. Inferior vena cava compression reduces venous return to the heart (reduced preload). Perfusion to visceral organs is reduced causing acidosis and renal dysfunction. Cardiac output drops due to decreased preload and increased afterload. Abdominal compartment syndrome is the most likely cause for this patient's clinical decline. If cardiomyopathy or hypovolemia with ARDS were the etiology, pulmonary edema would be expected to be greater. Infection would not be expected to cause high airway pressures unless the infectious source was pulmonary that would likely be visible on CXR. Pulmonary embolism would be a less likely cause of this patient's symptoms. (5:1394; 6:332, 2634-43)

473.   **(C)** This patient has heparin-induced thrombocytopenia (HIT) as a complication of therapy with low-molecular-weight-heparin (LMWH). The risk of HIT with LMWHs is about fivefold lower than with heparin, but HIT is still a risk of administration. In HIT, thrombocytopenia would be the only expected laboratory abnormality unless the patient developed bleeding. Gravid women have a number of risk factors for DIC, but the consumptive coagulopathy in DIC causes prolongation of the prothrombin and partial thromboplastin times as well as

thrombocytopenia. A patient with placental abruption may develop DIC. Fetal heart tones are often nonreassuring in this setting. HELLP syndrome consists of hemolysis, elevated liver enzymes, and low platelets in a preeclamptic patient. Vitamin B$_{12}$ deficiency would be expected to cause a megaloblastic anemia. *(5:215-6, 296, 1395, 1443; 6:862, 996)*

474. **(B)** Calcium concentrations are reduced in massive transfusion due to administration of citrated blood products. This effect is pronounced in patients with liver dysfunction as citrate is metabolized in the liver. Calcium is necessary for smooth muscle and myocardial contractility as well as for clotting. Hypocalcemia reduces vascular tone and myocardial inotropy. Reduced calcium levels may also worsen coagulopathy. Calcium may be repleted using intravenous calcium gluconate or calcium chloride. Calcium should not be given in an intravenous line being used for transfusion. Hypothermia is common in trauma patients and in patients receiving massive transfusion. Although hypothermia can decrease cardiac function, this is unlikely to occur at >35°C. There is little evidence that bicarbonate administration improves hemodynamics or vasopressor response, and bicarbonate has many negative effects. Bicarbonate is typically reserved for severe metabolic acidosis (pH < 7.2). Bicarbonate should not be given if the patient will be unable to increase minute ventilation in response to the expected rise in PaCO$_2$ produced by bicarbonate administration. Although increasing PEEP may improve oxygenation, it is unlikely to improve the hemodynamic picture is a patient with an SpO$_2$ of 95% and no evidence of volume overload on TEE. This patient has no evidence of hypovolemia and a hemoglobin of 8.9 g/dL. Transfusion of PRBC is unlikely to improve his hemodynamics. *(5:1074, 1451-2; 6:166, 2222, 2230)*

475. **(A)** A fibrinogen level < 100 mg/dL can lead to a significant coagulopathy. Fresh frozen plasma contains fibrinogen and would improve this patient's coagulopathy, but cryoprecipitate is the blood component containing the highest concentration of fibrinogen. Cryoprecipitate would be most likely to resolve a coagulopathy due to fibrinogen deficiency. Platelet transfusion is unlikely to improve clotting in a patient with a platelet count of >100,000/mm^3. Hypothermia-induced coagulopathy would be expected at temperatures below 35°C. DDAVP is used to treat bleeding due to some subtypes of von Willebrand disease or severe kidney disease. *(1:712-4; 5:209, 1443, 1446, 1451; 6:2316)*

476. **(A)** The mortality associated with renal failure in critically ill patients is 23-64%. This patient is at risk for prerenal, postrenal, and intrinsic causes of renal failure. Urinary obstruction is a less likely cause in a patient still making urine, but flushing or replacing the urinary catheter plus imaging could rule out this important etiology of renal failure. This patient has a FENA = 3%, a BUN/creatinine ratio < 20:1, a urine Na > 40 mEq/L, and a urine osmolality < 350 mOsmol/L H$_2$O. This set of laboratory values makes an intrinsic cause of renal failure more likely than a prerenal cause. Urinalysis without white or red blood cells (which might implicate glomerulonephritis or acute interstitial nephritis) plus the clinical circumstance of prolonged hypotension make acute tubular necrosis the most likely etiology for this patient's acute kidney injury. *(5:1365-6, 1395; 6:334-8)*

477. **(E)** There are four parts to the treatment of hyperkalemia. First, stabilize the irritable myocardium with calcium. Second, drive potassium intracellularly. Insulin + glucose or inhaled β$_2$ agonists may be used for this purpose. These are temporizing measures. Third, eliminate potassium from the body. Potassium-wasting diuretics, renal replacement therapy or cation exchange resins may reduce the total body potassium load. Fourth, treat the underlying cause of hyperkalemia. *(1:1291; 5:1074; 6:355-9)*

478. **(D)** Rhabdomyolysis is a cause of renal failure and electrolyte abnormalities in critically ill patients. Expected laboratory abnormalities include hyperkalemia and hyperphosphatemia due to release of intracellular potassium. Metastatic tissue deposition of

calcium phosphate results in hypocalcemia. *(5:148-9; 6:356, 362, 2303, 3089)*

479. **(D)** This patient presents with dyspnea, chest pain, and shock. The differential diagnosis for this constellation of symptoms and findings would be broad, including pneumonia, empyema, pulmonary embolism (PE), pneumothorax, myocardial ischemia, myocarditis, pericarditis/pericardial effusion with tamponade, esophageal or gastric perforation, pancreatitis, cholangitis, and aortic dissection. A normal temperature, an INR > 3, and an ECG without acute ST changes makes infection, PE, or myocardial ischemia unlikely. The patient's history of breast cancer makes malignant pericardial disease more likely. Echocardiography is the test most likely to identify pericardial effusion/tamponade as the source of this patient's shock. *(6:102-7, 2267-8)*

480. **(B)** The differential diagnosis for new-onset seizures in an adult includes trauma, alcohol withdrawal, illicit drug use, cerebrovascular disease, brain tumor, metabolic disorders, and neurodegenerative diseases. This patient was found to have a frontal mass on head CT. Patients with seizures due to symptomatic brain metastases should be treated with anticonvulsant therapy (to increase the seizure threshold) and dexamethasone (to reduce tumor related edema). CSF diversion, intubation and hyperventilation, mannitol, and decompressive craniectomy would be treatments for increased intracranial pressure (ICP). This patient is unlikely to have elevated ICP, as she has a normal neurologic examination and sharp optic disks. *(1:1755; 6:2271-2, 3258)*

481. **(A)** A sentinel article published in 2006 demonstrated that a bundle of the following five evidence based-procedures could reduce the incidence of central line-associated blood stream infections (CLABSI) in a sustained fashion: hand washing, use of full-barrier precautions during line insertion, chlorhexidine skin preparation, avoidance of femoral site, and removal of unnecessary central lines. While other measures may be useful at preventing CLABSI, the former bundle was shown effective across more than 100 ICU's and has been widely adopted in critical care units. *(5:226, 234, 1319; 6:1114, 1116)*

482. **(D)** This patient likely has propofol infusion syndrome, a rare but highly fatal and poorly understood complication of propofol. It has been most commonly described in critically ill children who are sedated on high doses of propofol for a prolonged period, although the exact dose and duration of propofol exposure to produce the syndrome is unknown. Characteristic features include rhabdomyolysis, metabolic acidosis, and worsening hypotension despite pressor/inotropic support. The course typically proceeds to cardiac, renal, and other organ failure before eventual death. Cardiac effects may manifest as dysrhythmias, including bradycardia. The pathophysiology is believed to involve propofol impairment of free fatty acid utilization by the mitochondria leading to failure of the electron transport chain, low cellular energy production, and cell death. Treatment is discontinuation of propofol, and support of organ failure. *(1:537; 5:693)*

483. **(C)** The figure depicts pressure control ventilation (PC). In this mode, the clinician sets a pressure limit, respiratory rate, and inspiratory time. Inspiratory flow occurs in an exponentially descending waveform and the pressure applied to the airway is constant. Tidal volume is the dependent variable such that diminished pulmonary compliance, as in the case of this patient with increasing abdominal distention, results in diminished minute ventilation. *(5:1406-9; 6:2211-2)*

484. **(D)** The disorder is characterized as a mixed respiratory acidosis and metabolic acidosis. The pH for a simple acute respiratory acidosis with a Pa_{CO_2} = 55 would be 7.28. This patient's pH is lower, suggesting a mixed respiratory and metabolic acidosis. In addition, the base deficit (or negative base excess) in the setting of ongoing bleeding likely represents unmeasured anions due to lactic acid. *(5:525-31; 6:364-6)*

485. **(B)** The difference between the two depicted values is pulse pressure variation, the difference between maximal and minimal pulse pressure values during one mechanical positive pressure breath divided by the mean of these two values. It is only one of the available dynamic indices that utilize arterial waveform contour during positive pressure mechanical ventilation as a predictor of cardiovascular response to fluid administration. Another index that has been studied is systolic pressure variation, the largest difference between the systolic pressure during one breath. Systolic pressure variation may be further characterized into "delta up," the difference between baseline systolic pressure during apnea and the highest systolic pressure occurring immediately after delivery of a positive pressure breath, and "delta down," the difference between baseline systolic pressure during apnea and the lowest systolic pressure occurring following the increased systolic pressure after one mechanical positive pressure breath. A hypovolemic patient will have a more exaggerated arterial waveform response to positive pressure ventilation because venous return is more impaired, more lung units behave as West Zone 1 (where airway pressure increases RV afterload), and the ventricles are more sensitive to preload changes when operating on the steep part of the Starling curve (such as is generally present with hypovolemia). *(5:425-6; 6:2199; Michard, F. Anesthesiology 2005; 103:419-28)*

486. **(E)** The pulse pressure variation in this patient is greater than 12% that suggests that the patient is fluid responsive, i.e., fluid administration is expected to result in an increase in stroke volume. Whether or not fluid should be administered depends on the clinical context and the risks of fluid administration in the individual patient. In this case, the patient has ongoing bleeding, hypotension, and evidence of abdominal compartment syndrome (tense abdomen, oliguria, and diminished pulmonary compliance). Fluid administration is reasonable until more definitive treatment of abdominal compartment syndrome (e.g., surgical decompression) is performed. Support of the blood pressure with a vasopressor while fluid resuscitation is undertaken is reasonable

if necessary to prevent precipitous decline in perfusion, but vasopressors should be viewed as only temporizing in treatment of hypovolemia. *(5:424-8; 6:425, 1394)*

487. **(A)** The Fisher Grading Scale describes the amount of intracranial blood seen on head CT scan after subarachnoid hemorrhage (SAH). Progression from Fisher Grade 2 to Fisher Grade 3 describes an increase in subarachnoid blood, likely due to rebleeding. Rebleeding is a poor prognostic sign in patients with subarachnoid hemorrhage due to aneurysmal rupture. Risk of rebleeding is highest in the first 24 h (up to 8%), and the associated mortality is greater than 50%. Hypertension is a risk factor for rebleeding. Even transient hypertension during intubation can be devastating. As a result, hypertension during laryngoscopy should be avoided and aggressively treated. Elevated ICP, seizures, and vasospasm are other complications of SAH, but they would not cause an increase in intracranial hemorrhage. Vasospasm is usually not apparent until >72 h after the hemorrhage. *(5:885-7)*

488. **(C)** SIMV is a ventilatory mode that employs a combination of spontaneous breaths and ventilator delivered breaths. It may be either volume or pressure targeted. The clinician sets a rate and target on the ventilator and the ventilator aims to deliver the breath synchronized to patient inspiratory effort, i.e., the ventilator waits a set period of seconds and, if the patient triggers, the inspiration is timed to coordinate. If after the programmed wait period, no breath is detected, then a mandatory breath is delivered. Spontaneous breaths are not supported by the ventilator in this mode. Advantages include exercise of the diaphragm and, with diaphragmatic motion, better V/Q matching to West zone III lung. Additionally, SIMV may decrease mean intrathoracic pressure, thereby reducing RV afterload and improving cardiac output. One disadvantage to SIMV, however, is a demonstrated increased work of breathing, particularly as the set rate on the ventilator is diminished. Increased work of breathing during SIMV weaning is also associated with

patient-ventilator dyssynchrony. *(5:1410-1; 6:2211-2)*

489. (A) The patient's acid-base disorder is a mild metabolic acidosis without an increased anion gap. The most likely diagnosis is intraoperative resuscitation with 0.9% NaCl (normal saline) intravenous solution that is commonly used during neurosurgical procedures because it is slightly hypertonic compared to plasma and theoretically may provide benefit in diminishing brain edema. However, administration of large quantities of normal saline causes a hyperchloremic metabolic acidosis with normal anion gap as a result of dilutional acidosis. The clinical significance of this acid-base disorder remains to be elucidated, but likely does not carry as poor a prognosis as lactic acidosis. Loop diuretic administration generally causes a metabolic "contraction" alkalosis. Propofol infusion syndrome and cyanide toxicity due to nitroprusside both cause an elevated anion gap metabolic acidosis due to lactic acidosis. *(1:796; 5:508, 528, 535-6)*

490. (D) Dopamine is an adrenoceptor agonist that acts at α, β_1, and dopaminergic receptors. It is a recommended first-line agent for the treatment of fluid-resuscitated patients in septic shock. Although it has theoretical benefits of splanchnic and renal circulatory dilatation, it has not been shown to produce superior outcomes when compared to norepinephrine. Studies suggest, however, a higher incidence of tachycardia and dysrhythmia with dopamine compared to norepinephrine. Norepinephrine is a more potent adrenergic agonist than dopamine. *(1:288; 5:1373)*

491. (B) This patient is suffering from traumatic brain injury (TBI) with CT evidence of subarachnoid, epidural, and intraparenchymal hemorrhage. There is mass effect on the left lateral ventricle, and left to right midline shift, findings that suggest elevated intracranial pressure (ICP). Emergent treatment goals include avoidance of further elevation of ICP that might precipitate herniation, correction of hypotension and hypoxemia, and medical management of elevated ICP until more definitive surgical management can be employed.

Priorities for management include endotracheal intubation, carefully performed to avoid further exacerbation of hypotension, hypercarbia, or hypoxia. Hyperventilation may be employed for brief periods of time until definitive surgical management occurs, but significant cerebral vasoconstriction, which occurs with $PaCO_2 < 30$ mm Hg, may in fact worsen cerebral hypoperfusion, leading to poor outcomes. Optimal ventilation is to maintenance of $PaCO_2$ 35-40 mm Hg. Hemodynamic support for this patient should include crystalloid volume resuscitation, avoiding hypotonic solutions such as lactated Ringer solution that may worsen brain edema and ICP. 5% albumin should be avoided in the resuscitation of patients with traumatic SAH since it is associated with poor outcomes. Blood pressure should be supported with vasopressors (phenylephrine, norepinephrine) to cerebral perfusion pressure > 60 mm Hg. Hypertonic saline in 23.4% solution, administered over 10-30 min, can be used to urgently reduce elevated ICP. Head of bed elevation is important to facilitate venous drainage from the brain. While CPP = MAP − ICP under conditions of elevated intracranial pressure, under normal conditions, CPP = MAP − CVP. Thus, head of bed elevation should be employed, and Trendelenburg position avoided in patients at risk for intracranial hypertension. Unlike vasogenic edema due to tumors, glucocorticoids play no role in treatment of traumatic ICP elevation. In this case, neurosurgical treatment options include ventriculostomy to drain CSF and reduce ICP, and craniectomy with removal of bone flap to provide decompression of the swollen brain parenchyma. *(1:682; 5:537, 1360-1; 6:2221)*

492. (D) Septicemia is the presence of microbes or their toxins in blood. SIRS is present when there are two or more of the following: oral temperature > 38°C or < 36°C, respiratory rate > 24 breaths/min, heart rate > 90 beats/min, white blood cell count > 12,000 or < 4,000/mm³, or > 10% bands. SIRS may have a non-infectious etiology. Sepsis is SIRS with a proven or suspected microbial etiology. Severe sepsis is defined as sepsis with one or more signs of organ dysfunction. Septic shock is defined as sepsis plus hypotension/need for vasopressor support despite adequate fluid resuscitation. This patient has fever, leukocytosis, an infectious source, and neurologic and renal dysfunction, making severe sepsis the most appropriate diagnosis. *(6:2223)*

493. **(E)** This patient has oliguria despite an adequate blood pressure and CVP. Although it would be appropriate to initiate a work-up for his oliguria (including flushing the urinary catheter, urine studies, and renal ultrasound), the most appropriate next step in management is to start antibiotic treatment. Antibiotics would address the underlying cause of his sepsis with organ dysfunction and should be initiated without delay. It is appropriate to perform a neurologic evaluation and consider the possibility of an intracranial process in this confused patient, however, if delirium is the cause of his mental status changes, then neuroimaging may not be helpful. *(6:196-200, 579)*

494. **(B)** Volume resuscitation is an integral part of shock management. In addition to a variety of different crystalloids, gelatins, dextrans, albumin, starches, and blood components have been used to expand the intravascular volume. Debate continues over the most appropriate resuscitation fluid with differences in blood volume effect, edema formation, antiinflammatory effect, cost and risk of anaphylaxis, coagulopathy, renal failure, and pruritis dominating the debate. Hydroxyethyl starch solutions have been associated with an increased risk of acute renal failure in critically ill patients. *(6:1399-1400)*

495. **(E)** Decreased FRC and ERV are the most common PFT abnormalities in obese patients. Chest wall compliance is decreased in obese patients due to adipose tissue in the chest wall and abdomen. Diminished outward recoil of the chest results in diminished FRC and ERV. Diminished FRC can result in lung volumes less than closing capacity at normal tidal volume leading to atelectasis. These changes are exacerbated in the perioperative period by diaphragmatic dysfunction, pain with diminished cough and secretion clearance, and

hypoventilation due to sedative medications. RV is usually unchanged. TLC may be near normal in obesity, but diminishes with increasing BMI. FEV_1/FVC is normal since both values are diminished relatively equally in obesity. Diffusing capacity is usually preserved unless pulmonary hypertension is present in which case this value is reduced. *(5:302-3; 6:2093)*

496. **(C)** Atelectasis and hypoventilation are the most common causes of hypoxemia in the PACU. Obesity and abdominal surgery will both increase the risk. Supine positioning intraoperatively, postoperative diaphragmatic dysfunction, and painful respiration promote atelectasis. Opioid analgesics may worsen hypoventilation. Hypoventilation and provision of supplemental oxygen postoperatively further contribute to atelectasis. The wife's history suggests that this patient has a high likelihood of undiagnosed obstructive sleep apnea (OSA) based on the following 4 (of 8) risk factors identified in the "STOP-BANG" score: snoring, daytime sleepiness, BMI > 35, and male gender. The remaining risks assessed for in STOP-BANG are observed apneic periods during sleep, high blood pressure, age > 50, and neck circumference > 40 cm. Residual anesthetic agents and postoperative opioids contribute to upper airway obstruction in patients with OSA due to impaired pharyngeal dilator function that causes pharyngeal collapse. *(5:304-5; 6:2184)*

497. **(D)** These three measures are reasonable first management steps to see if the patient's hypoventilation and hypoxemia can be quickly reversed, potentially avoiding need for ICU management. The opioid antagonist naloxone in small, incremental doses (40 mcg IV) may be used to attempt to reverse respiratory depression without fully reversing analgesic effect. Flumazenil is a reversal agent for benzodiazepines, but, unlike naloxone, primarily reverses the CNS depressant effects with no or incomplete reversal of the respiratory depressant effects of benzodiazepines. In this case, therefore, where reversal of respiratory depression is the priority, naloxone should be the first

choice agent. A trial of NIPPV may be helpful to reverse hypoventilation if the patient will tolerate the tight-fitting mask and has intact protective airway reflexes. Head of bed positioning at 45 degrees, by utilizing gravity to reduce impingement of abdominal contents on the diaphragm, may improve lung and chest wall compliance, diminish atelectasis, and improve ventilation. Additionally, this position provides superior preoxygenation of obese patients compared to supine when preparing for anesthetic induction and it may be useful if the patient deteriorates, requiring endotracheal intubation. An ABG may be performed after initial steps are taken to correct the patient's hypoxemia. Similarly, nasogastric tube decompression may be performed later if gastric distention is deemed an important contributor to diminished pulmonary compliance. Hydromorphone carries similar respiratory depressant risks as morphine and should be avoided at present. *(1:511, 656; 5:312, 314-5, 699, 1287)*

498.   **(C)** The patient likely has cor pulmonale (pulmonary hypertension and right ventricular hypertrophy and dilation). This is could be attributable to obesity-hypoventilation syndrome (OHS) that affects approximately 10% of morbidly obese patients. OHS occurs in the setting of chronic hypoventilation that leads to pulmonary hypertension and RV failure. The acute deterioration occurring following endotracheal intubation is secondary to acutely decreased RV preload and increased RV afterload associated with positive pressure ventilation. Findings on TTE include evidence of RV hypertrophy and dilation, elevated estimated systolic pulmonary artery pressure, paradoxical motion of the intraventricular septum due to RV overload, and a small LV due to displacement of the intraventricular septum by the dilated RV. Although LV failure is the most common cause of cor pulmonale, if this were the case in this patient, one would expect to see radiographic evidence of pulmonary edema in this clinical setting. *(6:1913-15)*

499.   **(C)** This patient has septic shock, a form of distributive shock. Initiation of mechanical ventilation in this setting may be expected to worsen hypotension due to 1) reduced work of breathing diminishing endogenous catecholamine levels; 2) positive pressure ventilation reducing venous return; and 3) sedative drugs causing vasodilation or depressed myocardial contractility. Positive pressure ventilation increases right ventricular afterload, but reduces left ventricular afterload, potentially improving left ventricular stroke volume in patients with LV dysfunction. Ketamine does not cause histamine release *(1:539; 6:2199)*

500.   **(D)** Auto positive end-expiratory pressure ("auto-PEEP") is an alveolar pressure above the airway opening pressure. Causes include flow limitation, dynamic hyperventilation, and a high minute ventilation. Patients with COPD often have auto-PEEP that may impair triggering of the ventilator and may cause patient-ventilator dyssynchrony. *(5:1411, 1413, 1416, 1419)*

501.   **(E)** In pressure assist/control ventilation, tidal volume varies based on the peak pressure setting. Secretions that obstruct the endotracheal tube will result in a higher peak inspiratory pressure, thereby diminishing tidal volume. Assuming no change in respiratory rate, minute ventilation will decrease. *(5:1407)*

502.   **(D)** This patient has sepsis and, as is common in the presentation of sepsis, he is hypovolemic. To treat the hypotension, he should first be volume resuscitated, in this case using crystalloid to target a CVP of 8-12 mm Hg. There is evidence that outcome from septic shock is improved with "early goal-directed therapy" that employs a stepwise fashion of rapid interventions to address the hypoperfused state. Current recommendations by the Surviving Sepsis Campaign include initial fluid resuscitation with crystalloid to a minimum dose of 30 mL/kg and continued fluid challenge if there is improvement in dynamic or static hemodynamic parameters. Hydroxyethyl starches should not be used to resuscitate septic patients because these products are associated with an increased risk of kidney injury in this setting. Other recommendations include that norepinephrine be the initial vasopressor choice with epinephrine added

if the MAP goal of 65 mm Hg cannot be achieved with norepinephrine alone. Inotropic support should be initiated with dobutamine trial if the MAP goal has been achieved but there are ongoing signs of hypoperfusion. Blood transfusion is recommended to target a hemoglobin concentration of 7-9 g/dL in clinical circumstances where active hemorrhage or myocardial ischemia is not present. It is important to note that at the time of publication of this book, there are several multinational, multicenter trials ongoing to determine the adequacy of these goals and their impact on patient outcomes. Note that these recommendations may change during the publication cycle of this book. Current recommendations may be viewed at the website www.survivingsepsis.org. Current goals of resuscitation in septic shock include a mean arterial pressure (MAP) > 65 mm Hg, urine output > 0.5 mL/kg/h, and ScvO$_2$ > 70%. *(5:543; 6:2228-31)*

503. **(C)** Current Surviving Sepsis Campaign guidelines suggest that in this case, where the MAP goal has been achieved, but there are ongoing signs of hypoperfusion (low ScvO$_2$), a trial of inotropic support with dobutamine, up to 20 mcg/kg/min, should be added. Treatment of impaired contractility due to septic shock may be individualized to the patient but a few general principles apply. Increasing the norepinephrine dose is not recommended since the MAP goal has been achieved in this patient. Milrinone is a phosphodiesterase inhibitor that inhibits degradation of cAMP resulting in improved myocardial contractility and relaxation; it also reduces systemic and pulmonary vascular resistance, and thus decreases ventricular afterload. It is a useful drug for treatment of heart failure but may exacerbate hypotension in septic shock. Dobutamine is a β_1 and β_2 agonist ($\beta_1 \gg \beta_2$) that increases myocardial contractility and therefore increases cardiac output. Tachycardia from dobutamine is less common than with some other adrenergic agents, although tachydysrhythmias may be a side effect that requires dose reduction or discontinuation of the drug. Many patients in septic shock will require both a vasopressor (e.g., norepinephrine) for α_1-mediated vasoconstrictive effects, and an

inotrope (e.g., dobutamine) to enhance cardiac contractility. Vasopressin acts at peripheral vasopressin (V$_1$) receptors to cause vasoconstriction. It is effective despite acidosis and may be useful in septic shock. It may be also be beneficial in replenishing vasopressin levels in the relative vasopressin deficient state of sepsis. Generally, vasopressin may be added as a vasopressor when patients are receiving high doses of standard α-agonists without acceptable response of blood pressure or to diminish the dose of norepinephrine required to achieve the MAP goal. However, one study (VASST) suggested that the best benefit of vasopressin in the care of patients with septic shock may be in those with less severe shock. Epinephrine is an effective vasopressor and inotrope but is associated with significant risk of tachydysrhythmias and, perhaps, gut ischemia. For these reasons, it is not considered a first line therapy (as is norepinephrine) for treatment of septic shock. *(1:301, 322, 805; 5:1373; 6:1373, 2:2229-30)*

504. **(E)** The figure shows a large pericardial effusion with right atrial and right ventricular compression. Pulsus paradoxus > 12 mm Hg is an extremely sensitive indicator of pericardial tamponade in the presence of pericardial effusion. Tamponade is consistent with the patient's symptoms, vital signs, and echocardiographic findings. *(6:1830)*

505. **(C)** Immediate pericardiocentesis is the treatment for life-threatening pericardial tamponade. *(6:2268)*

506. **(D)** Aspiration may have no, mild, or severe effects depending on the quantity and character of the aspirated material, patient response, and underlying medical condition. In this case, aspiration of feculent material may be anticipated to provoke severe lung injury with systemic effects (e.g., hypotension). Since the aspirated contents are solid, bronchoscopy should be performed to remove the particulate. Bronchoalveolar lavage, however, is not recommended after aspiration. Prone ventilation may be beneficial in patients with ARDS, although a definitive outcome benefit

has not been proven. Chest CT is not likely to provide useful diagnostic information to change management and the transfer to the radiologic suite may be hazardous to the patient with her current cardiopulmonary instability. There is no role for hyperbaric oxygen in the treatment of aspiration. *(5:1288; 6:1334, 2137, 2141, 2205)*

507. **(C)** Unlike patients who aspirate liquid gastric contents, this patient should be treated with antibiotics due to the expected bacterial concentration of the small bowel contents. Sodium bicarbonate administration in this patient may worsen acidosis if the lung injury is severe enough to cause ventilation impairment. This is due to the conversion of sodium bicarbonate to CO_2 that is eliminated via the lungs. If severe acidosis requiring treatment exists in a patient with severe lung injury or ARDS, consideration should be given to using THAM (tromethamine), a hydrogen ion acceptor that functions as a buffering agent without producing CO_2. *(5:532, 1074, 1288)*

508. **(D)** Critical myocardial blood flow is associated with an aortic diastolic blood pressure > 40 mm Hg. CPR is unlikely to result in return of spontaneous of circulation if a diastolic blood pressure > 40 mm Hg is not achieved during chest compressions. *(5:1423, 1427)*

509. **(D)** Maintaining high quality, uninterrupted chest compressions is critical to the success of CPR. Current adult ACLS guidelines call for chest compressions that depress the sternum 2 inches (5 cm) with 50% compression time at a rate of 100 compressions/min. Interruptions in chest compressions should be minimized and should never be greater than 10 sec long. *(5:1423, 1428)*

510. **(D)** The only consistently successful treatment of ventricular fibrillation (VF) is defibrillation, and the earlier defibrillation occurs, the more likely the patient is to survive. As a result, the first priority for a patient in ventricular fibrillation should be defibrillation if it can be accomplished within 5 min of arrest. If greater than 5 min has lapsed since the patient arrested,

2-3 min of chest compressions should be performed prior to defibrillation. This will reduce the myocardial oxygen debt and increase the chances of successful defibrillation. Intubation should not delay defibrillation. Current energy recommendations for defibrillation are 360 J for a monophasic defibrillator. For a biphasic defibrillator, the appropriate energy is device specific, but 200 J is recommended if the device specific setting is unknown. A patient in ventricular fibrillation cannot be cardioverted as there is no organized rhythm. Epinephrine and amiodarone are reserved for after defibrillation has been attempted. Chest compressions should be resumed immediately after a defibrillation attempt (without pausing for a pulse/rhythm check). *(5:1430-1, 1433)*

511. **(B)** The low flow conditions of CPR result in low pulmonary blood flow and a substantial increase in dead space due to lack of perfusion to nondependent alveoli. This increased dead space will dilute the alveolar CO_2 of perfused lung units resulting in a low end-tidal CO_2 that correlates poorly with arterial CO_2. When flow increases (due to improved CPR), there is an increase in end-tidal CO_2 due to a decrease in dead space (more lung units are perfused). As a result, end-tidal CO_2 correlates well with cardiac output during CPR. Current ACLS guidelines recommend end-tidal CO_2 monitoring as a noninvasive means of monitoring the adequacy of chest compressions. An end-tidal CO_2 < 10 mm Hg is unlikely to result in successful resuscitation. An end-tidal CO_2 in this range is a marker of the need to improve the delivered chest compressions. An increase in end-tidal CO_2 can also act as an early sign of return of spontaneous circulation. *(5:1423, 1427-8)*

512. **(D)** Current ACLS guidelines recommend 6-8 breaths/min (2 sec pause for 2 breaths after every 30 compressions) for patients receiving CPR without an advanced airway and 8-10 breaths/min (without interrupting chest compressions) for patients receiving CPR with an advanced airway. Hyperventilation inhibits effective chest compressions and should be avoided. *(5:1426)*

513. (B) Post-arrest care should focus on stabilizing the patient, on treating precipitating causes for the arrest, and on beginning therapeutic hypothermia in appropriate patients. Two studies have demonstrated improved neurologic outcomes when survivors who remain comatose after return of spontaneous circulation receive 12-24 h of therapeutic hypothermia. Hyperoxia and oxygen free radicals worsen brain reperfusion injury. As a result, FIO$_2$ should be titrated to the lowest level that allows maintenance of an oxygen saturation > 94%. If ischemia is suspected, cardiac catheterization should be scheduled promptly. It is not necessary to delay catheterization due to institution of therapeutic hypothermia. Neurologic prognosis is difficult to predict in the first 72 h post-arrest, and no clinical signs can reliably predict poor neurologic outcome in the first 24 h post-arrest. There is no role for mannitol, a treatment for increased intracranial pressure, in immediate post-arrest management. *(5:1423, 1435)*

514. (D) Cerebral salt wasting is a form of hypovolemic hyponatremia. Laboratory findings are notable for low serum sodium (< 135 mEq/L), low plasma osmolality, urine sodium > 40 mEq/L, high urine osmolality (>100 mOsm/kg). The mechanism of salt loss via the kidneys is poorly understood. Cerebral salt wasting most commonly occurs in patients with subarachnoid hemorrhage. *(6:345)*

515. (C) Congestive heart failure is associated with hypervolemic hyponatremia due to neurohumoral activation. Low cardiac output with a reduced effective circulatory volume to the kidneys causes renal sodium retention, but a proportionately greater increase in total body water that leads to hyponatremia. Urine sodium is low as the renal excretion of sodium is limited. In this circumstance, systolic pressure variation < 5 mm Hg is consistent with fluid nonresponsiveness. *(5:89, 425; 6:345)*

516. (G) Central diabetes insipidus (DI) may be seen in traumatic brain injury due to impaired ADH release from a damaged hypothalamus. It is a common feature seen in patients who are brain dead, characterized by an absence of brain stem reflexes, and absence of respiration on apnea testing. Characteristic laboratory features are hypernatremia, increased serum osmolality, and an inappropriately dilute urine (low urine osmolality). Without treatment with vasopressin or desmopressin (DDAVP), patients are at risk for severe hypovolemia with associated hemodynamic instability. *(5:516; 6:340)*

517. (E) This patient has evidence of hypovolemia based on hyponatremia, normal plasma osmolality, low urine sodium and, most sensitively, a pulse pressure variation > 12%. Pulse pressure variation (PPV) may be used as a determinant of fluid responsiveness in patients on positive pressure ventilation who have an arterial catheter monitoring blood pressure. PPV is measured during a single positive pressure breath, and is equal to the difference between maximal and minimal pulse pressure values divided by the mean of these maximum and minimum values. It is usually described as a percentage, and has the best discriminative ability for predicting fluid responsiveness among current respiratory variability-based indices (e.g., systolic pressure variation, delta down, stroke volume variation). *(5:425; 6:345)*

518. (B) Hepatorenal syndrome is a complication of hepatic cirrhosis with associated significant ascites. The pathophysiology involves severe renal vasoconstriction that produces oliguria and an elevated creatinine despite total body volume overload. Hyponatremia and urine sodium < 10 mEq/L are characteristic. When severe, prognosis for recovery is poor without liver transplantation. *(5:1052; 6:2306, 2601)*

519. (D) Severe burn injury (especially when TBSA burned exceeds 25%) results in significant tissue trauma, a generalized capillary leak syndrome, and hypovolemic shock. Although burn injury can also be complicated by myocardial depression, an elevated hematocrit acts as a marker for hypovolemia and suggests the need for significant resuscitation. A low central venous pressure, cardiac output, and venous oxygen saturation is consistent with hypovolemic shock. *(5:1334-5; 6:2219)*

520. (B) The differential diagnosis for postpartum hypotension includes infection, hypovolemia, pulmonary or venous air embolism, cardiomyopathy, and endocrine abnormalities. A central venous pressure of 15 mm Hg and a hemoglobin concentration of 9 g/dL make hypovolemia or underresuscitated septic shock less likely. A patient with hypotension, tachycardia, cool edematous extremities, and an elevated CVP could have an air embolism or a cardiomyopathy. An embolism causing this degree of hypotension, however, would be expected to have a greater effect on oxygenation. As a result, postpartum cardiomyopathy is a more likely cause of the patient's symptoms. *(6:1961, 2171-2)*

521. (F) The differential diagnosis for chest pain is broad, but the most likely diagnoses in a patient with acute onset of chest pain and dyspnea are acute coronary syndrome (ACS) and pulmonary embolism (PE). An ECG without ST changes does not support the diagnosis of ACS. This patient's clinical picture is consistent with PE. The incidence of DVT after hip replacement surgery in patients who do not receive thromboprophylaxis is estimated to be as high as 80-90% (with a 2% incidence of fatal PE). A large embolism burden is required to cause hypotension. As a result, a patient with PE causing hypotension would be expected to have a large A-a gradient and difficult to maintain oxygenation. Sinus tachycardia is the most frequent ECG abnormality in PE. *(5:1204; 6:102-7, 2170-2, 2177)*

522. (A) Children with spina bifida have a 28-67% incidence of latex allergy. Intraoperative exposure to surgical gloves can lead to anaphylaxis due to mucosal absorption of latex proteins. Cardiovascular collapse and respiratory distress are the most common signs of anaphylaxis in anesthetized patients. Bronchospasm results in increased airway pressures and reduced ventilation. Decreased minute ventilation and pulmonary edema (due to capillary leak) lead to hypoxemia. There is vasodilation and capillary leak, resulting in hypotension with a decrease in both preload and afterload.

CVP would be expected to be low. *(5:1478-89; 6:2709-11)*

523. (C) This patient has evidence of vasodilatory shock with hypotension and warm, well-perfused extremities. This patient will fulfill the clinical definition of septic shock, SIRS plus a proven or suspected microbial etiology plus hypotension, if he remains hypotensive after resuscitation. His clinical picture is consistent with aspiration pneumonia. *(6:1334-5, 2218-22, 2223)*

524. (E) The differential diagnosis for shock in trauma includes hemorrhage, SIRS, pericardial tamponade, tension pneumothorax, myocardial contusion, and neurogenic shock. The patient could also have shock that predated the trauma, perhaps causing the motor vehicle collision, fall, or other traumatic mechanism. This young patient has a negative initial trauma evaluation, warm feet and a low heart rate. Although bradycardia can occur in the setting of hemorrhage, it is far more common in neurogenic shock. The lack of motor response, despite eye opening to verbal stimuli, supports the diagnosis of high cervical spinal cord injury. High spinal cord injury results in neurogenic shock due to arteriolar and venodilation from interruption of sympathetic vasomotor input. *(6:2218-22)*

525. (B) Hypercarbia is the diagnosis in this woman with chronic COPD who underwent a surgical procedure involving carbon dioxide insufflation of the peritoneum. Abdominal distention has caused basilar atelectasis, worsened V/Q mismatch, and an increased fraction of dead space ventilation. Sedative medications administered during the anesthetic have exacerbated hypoventilation and baseline hypercarbia. This in combination with carbon dioxide absorption from the surgical procedure has resulted in severe acute superimposed on chronic hypercarbia with the neurologic finding of coma. *(5:2252)*

526. (H) The clinical presentation of head trauma with a period of lucidity then abrupt onset of coma is suggestive of epidural hematoma, perhaps due to skull fracture with injury to the middle meningeal artery. Treatment should consist of stat CT of the head followed by emergent neurosurgical decompression. *(6:2254, 3379)*

527. **(J)** A postseizure state may be a transient cause of coma. The etiology is thought to be due to release of toxic metabolites during the seizure or to temporary exhaustion of brain energy supplies. EEG performed during the coma may reveal a generalized slowing similar to toxic metabolic encephalopathy. *(6:2249)*

528. **(D)** A large infarct of a cerebral hemisphere, such as a middle cerebral artery stroke with resultant brainstem compression, may produce coma. Depending upon the size of the infarct, involvement of dominant or nondominant hemisphere, and neurologic prognosis, surgical intervention may be offered for decompression. *(6:2252)*

529. **(F)** The clinical picture, notable for high fever and severe leukocytosis, is most consistent with meningitis from an indwelling foreign body (external ventricular drain). Treatment includes immediate broad spectrum antimicrobials and removal of the drain. *(6:2252)*

530. **(E)** Septic shock or other severe infections can produce coma and is the most likely diagnosis in this immunosuppressed patient. *(6:2252)*

CHAPTER 19

Acute and Chronic Pain
Questions

DIRECTIONS (Questions 531-600): Each of the numbered items or incomplete statements in this section is followed by answers or by completions of the statement. Select the ONE lettered answer or completion that is BEST in each case.

531. A-δ fibers

    (A) are unmyelinated
    (B) are low-threshold mechanoreceptors
    (C) increase their firing as the intensity of the stimulus increases
    (D) do not respond to noxious stimuli
    (E) are thick nerves

532. In a patient with skeletal metastases, bisphosphonates have all of the following effects EXCEPT

    (A) inhibiting the recruitment and function of osteoclasts
    (B) inhibition of osteoblasts
    (C) they have their greatest effect in breast cancer and multiple myeloma
    (D) they have an acute pain-relieving effect

533. In the dorsal horn of the spinal cord,

    (A) cells from lamina I and II project to the hypothalamus
    (B) stimulation of lamina I and II produces pain
    (C) lamina I and II are found in the thoracic segment of the spinal cord only
    (D) discharge from lamina I and II decreases as a noxious stimulus increases
    (E) wide dynamic range (WDR) neurons are located predominantly in lamina I and II

534. Which one of the following is true regarding seizures as one of the multiple side effects from the use of opioids?

    (A) Morphine and related opioids can cause seizure activity when moderate doses are given.
    (B) Seizure activity is more likely with meperidine, especially in the elderly and with renal dysfunction.
    (C) Seizure activity is mediated through stimulation of N-methyl-D-aspartate (NMDA) receptors.
    (D) Naloxone is very effective in treating seizures produced by morphine and related drugs including meperidine.
    (E) Seizure activity is most likely related to the fact that opioids stimulate the production of γ-aminobutyric acid (GABA).

535. Windup is a phenomenon that occurs due to constant input of C-fiber activity to the spinal cord. This phenomenon defines

    (A) reduction in excitability of spinal neurons in the dorsal root ganglion
    (B) increase in excitability of spinal neurons in the dorsal root ganglion
    (C) reduction in excitability of spinal neurons in the dorsal horn
    (D) increase in excitability of spinal neurons in the dorsal horn

536. The cricoid cartilage corresponds with which vertebra?

(A) C1

(B) C3

(C) C5

(D) C6

(E) C8

537. The lumbar facet joints are oriented

(A) in a coronal plane

(B) in a sagittal plane

(C) 45° off the sagittal plane

(D) 20° off the coronal plane

(E) 20° off the sagittal plane

538. Vertebroplasty is indicated for all of the following conditions EXCEPT

(A) multiple myeloma

(B) chronic compression fractures of vertebral body

(C) osteolytic metastatic tumors

(D) facet arthropathy

539. Ziconotide, found in snail venom, acts primarily on which type of calcium channel?

(A) N-type

(B) T-type

(C) L-type

(D) P-type

(E) Q-type

540. Viscera are supplied by sympathetic nerves that contribute to pain generation and transmission. These nerves release all of the following chemical substances EXCEPT

(A) norepinephrine

(B) histamine

(C) serotonin

(D) epinephrine

541. Pretreatment with an NMDA antagonist prior to inflammation has been shown to

(A) enhance central sensitization

(B) attenuate central sensitization

(C) have no effect on central sensitization

(D) enhance peripheral sensitization

(E) attenuate peripheral sensitization

542. Indications for lumbar sympathetic blockade include all of the following EXCEPT

(A) acute herpes zoster

(B) phantom limb pain

(C) complex regional pain syndrome

(D) lumbar facet syndrome

(E) vascular insufficiency

543. NMDA receptor blockade in the spinal cord

(A) causes inhibition of pain modulation

(B) causes modulation of pain transmission

(C) does not have a role in pain transmission

(D) causes reduction in pain transmission

544. One important characteristic of methadone that has to be considered when prescribing it on an outpatient basis is

(A) there is usually a low chance for interactions on patients taking multiple medications

(B) withdrawal symptoms are as severe as with morphine

(C) it is rarely used in opioid addiction

(D) sedation and respiratory depression can outlast the analgesic action

(E) it allows rapid titration

545. With the use of intrapleural catheters for postoperative pain, all of the following statements are true EXCEPT

(A) the use of parenteral opioids is contraindicated

(B) pneumothorax can occur

(C) the usual dose is 20 to 30 mL 0.5% bupivacaine

(D) the mechanism of action is "unilateral intercostal nerve block"

546. A 35-year-old woman comes to your clinic complaining of pelvic pain. Which one of the following is important to consider during her evaluation?

(A) Endometriosis is the most common cause of pelvic pain in women.

(B) Endometriosis most likely does not have an inflammatory component.

(C) Endometriosis has been shown to be primarily dependent on the blood concentration of progesterone.

(D) An inflammatory process would be supported by findings of a decrease of interleukin-8 in testing of peritoneal fluid.

547. Which one of the following statements regarding fibromyalgia is true?

(A) Two central criteria for fibromyalgia are chronic widespread pain (CWP) defined as pain in all four quadrants of the body and the axial skeleton for at least two years, and the finding of pain by 25-kg pressure on digital palpation of at least 11 of the 18 defined tender points.

(B) It is generally agreed that abnormal CNS mechanisms are responsible for all of the symptoms of fibromyalgia.

(C) There are both primary and secondary fibromyalgia syndromes.

(D) Fibromyalgia symptoms generally resolve if a rheumatic process is identified and treated appropriately.

(E) Most fibromyalgia patients are male.

548. A recommended practice in the management of patients with cancer pain is

(A) less concern regarding side effects than in patients with nonmalignant pain

(B) dosing analgesics only on an as needed basis

(C) considering the use of adjuvant drugs

(D) avoiding opioid drugs due to the potential for development of tolerance

549. An 85-year-old woman comes into your clinic with chronic pain over her left breast for more than 1 year. The symptoms began after she broke out in a rash in the same distribution. Which one of the following statements is true?

(A) Zoster reactivation is always accompanied by a rash.

(B) Zoster reactivation may occur two to three times in a healthy individual.

(C) Post herpetic neuralgia (PHN) is pain that persists for more than 120 days.

(D) The incidence of PHN is expected to remain stable in the future.

(E) PHN should be treated with an antiviral agent like ganciclovir.

550. A 10-year-old boy with a diagnosis of sickle cell disease comes into your clinic. Which one of the following statements is true regarding his condition?

(A) A vaso-occlusive crisis commonly involves the back, legs, and eyes.

(B) Acute pain in patients with sickle cell disease is caused by ischemic tissue injury resulting from the occlusion of macrovascular beds by sickled erythrocytes during an acute crisis.

(C) When a vaso-occlusive crisis lasts longer than 7 days, it is important to search for other causes of bone pain.

(D) Patients with sickle cell disease have a lower incidence of vaso-occlusive disease than patients with β-thalassemia.

551. Complex regional pain syndrome type II (CRPS II) differs from CRPS I because in CRPS II there is

(A) allodynia
(B) movement disorder
(C) sudomotor and vasomotor changes
(D) evidence of major nerve damage
(E) severe swelling

552. What is the primary mechanism by which opioids produce analgesia?

(A) Coupling of opioid receptors to sodium and potassium ion channels, thereby inhibiting neurotransmitter release (presynaptic), and inhibiting neuronal firing (postsynaptically)

(B) Coupling of opioid receptor to potassium and calcium channels, thereby inhibiting neurotransmitter release (presynaptic), and inhibiting neuronal firing (postsynaptically)

(C) Coupling of opioid receptors to sodium and calcium channels, thereby inhibiting neurotransmitter release (presynaptic), and inhibiting neuronal firing (postsynaptically)

(D) Coupling of opioid receptors to potassium and calcium channels, thereby inhibiting neuronal firing (presynaptically), and inhibiting neurotransmitter release (postsynaptically)

(E) Coupling of opioid receptors to sodium and calcium channels, thereby inhibiting neuronal firing (presynaptically), and inhibiting neurotransmitter release (postsynaptically)

553. The definition of pain that is endorsed by the International Association for the Study of Pain is, "Pain is an unpleasant sensory and emotional experience associated with actual or potential tissue damage, or described in terms of such damage." There are a host of physiologic mechanisms by which injuries lead to nociceptive responses and ultimately to pain. However, not all nociceptive signals are perceived as pain and not every pain sensation originates from nociception. All of the following statements regarding pain are true EXCEPT

(A) two types of pain receptors are primarily activated by nociceptive input. These include low-threshold nociceptors that are connected to fast pain-conducting A-δ fibers, and high-threshold nociceptors that conduct impulses in slow (unmyelinated) C fibers

(B) neurotransmitters (e.g., glutamate and substance P) are able to modulate postsynaptic responses with further transmission to supraspinal sites (thalamus, anterior cingulate cortex, insular cortex, and somatosensory cortex) via ascending pathways

(C) prolonged or strong activity of dorsal horn neurons caused by repeated or sustained noxious stimulation may subsequently lead to increased neuronal responsiveness or central sensitization

(D) windup refers to a mechanism present in the peripheral nervous system in which repetitive noxious stimulation results in a slow temporal summation that is experienced in humans as increased pain

(E) substance P is an important nociceptive neurotransmitter. It lowers the threshold of synaptic excitability, resulting in the unmasking of normally silent interspinal synapses and the sensitization of second-order spinal neurons

554. A 32-year-old female develops severe stabbing, "like an ice pick," pain at the base of tongue after an infratemporal neurosurgical procedure. Pain comes in paroxysms and last a few seconds and is triggered by swallowing, yawning, and coughing. This patient most likely has

(A) trigeminal neuralgia

(B) geniculate neuralgia

(C) glossopharyngeal neuralgia

(D) migraine with atypical aura

(E) cluster headache

555. An advantage of transcutaneous electrical nerve stimulation (TENS) for postoperative pain is

(A) no patient instruction is needed

(B) the absence of opioid-induced side effects

(C) it can be used by patients with pacemakers

(D) it does not require any action on the part of the patient

556. A 31-year-old woman presents to your office with marked pain and swelling in her ankle 6 weeks after an open reduction and internal fixation with casting. On examination, the ankle is warm and erythematous. Lightly touching the ankle with a cotton swab evokes severe, lancinating pain. You suspect CRPS I. As a syndrome, CRPS is diagnosed by

(A) lumbar sympathetic block
(B) phentolamine infusion test
(C) triple phase isotope bone scan
(D) erythrocyte sedimentation rate
(E) history and physical examination

557. Which one of the following statements concerning central pain is true?

(A) Spinal cord injury is the leading cause of central pain in the United States.
(B) Lesions involving spinothalamocortical pathways are necessary and sufficient to cause central pain.
(C) Central pain is a common sequela following neurosurgical procedures.
(D) Motor cortex stimulation is an effective means to treat central pain.
(E) The most typical presentation of central pain is a spontaneous, burning sensation over the entire body contralateral to the lesion site.

558. Epidural steroid injections may be effective in which one of the following conditions?

(A) Herniated nucleus pulposus without neurologic deficit
(B) Ankylosing spondylitis
(C) Fibromyalgia
(D) Functional low back pain

559. A 42-year-old man underwent a celiac plexus block procedure with 20 mL of 50% alcohol. All of the following listed conditions are complications of this intervention EXCEPT

(A) genitofemoral neuralgia
(B) hypertension
(C) diarrhea

(D) paralysis
(E) infection

560. A patient who received 1 mL of 0.25% bupivacaine after negative aspiration following a selective cervical nerve root injection became agitated and then developed generalized tonic-clonic movements. Which one of the following is the most likely explanation?

(A) High spinal anesthetic from accidental intrathecal injection
(B) Anxiety attack from pain during injection
(C) Vertebral artery injection of local anesthetic
(D) Injection into spinal cord
(E) Hypoxia

561. Which one of the following is true regarding oxcarbazepine?

(A) It has more adverse effects than carbamazepine.
(B) It is a sodium channel blocker.
(C) A dose adjustment is unnecessary in a patient with renal insufficiency.
(D) Its most frequent adverse effects is weight loss and dizziness.

562. Spinal cord stimulation (SCS) has been used with success for the treatment of all of the following conditions EXCEPT

(A) failed back surgery syndrome
(B) complex regional pain syndrome
(C) angina
(D) peripheral vascular disease
(E) diffuse chronic pain syndromes

563. A patient with obstructive lung disease develops complex regional pain syndrome involving the right arm after an injury. Treatment of the syndrome may involve all of the following EXCEPT

(A) stellate ganglion block
(B) lumbar sympathetic block
(C) surgical sympathectomy
(D) TENS

564. As compared with somatic pain, all of the following are true about visceral pain, EXCEPT

(A) it may follow the distribution of a somatic nerve

(B) it is dull and vague

(C) it is often periodic and builds to peaks

(D) it is often associated with nausea and vomiting

(E) it is poorly localized

565. The following statements are true regarding preemptive analgesia, EXCEPT

(A) preemptive analgesia is helpful in reducing postoperative pain in part by reducing the phenomenon of central sensitization

(B) early postoperative pain is not a significant predictor of long-term pain

(C) local anesthetics, opioids, and COX inhibitors can be used for preemptive analgesia

(D) preemptive analgesia may have the potential to prevent the development of chronic pain states

(E) preemptive analgesia is thought to reduce neuroplastic changes in the spinal cord

566. All of the following statements about postherpetic neuralgia (PHN) are correct, EXCEPT

(A) a midthoracic dermatome is one of the most common sites for PHN

(B) men are affected more often than women in a ratio of 3:2

(C) the ophthalmic division of the trigeminal nerve is one of the most common sites for PHN

(D) PHN may occur in any dermatome

(E) PHN has an incidence of 9% to 14.3%

567. Which of the following statements is true regarding acetaminophen toxicity?

(A) Acetaminophen is nontoxic until undergoing metabolism.

(B) Oral glutathione is the antidote of choice.

(C) The antidote must be started within 6 h of ingestion in order to be effective.

(D) Vasodilatory β_2-adrenoceptor agonists potentiate the antidote efficacy.

568. Which one of the following is true regarding respiratory depression related to the use of opioids?

(A) Opioid agonists, partial agonists, and agonist/antagonists produce the same degree of respiratory depression.

(B) Opioids produce a leftward shift of the CO_2 responsiveness curve.

(C) Depression of respiration is produced by a decrease in respiratory rate, with a constant minute volume.

(D) Naloxone partially reverses the opioid-induced respiratory depression.

(E) The apneic threshold is decreased.

569. Of the two principal neurolytic agents, alcohol and phenol,

(A) alcohol has the greater tendency to produce neuritis

(B) alcohol is used in a 6% concentration

(C) phenol has the more rapid onset of action

(D) phenol is used in a 50% concentration

570. Pain theories currently being proposed postulate a

(A) straight stimulus-to-nervous system path

(B) system involving large fibers only

(C) system with inhibition exerted by small fibers

(D) system involving excitatory and inhibitory input with resulting sensation

571. Cluster headaches are characterized by

(A) lancinating unilateral headache that is commonly triggered by stress factors

(B) pain that is strictly unilateral and autonomic symptoms that occur ipsilateral to the pain

(C) slow onset with progressive worsening of the pain over several hours with an attack usually lasting 3 to 4 days

(D) the common use of melatonin as therapy for the acute attack

(E) a higher incidence in elderly patients

572. Which one of the following characterizes spontaneous intracranial hypotension (SIH)?

(A) It is the same entity as post–dural puncture headache (PDPH).

(B) The headache is consistently unilateral.

(C) Orthostatic headache is pathognomonic.

(D) Patients complain of bitemporal headache.

(E) To confirm the diagnosis, it is required that cerebrospinal fluid (CSF) opening pressures are below 60 mm H_2O.

573. Adverse effects of epidurally administered glucocorticoids include all of the following, EXCEPT

(A) Cushing syndrome

(B) osteoporosis

(C) avascular bone necrosis

(D) hypoglycemia

(E) suppression of the hypothalamic-pituitary axis

574. All of the following are true about chronic pain in the spinal cord injury (SCI) patient, EXCEPT

(A) approximately two-thirds of all SCI patients suffer from chronic pain

(B) approximately one-third of SCI patients with pain have severe pain

(C) pain in SCI patients may lead to severe depression and even suicide

(D) because of the overwhelmingly significant impairment of other important functions, pain is only a minor consideration in an SCI patient

(E) pain in SCI interferes with rehabilitation and activities of daily living (ADLs)

575. Which one of the following is true in relation to complex regional pain syndrome (CRPS)?

(A) Males are more commonly affected than females.

(B) CRPS II is more common than CRPS I.

(C) Three-phase bone scan showing unilateral periarticular uptake is mandatory to confirm CRPS diagnosis.

(D) The diagnosis of CRPS is mainly clinical.

(E) The mean age group is between 15 and 25 years.

576. In the neurolytic treatment of cancer pain, all of the following are true statements EXCEPT

(A) alcohol injections around a peripheral nerve may produce an uncomfortable neuritis.

(B) bowel and bladder function is almost always preserved.

(C) such treatment should be used only in those with terminal disease.

(D) absence of sensation may be perceived by the patient to be worse than the pain.

577. Advantages of intrathecal drug-delivery are all of the following EXCEPT

(A) the first-pass effect can be avoided

(B) intrathecal morphine is 300 times as effective as oral morphine for equivalent analgesia

(C) the number of CNS-associated side effects can be reduced

(D) the blood brain barrier does not interfere with the CNS uptake of the drug

(E) there is no systemic absorption of drugs administered via the intrathecal route

578. Which one of the following opioids does not produce dose-dependant bradycardia?

(A) Morphine

(B) Fentanyl

(C) Meperidine

(D) Sufentanil

(E) Alfentanil

579. The stellate ganglion is located between

(A) C6-C7

(B) C7-T1

(C) C5-C7

(D) C5-C6

(E) T1-T2

580. Which one of the following statements is false regarding tramadol?

(A) It has opioid characteristics.

(B) There is a dose limit of 400 mg/d.

(C) It is a centrally acting analgesic.

(D) There is no effect on norepinephrine or serotonin neurotransmission.

(E) The drug inhibits the reuptake of norepinephrine and serotonin.

581. The paroxysmal hemicranias are rare benign headache disorders that may typically be associated with all of the following EXCEPT

(A) conjunctival injection

(B) rhinorrhea

(C) ptosis

(D) eyelid edema

(E) monocular blindness

582. All of the following statements regarding the theory and use of acupuncture are true EXCEPT

(A) "qi" is the life force or energy that flows through the body

(B) "qi" influences our health at physical, mental, emotional, and spiritual levels

(C) any excess or deficiency of "qi" will contribute to our health problems

(D) blockage of "qi" may cause pain

(E) acupuncture should not be offered as part of comprehensive pain management until more clinical trials proving its efficacy have been completed

583. The gate control theory is one postulated mechanism of action for spinal cord stimulators (SCS). Which one of the following is the most accurate application of SCS to this postulated mechanism of action?

(A) Activation of large-diameter afferents thereby "closing the gate"

(B) Activation of large-diameter afferents thereby "opening the gate"

(C) Activation of small-diameter afferents thereby "closing the gate"

(D) Activation of small-diameter afferents thereby "opening the gate"

(E) Activation of both large- and small-diameter afferents equally

584. The duration of aspirin effect is related to the turnover rate of COX in different target tissues because aspirin

(A) competitively inhibits the active sites of COX enzymes

(B) nonirreversibly inhibits COX activity

(C) irreversibly inhibits COX activity

(D) noncompetitively inhibits the active sites of COX enzymes

(E) acetylates COX-1

585. Which one of the following best fits the pharmacologic mechanisms of action of traditional nonsteroidal antiinflammatory drugs?

(A) Inhibition of phospholipase A2

(B) Inhibition of COX-2

(C) Inhibition of lipoxygenase

(D) Inhibition of arachidonic acid

(E) Inhibition of prostaglandin G/H synthase enzymes

586. The following statements are true about methadone EXCEPT it

(A) has a highly variable oral bioavailability

(B) is a low cost medication

(C) has no known active metabolites

(D) has N-methyl-D-aspartate (NMDA) receptor agonist properties

(E) has high lipid solubility

587. Ketamine and memantine are NMDA receptor

(A) allosteric regulators

(B) agonists

(C) inverse agonists

(D) antagonists

588. Which one of the following is the correct statement regarding the pharmacologic properties of nonselective COX inhibitors?

(A) They readily cross the blood–brain barrier.

(B) Their chemical structure consists of aromatic rings connected to basic functional groups.

(C) They act mainly in the periphery.

(D) They have a high renal clearance.

(E) They are not metabolized by the liver.

589. Occipital neuralgia involves

(A) the greater occipital nerve

(B) the cervical plexus

(C) a pain distribution confined to the occipital area

(D) the scapular nerve

(E) trophic lesions of the skull

590. A tricyclic antidepressant in the secondary amine class is

(A) imipramine

(B) nortriptyline

(C) doxepin

(D) amitriptyline

(E) trazodone

591. Inhibitory substances that are believed to modulate the transmission of nociceptive signals in the dorsal horn of the spinal cord include all of the following EXCEPT

(A) substance P

(B) β-endorphin

(C) dopamine

(D) epinephrine

(E) adenosine

592. Which one of the following is a nociceptor?

(A) Meissner's corpuscles

(B) Pacinian corpuscles

(C) Merkel's disks

(D) Free nerve endings on A-delta and C fibers

(E) Golgi–Mazzoni endings

593. All of the following statements are true about myofascial pain EXCEPT

(A) it is dermatomal in distribution

(B) it should be treated early in the course of the disease

(C) injection of local anesthetic may provide relief

(D) the pain can occur in the back, neck, and shoulders

(E) it can sometimes be relieved by simply needling the affected area

594. All of the following are major anatomic structures in the transmission and relay of nociceptive information EXCEPT

(A) spinothalamic tract

(B) locus coeruleus

(C) thalamus

(D) reticular formation

(E) sensory cortex

595. Gabapentin

(A) is structurally unrelated to GABA

(B) acts directly at GABA-binding site in the CNS

(C) inhibits voltage-dependent calcium channels

(D) is the drug of choice for fibromyalgia

596. Advantages of patient-controlled analgesia (PCA) include all of the following EXCEPT

(A) high patient satisfaction

(B) elimination of painful injections

(C) no need to adjust dosing parameters with increasing age

(D) more consistent levels of analgesia

(E) the ability of the patient to titrate pain relief to painful procedures such as chest physical therapy

597. The effectiveness of a neurolytic agent is dependent on all of the following EXCEPT

(A) location of the injection

(B) concentration

(C) histology of the nerve

(D) volume

(E) needle size

598. If a patient undergoing thoracotomy receives intercostal blocks with bupivacaine, his postoperative period will

(A) be little different from controls

(B) show marked improvement in respiratory function over controls

(C) show little difference in vital capacity but marked pain relief

(D) be marked by hyperventilation

(E) be marked by increased incidence of atelectasis

599. The McGill Pain Questionnaire

(A) consists of three major measures

(B) was developed by McGill

(C) is not widely used

(D) is a single-dimensional pain scale

(E) does not ask about the location of pain

600. Which of the following is a true statement concerning the use of epidural morphine?

(A) A biphasic respiratory depression pattern can develop, with the initial phase within 30 min of the bolus dose and a second phase 2-4 h later.

(B) Spinal morphine solutions must be preservative-free while epidural morphine solutions may contain preservatives.

(C) Patients should be closely monitored for 48 hours after the administration of epidural morphine.

(D) Patients may ambulate with assistance after an injection of epidural morphine.

Answers and Explanations

531. **(C)** A-δ fibers are thin, myelinated fibers, hence they have a faster conduction velocity than C fibers. They are high threshold mechanoreceptors. They are associated with sharp pain, temperature, cold, and pressure sensations. *(7:13-4)*

532. **(B)** Bisphosphonates decrease resorption of bone directly, by inhibiting the recruitment and function of osteoclasts, and indirectly by stimulating osteoblasts. In patients with bony metastases, they are the standard therapy for hypercalcemia after rehydration, and have the greatest effect in patients with breast cancer and multiple myeloma. Bisphosphonates also have an acute pain-relieving effect that is thought to be derived from the reduction of various pain-producing substances. *(1:1294-6)*

533. **(B)** The Rexed laminae is a complex of 10 layers of grey matter located in the spinal cord. They are labeled as I to X. Laminae I to VI are in the dorsal horn and VII to IX are in the ventral horn. Lamina X borders the central canal of the spinal cord. Lamina I is also known as the posteromarginal nucleus. The neurons in lamina I receive input mainly from the Lissauer tract. They relay pain and temperature sensation. Lamina II is known as the substantia gelatinosa. The neurons contain κ- and μ-opioid receptors. C fibers terminate in the substantia gelatinosa. Laminae I and II are found along the entire spinal cord. The neurons in lamina I project to the thalamus. WDR neurons are concentrated in lamina V. *(7:17-9)*

534. **(B)** Extremely high doses of morphine and related opioids can produce seizures, presumably by inhibiting the release of GABA (at the synaptic level). Normeperidine, a metabolite of meperidine, is prone to producing seizures and tends to accumulate in patients with renal dysfunction and in the elderly. Naloxone may not effectively treat seizures produced by meperidine. *(1:494; 5:1302)*

535. **(D)** Windup refers to the progressive increase in the magnitude of C-fiber evoked responses of dorsal horn neurons produced by repetitive activation of C-fibers. Neuronal events leading to windup also produce some of the classical characteristics of central sensitization including expansion of receptive fields and enhanced responses to C but not A-δ fiber stimulation. *(7:22)*

536. **(D)** The carotid tubercle (Chassaignac tubercle) lies 2.5 cm lateral to the cricoid cartilage. It is a part of the transverse process of the C6 vertebra and can be easily palpated. The carotid tubercle is an important landmark for stellate ganglion blocks. *(5:254)*

537. **(C)** The cervical facet joints are oriented in a coronal plane to allow for extension, flexion, and lateral bending. The thoracic facets are oriented approximately 20° off the coronal plane. The lumbar facet joints are oriented 45° off the sagittal plane. *(7:285)*

538. (D) Vertebroplasty is best used for acute vertebral fracture where bone cement is percutaneously injected into a fractured vertebra in order to stabilize it. Alternatively, kyphoplasty involves placement of a balloon into a collapsed vertebra, followed by injection of bone cement to stabilize the fracture. It is not clear if one procedure has an advantage over the other. Both procedures may produce almost immediate pain relief. They are indicated for painful compression fractures because of osteoporosis and metastatic tumors. *(5:1610)*

539. (A) The nonopioid analgesic ziconotide has been developed as a new treatment for patients with severe chronic pain who are intolerant of and/or refractory to other analgesic therapies. Ziconotide is the synthetic equivalent of a 25-amino-acid polybasic peptide found in the venom of the marine snail *Conus magus*. In rodents, ziconotide acts by binding to neuronal N-type voltage-sensitive calcium channels, thereby blocking neurotransmission from primary nociceptive afferents. Ziconotide produces potent antinociceptive effects in animal models and its efficacy has been demonstrated in human studies. *(1:514)*

540. (D) In the viscera, sympathetic nerve terminals, mast cells, and epithelial cells, including enterochromaffin cells in the gastrointestinal tract, release a variety of bioactive substances, including norepinephrine, histamine, serotonin, adenosine triphosphate (ATP), glutamate, nerve growth factor (NGF), and tryptase. Resident leukocytes and macrophages attracted to an area of insult collectively contribute products of cyclooxygenase and lipoxygenase, including prostaglandin I_2, prostaglandin E_2, hydroxyeicosatetraenoic acids (HETEs), and hydroperoxyeicosatetraenoic (HPETEs), and a variety of cytokines, reactive oxygen species, and growth factors. Some of these chemicals can directly activate visceral afferent terminals (e.g., serotonin, ATP, and glutamate), whereas others probably play only a sensitizing role (e.g., prostaglandins, NGF, and tryptase). *(1:514)*

541. (B) Pretreatment with an NMDA antagonist attenuates the central sensitization from inflammation. *(7:24)*

542. (D) Lumbar sympathetic blockade has been shown to be effective in all of the pain syndromes listed except lumbar facet syndrome. Heat, COX inhibitors, and facet injections may be useful. *(1:1445-8; 5:1486)*

543. (B) NMDA receptor activation causes increased pain transmission whereas its blockade attenuates pain transmission. There are four receptor types for glutamate and aspartate in the somatosensory system. The class of receptors best activated by NMDA is termed the NMDA receptor. The NMDA receptor is usually considered as recruited only by intense and/or prolonged somatosensory stimuli. This characteristic is due to the NMDA receptor's well-known magnesium block that is only relieved by prolonged depolarization of the cell membrane. *(7:24)*

544. (D) Methadone, unlike morphine, is metabolized through N-demethylation by the hepatic cytochrome P450 enzyme system whose activity can vary widely in different people. Methadone should be administered with caution in patients receiving multiple medications, especially antivirals and antibiotics. Methadone's withdrawal symptoms tend to be less severe than morphine's; this and its long duration of action, good oral bioavailability, and high potency made it the maintenance drug or detoxification treatment of choice in opioid addiction. Methadone has biphasic elimination. A long terminal phase (ranging from 30-60 h) producing sedation and respiratory depression can outlast the analgesia that correlates with the redistribution phase (6-8 h). This biphasic pattern explains why methadone is used once a day for opioid maintenance therapy and every 4-8 h for analgesia. Rapid titration is not possible making this drug more useful for chronic pain. *(5:329-30; 704; 718)*

545. **(A)** The use of an intrapleural catheter can be effective for unilateral postoperative pain such as that following cholecystectomy. A pneumothorax can occur during catheter placement. Since only local anesthetic is injected, the use of parenteral opioids is not contraindicated. *(1:1327; 5:1829)*

546. **(A)** Endometriosis is the most common cause of chronic pelvic pain in women. It is characterized by the presence of uterine endometrial tissue outside the uterus, most commonly in the pelvic cavity. The disorder mainly affects women of reproductive age. Endometriosis has been described as a pelvic inflammatory process with altered function of immune cells and an increased number of activated macrophages in the peritoneal environment that secrete various local products such as growth factors and cytokines. Endometriosis is estrogen-dependent and traditional treatments have aimed to decrease production of estrogens such as estradiol. However, the exact mechanism by which estrogens promote endometriosis is unclear and suppression of estrogens has variable effects. Endometriotic lesions themselves secrete proinflammatory cytokines such as interleukin-8 (IL-8) that recruit macrophages and T-cells to the peritoneum and mediate inflammatory responses. *(6:387-8)*

547. **(C)** The two operational criteria are chronic widespread pain (CWP) defined as pain in all four quadrants of the body and the axial skeleton for at least three months, and the finding of pain by 4-kg pressure on digital palpation of at least 11 of 18 defined tender points. The exact pathogenesis of fibromyalgia has not been elucidated yet, but according to the currently held view a variety of biological, psychological, and social factors play a role in the manifestation of the disorder. Among other things, inflammatory, traumatic, and immunological processes;

static problems; endocrine disorders; and depression and anxiety disorders and stress factors are thought to trigger the syndrome. A dysfunction of the central affective and/or sensory pain memory may possibly be at work in the different illnesses mentioned above that then results in fibromyalgia pain. In principle, fibromyalgia can be categorized as primary or secondary fibromyalgia. In primary fibromyalgia, which is much more common than the secondary type, even the most careful work-up will not reveal any definitive organic factors triggering the syndrome. With secondary fibromyalgia, on the other hand, the underlying disease, such as inflammatory rheumatic processes or collagenosis can be diagnosed with relative ease. Symptoms associated with fibromyalgia often do not disappear when the rheumatic processes have subsided, suggesting that some central mechanisms may be responsible for the persistence of generalized pain and hyperalgesia, possibly due to a disorder of the central affective pain memory and/or the memory of sensory pain or else to latent peripheral immunological processes. It is precisely this coexistence of pain and hyperalgesia in secondary fibromyalgia associated with systemic inflammatory rheumatic diseases that proves that pain and sensitivity to pain cannot be separated strictly in fibromyalgia. *(6:2849-52)*

548. **(C)** Most published guidelines for the treatment of cancer pain include the concept of dosing medications, including opioids, to adequately treat pain on an around the clock basis. Respiratory depression is unusual in opioid-tolerant patients. The use of adjuvant drugs including antidepressants and anticonvulsants may be useful. Side effects such as nausea and constipation should be anticipated and treated. *(1:1451; 5:2770)*

549. (C) Reactivation of the varicella-zoster virus can cause dermatomal pain without a rash in a process termed "zoster sine herpete." This diagnosis cannot be made on the basis of clinical presentation alone and would require evidence of concurrent viral reactivation. Zoster reactivation typically occurs only once for an individual. Atypical manifestations that occur in immunocompromised patients include a prolonged course, recurrent lesions, and involvement of multiple dermatomes. Diagnostic laboratory tests are recommended when herpes simplex must be ruled out (e.g., recurrent rash or sacral lesions) and for patients with atypical lesions. Until recently, these definitions have been arbitrary, but the results of recent research now provide support for the validity of distinguishing between three phases of pain in affected and adjacent dermatomes: (1) herpes zoster acute pain (also termed acute herpetic neuralgia), defined as pain that occurs within 30 days after rash onset; (2) subacute herpetic neuralgia, defined as pain that persists beyond the acute phase but that resolves before the diagnosis of PHN can be made; and (3) PHN, defined as pain that persists 120 days or more after rash onset. It can also be predicted that the number of adults developing herpes zoster in the United States may increase as a consequence of reduced opportunities for subclinical immune boosting resulting from near-universal varicella vaccination of children. Recent data showing an increase in herpes zoster in the United States are consistent with this prediction. An increase in the incidence of herpes zoster could be offset by zoster vaccination, but the extent to which widespread herpes zoster vaccination will occur is presently unknown. *(7:417-9)*

550. (C) A vaso-occlusive crisis most commonly involves the back, legs, knees, arms, chest, and abdomen. The pain generally affects two or more sites. Bone pain tends to be bilateral and symmetric. Recurrent crises in an individual patient usually have the same distribution. Acute pain in patients with sickle cell disease is caused by ischemic tissue injury resulting from the occlusion of microvascular beds by sickled erythrocytes during an acute crisis. Acute bone pain from microvascular occlusion is a common reason for emergency department visits and hospitalizations in patients with sickle cell disease. Obstruction of blood flow results in regional hypoxemia and acidosis, creating a recurrent pattern of further sickling, tissue injury, and pain. The severe pain is believed to be caused by increased intramedullary pressure, especially within the juxtaarticular areas of long bones, secondary to an acute inflammatory response to vascular necrosis of the bone marrow by sickled erythrocytes. The pain may also occur because of involvement of the periosteum or periarticular soft tissue of the joints. When a vaso-occlusive crisis lasts longer than 7 days, it is important to search for other causes of bone pain, such as osteomyelitis, avascular necrosis, or compression deformities. When a recurrent bone crisis lasts for weeks, an exchange transfusion may be required to abort the cycle. Patients with sickle cell disease have a higher incidence of vaso-occlusive disease than patients with β-thalassemia. *(6:854-6)*

551. (D) CRPS I and CRPS II are clinically indistinguishable. The only difference is that in CRPS II there is evidence of major nerve damage. *(7:408)*

552. (B) Opioid receptors are coupled to G proteins that affect protein phosphorylation via a second messenger, thereby altering the conductance of potassium and calcium ion channels. These are believed to be the main mechanisms by which endogenous and exogenous opioids produce analgesia. The opening of potassium channels inhibits the release of neurotransmitters, including substance P and glutamate, if the receptors are presynaptic. Opioids also inhibit neuronal firing by hyperpolarization of the cell if the receptors are postsynaptic on the neurons. *(1:490-1)*

553. (D) Two types of pain receptors are primarily activated by nociceptive input. These include low-threshold nociceptors that are connected to fast conducting A-δ pain fibers, and high-threshold nociceptors that conduct impulses in slow, unmyelinated C fibers. Within the dorsal horn of the spinal cord, these pain fibers synapse with spinal neurons. Neurotransmitters (e.g., glutamate and substance P) are able to modulate the postsynaptic responses with further transmission to supraspinal sites (thalamus, anterior cingulate cortex, insular cortex, and somatosensory cortex) via the ascending pathways. The simplest form of plasticity in the nervous system is that repeated noxious stimulation may lead to habituation (decreased response) or sensitization (increased response). Prolonged or strong activity of dorsal horn neurons caused by repeated or sustained noxious stimulation may subsequently lead to increased neuronal responsiveness or central sensitization. Neuroplasticity and subsequent CNS sensitization include altered function of chemical, electrophysiological, and pharmacological systems. These changes cause exaggerated perception of painful stimuli (hyperalgesia), a perception of innocuous stimuli as painful (allodynia), and may be involved in the generation of referred pain and hyperalgesia across multiple spinal segments. While the exact mechanism by which the spinal cord becomes sensitized or in a "hyperexcitable" state currently remains somewhat unknown, some contributing factors have been proposed. Windup refers to a central spinal mechanism in which repetitive noxious stimulation results in a slow temporal summation that is experienced in humans as increased pain. In 1965, animal experiments showed for the first time that repetitive C-fiber stimulation could result in a progressive increase of electrical discharges from the second-order neuron in the spinal cord. This mechanism of pain amplification in the spinal cord is related to temporal summation of second pain or windup. Second pain, which is of dull quality and strongly related to chronic pain states, is transmitted through unmyelinated C fibers to dorsal horn nociceptive neurons. During the C-fiber's transmitted stimuli, NMDA receptors of second-order neurons become activated. It is well known that NMDA activation induces calcium entry into the dorsal horn neurons. Calcium entry into sensory neurons in the dorsal horn induces activation of nitric oxide (NO) synthase, leading to the synthesis of NO.

NO can affect the nociceptor terminals and enhance the release of sensory neuropeptides (in particular, substance P) from presynaptic neurons, therefore contributing to the development of hyperalgesia and maintenance of central sensitization. Substance P is an important nociceptive neurotransmitter. It lowers the threshold of synaptic excitability, resulting in the unmasking of normally silent interspinal synapses and the sensitization of second-order spinal neurons. Furthermore, substance P can extend for long distances in the spinal cord and sensitize dorsal horn neurons at a distance from the initial input locus. This results in an expansion of receptive fields and the activation of wide dynamic neurons by nonnociceptive afferent impulses. *(7:13-24)*

554. **(C)** Glossopharyngeal neuralgia is a disorder characterized by intense pain in the tonsils, middle ear, and back of the tongue. The pain can be intermittent or relatively persistent. Swallowing, chewing, talking, sneezing, or eating spicy foods may trigger the disorder. It is often the result of compression of the 9th nerve (glossopharyngeal) or 10th nerve (vagus), but in some cases, no cause is evident. Skull base surgery or surgeries in the infratemporal region may result in damage or irritation of the glossopharyngeal nerve. Conservative treatment includes using anticonvulsants. In refractory cases, glossopharyngeal nerve block may be helpful. Radiofrequency lesioning or neurolytic treatment should be reserved for resistant cases or ones associated with head and neck cancer. Surgical decompression should be reserved for nonresponders and resistant cases. *(7:248)*

555. **(B)** Transcutaneous electrical nerve stimulation (TENS) provides a "tingling" sensation that is not usually perceived as pain. Patients should be instructed in the use of the stimulator. It has the advantages of allowing the patient to participate in his or her therapy and the lack of opioid-induced side effects. The presence of a cardiac pacemaker is considered a relative contraindication. *(1:1424; 7:2777)*

556. (E) In the early 1990s, a panel of experts reached a consensus that the terms "reflex sympathetic dystrophy" and "causalgia" had lost their utility as clinical diagnoses and suggested a new nomenclature be adopted. The new terms designated for these conditions are "CRPS types I and II". According to the new diagnostic criteria, CRPS need not be maintained by sympathetic mechanisms. A three-phase isotope bone scan is often positive in CRPS, but a normal bone scan does not exclude the diagnosis. Erythrocyte sedimentation rate is a nonspecific test that is positive in many painful conditions including infection, inflammatory arthritides, and inflammatory myopathies. As a syndrome, CRPS is diagnosed by history and physical examination. For CRPS I, the diagnostic criteria include (1) an initiating noxious event; (2) spontaneous pain and/or allodynia occurring outside the territory of a single peripheral nerve that is/are disproportionate to the inciting event; (3) there is or has been evidence of edema, cutaneous perfusion abnormalities, or abnormal sudomotor activity in the region of pain since the inciting event; and (4) the diagnosis is excluded by the existence of any condition that would otherwise account for the degree of pain and dysfunction. *(7:410-1)*

557. (D) Owing to its high incidence, stroke is the leading cause of central pain in the industrialized world. The chance of developing central pain following spinal cord injury is higher than after stroke (30%-50% vs 8%), but the overall number of stroke patients with central pain is higher. Syringomyelia is the disorder with the highest incidence of central pain (60%-80%). According to neurosurgical studies conducted by V. Cassinari and C.A. Pagni in the 1960s, injury to spinothalamocortical pathways is necessary but not sufficient to cause central pain. The reason why some patients develop central pain but others with identical injuries do not is unknown. Central pain may occur after neurosurgical procedures and intracranial hemorrhage, but these are unusual occurrences. There are now several prospective studies showing motor cortex stimulation to be an effective treatment for central pain. There is

no typical presentation for central pain. While spontaneous pain is almost universal, allodynia also affects a majority of central pain patients. The time lag between the injury and onset of pain, and the location of central pain are extremely variable. *(7:394-400)*

558. (A) An indication for epidural steroid injections is nerve root irritation and accompanying inflammation. The use of epidural steroids in low back pain is an area of controversy. However, most experts agree that a trial of epidural steroids may be indicated in radicular pain of less than 12 months duration. Epidural steroid injections have been found to be ineffective in the relief of fibromyalgia, ankylosing spondylitis, and functional low-back pain. *(1:1443, 1448)*

559. (B) Celiac plexus block is both a diagnostic and therapeutic tool to help in managing upper abdominal pain arising from viscera. Pancreatic cancer is the leading diagnosis requiring neurolytic celiac plexus block; other conditions may include visceral pain arising from malignancies of the liver or GI tract. The procedure is performed either under fluoroscopic guidance or CT scan, though blind approaches have also been described. Both single transaortic as well bilateral needle approaches have been described. Complications include diarrhea, hypotension, genitofemoral neuralgia, infection, bleeding, damage to surrounding structures, and rarely paralysis. All complications mentioned above may occur except hypertension. *(7:703)*

560. (C) Selective cervical nerve root injection may be indicated for diagnosis and treatment of cervical radiculopathy. Complications other than infection, bleeding, and nerve damage include intravascular uptake into the vertebral artery or radicular arteries resulting in seizure, stroke, or paraplegia. Intraspinal spread into the epidural space or intrathecal spread is also possible, resulting in high spinal anesthesia. Damage to the spinal cord has also been reported with injection into the spinal cord. Considering the life-threatening complications, selective cervical nerve root block should only be performed by physicians well versed in this technique. *(5:853-4; 7:741-3)*

561. **(B)** Oxcarbazepine is an analogue of carbamazepine with a keto group at the carbon-10 position. It is roughly 50% protein bound in the plasma. The dose should be decreased at least by half if the patient has significant renal insufficiency. The most frequent adverse effects experienced include dizziness and vertigo, weight gain and edema, GI symptoms, fatigue, and allergic-type reactions. Allergic cross-sensitivity to carbamazepine occurs in about 25% of patients and may be severe. *(5:1560)*

562. **(E)** SCS has been utilized by clinicians for a variety of chronic pain issues. Although a large body of work has been published, precise mechanisms of action of SCS remain elusive. Animal studies suggest that SCS triggers release of serotonin, substance P, and γ-aminobutyric acid (GABA) within the spinal cord dorsal horn. Pain responds best to SCS when it is well localized, such as radicular pain in the upper or lower extremities. Diffuse pain may be impossible to treat with this modality because of the inability to get effective coverage with stimulation using SCS. *(5:1595; Kumar K, et al., Pain 2007; 132:179-88; Deer TR, et al., Curr Pain Heache Rep 2009; 131:18-23; Kemler MA, et al., J Neurosurg 2008; 108:292-8)*

563. **(B)** All of the options listed are important for the patient with complex regional pain syndrome. In the patient with obstructive lung disease, one may want to avoid the stellate ganglion approach, since there is a possibility of pneumothorax that could be life-threatening. A lumbar sympathetic block would not be used for pain in the upper extremity. *(1:1446)*

564. **(A)** The following are the usual features of somatic pain: well localized, sharp and definite, often constant (sometimes periodic); it is rarely associated with nausea except when it is deep somatic pain with bone involvement; and it may follow the distribution of a somatic nerve. In contrast, visceral pain: is poorly localized, diffuse, dull, and vague; it is often periodic and builds to peaks (sometimes constant); and it is often associated with nausea and vomiting. *(5:1601-2)*

565. **(B)** It has been demonstrated that early postoperative pain is a significant predictor of long-term pain. The rest of the answers are correct. *(5:1299)*

566. **(B)** PHN affects women more often than men, in a ratio of approximately 3:2. The rest of the answers are correct. *(5:417-9)*

567. **(A)** The liver receives the major insult from acetaminophen toxicity. When very large doses of acetaminophen exceed the liver's capacity to conjugate it to glucuronic acid or sulfate, it undergoes metabolism by CYP2E1 to a toxic metabolite that is scavenged by glutathione. Hepatic necrosis ensues when the supply of glutathione is exhausted. Exogenous administration of the glutathione analogue N-acetylcysteine scavenges the reactive metabolite and decreases the degree of cell death. N-acetylcysteine should be started within 36 h for greatest effectiveness. *(1:983-4; 5:191)*

568. **(E)** Opioids produce a dose-dependant respiratory depression by acting directly on the respiratory centers in the brainstem. Partial agonist and agonist-antagonist opioids are less likely to cause severe respiratory depression, as are the selective κ-opioid agonists. Therapeutic doses of morphine decrease minute ventilation by decreasing respiratory rate (as oppose to tidal volume). Opioids depress the ventilatory response to carbon dioxide; the carbon dioxide–response curve shows a decreased slope and rightward shift. The apneic threshold is decreased and the increase in ventilatory response to hypoxemia is blunted by opioids. Naloxone can effectively and fully reverse the respiratory depression from opioids. *(5:710)*

569. **(A)** Alcohol has a faster onset of action but a greater tendency to produce neuritis. It is used in concentrations of 50% to 100%. Phenol is used in concentrations of 5% to 20%. *(1:1453)*

570. (D) Current pain theories involve the small and large nerves and a path through the dorsal root. Both inhibitory and excitatory nerves are involved. *(1:1403; 5:2730; 7:2346)*

571. (B) The first statement better describes trigeminal neuralgia. Cluster headache affects more males than females with a 5:1 ratio and can begin at any age. Attacks are severe, stabbing, screwing, unilateral pain, occasionally preceded by premonitory symptoms, with sudden onset and rapid crescendo. Therapeutic interventions for the acute attack include oxygen, triptans, dihydroergotamine, ketorolac, chlorpromazine, or intranasal lidocaine, cocaine, or capsaicin. Melatonin has been found to be moderately effective as a preventive treatment in episodic and chronic cluster headache. *(7:212-4)*

572. (C) PDPH and SIH are two distinct clinical entities with similar presentations. The headache is always bilateral, located in the occipital and/or frontal area. Although low CSF pressure is often noted, it is not necessary to confirm the diagnosis. *(7:242)*

573. (D) The major theoretical complications of glucocorticoid administration include suppression of pituitary-adrenal axis, hypercorticism, Cushing syndrome, osteoporosis, avascular necrosis of bone, steroid myopathy, epidural lipomatosis, weight gain, fluid retention, and hyperglycemia. *(7:658-9)*

574. (D) Chronic pain is a major complication of SCI. Epidemiologic studies indicate that approximately two-thirds of all SCI patients suffer from chronic pain out of which one-third have severe pain. Pain interferes with rehabilitation, daily activities, quality of life, and may have significant influence on mood leading to depression and even suicide. *(7:394-5)*

575. (D) The diagnosis of CRPS I and II follows the IASP clinical criteria. Bone scintigraphy may be a valuable tool to rule out other conditions. CRPS I is more common than CRPS II and the female to male ratio is from 2:1 to 4:1. *(7:405-14)*

576. (B) In treating chronic pain, one must remember that the patient's perception of the pain may not be as bad as the loss of bowel and urinary control and the absence of sensation. This must be thoroughly discussed with the patient prior to proceeding. Most pain specialists believe that neurolytic blocks should be reserved for the patient with a short life expectancy. *(1:1453-4)*

577. (E) The premise behind intrathecal drug delivery is that by directly depositing drugs into the CSF, the first-pass effect is avoided. Intrathecal morphine is 300 times more effective than oral morphine on a dose basis. From spinal to epidural morphine the conversion is in the ratio of 1:10. From epidural to IV morphine the conversion is in the ratio of 1:10. From IV to oral morphine the conversion is in the ratio of 1:3, hence $10 \times 10 \times 3 = 300$. By the direct action of the medication, the number of CNS-associated side effects can be reduced. There is however, systemic uptake of drugs administered via the intrathecal route such as opioids, but in doses too low to result in analgesia. This is different from administration of opioids into the epidural space, where in the case of fentanyl for example, analgesia is mediated through systemic uptake and supraspinal effects. *(1:20-3; 5:798)*

578. (C) High doses of any opioid reduce sympathetic output allowing the parasympathetic output to predominate. The heart rate decreases by stimulation of the vagal center, especially with high doses. Meperidine has an atropine-life effect and may elevate the heart rate after IV administration. *(5:711)*

579. (B) The stellate ganglion is formed by the fusion of the inferior cervical ganglion resting over the anterior tubercle of C7 and first thoracic ganglion resting over the first rib. *(7:696-7)*

580. (D) Tramadol hydrochloride is a centrally-acting analgesic that is thought to provide analgesia via at least two mechanisms: some analgesia may be derived from the relatively weak interaction of tramadol with the μ-opioid receptor. The second and major mechanism, which is thought to account for at least 70% of tramadol's analgesic activity, is via inhibiting the reuptake of norepinephrine and serotonin. *(5:718)*

581. **(E)** Paroxysmal hemicranias may be chronic (CPH, e.g., daily) or episodic (EPH, e.g., discrete headache periods separated by periods of remission) characterized by severe, excruciating, throbbing, boring, or pulsatile pain affecting the orbital, supraorbital, and temporal regions. The pain tends to be associated with at least one of the following signs or symptoms ipsilateral to the painful side: conjunctival injection, nasal congestion, lacrimation, ptosis, rhinorrhea, or eyelid edema. Attacks may occur at any time, occasionally waking patients from sound sleep and tend to last for 2-25 min (although they may linger for hours). The patient generally has 1 to 40 attacks per day. Loss of sight is not associated with these headaches. *(7:221; 256)*

582. **(E)** According to traditional Chinese medicine, "qi" (pronounced "chee") is the life force or energy that flows through all living things. "Qi" affects our body at physical, mental, emotional, and spiritual levels. Any imbalance (deficiency or excess) or blockage of "qi" may result in disease or pain. Acupuncture treats disorders by influencing the flow of "qi," thus restoring the normal balance of organ systems. According to a 1998 NIH consensus panel, acupuncture may be included in a comprehensive management program for the treatment of a variety of conditions such as headache, fibromyalgia, lateral epicondylitis ("tennis elbow"), myofascial pain, low back pain, and osteoarthritis. *(5:1569)*

583. **(A)** Ronald Melzack and Patrick Wall published the landmark gate control theory in the journal *Science* in 1965. According to this theory, large and small fibers project to the substantia gelatinosa. The substantia gelatinosa exerts an inhibitory effect on afferent fibers. Large fibers increase the inhibitory effect, "close the gate," and decrease the afferent pain signal. Small fibers decrease the inhibitory effect, "open the gate," and increase the afferent pain signal. This gate control theory is commonly cited as the mechanism of action of SCS, but a 2002 review concludes that other mechanisms must also play a role. *(Oakley JC, Prager JP, Spine 2002; 27:2574-83; Melzack R, Wall PD, Science 1965; 150:3699)*

584. **(C)** Aspirin covalently acetylates COX-1 and COX-2, irreversibly inhibiting COX activity. This makes the duration of aspirin's effects related to the turnover rate of COX in different target tissues. Other COX inhibitors competitively inhibit the active site of COX enzymes that relate their duration more directly to the time course of drug disposition. *(1:964)*

585. **(E)** Traditional nonsteroidal antiinflammatory drugs inhibit the prostaglandin G/H synthase enzymes, colloquially known as COX, therefore inhibiting the synthesis of prostaglandin E, prostacyclin, and thromboxane. They inhibit the activity of not only COX-2 but also COX-1. Glucocorticoids inhibit phospholipase A2. *(1:959)*

586. **(D)** Methadone has a variable oral bioavailability between 41% and 99% and, therefore, should be started with extra caution (low initial dose and slow subsequent increases). Methadone differs from all other opioids by its noncompetitive antagonist activity at the NMDA receptors. Activation of NMDA receptors has been shown to play a role in development of tolerance to analgesic effects of opioids, as well as in the pathologic sensory states, such as neuropathic pain, inflammatory pain, ischemic pain, allodynia, and spinal states of hypersensitivity. *(1:506-7)*

587. **(D)** Both are clinically used NMDA receptor antagonists that produce analgesia. Clinically available compounds that are demonstrated to have NMDA receptor-blocking properties include ketamine, dextromethorphan, and memantine. Dextromethorphan, for example, is effective in the treatment of painful diabetic neuropathy and not effective in postherpetic neuralgia and central pain. NMDA receptor blockers may therefore offer new options in the treatment of pain. *(1:417; 1778)*

588. **(C)** The COX inhibitors are weak organic acids, consisting of one or two aromatic rings connected to an acidic functional group. They do not cross the blood–brain barrier, are 95% to 99% bound to albumin, are extensively metabolized by the liver, and have low renal clearance (< 10%). They act mainly in the periphery, but they may have a central effect. COX-2 induction within the spinal cord may play an important role in central sensitization. The acute antihyperalgesic action of COX inhibitors has been shown to be mediated by the inhibition of constitutive spinal COX-2 that has been found to be upregulated in response to inflammation and other stressors. *(5:1302-4)*

589. **(A)** Occipital neuralgia involves the greater occipital nerve and leads to a chronic headache that may extend to the shoulder or forward to the area around the eye. It may be due to compression of the occipital nerve within the skull. The scapular nerve is not involved nor is the cervical plexus. Occipital nerve block may be useful in diagnosis and treatment. *(1:721)*

590. **(B)** The tricyclic antidepressants (TCA's) can be divided into tertiary amines and their demethylated secondary amine derivatives. Examples of tertiary TCA's include amitriptyline, imipramine, clomipramine, and doxepin. Examples of secondary TCA's include nortriptyline, desipramine, and protriptyline. Trazodone is an atypical antidepressant. *(1:404)*

591. **(A)** All of choices listed are thought to be inhibitory modulators in the dorsal horn of the spinal cord with the exception of substance P. Substance P is found in the synaptic vesicles of unmyelinated C fibers. It has been shown to aggravate pain. *(1:1404)*

592. **(D)** Cutaneous nociceptors are defined by the fiber type and the type of stimuli to which they respond. Merkel's disks and Meissner's corpuscles are touch receptors. Pacinian corpuscles and Golgi-Mazzoni endings sense pressure. *(1:1435; 7:2346)*

593. **(A)** Symptoms of myofascial pain include pain in a nondermatomal distribution. The pain can be elicited by palpating the muscles near the affected area. A mainstay of treatment is the injection of local anesthetic into the "trigger point." *(1:1445; 5:2772)*

594. **(B)** Nociceptive information travels via the spinothalamic tract. The cell body of the primary afferent is located in the dorsal horn. From there the impulse travels via the spinothalamic tract. Branches may synapse in areas of the brain stem, including the periaqueductal gray and the nucleus raphe magnus. The thalamus and sensory cortex are also important in the pain pathway. *(1:1404; 5:2706)*

595. **(C)** Gabapentin has a chemical structure similar to GABA. It seems not to act directly at the GABA-binding site in the CNS, however. The mechanism of action is still unclear. It may enhance the release or activity of GABA and seems to inhibit voltage-dependent sodium channels. *(1:599)*

596. **(C)** The demand dose, lockout interval, and one-hour limit should be individually adjusted according to the patient's physiologic status and requirement for analgesia. *(5:2734; 7:2330)*

597. **(E)** The size of the needle used to deposit the neurolytic agent is not important. What is important are the location of the injection (proximity to the nerve), the concentration of the neurolytic agent, the volume of the agent, and the histology of the nerve. Smaller nerves are easier to block than larger nerves. *(1:1453; 5:2776)*

598. **(B)** There is some controversy concerning the usefulness of intraoperative intercostal blocks. Some reports did not demonstrate any difference in postoperative ventilation. Most current authors have found that the postoperative course is easier and shorter if blocks are done at the time of the thoracotomy. Most use bupivacaine. There is still a danger of a total spinal block and of administration of a toxic dose of the local anesthetic drug. *(1:730; 5:2743)*

599. **(A)** The McGill Pain Questionnaire was developed in 1975 by Ronald Melzack at McGill

University in Canada. It consists of three major measures: pain rating index, total number of words chosen, and the present pain intensity. This is a multidimensional scale for measurement of pain. The questionnaire tries to assess the three components of pain postulated by the gate theory: the sensory, the affective, and the evaluative dimensions. *(7:73)*

600. **(C)** The use of hydrophilic opioids like morphine in the epidural space produces a biphasic respiratory depression pattern. One portion of the initial bolus is absorbed systemically, accounting for the initial phase that usually occurs within 2 h of the bolus dose. The second phase occurs 6-12 h later owing to the slow rostral spread of the remaining drug as it reaches the brainstem. All medications injected neuraxially should be preservative-free. Epidural morphine does not cause lower extremity weakness. *(1:513-4)*

CHAPTER 20

Practice Test
Questions

DIRECTIONS (Questions 1-150): Each of the numbered items or incomplete statements in this section is followed by answers or by completions of the statement. Select the ONE lettered answer or completion that is BEST in each case.

1. A 58-year-old male is undergoing open repair of a 6.8 cm infrarenal aortic aneurysm. Preoperative CT-angiogram does not show any evidence of aortic occlusion. Clamping of the distal aorta in this patient will most likely be followed by

   (A) increased cardiac output
   (B) decreased arterial blood pressure
   (C) decreased systemic vascular resistance
   (D) increased stroke volume
   (E) stable heart rate

2. During surgery for strabismus in an otherwise healthy 3-year-old boy, you note that the patient is likely demonstrating the oculocardiac reflex and you inform the surgeon. All of the following are associated with the oculocardiac reflex EXCEPT

   (A) sinus tachycardia
   (B) sinus bradycardia
   (C) atrioventricular block
   (D) fatigability of the reflex
   (E) regional anesthesia

3. A 68-year-old female is admitted to the ICU for management of peritonitis from a perforated diverticulum demonstrated on CT scan of the abdomen. Her hemodynamic evaluation is consistent with a picture of septic shock.

Which one of the following statements regarding the use of hetastarch for volume expansion is most accurate?

   (A) Hetastarch is less likely than crystalloid solutions to cause renal insufficiency.
   (B) Hetastarch is a synthetic colloid.
   (C) Hetastarch is free of allergenic potential.
   (D) Hetastarch, when used in dose >20 mL/kg does not interfere with coagulation.
   (E) Hetastarch is metabolized in the liver to glucose monomers.

DIRECTIONS: Use the following scenario to answer Questions 4-5: A 27-year-old G1P0 patient presents at 39 weeks gestational age for induction of labor. Her prenatal course was complicated by a history of myasthenia gravis (MG). She is currently being treated with pyridostigmine.

4. True statements regarding myasthenia gravis in pregnancy include all of the following EXCEPT

   (A) smooth muscle and cardiac muscle are not affected by the disease
   (B) the disease affects twice as many women as men
   (C) the course of MG in pregnancy varies with one-third showing improvement of symptoms, one-third showing worsening of symptoms, and one-third showing no change
   (D) there is an association between MG and other autoimmune diseases
   (E) the first stage of labor is prolonged in patients with MG

5. The anesthetic management of this patient includes all of the following EXCEPT

   (A) opioids should be used cautiously in this patient

   (B) neuraxial anesthesia is the preferred method for pain management during labor

   (C) patients with severe bulbar involvement or respiratory compromise may require general anesthesia for cesarean section

   (D) succinylcholine should be avoided during emergent cesarean section

   (E) small doses of neostigmine may be used for reversal of neuromuscular blockade

6. A 2-year-old child weighing 12 kg is having a repair of an umbilical hernia and a right inguinal hernia. The surgeon asks you how many milliliters of 0.5% bupivacaine may be used for local infiltration at the incision sites. Which one of the following is the most appropriate dose for this patient?

   (A) 3 mL

   (B) 6 mL

   (C) 12 mL

   (D) 18 mL

   (E) 24 mL

7. An 18-year-old male takes atenolol daily to prevent cardiac arrhythmias following his diagnosis of congenital long QT syndrome. He is scheduled for outpatient arthroscopic surgery of the knee. He also has a history of severe rash following administration of beta lactam antibiotics. Appropriate perioperative antimicrobial therapy would be with

   (A) clindamycin

   (B) azithromycin

   (C) levofloxacin

   (D) gentamicin

   (E) tetracycline

DIRECTIONS: Use the following figure to answer Question 8:

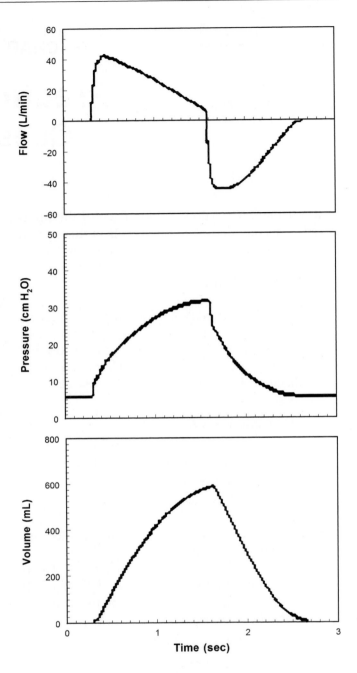

8. The figure depicts which mode of mechanical ventilation?

   (A) Pressure support

   (B) Pressure control

   (C) Volume control, constant waveform

   (D) Volume control, decelerating waveform

   (E) Airway pressure release ventilation

9. The Pa_{CO_2} of a patient on cardiopulmonary bypass

(A) is determined by the oxygen concentration of the fresh gas

(B) is generally adjusted through changes in fresh gas flow rate

(C) is generally adjusted through pulmonary ventilation

(D) should be maintained at less than 30 mmHg

(E) is determined by the type of oxygenator

10. A 5-year-old child presents for general anesthesia for closure of a severe scalp laceration. He ate a sandwich 2 h before his accident. He should

(A) have a rapid sequence induction with propofol and succinylcholine

(B) have a nasogastric tube passed to remove gastric contents before induction

(C) not be operated on for 6 h

(D) have vomiting induced

(E) be allowed to awaken with the endotracheal tube in place at the end of the procedure

11. You are seeing a pediatric patient preoperatively prior to surgery for correction of scoliosis. In order to be properly prepared for possible intraoperative blood loss and to plan for appropriate monitoring, you ask the family what type of scoliosis the patient has. All of the following types of scoliosis are associated with large expected amounts of intraoperative blood loss during scoliosis correction EXCEPT

(A) Duchenne muscular dystrophy

(B) spinal muscular atrophy

(C) arthrogryposis

(D) Marfan syndrome

(E) idiopathic infantile scoliosis

12. Well known respiratory physiologic changes that occur at term in pregnancy include all of the following EXCEPT

(A) a 40% rise in respiratory rate

(B) a 45% increase in tidal volume

(C) an increase in dead space of 45%

(D) a decrease in respiratory reserve volume of 15%

(E) a combined respiratory alkalosis and compensatory metabolic acidosis

13. Anesthesia for carotid endarterectomy generally involves all of the following EXCEPT

(A) hypercapnia

(B) normal or slightly increased arterial oxygen tension

(C) normal or slightly increased arterial pressure

(D) systemic heparinization

(E) normothermia

14. The primary mechanism of spinal opioid analgesia is via

(A) activation of presynaptic opioid receptors

(B) activation of postsynaptic opioid and GABA receptors

(C) activation of opioid receptors on the midbrain

(D) activation of opioid receptors on the rostral ventromedial medulla

(E) inhibition of small spinal interneurons

15. A 3-month-old, full term infant, weighing 5 kg presents for ventriculoperitoneal shunt placement. The patient is asymptomatic at this time. In reviewing labs for this patient, you note that the hematocrit is 30. Which one of the following statements is true?

(A) The hematocrit has reached its lowest post-delivery value.

(B) The patient is anemic and should receive a blood transfusion prior to surgery.

(C) The patient is anemic and surgery should be postponed until the hematocrit rises.

(D) The hematocrit is likely low due to dilution from IV fluid infusions.

(E) The patient is anemic and should be started on iron supplementation.

16. A 48-year-old, 111 kg female presents for surgical excision of a pheochromocytoma, for which she has already received a 14-d course of phenoxybenzamine. The patient is scheduled for a combined epidural and general anesthetic. The agent that should be avoided during maintenance of anesthesia is

   (A) nitrous oxide
   (B) propofol
   (C) desflurane
   (D) isoflurane
   (E) sevoflurane

17. When ventilating the patient with a head injury, all of the following statements are true EXCEPT

   (A) the patient should be kept supine
   (B) prolonged hyperventilation has diminished efficacy in reducing ICP
   (C) PEEP may be appropriate
   (D) hypoxia and hypercarbia should be avoided
   (E) coughing should be minimized

18. Esmolol

   (A) is a β_1-adrenoceptor agonist
   (B) has a half-life of 4 h
   (C) is contraindicated in the patient with AV block
   (D) is more likely than propranolol to cause bronchospasm
   (E) is metabolized in the liver

19. In the adult, the tracheobronchial tree

   (A) divides at an uneven angle, making foreign bodies more apt to go to the left side
   (B) divides into right and left bronchi, the left bronchus being narrower and longer
   (C) does not move with respiration
   (D) is lined with squamous epithelium
   (E) is protected by circular cartilaginous rings throughout

20. Which one of the following is most likely to result in an underestimation of the anion gap in critically ill patients?

   (A) Hyperchloremia
   (B) Lactic acidosis
   (C) Hyperphosphatemia
   (D) Hypoalbuminemia
   (E) Hypocapnia

21. Mannitol may lead to subdural hematoma by

   (A) increasing cerebral edema
   (B) interfering with the clotting mechanisms
   (C) leading to disruption of cortical veins
   (D) producing hypertension
   (E) direct passage through the vein wall

22. A patient is referred to you with facial pain. Which one of the following statements is true?

   (A) The pain of glossopharyngeal neuralgia is very similar to that of trigeminal neuralgia but affects the anterior two-thirds of the tongue, tonsils, and pharynx.
   (B) Giant cell arteritis is a vasculitic condition that can lead to visual loss but has never been reported in a case of stroke.
   (C) Cervical carotid artery dissection most commonly presents with neck, head, or facial pain.
   (D) Pure facial pain is rarely associated with sinusitis alone.

23. A 135 kg, 48-year-old female is scheduled for a laparoscopic cholecystectomy under general anesthesia. The factor most significant in affecting intraoperative arterial oxygenation is

   (A) body position
   (B) mode of ventilation
   (C) body weight
   (D) presence of pneumoperitoneum
   (E) lung compliance

24. Well known hematologic changes that occur in pregnancy include each of the following EXCEPT

(A) maternal blood volume increases by approximately 45% at term

(B) plasma cholinesterase levels decrease by about 25% resulting in a clinically relevant prolongation of paralysis after a single dose of succinylcholine

(C) plasma albumin levels drop during pregnancy

(D) the concentrations of most coagulation factors increase during pregnancy thus representing a relative hypercoagulable state

(E) red blood cell volume increases secondary to increased production of erythropoietin as well as the erythropoietin-like effects of progesterone, prolactin, and placental lactogen

DIRECTIONS: Use the following scenario to answer Questions 25-29: A 65-year-old male has a right hilar mass with postobstructive pneumonia.

25. In evaluating this patient's suitability for pneumonectomy, which one of these tests would be the LEAST useful?

(A) Pa_{CO_2}
(B) Pa_{O_2}
(C) FEV_1
(D) FVC
(E) Ventilation/perfusion scan (V/Q scan)

26. The patient is hypoxic on preoperative evaluation. Which therapy is LEAST likely to be effective?

(A) Lateral position
(B) Chest physical therapy
(C) Sodium nitroprusside
(D) Supplemental oxygen
(E) Pneumonectomy

27. The best method to provide good surgical exposure for a left lower lobectomy is

(A) using a large single-lumen endotracheal tube
(B) using an endotracheal tube with a ballooned catheter (Univent) placed on the operative side
(C) using a right sided double-lumen tube
(D) using a left sided double-lumen tube
(E) using an LMA

28. After induction of general anesthesia, the patient is intubated with a left-sided double-lumen tube. When the circuit is connected to the double-lumen tube, it is possible to ventilate the left lung, but not the right lung. Possible causes include all EXCEPT

(A) the tube is advanced too far
(B) the right mainstem bronchus is blocked by tumor
(C) the right lumen is blocked by secretions
(D) the tube is not advanced far enough
(E) the tube is in the wrong side

29. The patient underwent uneventful right pneumonectomy and remains intubated at the end of the procedure. On transferring the patient from the operating room table to the bed for transfer to the intensive care unit, there is a sudden decrease in blood pressure. Pulses are faint. Appropriate maneuvers include all of the following EXCEPT

(A) placing the patient laterally on his left side
(B) applying suction to the chest tube
(C) immediately reopening the wound and exploring the surgical field
(D) providing oxygen and managing the airway
(E) supporting cardiac function with an inotropic agent

30. A 32-year-old G1P0 patient presents for an anesthesia consult at 20 weeks gestational age. She has a history of tonic-clonic seizures that are well-controlled on phenytoin. You tell her all of the following statements about her condition are true EXCEPT

   (A) approximately 0.5% of all parturients have a chronic seizure disorder

   (B) single-agent anticonvulsant therapy is preferred over combination therapy

   (C) approximately one-third of patients will experience an increase in seizure frequency during pregnancy

   (D) there is no contraindication to neuraxial anesthesia

   (E) higher estrogen concentrations increase the seizure threshold during pregnancy

31. The agent with the highest ratio of β-adrenergic agonist to α-adrenergic agonist activity is

   (A) isoproterenol
   (B) dobutamine
   (C) epinephrine
   (D) norepinephrine
   (E) phenylephrine

DIRECTIONS: Use the following scenario to answer Questions 32-36: A 33-year-old multiparous female just delivered healthy twin girls vaginally. After delivery she has poor uterine tone, resulting in postpartum hemorrhage. Her mental status and blood pressure decline, and you are called to assist with management. You intubate the patient, place intravenous access, and resuscitate the patient with fluids and blood products while the obstetricians control the bleeding. Once stabilized, she is brought to the ICU for further care. Over the course of two hours, she develops worsening oxygenation. Her vital signs are T 37.3°C, HR 93, BP 113/64, SpO_2 92% on FIO_2 1.0. She is 5 feet, 2 inches and 76 kg. Her hemoglobin is 8 mg/dL. Chest x-ray shows bilateral diffuse infiltrates. A bedside echocardiogram is unremarkable.

32. Which one of the following is the most appropriate ventilator setting?

   (A) Volume control TV 250, RR 20, PEEP 5, FIO_2 1.0

   (B) Volume control TV 300, RR 20, PEEP 5, FIO_2 1.0

   (C) Volume control TV 300, RR 20, PEEP 12, FIO_2 1.0

   (D) Volume control TV 440, RR 20, PEEP 5, FIO_2 1.0

   (E) Volume control TV 440, RR 20, PEEP 12, FIO_2 1.0

33. Six hours later, she is hemodynamically stable and has required no further transfusions. Repeat hemoglobin is 7.8 g/dL. INR is 1.6. Platelet count is 86,000/mm^3. Which one of the following is the most appropriate therapeutic intervention?

   (A) No transfusion

   (B) Transfuse one unit of packed red blood cells

   (C) Transfuse two units of packed red blood cells

   (D) Transfuse one unit of fresh frozen plasma

   (E) Transfuse a single donor unit of platelets

34. Twenty four hours later, the patient has had a dramatic improvement in her pulmonary status, and she is extubated successfully. Which one of the following is the most likely cause of her respiratory failure?

   (A) Amniotic fluid embolism
   (B) Pneumonia
   (C) Pulmonary contusion
   (D) TRALI (transfusion related acute lung injury)
   (E) Volume overload

35. Mechanical ventilation with PEEP results in which one of the following?

   (A) Decreased preload and left ventricular afterload

   (B) Decreased preload and increased left ventricular afterload

   (C) Increased preload and decreased left ventricular afterload

(D)   Increased preload and left ventricular afterload

(E)   Increased preload and right ventricular afterload

36. Which one of the following has been shown to reduce the number of days that a patient requires mechanical ventilation?

(A)   Daily recruitment maneuvers

(B)   Daily spontaneous breathing trials

(C)   Prophylactic antibiotics

(D)   Scheduled suctioning

(E)   Volume control ventilation

37. The atypical antipsychotics like clozapine and olanzapine differ from antipsychotic agents like haloperidol and chlorpromazine in that they

(A)   cause less extrapyramidal effects

(B)   do not produce hypotension

(C)   do not cause weight gain and increased appetite

(D)   have less anticholinergic effects

(E)   have not been associated with a risk of new-onset type 2 diabetes

38. General anesthesia as compared to regional anesthesia in parturients is associated with all of the following EXCEPT

(A)   less hypotension

(B)   less cardiovascular instability

(C)   less uterine relaxation

(D)   more rapid induction

(E)   better control of the airway

39. A 2-year-old child is brought to the emergency department with a 6-d history of increasing cough and wheezing. Symptoms have not responded to bronchodilator therapy and broad-spectrum antibiotics. On examination, the child is agitated, tachypneic, and has a heart rate of 150 bpm. There are decreased breath sounds in the right lower zone of the lung fields. This clinical presentation is most consistent with

(A)   right lower lobe pneumonia

(B)   exacerbation of underlying asthma

(C)   inhaled foreign body

(D)   acute laryngotracheobronchitis

(E)   ruptured congenital bullus

40. The blood flow during total cardiopulmonary bypass

(A)   is not adjustable

(B)   is virtually nonpulsatile

(C)   provides a pulsatile pressure

(D)   is a pulsatile flow

(E)   mimics normal flow in all respects

41. In neurosurgical patients, dextrose containing solutions

(A)   are the fluids of choice

(B)   may cause excessive diuresis

(C)   may exacerbate hyperglycemia

(D)   may produce brain edema

(E)   lead to water retention

42. All of the following statements regarding headaches are true EXCEPT

(A)   the International Headache Society's diagnostic criteria for cervicogenic head-aches includes unilaterality of symptoms and relief of pain by diagnostic anesthetic blocks

(B)   migraine with aura is more common than migraine without aura

(C)   in chronic tension-type headaches, the average headache frequency is equal to or greater than 15 d per month

(D)   cluster headaches are more prevalent in men than in women

(E)   tricyclic antidepressants are a mainstay of treatment for both migraine and tension-type headaches

43. Dexmedetomidine

    (A) is a hypnotic agent used for the induction of general anesthesia

    (B) can markedly reduce the MAC of inhalational anesthetics

    (C) when given as an IV bolus of 2 mg/kg will result in an initial decrease in blood pressure and increase in heart rate

    (D) will result in adrenal suppression when infused continuously for postoperative sedation

    (E) causes more respiratory depression than opioids and benzodiazepines

44. Preeclampsia is associated with which one of the following findings?

    (A) Hypovolemia

    (B) Low serum creatinine

    (C) Low hematocrit

    (D) Decreased serum uric acid

    (E) Hypotension

45. Carbon dioxide is sometimes added to the fresh gas supply of the oxygenator during hypothermic cardiopulmonary bypass

    (A) to decrease pulmonary vascular resistance

    (B) to increase the affinity of hemoglobin for oxygen

    (C) to dilate coronary arteries

    (D) to maintain the corrected Pa_{CO_2} at 40 mm Hg

46. A relative, but not absolute, contraindication to an epidural steroid injections is

    (A) preexisting neurologic disorder (e.g., multiple sclerosis)

    (B) sepsis

    (C) therapeutic anticoagulation

    (D) localized infection at injection site

    (E) patient refusal

47. You are giving a talk to a group of pregnant women during a birthing class about the options of analgesia during labor. You specifically discuss epidural analgesia. In your discussion, you pull out a diagram of the lumbar spine and you specifically state that a catheter will be placed

    (A) below the dura

    (B) between the dural and the arachnoid

    (C) in the intrathecal space

    (D) between the dura and the pia

    (E) between the ligamentum flavum and the dura

48. A 74-year-old man is undergoing a transurethral resection of prostate with sorbitol irrigation under spinal anesthesia. Approximately 1 h after the beginning of the resection, he begins to complain of difficulty breathing. He becomes progressively more confused, tachycardic, and hypertensive. The serum sodium concentration is 114 mEq/L. While informing the surgeon and asking him to complete the procedure expeditiously, the most appropriate next step would be to

    (A) administer labetalol

    (B) ask the surgeon to change the irrigating solution to normal saline

    (C) administer furosemide

    (D) induce general endotracheal anesthesia

    (E) administer 3% sodium chloride

49. As the neurosurgeon manipulates tissue in the posterior fossa, there is sudden bradycardia. The anesthetist should

    (A) lower the head

    (B) administer lidocaine

    (C) inform the neurosurgeon

    (D) turn off all volatile anesthetics

    (E) administer naloxone to reverse effects of opioids

50. Prostaglandin E_1

    (A) is a potent vasoconstrictor

    (B) should be given by bolus

    (C) should always be stopped before inducing anesthesia

    (D) is useful in closing a patent ductus arteriosus

    (E) may cause hypotension

51. Post-herpetic neuralgia

   (A) is common in children and adolescents

   (B) is best treated with opioids

   (C) never responds to local application of counterirritants

   (D) usually responds to tricyclic antidepressants

   (E) is a difficult syndrome to treat and success is limited

52. A 61-year-old male with Marfan syndrome is referred for surgical repair of a 6.4 cm ascending aortic aneurysm that will include replacement of the aortic valve. The surgeon informs you that the repair will require deep hypothermic cardiac arrest with an expected duration of over 30 min. In addition to effective cooling of the patient to a core temperature of 25°C, the best strategy for the prevention of cerebral ischemia during surgery is which one of the following?

   (A) Ice packs around the patient's head

   (B) Selective antegrade cerebral perfusion with cold, oxygenated blood into a single aortic arch branch vessel

   (C) Administration of a barbiturate

   (D) Retrograde cerebral perfusion with cold, oxygenated blood into the superior vena cava (SVC)

   (E) Administration of high-dose glucocorticoids

DIRECTIONS: Use the following scenario to answer Questions 53-55: A 24-year-old female pedestrian was struck by a car 3 d ago. She was brought to the emergency department by emergency medical personnel, where she was intubated for confusion and combativeness. Her initial trauma evaluation revealed a positive FAST scan. She was taken emergently to the operating room where she underwent a splenectomy for a ruptured spleen. She subsequently underwent a more complete trauma evaluation that revealed a T10 burst fracture and an acetabular fracture. She has been intubated while awaiting repair of her fractures. You are called to the bedside because the patient has developed fever, tachycardia, hypoxia, and increased secretions. Chest x-ray shows a new pulmonary infiltrate. She has rhonchi but no other changes in her physical examination.

53. Which one of the following is the most appropriate next step in management?

   (A) Administer an antipyretic

   (B) Administer post-splenectomy vaccines

   (C) Begin chest physiotherapy

   (D) Obtain cultures

   (E) Start antibiotics

54. Which one of the following is the most appropriate pharmacotherapy?

   (A) Ceftriaxone

   (B) Levofloxacin

   (C) Linezolid + ertapenem

   (D) Vancomycin + ceftriaxone

   (E) Vancomycin + levofloxacin + cefepime

55. Forty-eight hours later, the patient is afebrile with decreased secretions and improved oxygenation. Sputum culture obtained before initiation of antibiotics revealed *Haemophilus influenzae*. What is the most appropriate next step in management?

   (A) Change antibiotics to ceftriaxone only

   (B) Change antibiotics to clindamycin only

   (C) Change antibiotics to vancomycin only

   (D) Continue current antibiotics

   (E) Discontinue all antibiotics

56. All of the following statements are true concerning somatosensory evoked potentials EXCEPT

   (A) waveform peaks are described in terms of amplitude, latency, and polarity

   (B) amplitude of evoked potentials is greater than those of the EEG

   (C) injury is manifested as an increase in latency and/or decrease in amplitude

   (D) brain stem potentials are more resistant to anesthetic influences than cortical potentials

   (E) volatile anesthetics produce dose-dependent alterations in evoked potentials

57. You are called to a delivery room where the obstetrician has decided to perform a low outlet forceps delivery in a patient. All of the following techniques are appropriate EXCEPT

   (A) bilateral pudendal block
   (B) paracervical block
   (C) subarachnoid block
   (D) caudal block
   (E) epidural block

58. Terbutaline

   (A) is an α-adrenergic agonist
   (B) is a selective β_2-adrenergic agonist
   (C) causes more tachycardia than isoproterenol
   (D) should be avoided in patients with heart disease
   (E) causes hyperkalemia

59. The one best block for pain secondary to pancreatic cancer is a(n)

   (A) stellate ganglion block
   (B) Bier block
   (C) block of the hypogastric plexus
   (D) celiac plexus block
   (E) intrathecal neurolysis

60. Pulmonary vascular resistance is increased by

   (A) sevoflurane
   (B) desflurane
   (C) isoflurane
   (D) nitrous oxide
   (E) oxygen

DIRECTIONS: Use the following figure to answer Questions 61-62:

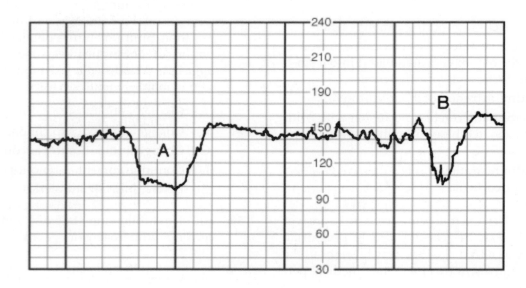

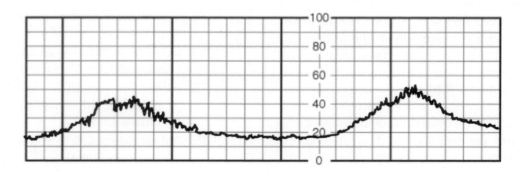

61. The tracing in the graph shows a pattern referred to as

(A) early deceleration
(B) late deceleration
(C) saltatory deceleration
(D) variable deceleration
(E) sinusoidal deceleration

62. This type of fetal heart rate pattern is usually associated with

(A) uteroplacental insufficiency
(B) head compression
(C) cord compression
(D) severe fetal asphyxia
(E) prematurity

63. Complications of spinal cord stimulation include all of the following EXCEPT

(A) lead migration
(B) increased risk of development of chordoma
(C) lead breakage
(D) bleeding

64. A 58-year-old otherwise healthy man is undergoing repair of an Achilles tendon rupture. The orthopedic surgeon asked that the lower extremity tourniquet remain inflated through the entire 2-h procedure. Upon release of the tourniquet, you will expect to see

(A) decreased end-tidal CO_2
(B) metabolic alkalosis
(C) increased blood pressure
(D) decreased body temperature
(E) increase in anesthetic requirements

65. A 72-year-old male with Parkinson disease on levodopa is scheduled for surgery. The anesthetic plan should include

(A) stopping levodopa for 24 h before induction
(B) avoidance of phenothiazines
(C) use of neuroleptanesthesia as the technique

(D) anticipated need for larger than usual doses of pressors
(E) use of high concentrations of a volatile agent in lieu of a nondepolarizing muscle relaxant

66. Acute treatment of cerebral edema includes all of the following EXCEPT

(A) osmotic diuretics
(B) loop diuretics
(C) glucocorticoids
(D) surgical decompression
(E) drainage of CSF

67. You are called to the labor and delivery suite to evaluate a patient who has just delivered. The obstetrician states the uterus is atonic. Each of the following may be used to treat the uterine atony EXCEPT

(A) uterine massage
(B) intramuscular methylergonovine
(C) intrauterine prostaglandin $F_{2\alpha}$
(D) intravenous methylergonovine
(E) intravenous oxytocin

DIRECTIONS: Use the following figure to answer Question 68:

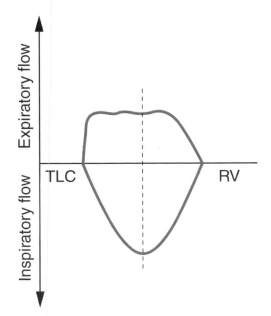

68. The flow/volume curve shows

(A) normal inspiratory and expiratory volume curves

(B) fixed intrathoracic or extrathoracic obstruction

(C) variable intrathoracic obstruction

(D) variable extrathoracic obstruction

69. A 6-month-old infant, born full term, presents for elective inguinal hernia repair. The infant is otherwise healthy, and in no acute distress. Which one of the following are normal heart rate, blood pressure and O_2 consumption for this patient?

(A) HR 120, BP 90/60, O_2 consumption 5 mL/kg

(B) HR 140, BP 90/60, O_2 consumption 10 mL/kg

(C) HR 140, BP 70/40, O_2 consumption 5 mL/kg

(D) HR 120, BP 90/60, O_2 consumption 15 mL/kg

(E) HR 120, BP 110/70, O_2 consumption 10 mL/kg

70. Diagnostic criteria for cervicogenic headache by the International Headache Society and the International Association for the Study of Pain (IASP) include all of the following EXCEPT

(A) unilateral headache

(B) relief of acute attacks by blocking the V2 branch of the trigeminal nerve with local anesthetic

(C) aggravation of the headache with neck movements

(D) decreased range of neck motion

71. Upon doing a morning postoperative check on a patient who underwent a total thyroidectomy for a longstanding multinodular goiter the previous afternoon, you notice he is somewhat stridorous, with sternal retractions. He asks why the anesthesia has made his fingers and toes tingle. On evaluation you note

(A) a positive Chvostek sign

(B) diminished reflexes

(C) a negative Trousseau sign

(D) edema of his upper extremities

(E) incisional swelling

72. α-adrenoceptors in the adrenergic nervous system

(A) are stimulated by isoproterenol

(B) are blocked by metoprolol

(C) cause vasoconstriction

(D) cause bronchial dilatation

(E) are found on adipocytes

73. Patients with acute subarachnoid hemorrhage may demonstrate all of the following EXCEPT

(A) ST segment elevation consistent with myocardial ischemia

(B) cardiac arrhythmia

(C) elevated cardiac enzymes

(D) depressed ventricular function

(E) pulmonary hypertension

74. All of the following are indicative of fetal well-being EXCEPT

(A) good long-term variability

(B) biophysical profile score of 8/10

(C) reactive non-stress test

(D) a positive oxytocin contraction stress test

(E) fetal scalp pH of 7.27

75. A healthy 29-year-old woman delivers a healthy full term neonate. There have been no problems or complications during pregnancy or labor and delivery. The neonate's 1- and 5-min Apgar scores were 8 and 9, respectively. Both mother and infant are doing well. All of the following would be expected to occur in the first 24 h of life of this neonate EXCEPT

(A) functional closure of the foramen ovale

(B) functional closure of the ductus arteriosus

(C) decrease in afterload on the left ventricle

(D) increase in pulmonary blood flow

(E) large increase in volume load on left ventricle

76. In terms of complex regional pain syndrome (CRPS), which one of the following statements is true?

    (A) The incidence of CRPS is 20% after brain lesion.
    (B) Extremities affected by a brain injury are at higher risk of developing CRPS than unaffected extremities.
    (C) CRPS following spinal cord injury is frequent.
    (D) Lower extremities are more commonly affected than upper extremities.

77. A patient is scheduled for a CO_2 laser ablation of a laryngeal tumor. The risk of airway fire is decreased by

    (A) a fresh gas flow less than 2 L/min
    (B) use of a clear PVC endotracheal tube
    (C) use of a petroleum-based lubricant
    (D) substitution of helium for N_2O
    (E) use of the laser in continuous mode

78. In preeclamptic or eclamptic patients

    (A) regional anesthesia is contraindicated
    (B) hyporeflexia is common
    (C) fluid restriction is necessary because of the presence of pulmonary edema in a majority of patients
    (D) resistance to vasopressors is common
    (E) significant coagulopathies may occur

79. An 81-year-old woman slipped on a piece of ice and in the process sustained an open right distal ulna fracture in her outstretched hand. All of the following are reasonable regional anesthetic blocks for surgeries distal to the elbow EXCEPT a(n)

    (A) axillary block
    (B) supraclavicular block
    (C) infraclavicular block
    (D) interscalene block

80. A 6-year-old patient is undergoing a craniotomy in the prone position for removal of a posterior fossa tumor. You are concerned about venous air embolism and hemodynamic instability during this surgery so you are using multiple monitors during this surgery in addition to the standard ASA monitors. These include an arterial catheter, end-tidal nitrogen, and esophageal stethoscope. Of the following monitors, which one is the most sensitive indicator of a venous air embolism?

    (A) End-tidal nitrogen
    (B) Blood pressure
    (C) End-tidal carbon dioxide
    (D) Change in ECG
    (E) Esophageal stethoscope

81. A 1-month-old infant presents for exploratory laparotomy for symptoms of bowel obstruction. The initial temperature after induction is noted to be 35.6°C. At the time of incision, the temperature is noted to be 34.9°C. All of the following are mechanisms by which an infant under anesthesia loses body heat EXCEPT

    (A) the metabolism of brown fat
    (B) breathing dry gases
    (C) conduction to cold surroundings
    (D) cold skin preparation solutions
    (E) exposure of abdominal contents

82. Which one of the following is a possible advantage of acupuncture over other methods of pain therapy?

    (A) Safety, since the physiology of the patient is not disturbed
    (B) A tonic or regulatory effect on the body
    (C) Long-lasting residual effects
    (D) An anti-inflammatory effect

83. A 72-year-old patient with a history of closed angle glaucoma presents for cataract surgery. In order to prevent an increase in intraocular pressure, one should avoid

    (A) hypothermia
    (B) hypercarbia
    (C) intravenous acetazolamide
    (D) hypotension
    (E) topical timolol

84. A 68-year-old male is scheduled to have endo-vascular stent graft repair of a 7.4 cm descending thoracic aortic aneurysm. The patient's past medical history is significant for insulin dependent diabetes, hypertension, hypercholesterolemia, and myocardial infarction. The patient's past surgical history is significant for infrarenal aortic aneurysm repair. In order to decrease the risk of spinal cord ischemia, the patient will undergo preoperative placement of a lumbar drain for CSF drainage. Which one of the following additional interventions is most appropriate to decrease the risk of spinal cord ischemia in this patient?

    (A) Deep hypothermic circulatory arrest (DHCA)
    (B) Pulse dose glucocorticoid therapy
    (C) High-dose opioid anesthesia technique
    (D) Deliberate mild to moderate systemic hypothermia
    (E) Deliberate mild to moderate hypotension

85. β_2-adrenoceptors in the autonomic nervous system

    (A) are stimulated by isoproterenol
    (B) are antagonized by esmolol
    (C) are activated by clonidine
    (D) cause vasoconstriction
    (E) are the principal prejunctional receptors that inhibit sympathetic neurotransmitter release

DIRECTIONS: Use the following scenario to answer Questions 86-87: A 67-year-old woman with COPD is admitted to the ICU with pneumonia and respiratory failure several days following video-assisted thoracoscopic lung resection of squamous cell carcinoma. Her height is 63 inches, weight 80 kg (ideal body weight 52 kg). Vital signs are T 38.2°C, HR 98, BP 110/72, RR 36, SpO_2 96% while mechanically ventilated with FIO_2 1.0. Sputum cultures reveal abundant growth of *Streptococcus pneumoniae*.

86. Which one of the following ventilator settings is most likely beneficial in preventing ventilator induced lung injury?

    (A) Tidal volume 520 mL
    (B) PEEP equal to 0 cm H_2O
    (C) Inspiratory time < 1 sec
    (D) Plateau pressure < 30 cm H_2O
    (E) Recruitment maneuver with CPAP = 40 cm H_2O

87. After 24 h of mechanical ventilation, a spontaneous breathing trial (SBT) is conducted. Which one of the following combinations of criteria during the SBT suggest that extubation should be considered?

    (A) RR 36, SpO_2 95%, HR 88
    (B) RR 18, SpO_2 91%, HR 90
    (C) Patient requesting to be extubated, SBP 200 mm Hg, HR 150
    (D) RR 32, SpO_2 96%, patient reporting shortness of breath and anxiety
    (E) RR 12, SpO_2 89%, HR 87

88. Increased neonatal depression has been observed after nonurgent cesarean delivery in which one of the following circumstances?

    (A) General anesthesia compared to regional anesthesia
    (B) An elapsed time of 8 min between induction and delivery
    (C) Use of a volatile agent
    (D) An elapsed time of 4 min between uterine incision and delivery
    (E) epidural versus spinal anesthesia

89. Concerning induced hypotension in neurosurgery

    (A) induced vasodilation may facilitate perfusion during ischemia
    (B) is best provided with phenoxybenzamine
    (C) may be required for brief periods
    (D) may decrease physiologic dead space
    (E) is relatively contraindicated for any length of time during intracranial surgery

DIRECTIONS: Use the following scenario to answer Questions 90-91: A-22 year-old male presents for left shoulder arthroscopy with a rotator cuff repair after sustaining a basketball injury. The following ultrasound-guided nerve block was performed for postoperative analgesia.

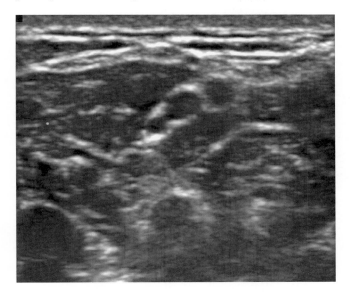

90. The nerve that will most likely be spared is the

    (A) phrenic nerve
    (B) musculocutaneous nerve
    (C) ulnar nerve
    (D) suprascapular nerve
    (E) radial nerve

91. Thirty minutes after the block is performed the patient is noted to have sensation on the cape of the ipsilateral shoulder. The most likely reason for this is failure to

    (A) block the axillary nerve
    (B) block the superficial cervical plexus
    (C) anesthetize the suprascapular nerve
    (D) anesthetize the musculocutaneous nerve
    (E) perform a T1 paravertebral block

92. A 5-year-old boy presents for elective outpatient repair of an inguinal hernia. His parents inform you that he has a runny nose with yellow nasal discharge and a mild occasional wet cough. They deny any fevers. He has been eating and drinking normally and has been active as usual. Lungs are clear to auscultation bilaterally. You inform the parents that you will

    (A) proceed with surgery today
    (B) prescribe antibiotics for the patient
    (C) admit to the floor postoperatively for overnight monitoring
    (D) postpone surgery for 2-4 weeks
    (E) administer an albuterol nebulizer preoperatively and postoperatively as needed

93. An advantage of selective COX-2 inhibitors over nonselective COX inhibitors is

    (A) protective renal effects
    (B) protective cardiovascular effects
    (C) inhibit production of thromboxane A2
    (D) fewer GI side effects

94. The medication occasionally used as a bedtime sedative that is associated with CNS excitation a few hours after taking it is

    (A) diphenhydramine
    (B) ethanol
    (C) pentobarbital
    (D) eszopiclone
    (E) melatonin

95. What is the meaning of the term "left dominant" on a cardiac catheterization report?

    (A) It refers to the blood supply of the sinus node by the left circumflex artery.
    (B) It indicates that the patient has left ventricular hypertrophy.
    (C) It indicates that the entire left ventricle is supplied by the left coronary artery.
    (D) It indicates that the posterior descending artery is supplied by the left circumflex artery.
    (E) It indicates a large left anterior descending artery.

96. Complex regional pain syndrome is characterized by all of the following EXCEPT it

(A) may result from a gunshot wound

(B) is generally less severe in persons with underlying anxiety or depression

(C) can respond to sympathectomy

(D) is often accompanied by dystrophic changes of bone

97. Seizures

(A) produce cerebral alkalosis

(B) are terminated by isoflurane anesthesia at 1 MAC

(C) generate burst activity on EEG

(D) reduce regional cerebral blood flow and metabolism

(E) are initiated by most general anesthetics

98. A 5-week-old infant presents for pyloromyotomy. The anesthetic plan includes a rapid sequence induction and intubation. Several steps in positioning and equipment selection are taken to aid in securing the airway as rapidly as possible. All of the following are true of the infant's airway relative to an adult's airway EXCEPT

(A) the infant has a more cephalad-placed larynx

(B) the infant's epiglottis is long and omega shaped

(C) the infant's vocal cords are slanted down and anteriorly

(D) the narrowest area of the infant's airway is at the rima glottidis

(E) the infant's tongue is larger relative to the rest of the airway

99. A 30-year-old G4P0 patient with a history of antiphospholipid syndrome and recurrent pregnancy loss presents at 20 weeks gestational age for an anesthesia consult. She is currently on aspirin and a prophylactic dose of low molecular weight heparin (LMWH) once daily. She asks about her disease and pregnancy. You tell her that

(A) epidural anesthesia is contraindicated secondary to the increased risk of bleeding with lupus anticoagulant present

(B) she must wait 24 h from the last dose of LMWH to receive neuraxial anesthesia

(C) most infants of women with antiphospholipid syndrome have an increased rate of neonatal or childhood complications

(D) lupus anticoagulant and anticardiolipin antibody are associated with both venous and arterial thrombotic events

(E) women diagnosed with antiphospholipid syndrome on the basis of a history of recurrent pregnancy loss and evidence of antiphospholipid antibody, but without prior thrombotic events, often suffer thrombotic events during pregnancy

100. Arrhythmia is associated with all of the following EXCEPT

(A) orbital decompression

(B) tentorial manipulation

(C) spinal cord rhizotomy

(D) arterial venous malformation embolization

(E) carotid artery balloon angioplasty

101. Preeclampsia is characterized by all of the following EXCEPT

(A) intravascular volume depletion

(B) proteinuria

(C) occurrence anytime time pregnancy

(D) no change in placental perfusion

(E) decreased production of renin

102. An active agent useful in the performance of a neurolytic block is

(A) 40% potassium hydroxide

(B) 10% glycerin

(C) 50% alcohol

(D) 100% phenol

103. A major side effect of valproic acid is

   (A) decreased renal function
   (B) elevation in liver enzymes
   (C) potentiation of muscle relaxants
   (D) arrhythmias
   (E) anemia

DIRECTIONS: Use the following scenario to answer Questions 104-106: A 42-year-old female with a longstanding history of type I diabetes and end-stage renal disease requiring dialysis has received the call that an appropriate kidney is now available for transplant. She is scheduled for immediate transplant, and arrives, quite anxious, directly from dialysis to the preoperative area. She has been NPO for 4 h. Preoperative labs include Hgb of 8.4 g/dL, glucose 183 mg/dL, and $[K^+]$ 5.3 mEq/L. Her vital signs are BP 112/62, HR 104 bpm, SpO_2 97%. The anesthetic plan is for general anesthesia.

104. The anesthetic agent best avoided in this patient is

   (A) etomidate
   (B) N_2O
   (C) succinylcholine
   (D) sevoflurane
   (E) vecuronium

105. The surgeon is concerned about the risk of a postoperative epidural hematoma, and asks that you use parenteral opioids for postoperative analgesia rather than place an epidural catheter. As he completes the procedure, the surgeon expresses concern about the functioning of the transplanted kidney. The opioid that would be affected the most by this patient's renal dysfunction is

   (A) fentanyl
   (B) hydromorphone
   (C) morphine
   (D) sufentanil

106. Which one of the following maneuvers is the most effective means to prevent acute tubular

necrosis and thereby facilitate immediate graft function in this patient?

   (A) Volume expansion with saline, albumin and/or blood
   (B) Volume expansion plus mannitol
   (C) Addition of cyclosporine
   (D) Volume expansion plus furosemide

107. A 27-year-old G1P0 patient presents for an anesthesia consult at 20 weeks gestational age. Her prenatal course is notable for a history of corrected idiopathic scoliosis. True statements regarding her disease in pregnancy include all of the following EXCEPT

   (A) pregnant women with corrected idiopathic scoliosis tolerate pregnancy, labor, and delivery well
   (B) insertion of an epidural needle in the fused area may not be possible
   (C) the spread of injected local anesthetic may be altered resulting in an increased incidence of inadequate analgesia after epidural placement
   (D) 80% of patients undergo fusion to the lowest lumbar levels, limiting the potential for neuraxial anesthesia
   (E) there is a higher incidence of dural puncture

108. A 72-year-old female patient is undergoing right pneumonectomy for lung cancer. After starting one-lung ventilation with oxygen and isoflurane, a tidal volume of 500 mL, and a rate of 10 breaths per minute, the patient's oxygen saturation starts to fall as the surgeon is opening the chest. The most effective means of improving the oxygen saturation is

   (A) increasing oxygen flow to the anesthesia circuit
   (B) adding 10 cm H_2O PEEP to the ventilated lung
   (C) clamping the right pulmonary artery
   (D) starting intravenous nitroglycerin
   (E) increasing the concentration of isoflurane

109. A 35-year-old G1P0 patient with a history of chronic hypertension who takes lisinopril presents for her first prenatal visit at 12 weeks gestational age. The obstetrician calls and asks your opinion regarding her medication. You advise the obstetrician that which one of the following drugs has the best safety profile in pregnancy?

(A) Labetalol
(B) Nifedipine
(C) Methyldopa
(D) Furosemide
(E) Captopril

110. Management of the airway during induction of general anesthesia in a patient in a halo brace for a nondisplaced unstable fracture of C6 incurred in a high-speed motor vehicle accident includes all of the following EXCEPT

(A) assessment for injuries of the face
(B) awake fiberoptic intubation
(C) adequate anesthesia of the trachea to prevent coughing
(D) removal of the cervical brace for intubation
(E) nasal or oral route of intubation

111. An elderly gentleman presenting to the pain clinic complains of right-sided thoracic pain. He developed a very painful rash that started about 6 months ago. The lesions are now gone, but he states that the pain is persistent. A beneficial therapy modality is

(A) high-dose aspirin
(B) TENS (transcutaneous electrical nerve stimulation)
(C) tricyclic antidepressants
(D) opioids

112. A 3-year-old, previously healthy child, presents for an urgent left sided VATS procedure and chest tube placement for a parapneumonic effusion. The child is on 3 liters of oxygen by nasal cannula with SpO2 of 92-95%. She is tachypneic, but does not appear to be in distress and is hemodynamically stable.

Which one of the following is true regarding management of ventilation in this patient?

(A) Use of a double lumen tube would be the best way to provide lung isolation in this case.
(B) Because the blocker tube is attached to the main endotracheal tube in a Univent tube, there is greater chance of displacement of the blocker than when other blockers are used.
(C) Lung isolation is not likely to be necessary for this procedure.
(D) An arterial catheter will be necessary to guide ventilation management.
(E) If a bronchial blocker is used to provide lung isolation for this procedure, a larger endotracheal tube will be required in order to allow the passage of the fiberoptic bronchoscope and the bronchial blocker.

113. The neural pathways that are responsible for the transmission of pain during the first and second stages of labor are

(A) T6 – T12 and S1 – S4
(B) T8 – L2 and S1 – S3
(C) T10 – L1 and S2 – S4
(D) T10 – L5
(E) T12 – L3 and S2 – S5

114. A 38-year-old woman presents with palpitations and is found to be in atrial fibrillation. She is otherwise healthy and active. An echocardiogram is performed that reveals a congenital cardiac lesion. The most likely diagnosis in this patient is

(A) ventricular septal defect
(B) atrial septal defect
(C) coarctation of the aorta
(D) patent ductus arteriosus
(E) pulmonary stenosis

DIRECTIONS: Use the following scenario to answer Questions 115-116: A 65-kg patient presents for elective CABG. Induction of anesthesia is facilitated with fentanyl 15 mcg/kg, midazolam 150 mcg/kg, propofol 0.8 mg/kg, and rocuronium 0.8 mg/kg.

Anesthesia is maintained with isoflurane 0.7 MAC in oxygen and air, and initial minute ventilation is set at 4 L/min. During the prebypass period the patient develops tachycardia, hypotension, and subsequent ST elevations in lead V, as well as a rise in the pulmonary artery (PA) pressure.

115. The rise in PA pressure is most likely caused by

(A) myocardial ischemia

(B) pulmonary embolism

(C) hypoventilation

(D) hypovolemia

(E) light anesthesia

116. Administration of which one of the following agents is most appropriate in this situation?

(A) Epinephrine

(B) Glycopyrrolate

(C) Phenylephrine

(D) Sodium nitroprusside

(E) Nicardipine

DIRECTIONS: Use the following scenario to answer Questions 117-118: A 2-year-old child presents for strabismus repair. The child is otherwise healthy. After an uneventful induction and intubation, surgery begins. During the procedure the patient's heart rate acutely decreases from sinus rhythm at 110 bpm to sinus rhythm at 50 bpm. The blood pressure is normal and stable.

117. Which one of the following is the best treatment for this?

(A) Preoperative atropine

(B) A retrobulbar block

(C) Inform the surgeon and request that he/she stop until the heart rate recovers

(D) Administration of vecuronium

(E) Administration of neostigmine

118. Which one of the following are the respective afferent and efferent limbs of the reflex that resulted in the patient's bradycardia?

(A) Ciliary nerve and vagus nerve

(B) Trigeminal nerve and facial nerve

(C) Trigeminal nerve and vagus nerve

(D) Vagus nerve and ophthalmic nerve

(E) Ciliary nerve and facial nerve

119. A 30-year-old G2P1 patient presents for an anesthetic consultation at 20 weeks gestational age. Her prenatal course is complicated by Graves disease. She has not undergone radioactive iodine treatment to date and is currently on methimazole. True statements regarding her care include all of the following EXCEPT

(A) radioactive iodine is contraindicated during pregnancy

(B) the mainstay of treatment for hyperthyroidism during pregnancy is the use of antithyroid medication

(C) methimazole does not cross the placenta in appreciable amounts.

(D) thyroid storm occurs in 2-4% of pregnant patients with hyperthyroidism

(E) hyperthyroid patients should receive glucocorticoid supplementation

120. In comparing zaleplon and triazolam, which one of the following adverse effects is LEAST likely to occur with zaleplon although it commonly occurs with the use of triazolam?

(A) Prolonged sedation

(B) Abolition of REM sleep

(C) Extrapyramidal effects

(D) Ventilatory depression

(E) Amnesia

121. Therapy for a patient with closed head trauma and elevated intracranial pressure may include

(A) avoidance of sedation to maintain an unequivocal neurological exam

(B) use of pressors to maintain cerebral perfusion pressure at 80 mm Hg or above

(C) head down position to improve perfusion

(D) endotracheal intubation and mechanical ventilation for hypoxemia

(E) routine hyperventilation

122. A newborn is noted to have aspirated meconium. The oropharynx is suctioned and the patient remains stable with oxygen administered by nasal cannula. Which one of the following is true of this patient?

(A) This patient was likely born prematurely.

(B) The long-term outcome for this patient is poor.

(C) Chest physical therapy is not indicated.

(D) This patient most likely had in utero stress and fetal hypoxia.

(E) Vagal stimulation may cause passage of meconium in utero.

123. α1-antitrypsin deficiency is

(A) a nonvascular lung disease

(B) determined by a serum assay

(C) nonfamilial

(D) due to a lack of an enzyme produced by the lung

(E) the most common cause of COPD

124. The prevalence of obesity in the general population has been growing at an alarming rate and is reaching epidemic proportions. All of the following are true statements regarding morbid obesity in pregnancy EXCEPT

(A) there is a significantly higher failure rate of epidural blocks

(B) longer-than-normal spinal needles are more frequently required for neuraxial anesthesia than longer-than-normal epidural needles

(C) morbid obesity further increases the risks of maternal morbidity, fetal injury, and anesthesia-related maternal death during and after cesarean section

(D) there is a higher risk of both preterm delivery and delivery of a low-birth-weight infant

(E) morbidly obese patients who have undergone cesarean section should be monitored with continuous pulse oximetry after discharge from the post-anesthesia care unit

DIRECTIONS: Use the following scenario to answer Questions 125-126: A 52-year-old man is admitted to the ICU after he was rescued from a burning home. He was intubated without sedative medications in the emergency department and transferred to the ICU on mechanical ventilation. He has neither evidence of burns to his skin nor evidence of inhalation injury on external exam. He is comatose. Vitals show T 37.8°C, HR 122, BP 145/90, SpO_2 100% on FIO_2 1.0. A head CT scan is unremarkable.

125. Which one of the following is the most likely explanation for the normal oxygen saturation?

(A) Carboxyhemoglobin

(B) Sickle cell anemia

(C) Methemoglobinemia

(D) Methylene blue administration

(E) High FIO_2

126. The patient is transported to the hyperbaric oxygen (HBO) chamber for therapy. Which one of the following complications of HBO treatment may be seen in the chamber?

(A) Bradycardia

(B) Skin erythema

(C) Euphoria

(D) Seizures

(E) Chest pain

127. You are called to help resuscitate a newborn in the delivery room. The neonate is a 38-week gestational age female with an Apgar score of 4 at one minute. All of the following are appropriate interventions EXCEPT

(A) clearing of the airway with a bulb syringe

(B) intubation immediately

(C) bag mask ventilation of lungs at 60 breaths/min

(D) stimulation of the neonate

128. Which one of the following medications is MOST selective for inhibiting COX-2?

    (A) Celecoxib
    (B) Ibuprofen
    (C) Indomethacin
    (D) Ketorolac
    (E) Acetaminophen

129. When properly positioned, a left-sided double-lumen tube will have its lumens ending

    (A) in the left bronchus and the right bronchus
    (B) in the left bronchus and in the trachea
    (C) in the right bronchus and in the trachea
    (D) in the left upper lobe bronchus and in the left lower lobe bronchus
    (E) both in the trachea

130. A 68-year-old patient is on long term COX inhibitor therapy as part of her treatment for severe rheumatoid arthritis. The most common adverse effect of this class of drugs is

    (A) gastric side effects
    (B) ischemic heart disease
    (C) blood pressure elevation
    (D) analgesic nephropathy
    (E) hypersensitivity

131. A 3-year-old child experiences burn injuries to 50% of her body surface area. She also has significant inhalation injury. Which one of the following statements is true?

    (A) Within 4 d an amount of albumin equal to about the total body plasma content is lost through the wound.
    (B) Immediately after injury, cardiac output is increased.

    (C) The use of pulse oximetry is mandatory in monitoring the patient if carbon monoxide poisoning is suspected.
    (D) Evaporative fluid losses are approximately 4 liters for each square meter of burned surface per day.
    (E) Intubation should be avoided in this patient.

132. An anesthesiologist has a drinking problem. After coming to work on several occasions with alcohol on his breath, he was confronted by the Physicians' Health Committee and convinced to seek treatment. Which one of the following actions that he might take would be least effective in helping him maintain sobriety?

    (A) He gets an injection of naltrexone every two weeks.
    (B) He takes a disulfiram tablet each day.
    (C) He attends a meeting of Alcoholics Anonymous several times per week
    (D) He has blood drawn randomly once or twice a week for measurement of alcohol concentration.
    (E) He has a 50-min counseling session with his therapist once weekly.

133. Spinal cord stimulation

    (A) requires an external generator
    (B) involves an electrical stimulator placed in the subarachnoid space
    (C) is useful for postoperative pain management
    (D) may be helpful in patients with intractable back pain

134. At the molecular level, the effect of benzodiaz-epines is most accurately described as increasing

   (A) sodium conductance
   (B) potassium conductance
   (C) chloride conductance
   (D) endozepine binding to its receptor
   (E) acetylcholine binding to its receptor

135. You suspect nerve root impingement in the lumbar spine in a patient. Which one of the following physical findings would support this diagnosis?

   (A) You suspect L2 nerve root involvement and the patient has weakness of hip flexion and sensory loss on the lateral aspect of the calf.
   (B) You suspect L4 nerve root involvement and the patient has weakness of leg extension and loss of patellar reflex.
   (C) You suspect L5 nerve root involvement and the patient cannot dorsiflex his big toe and has a loss of the Achilles reflex.
   (D) You suspect S3 nerve root involvement and the patient has loss of sensation over the bottom of the foot. The Achilles tendon reflex is normal.

136. Fetal hemoglobin is necessary to allow transfer of oxygen from mother to fetus. Which one of the following is the reason why this transfer is able to occur?

   (A) Fetal hemoglobin has a dissociation curve shifted to the right relative to that for adult hemoglobin.
   (B) Fetal hemoglobin interacts with 2,3-diphosphoglycerate.
   (C) Fetal hemoglobin has a greater P_{50} value than adult hemoglobin.
   (D) Fetal hemoglobin has a greater affinity for oxygen than adult hemoglobin at any given partial pressure.

137. A 3-month-old infant, 46 weeks post-conceptual age, requires an inguinal hernia repair. The child was born by a spontaneous vaginal delivery, had an uncomplicated perinatal course, and was discharged home 2 weeks later. Which one of the following statements is true?

   (A) In order to minimize disruption of feeding and sleep, the infant should be operated on as an ambulatory surgical patient.
   (B) Spinal anesthesia is not a suitable technique.
   (C) Induction of anesthesia with sevoflurane is inadvisable because of the relatively slow uptake of inhalational agents in infants.
   (D) Halothane may cause depression of the chemoreceptor pathways, but is a suitable choice of inhalational agent.
   (E) A caudal epidural injection should not be performed due to the more caudal location of the spinal cord in the neonate compared to adults and older children.

DIRECTIONS: Use the following scenario to answer Questions 138-139: A patient with a history of asymmetrical cardiac septal hypertrophy (HOCM) is undergoing a liver resection for hepatocellular carcinoma. During the case there is sudden large volume blood loss. In addition to volume replacement, the patient is started on phenylephrine, followed by addition of epinephrine due to persistent hypotension. Shortly after initiation of epinephrine infusion, the patient has visible cyanosis and worsening hemodynamic instability.

138. An emergent TEE performed intraoperatively is most likely to reveal which one of the following findings?

   (A) Dilated right atrium and ventricle, and collapsed left atrium and ventricle
   (B) Decreased left ventricular function
   (C) Severe mitral regurgitation
   (D) Large VSD
   (E) Aortic dissection

139. Which one of the following interventions is most likely to improve this patient's hemodynamic instability?

(A) Addition of milrinone

(B) Discontinuation of epinephrine

(C) Administration of IV calcium

(D) Discontinue volume replacement

(E) Addition of nitroglycerin

140. A 5-year-old child with obstructive sleep apnea presents for tonsillectomy and adenoidectomy. The child has no other past medical history. The parents note that the patient snores loudly and has frequent pauses in breathing when sleeping. All of the following are possible complications or necessary interventions in this child EXCEPT

(A) pharyngeal airway obstruction may occur on induction of anesthesia

(B) use of an oral airway may be necessary during induction of anesthesia

(C) continuous positive airway pressure should not be used as it may inflate the stomach and make the patient more likely to have postoperative nausea and vomiting

(D) smaller than expected doses of opioid may produce pronounced respiratory depression

(E) difficulty in proper placement of an LMA may be encountered

DIRECTIONS (Questions 141-142): Each group of items below consists of lettered headings followed by a list of numbered phrases or statements. For each numbered phrase or statement, select the ONE lettered heading or component that is most closely associated with it. Each lettered heading or component may be selected once, more than once, or not at all.

(A) Intraparenchymal hemorrhage

(B) Disseminated intravascular coagulation

(C) Hypothermia

(D) Liver failure

(E) Uremia

(F) Factor VIII deficiency

(G) Von Willebrand disease

(H) Salicylate toxicity

For each patient with head trauma, select the most appropriate diagnosis to explain the hemorrhage.

141. A middle-aged man is brought to the operating room emergently for open head injury after an assault that occurred at least three hours before presentation to the hospital. He has a depressed skull fracture and scalp laceration with exposed brain; he is bleeding actively from the scalp. No previous medical history is available. Blood alcohol content is 0.5% by volume. Heart rate is 128 and non-invasive blood pressure is 85/35; esophageal temperature is 32°C after induction of general anesthesia. During debridement of the brain there is a significant brain laceration and marked bleeding from the scalp requiring replacement with multiple units of packed red blood cells to support intravascular volume; hematocrit is normal after transfusion. Intraoperatively, the PT and aPTT are prolonged; fibrinogen and platelet count are reduced.

142. A 25-year-old male with kidney failure from glomerular nephropathy requiring dialysis three times weekly is brought to the operating room emergently for evacuation of a subdural hematoma that developed after a blow to the head during a softball game. The patient underwent dialysis 36 h earlier; BUN is 67 mg/dL and creatinine is 8.3 mg/dL. He presented to the emergency department with a headache but suffered a progressive decline in mental status. After successful induction of general anesthesia, the cranium was opened and the hematoma removed. Intraoperatively the PT, aPTT, and platelet counts are normal. Profuse bleeding from the scalp and dura, requiring transfusion of packed red blood cells, complicates closure.

DIRECTIONS (Questions 143-146): Each group of items below consists of lettered headings followed by a list of numbered phrases or statements. For each numbered phrase or statement, select the ONE lettered heading or component that is most closely associated with it. Each lettered heading or component may be selected once, more than once, or not at all.

(A)   Acute alcohol intoxication
(B)   Delirium
(C)   Delirium tremens
(D)   Dementia

For each patient with agitation, select the most likely diagnosis.

143.   A 32-year-old female is in the hospital recovering after repair of a right lower extremity fracture sustained three days ago after jumping off a trampoline. On morning rounds, the patient is disoriented, tremulous, and pulling at her gown and IV lines. Her vitals are T 37.7°C, HR 121, BP 164/89, RR 26, SpO_2 96%.

144.   An 83-year-old female is in the ICU recovering from a colon resection for diverticulitis. On morning rounds, you find the patient talking to her incentive spirometer. As you approach, she is startled and asks how you got into her house. Her vitals are T 37.3°C, HR 89, BP 142/73, RR 18, SpO_2 97% on 2 L O_2 via nasal cannula. When you return to see the patient with your attending, she greets you by name and recounts the final moments of last night's televised basketball game.

145.   A 74-year-old female is brought to her internist's office by her daughter. She has become concerned because her mother has gotten lost while in familiar environments and has forgotten to pay several bills over the last several months.

The patient is pleasant. When asked about her symptoms, she suggests that her daughter is overreacting. Her Mini Mental Status Exam score is 20. Her vitals are T 36.9°C, HR 72, BP 128/78, RR 16, SpO_2 98%.

146.   A 67-year-old female is brought to the Emergency Department by paramedics after a motor vehicle collision. She has a laceration of her left forearm. When she stands to change into the hospital gown, she is unsteady and nearly falls. She falls asleep on the stretcher. When the staff wakes her to assess her vitals, she is uncooperative and confused. She demands to be left alone.

DIRECTIONS (Questions 147-148): Each group of items below consists of lettered headings followed by a list of numbered phrases or statements. For each numbered phrase or statement, select the ONE lettered heading or component that is most closely associated with it. Each lettered heading or component may be selected once, more than once, or not at all.

(A)   Epinephrine
(B)   Sodium bicarbonate
(C)   Atropine
(D)   Calcium
(E)   Volume expander
(F)   Dobutamine
(G)   Milrinone
(H)   Albumin

For each patient, select the most appropriate medication or therapy.

147.   After birth, a newborn remains apneic with a heart rate of less than 60 beats per minute despite adequate ventilation and chest compressions.

148. This drug is no longer recommended during the resuscitation of the newborn.

DIRECTIONS (Questions 149-150): Each group of items below consists of lettered headings followed by a list of numbered phrases or statements. For each numbered phrase or statement, select the ONE lettered heading or component that is most closely associated with it. Each lettered heading or component may be selected once, more than once, or not at all.

(A) Mid-esophageal four chamber
(B) Mid-esophageal two chamber
(C) Mid-esophageal long axis
(D) Transgastric two chamber
(E) Transgastric mid-papillary short axis
(F) Mid-esophageal aortic valve short axis
(G) Mid-esophageal aortic valve long axis
(H) Mid-esophageal bicaval
(I) Mid-esophageal right ventricular inflow - outflow
(J) Deep transgastric long axis
(K) Upper esophageal aortic valve short axis
(L) Upper esophageal aortic valve long axis
(M) Transgastric long axis
(N) Mid-esophageal ascending aortic short axis
(O) Mid-esophageal ascending aortic long axis

For each photograph of a transesophageal echocardiogram, select the standard, two-dimensional tomographic view.

149.

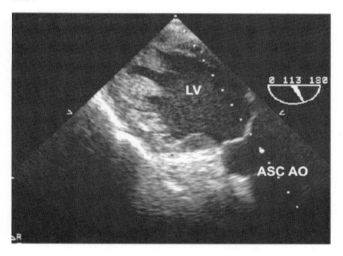

150.

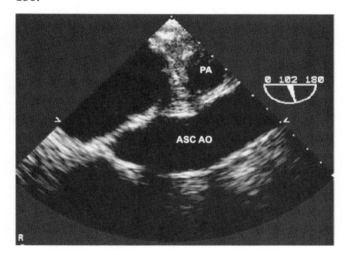

Answers and Explanations

1. **(E)** Clamping of the distal aorta in a patient with no preoperative aortic occlusion most likely leads to an increased vascular resistance and blood pressure and to decreased stroke volume and cardiac output. The heart rate usually is stable. *(5:1025-7)*

2. **(A)** The oculocardiac reflex (OCR) is associated with bradyarrhythmias. Traction on the extraocular muscles and pressure on the eye may cause the reflex. The reflex exhibits fatigability. Regional anesthesia may be used to prevent the OCR but it may also precipitate the reflex. *(5:1220)*

3. **(B)** Hetastarch is a synthetic colloid. Caution should be exercised when administering hetastarch solutions to patients with severe sepsis/septic shock, since it may increase the risk of acute kidney injury. The starch molecule is modified to resist metabolism by amylase to glucose monomers. The drug interferes with coagulation by diluting platelets and coagulation factors. The incidence of anaphylactoid reactions is about 1 in 1000. Hetastarch is eliminated primarily via the kidneys. *(5:541)*

4. **(E)** The uterus is composed of smooth muscle and therefore unaffected by MG. Therefore the first stage of labor should be unaffected. In contrast, the second stage of labor involves maternal expulsive efforts and may be affected by the disease process. MG is associated with other autoimmune diseases like rheumatoid arthritis and polymyositis. The course of MG during pregnancy is variable. *(2:1059-61; 5:995-6)*

5. **(D)** Patients with MG have a variable response to succinylcholine, but it is not contraindicated in parturients with MG. In general, there is a resistance to the paralytic effects of depolarizing neuromuscular agents and an increased sensitivity to nondepolarizing agents. Opioids should be used with caution as these patients may be more susceptible to respiratory depression. Neuraxial anesthesia is the preferred method of analgesia for labor and cesarean section, however, patients with severe disease with bulbar and respiratory involvement may not tolerate neuraxial anesthesia and may require general anesthesia to protect the airway and prevent aspiration. *(2:1060; 5:995-96)*

6. **(B)** Most dosage guidelines for pediatric patients have been derived from data extrapolated from adult studies. However, in a child the dose should not exceed a total dose of 3 mg/kg. In this case, the child is 12 kg, and could therefore receive up to 36 mg for local infiltration. The surgeon is using 0.5% bupivacaine, and so the maximum volume is 7 mL. *(5:846)*

7. **(A)** Azithromycin and levofloxacin are associated with prolonging the QT interval and are therefore contraindicated. Clindamycin is effective against the common skin pathogens and would be the preferred alternative to a first-generation cephalosporin. Gentamicin is generally not effective as a single agent against the common Gram positive skin pathogens, while tetracycline is too broad-spectrum to be used in routine perioperative prophylaxis. *(5:108, 232-4; 6:1897-8)*

8. **(D)** The volume control, decelerating waveform mode is shown. From top to bottom, the figure depicts flow, pressure and volume over time. Pressure support ventilation (PSV) requires patient inspiratory effort to trigger the breath and is seen as a negative deflection in the pressure waveform immediately preceding a breath; the inspiratory flow rate varies depending upon patient effort. Tidal volume in pressure support may be variable and is dependent upon the level of pressure support, rise time, inspiratory effort of the patient, and lung mechanics. Pressure control ventilation (PCV) requires the clinician to set a pressure and a respiratory rate. Tidal volume is variable. Inspiratory flow shows a descending waveform and is determined by the level of pressure control, respiratory compliance, and airway resistance. Volume control ventilation (VCV) requires the clinician to set a tidal volume, respiratory rate, flow waveform, and inspiratory time. Tidal volume is constant in this mode while pressure varies depending upon respiratory compliance and airway resistance. Inspiratory flow during VCV is fixed and may be set to a constant flow that creates a rectangular flow waveform or descending-ramp that creates a decelerating flow waveform as depicted in the figure. Airway pressure release ventilation (APRV) is a newer ventilator mode that is an adjunct to continuous positive airway pressure (CPAP). APRV adds alveolar ventilation to CPAP by transiently diminishing airway pressure to a lower level then restoring it to the higher level. This mode allows spontaneous breaths at both CPAP levels, but may be associated with dyssynchrony. A theoretic advantage to APRV is the potential recruitment of atelectatic lung units at lower pressure levels than conventional ventilator modes. Notably, newer ventilatory modes have not been convincingly shown to improve respiratory or mortality outcomes over properly employed conventional ventilation. *(5:1406-9, 1413; 6:2211-3)*

9. **(B)** Although carbon dioxide is sometimes added to the fresh gas during bypass, respiratory acidosis or alkalosis is generally corrected through changes in the fresh gas flow to the oxygenator. *(5:899)*

10. **(E)** The child should have an induction that is most appropriate for his clinical condition. If there has been a large amount of blood lost, a rapid sequence induction with propofol and succinylcholine may not be appropriate. Passing a nasogastric tube may not remove all of the stomach contents. The procedure should not be delayed to allow the stomach to empty. Once the injury has occurred, the stomach emptying probably stops, and the contents will still be there 6 h later. The child should be allowed to awaken with the endotracheal tube in place and be extubated once protective reflexes are intact. *(3:768-9)*

11. **(D)** Marfan syndrome is not associated with an elevated expected blood loss. The remaining types of scoliosis do have high expected blood loss. *(3:636)*

12. **(A)** There is no significant change in the respiratory rate at term. The increase in minute ventilation is almost entirely related to the increase in tidal volume. *(2:19-21; 5:290-91)*

13. **(A)** Maintenance of normocarbia is recommended during carotid endarterectomy. While hypocapnia can cause cerebral vasoconstriction, hypercapnia with resulting cerebral vasodilatation could cause steal phenomena. Vasodilatation has not proven to be helpful. Oxygen tension and blood pressure are kept at levels that are normal or slightly above normal. Normothermia is used, as is systemic heparinization. *(5:1018-21)*

14. **(A)** The different types of opioid receptors contribute in different proportions to the total opioid receptors in the spinal cord. μ-opioid receptors constitute 70%, κ-opioid receptors 24%, and δ-opioid receptors 6%. The main mechanism of spinal opioid analgesia is through presynaptic activation of opioid receptors. Opioid receptors are synthesized in small diameter dorsal root ganglion cell bodies and transported centrally and peripherally. They are mainly (70%) located presynaptically on small diameter nociceptive primary afferents (C and A-δ fibers). *(1:491)*

15. **(A)** The hematocrit reaches the lowest value between 8 and 12 weeks of age in full term infants. This is normal and does not require a blood transfusion or iron supplementation, and it is not due to hemodilution. This surgery, though not emergent, is not a procedure that needs to be delayed until the hematocrit increases. It may be best to avoid certain elective procedures that may result in significant blood loss at this time. *(5:257-8)*

16. **(C)** Although no specific anesthetics are indicated or contraindicated, those medications that cause release of catecholamines should be avoided if possible. Marked increases in heart rate are noted during induction with desflurane anesthesia or abrupt increases in the delivered concentrations of desflurane due to stimulation of the sympathetic nervous system. *(1:545; 5:1125-6)*

17. **(A)** Ventilation of the patient with a head injury requires meticulous attention. Head elevation reduces cerebral venous congestion and thereby lowers ICP. After prolonged hyperventilation the efficacy at reducing ICP is reduced as the pH of CSF returns to normal. While increases in intrathoracic pressure should be avoided, PEEP is useful when used judiciously to maintain oxygenation and avoid hypoxia and hypercarbia. The use of PEEP should be weighed against the potential to increase intracranial pressure. *(5:880, 1360-1; 6:3377)*

18. **(C)** Esmolol is a β_1-adrenoceptor antagonist and is contraindicated in the patient with AV block. Its half-life is less than 15 min. It is less likely than propranolol to cause bronchospasm, since it blocks β_1-adrenoceptor receptors, not β_2-adrenoceptor receptors. *(1:327)*

19. **(B)** The bronchial tree divides into right and left bronchi, the left bronchus being narrower and longer. Foreign bodies are more apt to go to the right side. The trachea moves during respiration and with movement of the head. It is lined with pseudostratified columnar epithelium. The rings of cartilage do not completely encircle the trachea; the posterior wall is membranous for all the rings except the cricoid. *(5:965)*

20. **(D)** Hypoalbuminemia, which is a common finding in critically ill patients, can lead to underestimation of the anion gap and a missed diagnosis of an increased anion gap metabolic acidosis. Albumin is a strong anion; a reduction in serum albumin level through dilution, capillary leak, or decreased hepatic production results in a metabolic alkalosis. Consequently, calculation of the anion gap without accounting for the abnormal albumin level may result in an anion gap in the "normal" range and a failure to appreciate unmeasured anions. To account for this flaw in the anion gap approach to assessing metabolic acidosis, an equation for the corrected anion gap has been suggested:

$$\text{Anion Gap}_{corrected} = \text{Anion Gap}_{calculated} + 2.5 \times (\text{Normal albumin g/dL} - \text{Observed albumin g/dL})$$

Because the Stewart-Fencl (strong ion difference) approach to acid-base assessment incorporates albumin into calculations, it may be a more useful tool for critically ill patients. *(5:365; 6:526-7, 530-1)*

21. **(C)** Mannitol, by decreasing brain size, may produce traction and even tearing of subdural veins that result in hematoma formation. This is more of a problem in the elderly. Mannitol may also lead to cerebral edema when the blood–brain barrier is disrupted. *(1: 681-2; 5:880; 6:2255-7)*

22. **(C)** The pain of glossopharyngeal neuralgia is very similar to that of trigeminal neuralgia but affects the posterior third of the tongue, tonsils, and pharynx. Giant cell arteritis is a common systemic vasculitis in the elderly. It is commonly associated with visual loss and strokes, so it must be diagnosed and treated aggressively. Temporal artery biopsy is the gold standard in the diagnosis of giant cell arteritis. Glucocorticoids are a common mode of treatment. Cervical carotid artery dissection most commonly presents with head, facial, or neck pain. Other commonly seen symptoms include

Horner syndrome, pulsatile tinnitus, and cranial nerve palsy. Pure facial pain is most often caused by sinusitis and the chewing apparatus, but also a multitude of other causes. *(7:246-9)*

23. **(C)** Larger tidal volumes increase airway pressures and lung compliance without significantly improving arterial oxygen tension but result in severe hypocarbia that increases shunt fraction at a Pa_{CO_2} less than 30 mm Hg. Arterial oxygenation during laparoscopy in morbidly obese patients is affected mainly by body weight and not body position, pneumoperitoneum, or mode of ventilation. PEEP is the only ventilatory parameter that has been shown to improve respiratory function in obese patients, but it may decrease venous return, cardiac output, and subsequent oxygen delivery. *(5:314)*

24. **(B)** Although plasma cholinesterase levels do decrease by roughly 25% before delivery and by 33% on postpartum day three, this usually does not result in a clinically relevant prolongation of paralysis from a single dose of succinylcholine. This may in part be due to the larger volume of distribution in pregnancy. The increase in blood volume is due to both an increase in plasma and red cell volume. The greater increase in plasma volume (55%) versus red cell volume (30%) results in the physiologic anemia of pregnancy. *(2:21-3)*

25. **(B)** An FEV_1 of less than 800 mL and an FVC of less than 2000 mL are associated with higher morbidity and poorer functional outcome. Regional function studies, like the V/Q scan, can show what fraction of the preoperative lung function comes from the area to be resected. Patients with an elevated Pa_{CO_2} are already in a state of chronic respiratory failure. Low Pa_{O_2} can reflect either poor underlying pulmonary function, or a shunting of blood through the diseased and nonventilated lung regions. When this area is resected, hypoxemia may resolve. *(5:952-5; 6:2087-91)*

26. **(C)** Hypoxia is likely caused by high physiologic shunt in the diseased lung. Physical therapy may help clear secretions and improve oxygenation. Supplemental oxygen will improve delivery to the good lung and reverse some hypoxic vasoconstriction on that side. Lateral position will improve flow to the good lung, as long as it doesn't increase soilage from the diseased side. Pneumonectomy will remove the diseased lung and eliminate blood flow to that side. An intravenous vasodilator, like sodium nitroprusside, will exacerbate shunting by inhibiting hypoxic pulmonary vasoconstriction. *(5:967-70)*

27. **(D)** A double lumen endotracheal tube fulfills several functions in a case that requires one-lung ventilation: 1. isolation of the operative side; 2. the possibility of application of mild CPAP to the operative lung in order to maintain oxygenation (and therefore limiting interruptions of the surgical procedure due to reinflation of the operative lung); and 3. the possibility of suctioning both the operative and non-operative lung. For these reasons, a left sided tube is preferred since it is unlikely to interfere with a lobectomy and its placement is significantly easier and more predictable due to the increased length between carina and left upper lobe bronchus as compared to the right side. Neither a single-lumen endotracheal tube, nor an LMA provide lung isolation, however a single-lumen tube with a balloon catheter (Univent) is an acceptable alternative to a double-lumen tube however it does not allow for CPAP and suctioning of the operative lung. *(5:963-7)*

28. **(E)** If the right side cannot be ventilated, there must be no clear channel from the right lung to the anesthesia circuit. Tumor or secretions could obstruct the lumen. The bronchial cuff could block the right side if the tube is not advanced far enough. The right tube lumen might be in the left mainstem bronchus if the tube is advanced too far. Placing the tube into the right side should not stop right-sided ventilation. *(5:963-5)*

29. **(B)** Particularly likely causes of this scenario are massive hemorrhage from the pulmonary artery stump or other great vessel, herniation of the heart through a pericardial window, or arrhythmia from cardiac irritation, hypoxia, or right heart failure. Applying suction to the chest tube could exacerbate the mediastinal shift, vascular compromise, and cardiac herniation (tension vacuthorax), as well as speed the hemorrhage. Surgical exploration is urgently needed, and the patient should also receive appropriate supportive care. *(5:1004-6)*

30. **(E)** A history of seizure disorder occurs in approximately 0.5% of parturients. One-third of these patients will experience an increase in seizure frequency during pregnancy. Proposed mechanisms include a decreased anticonvulsant drug concentration secondary to a larger volume of distribution, poor compliance, and a greater clearance of the drug during pregnancy. A high estrogen concentration is also known to lower the seizure threshold. Drug concentrations should be checked and the anticonvulsant drug continued, preferably in the parenteral form, in the peripartum period. Drugs such as ketamine and meperidine should be avoided as these are known to lower the seizure threshold. *(2:1061-3)*

31. **(A)** The agents are listed in decreasing order of β-adrenoceptor to α-adrenoceptor activity. *(1:201,206; 5:1401)*

32. **(C)** This patient has developed a severe A-a gradient with a PaO_2/FIO_2 ratio of < 100. Since there is no evidence of cardiogenic pulmonary edema, this is consistent with ARDS. Ventilatory strategies in patients with ARDS aim to support the patient without increasing lung injury through alveolar overdistension or recurrent alveolar collapse. The ARDSnet study published in 1999 demonstrated reduced mortality when patients with ARDS are ventilated with "lung-protective ventilation," including low (6 mL/kg ideal body weight) tidal volumes.

PEEP is titrated to minimize FIO_2, maximize PaO_2, and optimize alveolar recruitment. This typically occurs at >10 mm Hg. This patient has an ideal body weight of 50 kg.

Male ideal body weight (in kg) = 50 + 2.3 × (height in inches − 60)

Female ideal body weight (in kg) = 45.5 + 2.3 × (height in inches − 60)

(5:1392, 1412, 1415, 1418, 1420; 6:2207-8)

33. **(A)** This patient is hemodynamically stable. Although the debate over transfusion triggers continues, there is no evidence that supports transfusion of an otherwise healthy critically ill patient with a hemoglobin >7 g/dL and no evidence of hypoperfusion. The Transfusion Requirements in Critical Care (TRICC) trial did not demonstrate a benefit for a more liberal transfusion strategy in the study population. Transfusion of fresh frozen plasma (FFP) is necessary to avoid coagulopathy during massive transfusion. Once bleeding and transfusion requirements have stopped, however, the need for FFP is substantially reduced. Prothrombin time is a poor predictor of surgical bleeding, and large volumes of FFP may be required to improve a mildly elevated INR. A platelet count of >50,000/mm^3 is the usual target level for invasive procedures. *(5:201-3, 1394-5, 1442-3; 6:953)*

34. **(D)** The differential diagnosis for non-cardiogenic pulmonary edema in an intubated patient includes aspiration pneumonitis, pneumonia, transfusion related acute lung injury (TRALI), pulmonary embolism, or sepsis. This patient's normal echo and hemodynamics, rapid recovery, lack of fever, and substantial exposure to blood products makes TRALI the most likely etiology. TRALI presents as respiratory distress and noncardiogenic pulmonary edema that begins during, or within 4-6 h of a transfusion. Plasma is generally the culprit blood product. Treatment is supportive, and patients usually recover within 48 h. TRALI is

the leading cause of transfusion-related mortality. This patient did not have a history of trauma that would make pulmonary contusion likely. *(5:203-4, 1400; 6:280-1, 955)*

35. **(A)** Positive end-expiratory pressure (PEEP) reduces preload and left ventricular afterload by increasing intrathoracic pressure. *(6:2237)*

36. **(B)** Daily interruption of sedation and spontaneous breathing trials have been shown to reduce the number of days requiring mechanical ventilation and ICU care in eligible patients. Lung recruitment maneuvers have been shown to open the lungs in ARDS patients, but this has not resulted in an outcome benefit. Prophylactic antibiotics put the patient at higher risk of colonization with pathogens and have not been shown to reduce ventilator associated pneumonia. Suctioning can damage the tracheal mucosa, increasing the risk of tracheal colonization. Suctioning may also cause auto-inoculation from the endotracheal tube biofilm to the more distal airways. None of the ventilator modes have been shown to improve outcome. *(5:1406, 1418, 1421-2; 6:1115, 2138, 2200-1, 2213-4)*

37. **(A)** The atypical antipsychotics have less risk of extrapyramidal effects. They can cause hypotension and clozapine, olanzapine and quetiapine have been associated with an increased risk of new-onset type 2 diabetes as well as increased appetite and weight gain. Anticholinergic effects are least frequently caused by potent antipsychotics like haloperidol. *(1:359, 440-1)*

38. **(C)** General anesthesia provides a rapid induction with less hypotension and less cardiovascular instability and a more secure airway once it is established. An increased risk of aspiration and the potential for a difficult intubation limit general anesthesia to situations in which regional anesthesia is not optimal, such as when there is a need for emergent delivery in a patient without an epidural in place or the need for uterine relaxation (e.g., difficult breech extraction, replacement of uterine inversion). *(2:534-5; 5:1158)*

39. **(C)** A bacterial infection is likely to have responded to antibiotic therapy. A wheezy child may not be "asthmatic" but may have aspirated a foreign body. In a 2-year-old child this diagnosis should always be considered a possibility even if there is no clear history of aspiration. A child presenting with these symptoms and signs requires emergency therapy whatever the diagnosis. Agitation may be misinterpreted as emotional upset when it is due to serious underlying hypoxemia. If the child is stable, x-rays may be helpful in making the diagnosis and in identifying and localizing the foreign body. However, if the child is severely distressed, oxygen should be administered by face mask and immediate plans made for removal of the foreign body in the operating room. *(5:1002, 1250)*

40. **(B)** The flow during bypass is virtually non-pulsatile in both flow and pressure. This has been studied to determine if a more physiologic pattern would be beneficial. *(5:899)*

41. **(C)** Generally, solutions containing dextrose are not administered during neurosurgery unless indicated for treatment of hypoglycemia. Hyperglycemia has been implicated in animal experiments in worsening neurologic outcomes after ischemia. A plasma glucose concentration in excess of 300 mg/dL can produce an osmotic diuresis. Dextrose containing solutions do not lead to fluid retention. *(5:1471-2)*

42. **(B)** In population-based studies, migraine without aura is about twice as frequent as migraine with aura. Major criteria for the diagnosis of cervicogenic headache include signs and symptoms of neck involvement such as the precipitation of head pain by neck movement or external pressure over the upper cervical or occipital region, restricted range of motion in the neck, unilaterality of head pain with or without shoulder or arm pain, and confirmatory evidence by diagnostic anesthetic blocks. Chronic tension-type headache differs from episodic tension-type headache in that the average headache frequency is equal to or greater than 15 d per month or 180 d per year. A shift from peripheral to central mechanisms is believed to play a role in the evolution of episodic to chronic tension-type headache. Cluster headaches typically present as a series of intense unilateral headaches occurring over a period of 2 weeks to 3 months. They are associated with unilateral autonomic features such as nasal congestion, rhinorrhea, miosis, or lacrimation. The attacks are usually brief, lasting 150-180 min, and occur in the orbital, supraorbital and/or temporal regions. Unlike migraine headaches, tension-type headaches, temporal arteritis, and cervicogenic headaches, cluster headaches are more frequent in men, with an average male to female ratio of 5 to 1. Tricyclic antidepressants have been shown in numerous clinical trials to be effective in the prevention of both migraine and tension-type headaches. *(7:194-201)*

43. **(B)** Dexmedetomidine is an α_2-adrenoceptor agonist with 1600-fold greater selectivity for the α_2- than for the α_1-receptor. It is approved for short term sedation (≤ 24 h) but can be used as an adjunct for general anesthesia as well where it can markedly reduce the MAC of inhalational anesthetics. It causes less respiratory depression than opioids and benzodiazepines, and has not been associated with adrenal suppression. When administered as an intravenous bolus, it will cause an initial increase in blood pressure and decrease in heart rate. Dexmedetomidine is not indicated for the induction of general anesthesia. *(1:548-9; 5:701)*

44. **(A)** Preeclamptic patients are intravascularly volume depleted despite the fact that they may exhibit edema and weight gain. This may be due to a variety of reasons including a decreased colloid osmotic pressure and an increased vascular permeability from capillary leakage. Glomerular filtration rate (GFR) normally increases during pregnancy, thus lowering concentrations of serum markers of renal clearance (e.g., creatinine). In preeclampsia, GFR is decreased resulting in an increase in creatinine concentrations. Elevated uric acid concentrations reflect renal involvement with decreased renal clearance. The hematocrit is falsely elevated due to a reduction in plasma volume. *(2:983-4)*

45. **(D)** Carbon dioxide is sometimes added when the pH-stat strategy is used to adjust Pa_{CO_2} during hypothermia. *(5:532)*

46. **(A)** Absolute contraindications to epidural steroid injections include sepsis, infection at injection site, therapeutic anticoagulation, and patient refusal. Relative contraindications include preexisting neurologic conditions, prophylactic low-dose heparin, thrombocytopenia, and uncooperative patients. *(Abdi S, et al., Pain Physician 2007; 10:185-212; Cannon DT, et al., Arch Phys Med Rehabil 2000; 81:S-92)*

47. **(E)** When advancing with a needle, the ligamentum flavum feels firm and crunchy in the midline. When the needle passes through the ligamentum flavum, the epidural space is encountered as a distinct loss of resistance. *(5:793)*

48. **(C)** TURP is performed by resecting prostatic tissue with a cautery loop introduced through a special cystoscope. During the resection, venous sinuses are opened, and the irrigation fluid can be absorbed into the systemic circulation. As a result, a complication known as TURP syndrome may develop, with symptoms related to fluid overload, hypoosmolality, and hyponatremia. During TURP, systemic absorption of the irrigating solutions is influenced by the duration of exposure, the number and size

of venous sinuses opened, extravasation of the fluid into tissues outside the bladder or prostatic capsule, and the hydrostatic pressure of the fluid. When large volumes of fluid are absorbed, severe hyponatremia leading to cerebral edema may ensue. Additionally, neurologic manifestations may also occur due to direct toxic actions of some of the solutes used in irrigation. When TURP syndrome is suspected, the procedure should be stopped. Serum sodium, potassium, and osmolality should be measured in order to differentiate between true hypoosmolality and hyponatremia in the presence of circulating solutes such as glycine. Hemoglobin should be measured, because it is an index of the extent of fluid absorption. Hyponatremia does not need to be treated aggressively when it is not accompanied by hypoosmolality or in the absence of neurologic symptoms. If hyponatremia needs to be treated, rapid correction should be avoided because it can cause pontine myelinolysis. Hypertonic saline should be used only in the presence of life-threatening manifestations such as coma and seizures. Otherwise, sodium levels can be increased by administration of normal saline in combination with a loop diuretic or mannitol. Sodium correction should never exceed 1 to 1.5 mEq/L/h. *(5:1139-40, 514-5)*

49. **(C)** Traction on a number of structures in the posterior fossa may lead to arrhythmias, the most common of which is bradycardia. The surgeon should be informed immediately. If the bradycardia persists, atropine or glycopyrrolate may be indicated. Air embolism is more commonly associated with atrial and ventricular irritability and lidocaine may be necessary to treat frequent premature ventricular systoles or ventricular tachycardia associated with air embolism. Although it may be necessary to change the anesthetic or lower the head if air embolism is suspected, the first maneuver is to inform the surgeon of the problem and suspected diagnosis. *(5:893)*

50. **(E)** Prostaglandin E$_1$ may cause hypotension due to vasodilation. The drug should not be stopped before induction, since it may be required to keep a ductus arteriosus open. The drug is administered by infusion, since it has a short duration. *(1:948; 5:251)*

51. **(E)** Post-herpetic neuralgia most frequently occurs in elderly patients due to reactivation of the varicella zoster virus. It is usually refractory to opioids. Some patients respond to tricyclic antidepressants or to the topical administration of capsaicin that causes depletion of Substance P. *(1:1448)*

52. **(B)** Given that the duration of surgery is predicted to be greater than 30 min, option B is likely to be most efficacious. Retrograde perfusion is a suitable alternative for cases lasting less than 30 min. None of the pharmacological strategies listed is proven to be neuroprotective against cerebral ischemia during operative repairs of the aortic arch. While packing the patient's head in ice is routinely performed during deep hypothermic cardiac arrest, it is not sufficient in isolation to protect the brain from ischemia. *(5:916-7)*

53. **(D)** This patient has the clinical features of ventilator-associated pneumonia (VAP). VAP is a serious infection with high attributable mortality. The most important first steps in management of a patient with suspected VAP is to obtain specimens for culture, then begin appropriate antibiotic coverage. If cultures are not obtained, clinicians will be unable to narrow antibiotics, increasing the risk for selecting for multidrug-resistant organisms. If antibiotics are given before cultures are performed, the cultures may be inaccurate. Postsplenectomy vaccines are a standard part of post-splenectomy care, and may reduce the risk of future infection with encapsulated organisms in this vulnerable patient population. Vaccination would not be helpful, however, in the acute setting. Chest physiotherapy can be helpful in the treatment of patients with respiratory failure, but it is not the first priority in management. *(6:1026, 1115-6, 2130, 2137-41, 2200)*

54. (E) Patients with VAP should receive early broad spectrum antibiotics targeted at likely pathogens. Inappropriate selection of the initial antibiotic regimen has been associated with higher mortality. This patient has been in the hospital for >48 h and has had prior antibiotic exposure, two risk factors for infection with multidrug-resistant (MDR) bacteria. The initial antibiotic regimen should cover MRSA and MDR gram-negative rods such as *Pseudomonas* and *Acinetobacter*. Vancomycin or linezolid will cover MRSA. Levofloxacin or cefepime will cover MDR gram-negative rods. *(6:1115-6, 2130, 2137-41)*

55. (A) Tailoring antibiotics based on culture results reduces selection pressure for development of MDR bacteria and decreases the patient's exposure to drugs with potential side effects. This patient has had a clinical response and has a sputum culture that is positive for *Haemophilus influenzae*. Broad spectrum antibiotic coverage should be discontinued and she should be placed on a single antibiotic that will cover the causative organism at the site of infection. Third generation cephalosporins (including ceftriaxone) are the drugs of choice for serious infections due to *Haemophilus*. *(1:1499; 6:1115-6, 2130, 2137-41)*

56. (B) Because the amplitude of evoked potential responses is small (0.1–20 mV) as compared to the standard EEG (>50 mV), signal averaging is required to eliminate background noise. Multiple factors influence evoked responses including anesthetics and temperature. Resistance to these effects varies among the various potentials measured. *(5:484-9)*

57. (B) A paracervical block is effective for the first stage of labor since it helps with the pain associated with cervical dilatation. However, paracervical block has been largely abandoned in the United States due to a high incidence of reported fetal complications and the availability of other techniques with a lower complication rate. A pudendal block will provide anesthesia for the second stage and is appropriate for low forceps delivery and episiotomy. A subarachnoid block, caudal block, or epidural block is also appropriate. *(2:493-501)*

58. (B) The bronchodilator terbutaline is a selective β_2-adrenoceptor agonist. It causes less tachycardia than isoproterenol. It is preferred in the patient with heart disease compared to nonselective β-adrenoceptor agonists. *(1:293)*

59. (D) The celiac plexus block is useful for pain associated with upper abdominal malignancy. The most common complication is hypotension. *(1:735; 5:1711)*

60. (D) Factors increasing pulmonary resistance include nitrous oxide, hypoxia, and hypercarbia. *(1:547; 5:949)*

61. (D) There are three major types of fetal decelerations. Early decelerations demonstrate a slow drop in heart rate beginning with the uterine contraction (UC) with the nadir coinciding with the peak of the UC. It returns to baseline by the end of the UC. It is a result of vagal stimulation secondary to head compression and is not indicative of fetal asphyxia. Late decelerations begin after the UC and return to baseline after the end of the UC. They are often repetitive and associated with decreased fetal heart rate variability. They are associated with uteroplacental insufficiency. Variable decelerations are variable in configuration and bear no consistent temporal relationship to the onset of the UC. They are thought secondary to cord compression and unless severe and repetitive are not thought to be indicative of fetal compromise. *(2:145-6)*

62. (C) See the explanation for Question 61.

63. (B) Breakage and migration of the leads and bleeding at the site have all been reported. There is no increased risk of developing a spinal cord tumor. *(1:1457; 5:2774)*

64. (D) Reperfusion of an extremity after tourniquet deflation typically is associated with a decrease in core temperature of up to 1.0°C. Additionally, both preload and afterload decrease as blood reenters the affected extremity, often producing hypotension. During limb ischemia, carbon dioxide and lactic acid levels increase as ischemic tissues convert to anaerobic metabolism, with an incremental decrease in pH of the ischemic limb. After tourniquet deflation, aerobic metabolism resumes, with increases in oxygen consumption and carbon dioxide production. The systemic partial pressure of carbon dioxide increases, and pH transiently decreases as a result of combined metabolic and respiratory acidosis. During a general anesthetic, tourniquet pain manifests as increases in heart rate and blood pressures 45-60 min after tourniquet inflation. Increasing the depth of anesthesia or administering additional analgesics provides little relief. Tourniquet deflation is the only factor that eliminates tourniquet pain, thus decreasing anesthetic requirements. *(5:1202-3)*

65. **(B)** The patient with Parkinson disease has a deficiency in central dopaminergic activity. Thus, phenothiazines and neuroleptanesthesia (which employ a dopaminergic antagonist) are relatively contraindicated. There is no contraindication to muscle relaxants and the response to pressors is not abnormal. Since levodopa has a short duration of action, it should be continued up until the time of surgery. *(5:149)*

66. **(E)** Treatment of cerebral edema includes osmotic diuretics, loop diuretics, glucocorticoids, and surgical decompression. CSF drainage will reduce ICP and improve perfusion but has no effect on the edema. *(5:880-1; 6:2264-5)*

67. **(D)** Methylergonovine is not approved for intravenous injection and is usually given intramuscularly or intramyometrially. It should not be used intravenously except in severe cases of life-threatening hemorrhage as it may cause severe hypertension. If given intravenously as a lifesaving measure, it should be administered slowly over at least 60 sec with close monitoring of blood pressure. All other agents are useful to treat uterine atony. Rapid infusion of oxytocin can cause hypotension and prostaglandin $F_{2\alpha}$ can cause bronchoconstriction and hypertension. *(2:367-8; 5:1157)*

68. **(C)** A variable intrathoracic obstruction limits expiratory flow while preserving total lung volume and inspiratory flow. Forced expiration in variable intrathoracic obstruction results in a very positive pleural pressure that is greater than the slightly positive intratracheal pressure, resulting in an increase of the obstruction and narrowing of the airway. Forced inspiration in this situation will decrease the obstruction because of airway dilatation. *(5:997)*

69. **(A)** At the age of 6 months, a normal infant might be expected to have: a heart rate of 120 ± 20, blood pressure $90/60 \pm 30/10$, O_2 consumption of 5 ± 0.9 mL/kg. *(5:250; 357-8)*

70. **(B)** Cervicogenic headache is defined as headache that arises from painful disorders of structures in the upper neck that generates irritation of the upper cervical roots or their nerve branches. The current classification by the IHS and the IASP accepts these headaches to be unilateral or bilateral. Pain relief may be obtained by blocking the greater occipital nerve. The other options in the question are true. *(7:263-4)*

71. **(A)** Patients with acute hypocalcemia can present with paresthesias, muscle cramps, stridor, and positive Chvostek and Trousseau signs. Tracheomalacia, although rarely seen, may result from long-standing compression of the trachea by a large goiter that, when removed, may obstruct the trachea upon extubation. A major complication of thyroid surgery that usually appears early (immediately or within hours) in the postoperative period is airway obstruction attributable to recurrent laryngeal nerve (RLN) injury with resultant narrowing of the glottic opening. A unilateral RLN palsy would not produce significant respiratory compromise as long as the contralateral nerve and vocal apparatus function normally. However, bilateral nerve palsy, as from a new unilateral RLN injury in the setting of a preexisting deficit on the other side, can produce complete closure of the glottis and respiratory obstruction. Rapid onset of life threatening airway obstruction due to hematoma is a known complication of thyroid (and parathyroid) surgery. *(5:520, 1246)*

72. (C) α-adrenoceptors are stimulated by norepinephrine causing vasoconstriction. Isoproterenol is a nonspecific β-adrenoceptor agonist. Metoprolol is a β_1-selective antagonist. Bronchioles are not affected by α-adrenoceptor receptor agonists. Adipocytes carry β_3 receptors. *(1:203-4, 278, 311)*

73. (E) After subarachnoid hemorrhage ECG changes consistent with ischemia are common. A subpopulation of these patients demonstrate elevated cardiac enzymes including CK, CK-MB, and troponin and reduced ventricular contractility with low ejection fraction. Pulmonary hypertension is not part of the syndrome. *(5:885-7; 6:2261)*

74. (D) An oxytocin contraction test (OCT) involves the stimulation of uterine contractions with either oxytocin or breast stimulation. The presence of repetitive late decelerations represents a positive OCT, indicative of uteroplacental insufficiency and fetal compromise. Long-term variability implies an intact fetal sympathetic/parasympathetic nervous system. A biophysical profile (BPP) is an ultrasound that incorporates fetal movement, tone, breathing motion and amniotic fluid combined with a non-stress test to assess fetal wellbeing. A BPP of 8 or more is reassuring. A non-stress test involves the observation of two fetal heart rate accelerations within a 20-30 min period to assess fetal wellbeing. A reactive non-stress test is reassuring. Fetal scalp pH testing involves the assessment of fetal blood pH during labor. A fetal pH greater than or equal to 7.25 is reassuring. *(2:94-102; 5:292-3)*

75. (C) At birth, pulmonary vascular resistance declines rapidly in response to lung expansion and exposure of pulmonary resistance vessels to alveolar oxygen. At the same time, systemic vascular resistance increases. Pulmonary blood flow and venous return to the left atrium increase, and closure of the foramen ovale occurs when mean left atrial pressure exceeds mean right atrial pressure. Functional closure of the ductus arteriosus occurs in response to a rise in arterial oxygen saturation in the first 24 h after birth. Anatomic closure of both the ductus arteriosus and the foramen ovale occurs much later. *(5:250-1)*

76. (B) It is estimated that the risk of CRPS after fractures is 1% to 2% and the risk increases to 12% after brain lesions. Retrospective studies in large cohorts shows a distribution in the upper and lower extremity from 1:1 to 2:1. CRPS following SCI are rare. Extremities affected by a brain injury are at higher risk of developing CRPS than unaffected extremities. *(5:1542-3; 6:3358-9)*

77. (D) An appropriate laser endotracheal tube, such as metal, or a metal-taped PVC tube, should be used. Inspired oxygen should be reduced as tolerated by the patient to less than 30% but ideally 21%. Because N_2O supports combustion, either air or helium should be used to dilute the oxygen. The ETT cuff should be filled with a saline–dye mixture or lidocaine jelly. H_2O-based ointments should be used as lubricants, as petroleum-based ointments are flammable. Duration and intensity of laser exposure should be limited; continuous mode allows heat buildup. The fresh gas flow has no effect on prevention of airway fire. *(5:1238-9)*

78. (E) Preeclampsia can involve all organ systems with associated decreased platelets, abnormal clotting studies, and abnormal liver function tests. A combination of decreased plasma colloid osmotic pressure and increased vascular permeability results in decreased intravascular volume and extravascular water and sodium retention. Patients are usually hyperreflexic and hypertensive but intravascularly depleted with increased sensitivity to vasopressors. There is no contraindication to regional anesthesia if no coagulopathy exists and the patient is properly monitored. Pulmonary edema is rare, occurring in approximately 3% of women with preeclampsia. *(2:982-7)*

79. (D) The interscalene block will not reliably block the C8-T1 distribution of the brachial plexus. This will result in inadequate blockade of the ulnar nerve, medial brachial cutaneous nerve of the arm, and medial antebrachial cutaneous nerve of the forearm. *(5:831)*

80. **(A)** End-tidal nitrogen is the most sensitive monitor followed by end-tidal carbon dioxide, then blood pressure, then esophageal stethoscope, then ECG. *(3:519-20)*

81. **(A)** The metabolism of brown fat is a heat-producing mechanism. All of the other options are common methods of losing heat in an operating room. The temperature must be monitored and methods initiated to prevent heat loss. A warming blanket placed under the infant minimizes heat loss by conduction. *(5:251-2)*

82. **(A)** Acupuncture, the insertion of needles into specific points in the body, has the advantage of being a relatively benign mode of therapy for pain. It has been shown to have effects on the brain and endocrine system. *(5:612; 7:2366)*

83. **(B)** Whereas hypotension, hyperventilation, and hypothermia all decrease IOP, hypoventilation, hypoxia, and venous obstruction increase IOP. Hypertension may marginally increase IOP. Most drugs used in anesthesia either have minimal effect on or decrease IOP. Inhalational and intravenous (IV) drugs have the most rapid and pronounced effect. Most sedatives and induction agents (e.g., propofol and thiopental) reduce IOP in a dose-related manner. Succinylcholine has been reported to increase IOP by 6 to 12 mm Hg, but straining or coughing raises IOP much more. Acetazolamide (given IV) causes carbonic anhydrase inhibition and interferes with the formation of aqueous humor and lowers IOP. β-adrenoceptor antagonist (e.g., timolol) topical solutions are used in the treatment of glaucoma. This class of medication acts to reduce aqueous humor secretion *(5:1210-1, 1221)*

84. **(D)** Strategies to mitigate the risk of spinal cord ischemia in this high-risk patient include placement of a lumbar drain as well as neurophysiologic monitoring such as SSEP's and/or MEP's. Mild to moderate systemic hypothermia defined as core body temperature of 32-35°C is an additional established technique to protect against neuronal ischemia. Hypotension is to be avoided since it would increase the risk of ischemia. DHCA is a technique employed during open repair or replacement of the thoracic aorta. Patients undergoing successful stent graft repair of the thoracic aorta are routinely extubated at the end of the procedure, and a high-dose opioid technique does not provide spinal cord protection. *(5:915, 940, 1019).*

85. **(A)** β_2-adrenoceptors are stimulated by isoproterenol that results in peripheral vasodilation and increased skeletal muscle glycogenolysis. Esmolol is a selective β_1-adrenoceptor antagonist. Clonidine is an agonist at α_2-adrenoceptors that are the principal prejunctional receptors that inhibit sympathetic neurotransmitter release. *(1:179, 222, 278)*

86. **(D)** Mechanically ventilated patients are susceptible to ventilator-induced lung injury that is believed due to overdistention of lung units, repeated opening and closing of atelectatic lung, and likely inflammatory mediators released from injured lung. In patients with ARDS, a mortality benefit has been shown from a protective strategy using lower tidal volumes for ventilation, in the range of 6-7 mL/kg (calculated based on predicted body weight). Maintenance of plateau pressures < 30 cm H_2O are also recommended to reduce lung overdistention. Zero PEEP has been shown to be harmful in experimental rat models of mechanical ventilation. In humans with ARDS, the necessity of PEEP to prevent or reduce lung derecruitment is undisputed. The best method to determine the optimal PEEP level, however, does not have consensus agreement. Despite some strong individual preferences, no specific ventilator mode has been demonstrated superior to another based on outcome data for ARDS. *(5:1417-20)*

87. **(B)** Criteria for failure of a spontaneous breathing trial have been published by the American College of Chest Physicians. They are respiratory rate > 35, SpO2 < 90%, pulse > 140 bpm or sustained increase by 20%, SBP > 180 mm Hg or DBP > 90 mm Hg, and increased anxiety or diaphoresis. If any of these criteria exist, consideration of extubation should be delayed until a further evaluation of the patient and/or criteria occurs. *(5:1421)*

88. (D) There is no significant difference between general and regional anesthesia in neonatal condition after nonurgent cesarean section. No neonatal depression is demonstrated if delivery is within 10 min of induction or if less than 3 min elapses between uterine incision and delivery. *(2:534-5; 5:1159)*

89. (C) Induced hypotension may be necessary for short periods of time during a neurosurgical procedure. Thus, a short-acting drug, such as sodium nitroprusside or nicardipine, is ideal. The use of hypotension may produce an increase in dead space. Hypotension is not contraindicated in the neurosurgical patient. Hypotension never improves ischemia. *(5:892)*

90. (C) This is an ultrasound image of an interscalene nerve block. The C8-T1 nerve roots are usually spared. Therefore the ulnar nerve (C8-T1) is usually spared. *(5:831)*

91. (C) The supraclavicular nerves via the superficial cervical plexus innervate the cape of the shoulder. When performing an interscalene block, these nerves are usually anesthetized via indirect spread of local anesthetic. However, depending on the techniques employed and the volume of local anesthetic administered, these nerves may be occasionally spared. *(5:828)*

92. (D) The child with an upper respiratory tract infection (URI) is a dilemma. It has consistently been observed that the likelihood of laryngospasm, bronchospasm, and desaturation is increased when a patient has a mild URI, especially if an endotracheal tube is used. In the case of an acute URI the risk of the above may be greater. Most institutions will postpone elective surgery if the patient has signs and symptoms of an acute URI, especially if nasal discharge is purulent, a productive cough is present, the patient is febrile, or auscultation of the lungs reveals rales, rhonchi, or wheezing. The duration of postponing is another dilemma, however, 2 to 4 weeks is the usual time to wait for rescheduling surgery. *(3:226-9)*

93. (D) Selective COX-2 inhibitors do not have any advantages in terms of renal effects. COX-2 inhibitors are associated with less GI toxicity than nonselective COX inhibitors but they are more expensive. There is a possible increased risk of myocardial infarction (MI) and thrombotic stroke events associated with the continuous long-term use of selective COX-2 inhibitors. Those concerns led to rofecoxib and valdecoxib being withdrawn from the market in the years 2004 and 2005, respectively. Nonselective COX inhibitors inhibit the synthesis of TXA_2 by inhibiting COX-1 that is spared with the use of COX-2 inhibitors. *(5:1303)*

94. (B) Although many people self-administer ethanol as a bedtime sedative, and sedation is a prominent effect shortly after the ingestion of moderate amounts of ethanol, persons drinking ethanol just before bedtime often awaken a few hours later and have difficulty falling asleep again. *(1:634)*

95. (D) The blood supply of the posterior descending artery determines the pattern of coronary dominance: right coronary artery for right dominance and left circumflex artery for left dominance. Most patients have a right-dominant, or balanced, pattern of blood supply to the posterior descending artery. *(5:902)*

96. (B) Causalgia is the term that is sometimes used to indicate "sympathetically maintained pain" in association with a major nerve injury. "Complex regional pain syndrome" is now the accepted term. *(1:1444)*

97. (B) Despite increased blood flow accompanying elevated metabolic activity during generalized seizures, cerebral acidosis develops. The mechanism underlying this phenomenon is unclear. Most general anesthetics suppress seizure activity, including barbiturates, benzodiazepines, and volatile anesthetics. Prolonged anesthesia with isoflurane has been used to treat refractory seizures. *(5:875-8; 6:3267-8)*

98. (D) The infantile airway has a more cephalad-placed larynx, vocal cords that are slanted, and a large tongue in a relatively small jaw. The epiglottis is long and narrow and omega shaped. The narrowest portion of the infant airway is at the level of the cricoid cartilage. *(5:254)*

99. (D) The term lupus anticoagulant is a misnomer as lupus anticoagulant has no true anticoagulant activity *in vivo*. Therefore, neuraxial anesthesia is not contraindicated. The syndrome is characterized by recurrent pregnancy loss and/or recurrent venous or arterial thrombosis as well as laboratory evidence of either anticardiolipin antibody or lupus anticoagulant. Pregnant patients may be treated with low-dose aspirin therapy and heparin in order to improve fetal survival and decrease maternal thrombotic risk. Venous (e.g., deep venous thrombosis) and arterial (e.g., cerebral and myocardial infarction) thrombotic events occur in patients with antiphospholipid syndrome. A patient receiving a once daily prophylactic dose of LMWH should wait at least 12 h prior to placement of neuraxial anesthesia. *(2:872-4; 5:216)*

100. (D) The oculocardiac reflex may be initiated by manipulation of any of the structures of the afferent pathway, including the globe, orbital contents, ophthalmic division of cranial nerve V, and trigeminal ganglion and nerve. Tentorial manipulation can produce bradycardia and asystole. Spinal cord rhizotomy may produce bradyarrhythmias. Manipulation of the carotid sinus activates afferents of the baroreflex and can induce profound alterations in heart rate. Simple occlusion of an arteriovenous malformation is not associated with cardiac symptoms. *(5:887-93; 1206)*

101. (C) Preeclampsia occurs after the 20th week of gestation and requires at least two of the following: systolic blood pressure greater than 140 mm Hg or 30 mm Hg above prepregnancy values, diastolic blood pressure greater than 90 mm Hg or 15 mm Hg above prepregnancy values, generalized edema, or proteinuria. It can involve all organ systems. Its etiology remains unknown. *(2:975-98; 5:294-6)*

102. (C) Alcohol (50% to 100%) and phenol (5% to 20%) are both neurolytic agents. Glycerin is often added to phenol to make its specific gravity greater than that of cerebrospinal fluid when used for a hyperbaric spinal technique. *(1:1453; 5:2775)*

103. (B) Valproic acid commonly causes elevation of hepatic enzymes in plasma. *(1:596-7)*

104. (D) Sevoflurane is rarely used for renal transplantation due to concerns of fluoride and compound A toxicity. Although most human studies have not demonstrated deleterious effects of sevoflurane on the kidney, many authors feel, given the uncertainty surrounding the agent, as well as the safe alternatives available, that it should be avoided in renal transplant patients. It should be noted that sevoflurane has been demonstrated to have antiinflammatory effects on renal tissue that may be protective against ischemia reperfusion injury. Etomidate is well tolerated in hemodynamically compromised patients, particularly important in diabetic patients with autonomic neuropathy. Nitrous oxide has minimal side effects of concern in these patients, with no renal toxicity and rapid elimination. Succinylcholine can be used to facilitate a rapid sequence induction in patients with full stomach, gastroparesis, or acid reflux disease. Because the serum [K+] can increase 0.5 mEq/L with its administration, it should be used with caution in patients with renal failure who have an elevated preoperative potassium concentration (>5.5 mEq/L). Maintenance of skeletal muscle relaxation can be provided with nondepolarizing muscle relaxants that do not depend on the kidney for elimination, such as cisatracurium, rocuronium, or vecuronium. Although metabolized in the liver, accumulation of metabolites excreted by kidney may prolong their duration if large doses are used. *(5:1097-8)*

105. (C) All opioids must be used cautiously in renal transplant recipients, particularly if the graft is not functioning properly. A metabolite of morphine, morphine-6-glucuronide, has opioid agonist activity and is excreted by the kidneys. It can accumulate in renal failure and cause respiratory depression with long-term use. The metabolism of hydromorphone produces a neuroexcitatory compound that can accumulate in renal failure. However, hydromorphone has been used extensively in renal failure patients with no adverse effects. In contrast, a metabolite of meperidine, normeperidine, can accumulate in significant amounts in patients with renal failure, and this compound can cause seizures. The pharmacokinetics and pharmacodynamics of fentanyl, sufentanil, alfentanil, and remifentanil are not significantly altered by kidney disease. *(5:1098)*

106. (B) Immediate graft function leads to improved graft and patient survival. Volume expansion, maintenance of peripheral vascular resistance with vasopressors, and diuresis, are all helpful. Mannitol, when combined with volume expansion, has been shown to decrease the incidence of acute tubular necrosis in the transplanted kidney. The mechanism by which it does this may be related to decreasing tubular swelling by its osmotic effect, its action as a free-radical scavenger, or by flushing away sloughed renal tubule cells before they can cause injury by secondary obstruction. Although furosemide can be administered to enhance diuresis, it has not been shown to reduce the incidence of acute necrosis in the transplanted kidney. *(5:1099)*

107. (D) Only 20% of patients undergo fusion to the lowest lumbar levels. Complications seem to occur more in this patient population than in patients where the fusion ends in the upper lumbar spine. Pregnant women who have had surgically corrected scoliosis and are without significant respiratory or cardiac involvement tend to do well. Obliteration or scarring of the epidural space from trauma to the ligamentum flavum during corrective surgery can alter the spread of local anesthetic. This can lead to a higher incidence of failed or inadequate block and unintentional dural puncture. *(2:1038-43)*

108. (C) As oxygen is absorbed from the nonventilated lung, it becomes atelectatic. Persistent blood flow through that lung is then not oxygenated and contributes to shunt. Methods of improving oxygenation include decreasing the shunt or increasing mixed venous oxygen concentration. The most direct method of decreasing shunt is to mechanically stop blood flow to the atelectatic lung. Increasing oxygen flow to the circuit will not increase the F_{IO_2} so it will be ineffective. Nitroglycerin, or increased isoflurane, will impair hypoxic pulmonary vasoconstriction. PEEP may improve V/Q matching in the ventilated lung, but may also shift blood flow to the nonventilated lung. *(5:971-3)*

109. (C) Of all the drugs listed, methyldopa is the drug most studied in pregnancy and the only Category B (see list below) drug. Labetalol and nifedipine are Category C drugs that are often used in pregnancy but have not been studied as extensively as methyldopa. Diuretics are not commonly used in pregnancy and captopril is a category D drug. *(1:773-4, 1846-7)*

Category A: Controlled studies show no risk. Adequate, well-controlled studies in pregnant women have failed to demonstrate a risk to the fetus in any trimester of pregnancy.

Category B: No evidence of risk in humans. Adequate, well-controlled studies in pregnant women have not shown an increased risk of fetal abnormalities despite adverse findings in animals, or, in the absence of adequate human studies, animal studies show no fetal risk. The chance of fetal harm is remote, but remains a possibility.

Category C: Risk cannot be ruled out. Adequate, well-controlled human studies are lacking, and animal studies have shown a risk to the fetus or are lacking as well. There is a chance of fetal harm if the drug is administered during pregnancy, but the potential benefits may outweigh the potential risk.

Category D: Positive evidence of risk. Studies in humans, or investigational or post-marketing data, have demonstrated fetal risk. Nevertheless, potential benefits from the use of the drug may outweigh the potential risk. For example, the drug may be acceptable if needed in a life-threatening situation or serious disease for which safer drugs cannot be used or are ineffective.

Category X: Contraindicated in pregnancy. Studies in animals or humans, or investigational or post-marketing reports, have demonstrated positive evidence of fetal abnormalities or risk that clearly outweighs any possible benefit to the patient.

110.   **(D)** A halo device can limit neck motion necessary for direct laryngoscopy significantly. This necessitates alternative methods of airway management, including awake fiberoptic intubation by either a nasal or oral route. If the cervical spine is unstable, removal of the halo device is not recommended. The traumatized patient with a neck injury may have other associated injuries, including facial fractures and closed head injury. Anesthetizing the trachea is necessary before placement of the endotracheal tube to prevent coughing and straining. *(5:1361-2; 6:139)*

111.   **(C)** This patient has post-herpetic neuralgia. Tricyclic antidepressants are often the most effective drugs in treating this difficult condition. The anticonvulsant gabapentin has also been shown to be useful. The use of TENS or opioids is helpful in the occasional patient, but usually the results are disappointing. *(1:1448)*

112.   **(C)** For many thoracic procedures in pediatric patients such as this one, lung isolation is not necessary. If it is necessary, either a Univent tube, bronchial blocker, or mainstem intubation may be used to provide lung isolation. Double lumen tubes (DLT) are not available in a size small enough for this patient. The smallest DLT available in the United States is size 26-French that may be used in children as young as 8 years of age. With the Univent tube, the blocker is less likely to become dislodged because it is attached to the main endotracheal tube. An arterial catheter is not likely necessary in this patient as the patient is otherwise healthy, is not in distress, and is hemodynamically stable. If a bronchial blocker is used, it

may be passed inside of the tube with fiberoptic assistance, or, if the tube is too small, fluoroscopy may be used to guide placement, or the catheter may be placed with fiberoptic assistance outside of the endotracheal tube. Using a larger tube than is appropriate for the patient is not recommended as this could result in airway swelling and inflammation. *(3:281-6)*

113.   **(A)** Neural pathways responsible for the transmission of pain during the first stage of labor are visceral in nature and involve afferent pathways from T10 – L1. The pathways involved for the second stage of labor are somatic and produced by the distension of the perineum and stretching of the fascia, skin, and subcutaneous tissues and involve afferent pathways from S2 – S4 via the pudendal nerves. *(2:223-4)*

114.   **(B)** This is a common late presentation of an atrial septal defect. The other defects do not cause right atrial dilation that leads to atrial fibrillation. *(3:479)*

115.   **(A)** The most likely diagnosis is acute myocardial ischemia usually manifested by ST-segment changes, a rise in PA pressures, and new wall motion abnormalities on TEE. Promoting factors for myocardial ischemia include tachycardia, hypotension, a rise in left ventricular end diastolic pressure (that results in a rise in pulmonary capillary wedge and pulmonary artery pressures), severe anemia, and hypoxemia. While options B, C, and E might also lead to elevated PA pressures, they are less likely based on the information provided. Option D usually results in decreased PA pressures. *(5:908-9)*

116.   **(C)** Prompt treatment of hypotension is mandatory to restore coronary perfusion pressure and alleviate myocardial ischemia. Administration of the α-adrenoceptor agonist phenylephrine is the best option given; norepinephrine would be an alternative. While epinephrine can treat hypotension, it is likely to cause tachycardia and thus exacerbation of ischemia. Glycopyrrolate would cause tachycardia without associated rise in blood pressure. Arterial vasodilators are not indicated in this situation. *(1:295; 5:902-7)*

117. **(C)** If the patient is otherwise stable, the best treatment is to inform the surgeon and request that he/she stop the stimulus that precipitated the oculocardiac reflex. After a brief pause in which the heart rate is allowed to recover, the surgeon may resume surgery. The reflex does fatigue early and usually is not persistent. Preoperative atropine or a regional block of the orbit are methods of preventing the OCR, but are not treatments for it. There is some concern that the preoperative administration of atropine may lead to an increased incidence of intraoperative arrhythmias. Intravenous atropine is more effective than intramuscular or oral atropine in preventing this reflex. It is important to inform the surgeon as soon as bradycardia is seen. *(3:696; 5:1206, 1220)*

118. **(C)** The afferent limb of the oculocardiac reflex is the trigeminal nerve. The efferent limb is the vagus nerve. *(5:1220)*

119. **(C)** Methimazole does cross the placenta. This can result in fetal hypothyroidism and goiter formation. Fetal goiter can be diagnosed in utero with ultrasound. Hyperthyroid patients have decreased glucocorticoid reserves and should receive supplementation. Radioactive iodine is contraindicated during pregnancy. Undiagnosed or undertreated pregnant patients with Graves disease are at increased risk for thyroid storm and precipitating factors include infection, thyroid cancer, normal labor, hemorrhage, cesarean delivery, and eclampsia. Physicians should be prepared to treat thyroid storm should it occur during pregnancy. *(2:923-8)*

120. **(E)** Both drugs are short-acting and do not produce prolonged sedation and both drugs have little effect on REM sleep. Triazolam, like other benzodiazepines, produces anterograde amnesia. *(1:463, 465, 467)*

121. **(D)** Hypoxemia and intracranial hypertension are common problems after closed head trauma. Securing the airway and initiating mechanical ventilation may be required to maintain adequate oxygenation. Sedation, which decreases cerebral metabolic rate, is useful to reduce ICP but does obscure the neurological exam. Routine hyperventilation has been found not to be of benefit to outcome and is no longer recommended. The recommended lower limit for CPP is 60 mm Hg. *(5:1380, 1466-72; 6:2256-8)*

122. **(E)** Meconium aspiration usually occurs in full-term babies and is rare in those weighing less than 2 kg at birth. Regular chest physical therapy and postural drainage are recommended to clear residual meconium from the lungs. Long-term outcome is good, in terms of intellectual development and pulmonary function, unless asphyxia occurred in the perinatal period. Passage of meconium may occur in the presence or absence of fetal distress. *(5:247-8)*

123. **(B)** α_1-antitrypsin deficiency leads to airway disease that is familial and is determined by serum assay. The assay measures the level of a protective enzyme produced by the liver that acts to prevent autodigestion of lung tissue by the proteolytic enzymes of phagocytic cells. Only 1-2% of COPD patients are found to have severe α_1-antitrypsin deficiency as a contributing cause to their disease. *(5:188, 1090; 6:2152)*

124. **(D)** The morbidly obese patient is at a higher risk of having a macrosomic infant and a lower risk of preterm delivery. A higher initial failure rate of epidural placement has been reported and the need for placement of a second or third catheter is more common. Morbidly obese parturients are at higher risk for undiagnosed obstructive sleep apnea (OSA). Although the ASA guidelines for the perioperative management of patients with OSA was not intended specifically for pregnant patients, they do provide some guidance for the management of the obese parturient undergoing cesarean delivery. *(2:1081-90)*

125. **(A)** Carboxyhemoglobin, which is present in cases of carbon monoxide poisoning, may cause a normal pulse oximetry reading. The history of this patient who was trapped in a burning structure without burn injury and who is now comatose suggests carbon monoxide poisoning with neurologic impairment. Because the absorbance spectrum of carboxyhemoglobin is similar to that of oxyhemoglobin, most pulse oximeters will not discriminate carboxyhemo-globin from oxyhemoglobin and oximetry readings may be normal. An arterial blood gas will reflect a normal PaO_2 since the PaO_2 does not reflect the amount of oxygen bound to hemo-globin. *(6:1336)*

126. **(D)** Seizures are a known complication of hyperbaric oxygen therapy. Treatment is rapid decompression and removal from the chamber. *(Weaver L. Crit Care Med 2011; 39:1784-91)*

127. **(B)** An Apgar score of 7 to 10 indicates a healthy infant, who cries after delivery, maintains tone and color, has a heart rate above 100 beats/min and requires only routine care. An infant with an Apgar of 4 to 6 is depressed, may not breathe immediately and should be stimulated and have the airway cleared with a bulb and syringe. If the heart rate is less than 100 beats/min the infant should be ventilated with a bag and mask at a rate of 60/min. Long inflations rather than short, fast ones are optimal. An infant with an Apgar of 0 to 3 is flaccid, apneic, pale, and unresponsive. The ones that don't respond to bag and mask ventilation should be intubated, and if the heart rate remains less than 100/min, chest massage is initiated. *(3:834-5)*

128. **(A)** Celecoxib is selective for COX-2, while ketorolac and indomethacin are more selective for COX-1. Ibuprofen and acetaminophen have little selectivity. *(1:962)*

129. **(B)** Double-lumen tubes have one lumen in the trachea and one lumen in a mainstem bronchus. The handedness of the tube reflects the bronchus intubated. *(5:964)*

130. **(A)** The most common side effects of chronic COX inhibitor therapy are gastric in nature such as anorexia, nausea, dyspepsia, abdominal pain, and diarrhea. In addition, 15-30% of chronic users will develop gastric ulcers. All other conditions listed are side effects that are observed less frequently. Chronic use of COX inhibitors in the elderly must be accompanied by vigilance in monitoring for the various side effects. This vigilance includes determining (when appropriate) liver function tests, hematocrit, renal function, and occult blood in stool. Long-term use should probably also include use of misoprostol that can reduce the incidence of COX inhibitor-induced ulcers; empirical data suggest that other drugs (histamine H_2 antagonists, sucralfate, antacids, and proton pump inhibitors) may have similar effects. *(1:973-4)*

131. **(D)** Following a burn injury of this magnitude, vast amounts of fluid are lost from the circulation into the burned tissue, and thereafter are sequestered outside the circulation even in nonburned tissues. Albumin loss is usually at least twice the total body plasma content. Cardiac output is strikingly decreased immediately after injury because of the rapid reduction in circulating blood volume or the severe compressive effects of circumferential burns on the abdomen and chest impairing venous return. This is despite a large increase in circulating catecholamines. Evaporative fluid losses are about 4 liters per square meter per day. Pulse oximetry is not useful in monitoring oxygenation in carbon monoxide poisoning because carboxyhemoglobin produces an overestimation of oxygen saturation; the photodetector does not differentiate between oxyhemoglobin and carboxyhemoglobin. In contrast, transcutaneous oxygen analyzers are useful. As this patient has experienced significant inhalation injury, treatment involves intubation and mechanical ventilation with aggressive pulmonary toilet. *(5:1335-7)*

132. **(A)** The efficacy of the injected depot formulation of naltrexone in maintaining abstinence from ethanol is surprisingly modest. All of the other modalities have higher efficacy. *(1:642-4; 654-6; Pettinati HM, et al., Alcohol Clin Exp Res 2011; 35:1804-11)*

133. **(D)** Spinal cord stimulation involves the placement of stimulating electrodes in the epidural space. Typically the generators are implanted. With proper patient selection, it has been shown to be useful in several chronic pain conditions, including ischemic pain and "failed back syndrome" with a radicular component. *(1:1457; 5:2774)*

134. **(C)** Benzodiazepines bind to the GABA receptor, a chloride channel, and increase its affinity for GABA thereby increasing chloride conductance. *(1:461)*

135. **(B)** The expected effects of nerve root impingement are:

    L2 nerve: weakness of hip flexion (iliopsoas) and sensory loss on anterior groin and thigh. No deep tendon reflex

    L4 nerve: weakness of leg extension (quadriceps), ankle dorsiflexion (tibialis anterior); sensory loss medial calf/foot; loss of patellar reflex

    L5 nerve: weakness of dorsiflexion of big toe (EHL) sensory loss lateral aspect of calf and dorsum of foot. No deep tendon reflex

    S3 nerve: weakness of the anal and/or urinary sphincters and pain or sensory loss in the distribution of the pudendal nerve

    (7:275)

136. **(D)** Neonates have 60% to 90% hemoglobin F, and it is not until they are about 6 months of age that the adult hemoglobin A to hemoglobin F ratio is achieved. Hemoglobin F has a high affinity for oxygen, and the oxygen dissociation curve is shifted to the left, resulting in decreased oxygen delivery to the tissues at a given oxygen tension, and a lower P_{50} value compared to adult hemoglobin. 2,3-diphosphoglycerate interacts with hemoglobin A resulting in decreased affinity for oxygen. It does not interact with hemoglobin F. *(5:1175)*

137. **(C)** Infants of up to 50 weeks post-conceptual age are at risk of postoperative apnea, even if they have no history of previous apneic episodes. Therefore, they are usually kept in the hospital for the first postoperative night for close apnea monitoring and are not operated on as ambulatory surgery patients. Halothane has been shown to decrease chemoreceptor sensitivity and is therefore implicated in postoperative apnea, but with appropriate monitoring its use is not contraindicated. Spinal anesthesia can be used as the sole technique for this procedure, but should not be combined with a sedative agent because of the risk of postoperative apnea. Infants have a relatively rapid uptake of volatile agents because of decreased blood–gas partition coefficients, decreased MAC, increased cardiac output per kg body mass, and relatively high blood flow to the brain. Caudal epidural injection typically as an adjunct to general anesthesia is a reasonable technique. *(5:1187-9)*

138. **(C)** The most likely finding on TEE based on the patient's symptoms is severe mitral regurgitation (MR). MR in patients with HOCM occurs as a consequence of systolic anterior motion (SAM) of the anterior mitral valve leaflet, thus acutely narrowing the left ventricular outflow tract. This condition is exacerbated by states of increased contractility, in this case due to the infusion of epinephrine, and hypovolemia, for example due to sudden large volume blood loss. None of the other options listed would explain worsening hemodynamics in response to epinephrine infusion. TEE findings as described in option A can be expected in acute pulmonary embolus. *(5:449, 910; 6:1934, 1967)*

139. **(B)** States of increased contractility worsen left ventricular outflow tract obstruction as described in the explanation to the previous question. Epinephrine should therefore be discontinued immediately. Milrinone and calcium would have the same effect and likely worsen this patient's hemodynamics. The goal of therapy is restoration of preload with volume infusion and afterload support if indicated with pure α-adrenoceptor agonists such as phenylephrine. Nitroglycerin, due to the associated reduction in preload would likely worsen hemodynamics. *(5:449, 910; 6:1934, 1967)*

140. **(C)** Patients with obstructive sleep apnea (OSA) may have pronounced pharyngeal obstruction during induction of anesthesia requiring the placement of an oral or nasopharyngeal airway and/or CPAP to maintain a patent airway. These patients have greatly increased sensitivity to opioids, should be monitored carefully, and when necessary admitted for observation with apnea monitoring. Due to

the small oropharynx and adenotonsillar hypertrophy, placement of an LMA could be difficult. *(3:666-8)*

141. **(B)** Laceration of the brain commonly permits spilling of brain tissue thromboplastin into the systemic circulation. This can produce the rapid appearance of disseminated intravascular coagulation. Coagulation studies typically demonstrate a prolonged PT and aPTT with reduced fibrinogen and platelet counts. D-dimers may also be elevated. *(5:217; 6:978)*

142. **(E)** Uremia from kidney failure is associated with platelet dysfunction that can cause significant bleeding during surgery. Coagulation studies are typically normal. *(5:1330, 1444; 6:460, 2203)*

143. **(C)** Delirium tremens is characterized by delirium, tremors, and overactivity of the autonomic nervous system. Symptoms begin within 5-10 h of decreased alcohol intake and peak on day 2-3. *(6:3551)*

144. **(B)** Delirium is defined as a disturbance of consciousness or cognition that has developed over a short period of time and is caused by direct physiologic consequences of a general medical condition. The hallmark symptom is a deficit of attention that fluctuates over hours or days. The patient may also have altered sleep-wake cycles, hallucinations and affect changes. Heart rate and blood pressure instability may occur. Delirium is an underdiagnosed, though common, finding in hospitalized patients (14-56%, with higher estimates in ICU patients). Mortality is estimated at 25-33% among delirious inpatients. *(5:1390-1; 6:196-201)*

145. **(D)** Dementia is defined as an acquired deterioration in cognitive abilities that impairs the successful performance of activities of daily living. Memory is the most common, but not the only cognitive ability that may be lost. Most forms of dementia are progressive. The Mini-Mental Status Examination is a screening tool used to confirm that a patient has cognitive impairment. *(6:3300-16)*

146. **(A)** Symptoms of acute alcohol intoxication include decreased inhibitions, a decrease in complex cognitive functions, slurred speech, motor irritability, and poor judgment. *(6: 3546-52)*

147. **(A)** Epinephrine is considered the drug of choice for the treatment of fetal bradycardia during the resuscitation of the newborn. It is recommended if the fetal heart rate remains less than 60 beats per minute after 30 sec of adequate ventilation and chest compressions. A dose of 0.01-0.03 mg/kg (or 0.1-0.3 mL/kg of a 1:10,000 solution) is recommended every 3-5 min. *(2:164-70)*

148. **(C)** See explanation to Question 147. Atropine is no longer recommended for use during the resuscitation of the newborn. Epinephrine is considered the drug of choice for the treatment of bradycardia in the newborn. *(2:169)*

149. **(M)** *(Lauer R, Mathew JP. Transesophageal tomographic views. In: Mathew JP, et al., eds., Clinical Manual and Review of Transesophageal Echocardiography, 2nd ed., New York: McGraw-Hill, 2010, Figure 5-21)*

150. **(O)** *(Lauer R, Mathew JP. Transesophageal tomographic views. In: Mathew JP, et al., eds., Clinical Manual and Review of Transesophageal Echocardiography, 2nd ed., New York: McGraw-Hill, 2010, Figure 5-32)*

References

1. Brunton LL, Chabner BA, Knollmann BC, eds. *Goodman and Gilman's The Pharmacological Basis of Therapeutics*, 12th ed. New York: McGraw Hill, 2011.

2. Chestnut DH, et al., eds. *Chestnut's Obstetric Anesthesia: Principles and Practice*, 4th ed. St. Louis: C. V. Mosby, 2009.

3. Coté CJ, Lerman J, Todres ID, eds. *A Practice of Anesthesia for Infants and Children*, 4th ed. Philadelphia: W.B. Saunders Co., 2008.

4. Hadzic A, ed. *NYSORA Textbook of Regional Anesthesia and Acute Pain Management*, New York: McGraw-Hill, 2007.

5. Longnecker DE, et al., eds. *Anesthesiology*, 2nd ed. New York: McGraw-Hill, 2012.

6. Longo, DL, et al., eds. *Harrison's Principles of Internal Medicine*, 18th ed. New York: McGraw-Hill, 2012.

7. Warfield CA, Bajwa ZH, eds. *Principles and Practice of Pain Medicine*, 2nd ed. New York: McGraw-Hill, 2004.

Index

The Roman numerals following the topic refer to Parts I or II of the book, and the numbers refer to specific questions in that Part. When a "t" follows the number, it denotes a question in one of the Practice Tests, Chapters 10 or 20 in Parts I or II, respectively.

Sympathetic nervous system, I:238, II:540

Synchronized intermittent mandatory ventilation (SIMV), I:179, II:488

Syncope, I:84t

Syndrome of inappropriate secretion of antidiuretic hormone (SIADH), I:344

Syphilis, I:299

Systemic lupus erythematosus, II:504–505

Systemic sequelae, II:185

Systemic toxicity, I:572

Systemic vascular resistance (SVR), II:465

T

T waves, II:477

Tachycardia, I:5t, I:68t, I:136, I:140, I:404, I:458–459, II:24–25, II:53t–55t, II:135–136, II:139

Tachyphylaxis, II:28

Tachypnea, I:117t, II:106–107

Taylor approach, I:562

TBW. *See* Total body water

Tec 5 vaporizer, I:69t

TEF. *See* Tracheoesophageal fistula

TEG. *See* Thromboelastogram

Temperature, I:60t, I:124t–126t, I:236, II:81t, II:175, II:333, II:428

TENS. *See* Transcutaneous electrical nerve stimulation

Terbutaline, II:58t, II:246, II:274

Terminal half-life of drug, I:442

Tetanus, I:33t, I:39t

Tetracaine, I:449, I:582

Tetralogy of Fallot, I:93t, I:137, II:336

Thalamus, I:247, I:249

Therapeutic hypothermia, II:513

Thermoregulation, II:347, II:445

Theta wave, I:251

Thiamine deficiency, I:294

Thiazide diuretics, I:416

Thiopental, I:21t, I:138t, I:369, I:389, I:412, I:445

Thoracic deformities, I:175

Thoracic dermatome, I:144t

Thoracoabdominal aneurysm, II:148

Thoracotomy, II:598

Thrombin inhibition, I:414

Thrombocytopenia, I:495

Thromboelastogram (TEG), II:154

Thrombophlebitis, I:556

Thyroid isthmus, II:155

Thyroidectomy, I:290, I:355

Thyrotropin, I:255

Tidal volume, I:50, I:230, II:294

TIPS. *See* Transjugular intrahepatic portosystemic shunt

Tissue water, I:237

TNS. *See* Transient neurological symptoms

Tobacco, I:97t, I:293. *See also* Smoking

Tonic-clonic movements, II:560

Tonic-clonic seizures, II:30t

Tonsillectomy, I:40t, I:286, II:140t

Tooth extraction, I:40t

Torsades des pointes, I:93

Total body tissue perfusion, II:468

Total body water (TBW), II:361

Total parenteral nutrition, II:38

Total pulmonary compliance, I:235

Tourniquet, I:593, II:64t, II:427

Toxic goiter, I:355

T-piece, I:39

Trachea, II:155

Tracheal collapse, II:152

Tracheal edema, I:4, I:10

Tracheal extubation, I:486

Tracheobronchial tree, II:19t

Tracheoesophageal fistula (TEF), II:346, II:379

Train-of-four stimulus, I:410, I:411

Tramadol, II:580

Tranexamic acid, I:89

Transcatheter aortic valve implantation, II:151

Transcranial Doppler, II:217

Transcutaneous electrical nerve stimulation (TENS), II:554

Transdermal scopolamine, I:43t, I:374

Transesophageal echocardiography, II:116, II:139, II:149t-150t, II:165-173, II:205

Transfusion risk, II:442

Transgastric long axis, II:149t

Transgastric mid-papillary short axis, II:168

Transgastric two chamber, II:167

Transient neurological symptoms (TNS), I:566

Transjugular intrahepatic portosystemic shunt (TIPS), II:444

Transmembrane transport mechanism, I:493

Transposition of great arteries, II:382

Transpulmonary pressure, I:127t, I:225

Transsphenoidal hypophysectomy, I:329, II:220

Transthoracic echocardiogram, II:137

Transurethral resection, II:419–420

Transverse process, II:71

Trauma patient, I:324

Trendelenburg position, I:55, II:240, II:279